Concise
Medical
Encyclopedia

MARTIN S. LIPSKY, MD, Medical Editor

The essential A-Z guide to
3,000+ medical terms—
including symptoms, diseases,
drugs, and treatments—from
America's top medical authority

**Random House
Reference**

New York   Toronto   London   Sydney   Auckland

Library of Congress Cataloging-in-Publication Data

American Medical Association concise medical encyclopedia / Martin S. Lipsky, medical editor.—1st ed.
    p. cm.
    Based on: American Medical Association complete medical encyclopedia / medical editors, Jerrold B. Leikin, Martin S. Lipsky. c2003.
    Includes index.
    ISBN-13: 978-0-375-72180-9
    ISBN-10: 0-375-72180-0
    1. Medicine, Popular—Encyclopedias. I. Lipsky, Martin S. II. American Medical Association. III. American Medical Association complete medical encyclopedia. IV. Title: Concise medical encyclopedia.
    [DNLM: 1. Medicine—Encyclopedias—English. W 13 A5119 2006
    RC81.A2A498 2006
    610.3—dc22
                                           2006050740

HOW TO USE THIS BOOK

The *American Medical Association Concise Medical Encyclopedia* is positioned as the one book that helps doctors help patients find definitive information about their family's health-related questions and concerns. This book has been planned to provide the reliable, clear, objective health care information that American consumers have come to expect from the American Medical Association. Featuring more than 3,000 entries and 100 illustrations, it is intended to be a comprehensive, medically accurate, and up-to-date source of consumer medical information.

This authoritative, single-volume resource will not only help you safeguard and improve your health, but it will also empower you to communicate more effectively with your doctor. For quick and easy access, the entries in the **Alphabetical encyclopedia of medicine** are arranged alphabetically. Longer entries are logically divided into subsections. With ease of reading in mind, thumbnail definitions of complex medical terms are provided parenthetically as you encounter them. Terms in SMALL CAPITAL LETTERS are cross-references; these point you to other entries for additional information. If you do not find the main entry topic or term you are looking for, consult the comprehensive **Index** at the back of the book.

AMERICAN MEDICAL ASSOCIATION

Michael D. Maves, MD	Executive Vice President, Chief Executive Officer
Bernard L. Hengesbaugh	Chief Operating Officer
Robert A. Musacchio, PhD	Senior Vice President, Publishing and Business Services
Anthony J. Frankos	Vice President, Business Products
Mary Lou White	Executive Director, Editorial and Operations

EDITORIAL STAFF

Martin S. Lipsky, MD	Medical Editor Regional Dean University of Illinois College of Medicine, Rockford
Patricia Dragisic	Senior Managing Editor
Mary Ann Albanese	Art·Editor
George Kruto	Indexer
Coralee Montes	Editorial Assistant

This book is based on the *American Medical Association Complete Medical Encyclopedia*, published by Random House Reference in 2003; medical editors Jerrold B. Leikin, MD, and Martin S. Lipsky, MD.

Editors of *American Medical Association Complete Medical Encyclopedia* included Claudia Appeldorn, Robin F. Husayko, and Eileen Norris.

CONTENTS

SYMPTOM CHARTS

Symptom charts help identify the possible causes of many common symptoms, for example, chest pain or diarrhea. After answering "yes" or "no" to the questions on the chart, follow the directional arrows, which lead you to a likely diagnosis. The terms in the boxes that appear in small capital letters (for example, HEADACHE) are cross-references to direct you to main entries in the alphabetical encyclopedia of medicine with more information. **Warning:** These symptom charts are designed to help diagnose the most common causes of some common symptoms. They are not intended to be exhaustive or to replace medical care by a physician. If any uncertainty remains regarding a diagnosis after consulting a particular chart, be sure to contact your doctor.

To help you determine what to do about various symptoms and whether medical help is needed urgently, the charts use the following language:

- EMERGENCY! Get medical help now! A diagnosis that appears with this heading may be life-threatening if prompt medical attention is not obtained. Calling 911 or your local emergency number is usually the best way to secure prompt medical attention.

- Contact your doctor immediately. A diagnosis that appears in this box may be serious and require urgent medical attention. Medical advice should be sought immediately. Call your doctor or triage nurse and ask for help in determining what to do next.

- Contact your doctor. A diagnosis that appears in this box is not usually life-threatening. Nevertheless, medical advice is recommended. Make an appointment to see your doctor for a consultation.

SYMPTOM CHART TOPICS

Abdominal pain

Pain experienced in the area of the trunk below the lower edge of the rib cage and above the groin.

START

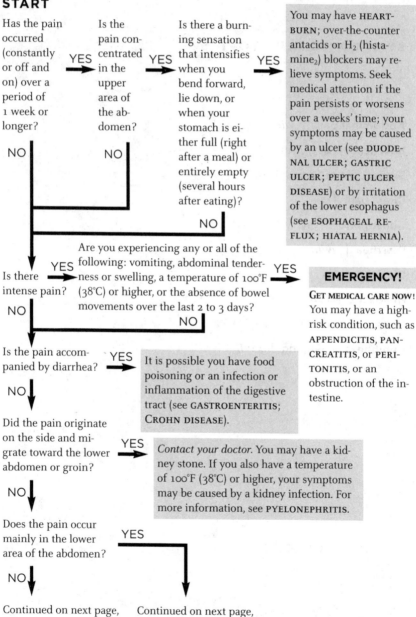

Has the pain occurred (constantly or off and on) over a period of 1 week or longer?

YES → Is the pain concentrated in the upper area of the abdomen?

YES → Is there a burning sensation that intensifies when you bend forward, lie down, or when your stomach is either full (right after a meal) or entirely empty (several hours after eating)?

YES → You may have HEARTBURN; over-the-counter antacids or H₂ (histamine₂) blockers may relieve symptoms. Seek medical attention if the pain persists or worsens over a weeks' time; your symptoms may be caused by an ulcer (see DUODENAL ULCER; GASTRIC ULCER; PEPTIC ULCER DISEASE) or by irritation of the lower esophagus (see ESOPHAGEAL REFLUX; HIATAL HERNIA).

NO **NO** **NO**

Is there intense pain?

YES → Are you experiencing any or all of the following: vomiting, abdominal tenderness or swelling, a temperature of 100°F (38°C) or higher, or the absence of bowel movements over the last 2 to 3 days?

YES →

EMERGENCY!

GET MEDICAL CARE NOW! You may have a high-risk condition, such as APPENDICITIS, PANCREATITIS, or PERITONITIS, or an obstruction of the intestine.

NO **NO**

Is the pain accompanied by diarrhea?

YES → It is possible you have food poisoning or an infection or inflammation of the digestive tract (see GASTROENTERITIS; CROHN DISEASE).

NO

Did the pain originate on the side and migrate toward the lower abdomen or groin?

YES → *Contact your doctor.* You may have a kidney stone. If you also have a temperature of 100°F (38°C) or higher, your symptoms may be caused by a kidney infection. For more information, see PYELONEPHRITIS.

NO

Does the pain occur mainly in the lower area of the abdomen?

YES

NO

Continued on next page, first column

Continued on next page, second column

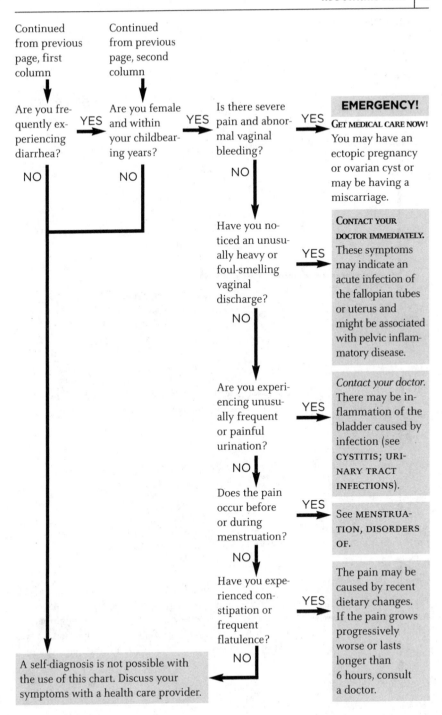

Continued from previous page, first column

Continued from previous page, second column

Are you frequently experiencing diarrhea?

YES →

Are you female and within your childbearing years?

YES →

Is there severe pain and abnormal vaginal bleeding?

YES →

NO

NO

NO

EMERGENCY!
GET MEDICAL CARE NOW! You may have an ectopic pregnancy or ovarian cyst or may be having a miscarriage.

Have you noticed an unusually heavy or foul-smelling vaginal discharge?

YES →

NO

CONTACT YOUR DOCTOR IMMEDIATELY. These symptoms may indicate an acute infection of the fallopian tubes or uterus and might be associated with pelvic inflammatory disease.

Are you experiencing unusually frequent or painful urination?

YES →

NO

Contact your doctor. There may be inflammation of the bladder caused by infection (see CYSTITIS; URINARY TRACT INFECTIONS).

Does the pain occur before or during menstruation?

YES →

NO

See MENSTRUATION, DISORDERS OF.

Have you experienced constipation or frequent flatulence?

YES →

NO

The pain may be caused by recent dietary changes. If the pain grows progressively worse or lasts longer than 6 hours, consult a doctor.

A self-diagnosis is not possible with the use of this chart. Discuss your symptoms with a health care provider.

Backache

Pain or stiffness that may include tenderness and may be experienced continuously or intermittently.

START

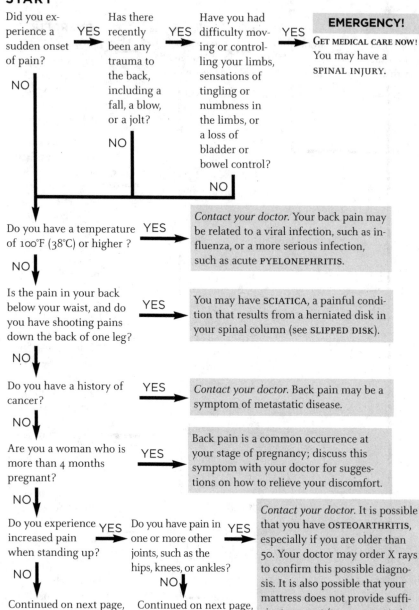

Did you experience a sudden onset of pain?

YES → Has there recently been any trauma to the back, including a fall, a blow, or a jolt?

YES → Have you had difficulty moving or controlling your limbs, sensations of tingling or numbness in the limbs, or a loss of bladder or bowel control?

YES →

EMERGENCY!
GET MEDICAL CARE NOW! You may have a SPINAL INJURY.

NO / **NO** / **NO**

Do you have a temperature of 100°F (38°C) or higher ? **YES** → *Contact your doctor.* Your back pain may be related to a viral infection, such as influenza, or a more serious infection, such as acute PYELONEPHRITIS.

NO

Is the pain in your back below your waist, and do you have shooting pains down the back of one leg? **YES** → You may have SCIATICA, a painful condition that results from a herniated disk in your spinal column (see SLIPPED DISK).

NO

Do you have a history of cancer? **YES** → *Contact your doctor.* Back pain may be a symptom of metastatic disease.

NO

Are you a woman who is more than 4 months pregnant? **YES** → Back pain is a common occurrence at your stage of pregnancy; discuss this symptom with your doctor for suggestions on how to relieve your discomfort.

NO

Do you experience increased pain when standing up? **YES** → Do you have pain in one or more other joints, such as the hips, knees, or ankles? **YES** → *Contact your doctor.* It is possible that you have OSTEOARTHRITIS, especially if you are older than 50. Your doctor may order X rays to confirm this possible diagnosis. It is also possible that your mattress does not provide sufficient support (see BACK PAIN).

NO

Continued on next page, first column

NO

Continued on next page, second column

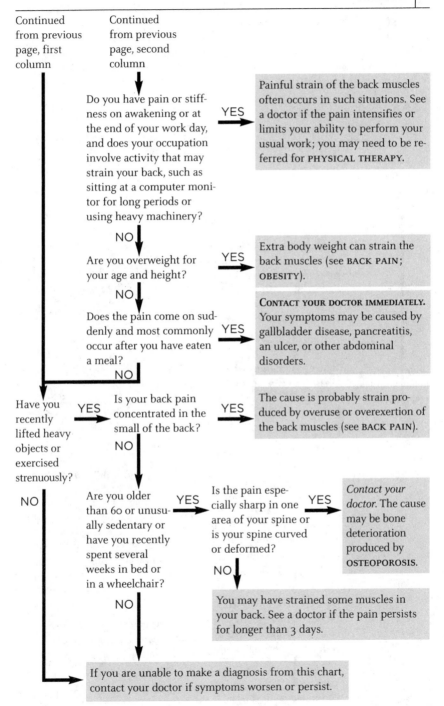

Continued from previous page, first column

Continued from previous page, second column

Do you have pain or stiffness on awakening or at the end of your work day, and does your occupation involve activity that may strain your back, such as sitting at a computer monitor for long periods or using heavy machinery?

YES → Painful strain of the back muscles often occurs in such situations. See a doctor if the pain intensifies or limits your ability to perform your usual work; you may need to be referred for PHYSICAL THERAPY.

NO

Are you overweight for your age and height?

YES → Extra body weight can strain the back muscles (see BACK PAIN; OBESITY).

NO

Does the pain come on suddenly and most commonly occur after you have eaten a meal?

YES → CONTACT YOUR DOCTOR IMMEDIATELY. Your symptoms may be caused by gallbladder disease, pancreatitis, an ulcer, or other abdominal disorders.

NO

Have you recently lifted heavy objects or exercised strenuously?

YES → Is your back pain concentrated in the small of the back?

YES → The cause is probably strain produced by overuse or overexertion of the back muscles (see BACK PAIN).

NO

Are you older than 60 or unusually sedentary or have you recently spent several weeks in bed or in a wheelchair?

YES → Is the pain especially sharp in one area of your spine or is your spine curved or deformed?

YES → *Contact your doctor.* The cause may be bone deterioration produced by OSTEOPOROSIS.

NO

You may have strained some muscles in your back. See a doctor if the pain persists for longer than 3 days.

NO

NO

If you are unable to make a diagnosis from this chart, contact your doctor if symptoms worsen or persist.

Breast pain or lumps

Pain, aching, or tenderness in one or both breasts that may commonly occur during pregnancy, within 4 months postpartum, or during breastfeeding or may be associated with the menstrual cycle or with menopause. Lumps are masses that can be felt during examination of the breast tissues.

START

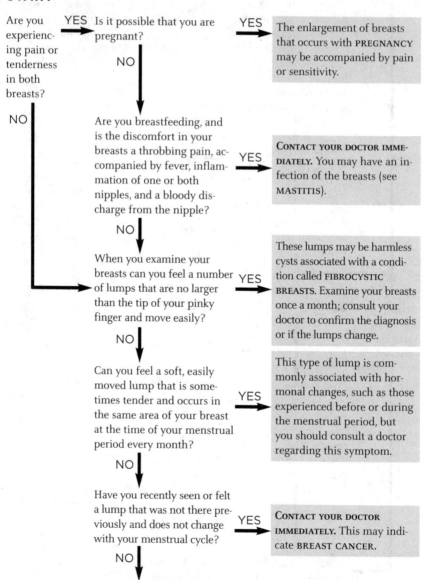

Are you experiencing pain or tenderness in both breasts?

YES → Is it possible that you are pregnant?

YES → The enlargement of breasts that occurs with PREGNANCY may be accompanied by pain or sensitivity.

NO

Are you breastfeeding, and is the discomfort in your breasts a throbbing pain, accompanied by fever, inflammation of one or both nipples, and a bloody discharge from the nipple?

YES → **CONTACT YOUR DOCTOR IMMEDIATELY.** You may have an infection of the breasts (see MASTITIS).

NO

When you examine your breasts can you feel a number of lumps that are no larger than the tip of your pinky finger and move easily?

YES → These lumps may be harmless cysts associated with a condition called FIBROCYSTIC BREASTS. Examine your breasts once a month; consult your doctor to confirm the diagnosis or if the lumps change.

NO

Can you feel a soft, easily moved lump that is sometimes tender and occurs in the same area of your breast at the time of your menstrual period every month?

YES → This type of lump is commonly associated with hormonal changes, such as those experienced before or during the menstrual period, but you should consult a doctor regarding this symptom.

NO

Have you recently seen or felt a lump that was not there previously and does not change with your menstrual cycle?

YES → **CONTACT YOUR DOCTOR IMMEDIATELY.** This may indicate BREAST CANCER.

NO

Continued on next page

Continued from previous page

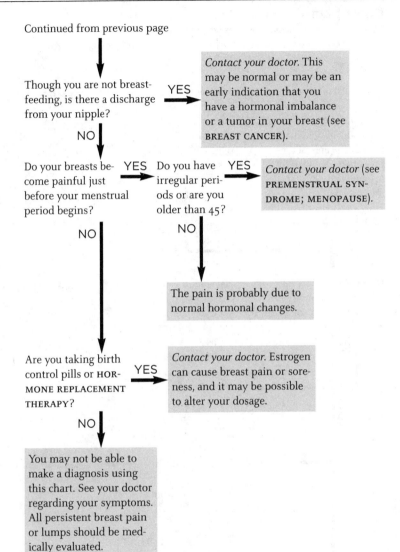

Though you are not breast-feeding, is there a discharge from your nipple?

YES → *Contact your doctor.* This may be normal or may be an early indication that you have a hormonal imbalance or a tumor in your breast (see BREAST CANCER).

NO ↓

Do your breasts become painful just before your menstrual period begins?

YES → Do you have irregular periods or are you older than 45?

YES → *Contact your doctor* (see PREMENSTRUAL SYNDROME; MENOPAUSE).

NO ↓

The pain is probably due to normal hormonal changes.

NO ↓

Are you taking birth control pills or HORMONE REPLACEMENT THERAPY?

YES → *Contact your doctor.* Estrogen can cause breast pain or soreness, and it may be possible to alter your dosage.

NO ↓

You may not be able to make a diagnosis using this chart. See your doctor regarding your symptoms. All persistent breast pain or lumps should be medically evaluated.

Chest pain

Pain that occurs in the area between the neck and the bottom of the rib cage and may be experienced as mild, aching, dull, and pressing or as severe, stabbing, burning, or crushing.

START

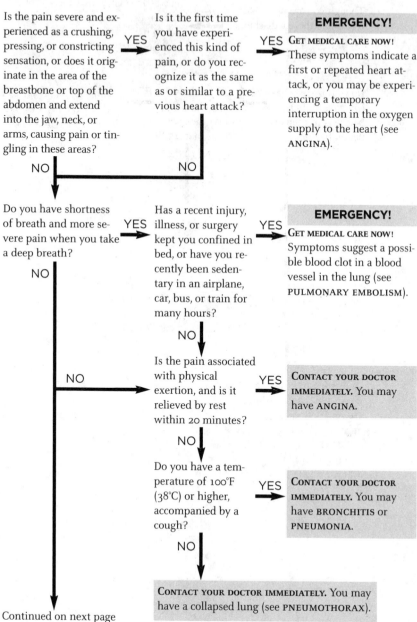

Is the pain severe and experienced as a crushing, pressing, or constricting sensation, or does it originate in the area of the breastbone or top of the abdomen and extend into the jaw, neck, or arms, causing pain or tingling in these areas?

YES → Is it the first time you have experienced this kind of pain, or do you recognize it as the same as or similar to a previous heart attack?

YES →

EMERGENCY!
GET MEDICAL CARE NOW! These symptoms indicate a first or repeated heart attack, or you may be experiencing a temporary interruption in the oxygen supply to the heart (see ANGINA).

NO

NO

Do you have shortness of breath and more severe pain when you take a deep breath?

YES → Has a recent injury, illness, or surgery kept you confined in bed, or have you recently been sedentary in an airplane, car, bus, or train for many hours?

YES →

EMERGENCY!
GET MEDICAL CARE NOW! Symptoms suggest a possible blood clot in a blood vessel in the lung (see PULMONARY EMBOLISM).

NO

NO

Is the pain associated with physical exertion, and is it relieved by rest within 20 minutes?

NO

YES → **CONTACT YOUR DOCTOR IMMEDIATELY.** You may have ANGINA.

NO

Do you have a temperature of 100°F (38°C) or higher, accompanied by a cough?

YES → **CONTACT YOUR DOCTOR IMMEDIATELY.** You may have BRONCHITIS or PNEUMONIA.

NO

CONTACT YOUR DOCTOR IMMEDIATELY. You may have a collapsed lung (see PNEUMOTHORAX).

Continued on next page

Continued from previous page

Do you experience a burning sensation in your chest, do you feel bloated, have you been belching, or does the pain become more intense when you bend forward or lie down?

 YES

This may indicate ESOPHAGEAL REFLUX (see also HEARTBURN; HIATAL HERNIA). See a doctor if symptoms persist.

NO

Is the pain more severe when you swallow?

NO

Is the pain on only one side of the chest?

YES

Have you recently injured your chest, undergone chest surgery, or had one or more episodes of severe coughing?

YES

Contact your doctor if pain persists. You may have a pulled muscle or a rib fracture.

NO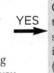

Is the main source of discomfort a burning or itching sensation in the skin of the chest, which is not affected by chest movement during breathing, or do you have blisters on the skin of your chest?

YES ➡

Contact your doctor if this symptom persists. You may have an infection of the nerves (see SHINGLES).

NO

If you cannot identify all your symptoms using the information on this chart, consult a doctor as soon as possible.

Constipation

Infrequent bowel movements (fewer than 3 per week), painful bowel movements, or uncomfortable bowel movements that produce dry or hard stools in adults.

START

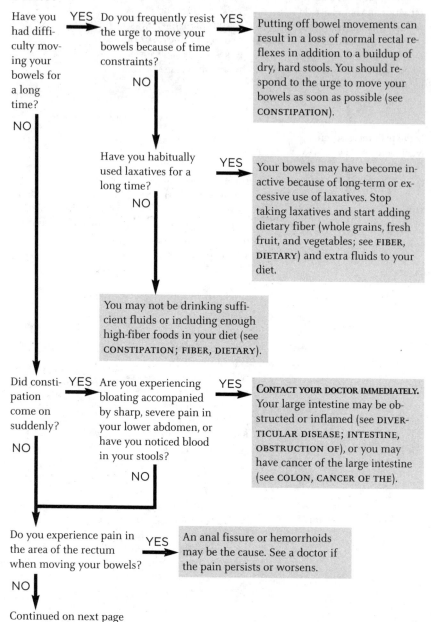

Have you had difficulty moving your bowels for a long time?

YES → Do you frequently resist the urge to move your bowels because of time constraints?

YES → Putting off bowel movements can result in a loss of normal rectal reflexes in addition to a buildup of dry, hard stools. You should respond to the urge to move your bowels as soon as possible (see CONSTIPATION).

NO ↓

Have you habitually used laxatives for a long time?

YES → Your bowels may have become inactive because of long-term or excessive use of laxatives. Stop taking laxatives and start adding dietary fiber (whole grains, fresh fruit, and vegetables; see FIBER, DIETARY) and extra fluids to your diet.

NO ↓

You may not be drinking sufficient fluids or including enough high-fiber foods in your diet (see CONSTIPATION; FIBER, DIETARY).

NO (from first question) ↓

Did constipation come on suddenly?

YES → Are you experiencing bloating accompanied by sharp, severe pain in your lower abdomen, or have you noticed blood in your stools?

YES → **CONTACT YOUR DOCTOR IMMEDIATELY.** Your large intestine may be obstructed or inflamed (see DIVERTICULAR DISEASE; INTESTINE, OBSTRUCTION OF), or you may have cancer of the large intestine (see COLON, CANCER OF THE).

NO ↓

NO ↓

Do you experience pain in the area of the rectum when moving your bowels?

YES → An anal fissure or hemorrhoids may be the cause. See a doctor if the pain persists or worsens.

NO ↓

Continued on next page

Continued from previous page

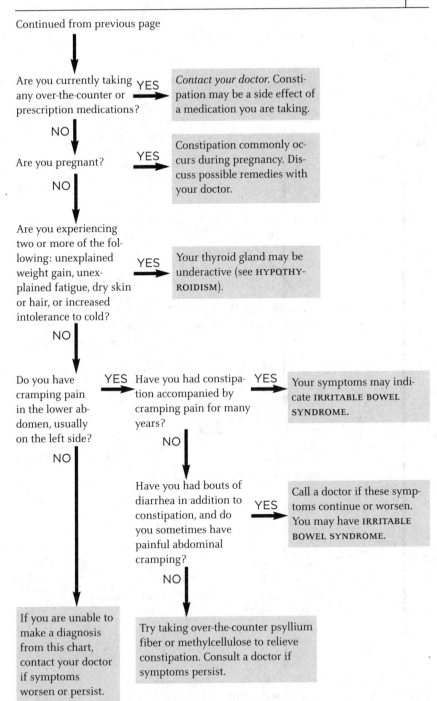

Are you currently taking any over-the-counter or prescription medications? **YES** → *Contact your doctor.* Constipation may be a side effect of a medication you are taking.

NO ↓

Are you pregnant? **YES** → Constipation commonly occurs during pregnancy. Discuss possible remedies with your doctor.

NO ↓

Are you experiencing two or more of the following: unexplained weight gain, unexplained fatigue, dry skin or hair, or increased intolerance to cold? **YES** → Your thyroid gland may be underactive (see HYPOTHYROIDISM).

NO ↓

Do you have cramping pain in the lower abdomen, usually on the left side? **YES** → Have you had constipation accompanied by cramping pain for many years? **YES** → Your symptoms may indicate IRRITABLE BOWEL SYNDROME.

NO ↓

Have you had bouts of diarrhea in addition to constipation, and do you sometimes have painful abdominal cramping? **YES** → Call a doctor if these symptoms continue or worsen. You may have IRRITABLE BOWEL SYNDROME.

NO ↓

NO (left branch) ↓ If you are unable to make a diagnosis from this chart, contact your doctor if symptoms worsen or persist.

Try taking over-the-counter psyllium fiber or methylcellulose to relieve constipation. Consult a doctor if symptoms persist.

Diarrhea

Frequent passing of loose or watery bowel movements.

START

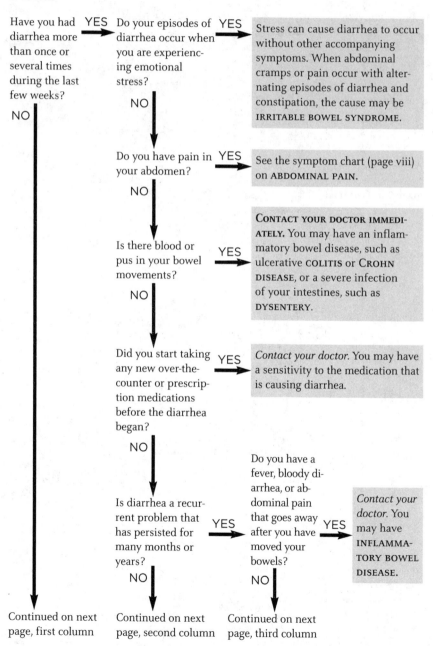

Have you had diarrhea more than once or several times during the last few weeks?

YES → Do your episodes of diarrhea occur when you are experiencing emotional stress?

YES → Stress can cause diarrhea to occur without other accompanying symptoms. When abdominal cramps or pain occur with alternating episodes of diarrhea and constipation, the cause may be IRRITABLE BOWEL SYNDROME.

NO ↓

Do you have pain in your abdomen?

YES → See the symptom chart (page viii) on ABDOMINAL PAIN.

NO ↓

Is there blood or pus in your bowel movements?

YES → CONTACT YOUR DOCTOR IMMEDIATELY. You may have an inflammatory bowel disease, such as ulcerative COLITIS or CROHN DISEASE, or a severe infection of your intestines, such as DYSENTERY.

NO ↓

Did you start taking any new over-the-counter or prescription medications before the diarrhea began?

YES → *Contact your doctor.* You may have a sensitivity to the medication that is causing diarrhea.

NO ↓

Is diarrhea a recurrent problem that has persisted for many months or years?

YES → Do you have a fever, bloody diarrhea, or abdominal pain that goes away after you have moved your bowels?

YES → *Contact your doctor.* You may have INFLAMMATORY BOWEL DISEASE.

NO ↓

NO ↓

Continued on next page, first column

Continued on next page, second column

Continued on next page, third column

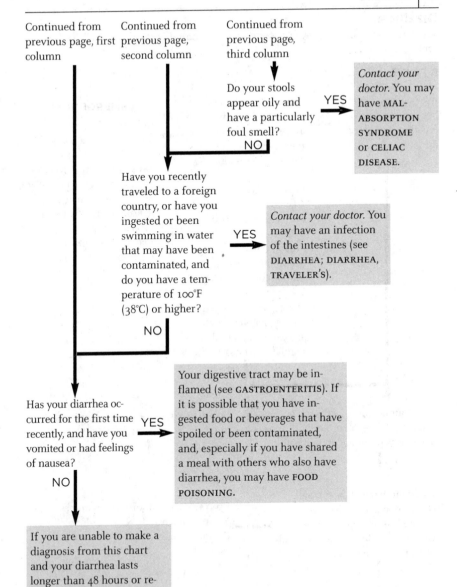

Continued from previous page, first column

Continued from previous page, second column

Continued from previous page, third column

Do your stools appear oily and have a particularly foul smell?

YES → *Contact your doctor.* You may have MAL-ABSORPTION SYNDROME or CELIAC DISEASE.

NO

Have you recently traveled to a foreign country, or have you ingested or been swimming in water that may have been contaminated, and do you have a temperature of 100°F (38°C) or higher?

YES → *Contact your doctor.* You may have an infection of the intestines (see DIARRHEA; DIARRHEA, TRAVELER'S).

NO

Has your diarrhea occurred for the first time recently, and have you vomited or had feelings of nausea?

YES → Your digestive tract may be inflamed (see GASTROENTERITIS). If it is possible that you have ingested food or beverages that have spoiled or been contaminated, and, especially if you have shared a meal with others who also have diarrhea, you may have FOOD POISONING.

NO

If you are unable to make a diagnosis from this chart and your diarrhea lasts longer than 48 hours or recurs, see a doctor for a medical evaluation.

Dizziness

A spinning sensation that may be accompanied by a dazed, unsteady feeling or a sense of light-headedness.

START

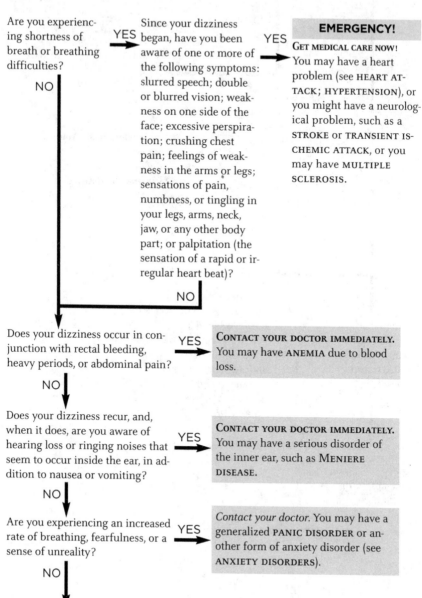

Are you experiencing shortness of breath or breathing difficulties?

YES → Since your dizziness began, have you been aware of one or more of the following symptoms: slurred speech; double or blurred vision; weakness on one side of the face; excessive perspiration; crushing chest pain; feelings of weakness in the arms or legs; sensations of pain, numbness, or tingling in your legs, arms, neck, jaw, or any other body part; or palpitation (the sensation of a rapid or irregular heart beat)?

YES → **EMERGENCY!**

GET MEDICAL CARE NOW! You may have a heart problem (see HEART ATTACK; HYPERTENSION), or you might have a neurological problem, such as a STROKE or TRANSIENT ISCHEMIC ATTACK, or you may have MULTIPLE SCLEROSIS.

NO ↓

NO

Does your dizziness occur in conjunction with rectal bleeding, heavy periods, or abdominal pain?

YES → CONTACT YOUR DOCTOR IMMEDIATELY. You may have ANEMIA due to blood loss.

NO ↓

Does your dizziness recur, and, when it does, are you aware of hearing loss or ringing noises that seem to occur inside the ear, in addition to nausea or vomiting?

YES → CONTACT YOUR DOCTOR IMMEDIATELY. You may have a serious disorder of the inner ear, such as MENIERE DISEASE.

NO ↓

Are you experiencing an increased rate of breathing, fearfulness, or a sense of unreality?

YES → *Contact your doctor.* You may have a generalized PANIC DISORDER or another form of anxiety disorder (see ANXIETY DISORDERS).

NO ↓

Continued on next page

Continued from previous page

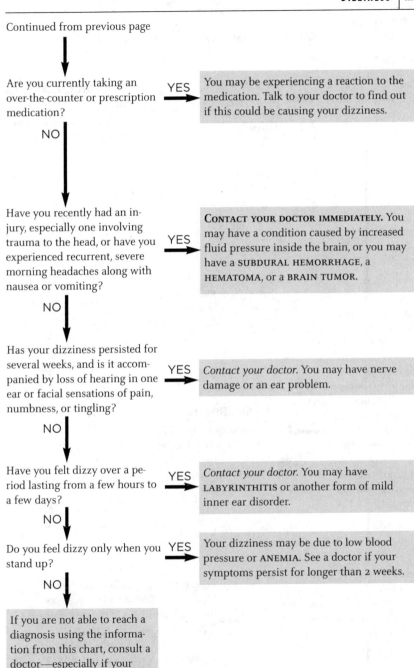

Are you currently taking an over-the-counter or prescription medication?

YES → You may be experiencing a reaction to the medication. Talk to your doctor to find out if this could be causing your dizziness.

NO

Have you recently had an injury, especially one involving trauma to the head, or have you experienced recurrent, severe morning headaches along with nausea or vomiting?

YES → **CONTACT YOUR DOCTOR IMMEDIATELY.** You may have a condition caused by increased fluid pressure inside the brain, or you may have a SUBDURAL HEMORRHAGE, a HEMATOMA, or a BRAIN TUMOR.

NO

Has your dizziness persisted for several weeks, and is it accompanied by loss of hearing in one ear or facial sensations of pain, numbness, or tingling?

YES → *Contact your doctor.* You may have nerve damage or an ear problem.

NO

Have you felt dizzy over a period lasting from a few hours to a few days?

YES → *Contact your doctor.* You may have LABYRINTHITIS or another form of mild inner ear disorder.

NO

Do you feel dizzy only when you stand up?

YES → Your dizziness may be due to low blood pressure or ANEMIA. See a doctor if your symptoms persist for longer than 2 weeks.

NO

If you are not able to reach a diagnosis using the information from this chart, consult a doctor—especially if your dizziness gets worse or persists for longer than 2 weeks.

Headache

Any pain in the head that may range in severity from mild to incapacitating.

START

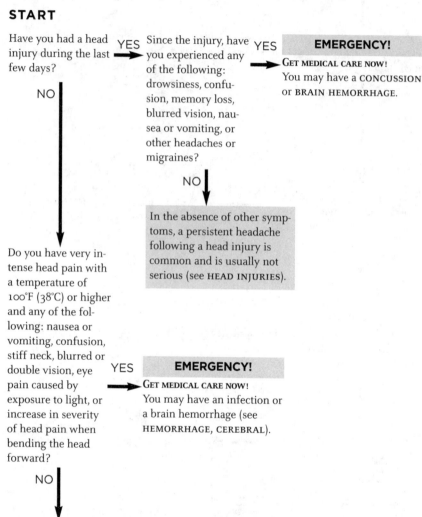

Have you had a head injury during the last few days?

YES → Since the injury, have you experienced any of the following: drowsiness, confusion, memory loss, blurred vision, nausea or vomiting, or other headaches or migraines?

YES →

EMERGENCY!

GET MEDICAL CARE NOW! You may have a CONCUSSION or BRAIN HEMORRHAGE.

NO ↓

In the absence of other symptoms, a persistent headache following a head injury is common and is usually not serious (see HEAD INJURIES).

NO ↓

Do you have very intense head pain with a temperature of 100°F (38°C) or higher and any of the following: nausea or vomiting, confusion, stiff neck, blurred or double vision, eye pain caused by exposure to light, or increase in severity of head pain when bending the head forward?

YES →

EMERGENCY!

GET MEDICAL CARE NOW! You may have an infection or a brain hemorrhage (see HEMORRHAGE, CEREBRAL).

NO ↓

In the absence of a fever, do you have severe pain in and around one eye or blurred vision in that eye, and have you vomited or felt nauseated?

YES →

CONTACT YOUR DOCTOR IMMEDIATELY. Raised pressure inside the eye may result in acute GLAUCOMA, or you may have a MIGRAINE, particularly if your vision was disturbed before the onset of your headache (see AURA).

NO ↓

Continued on next page

Continued from previous page

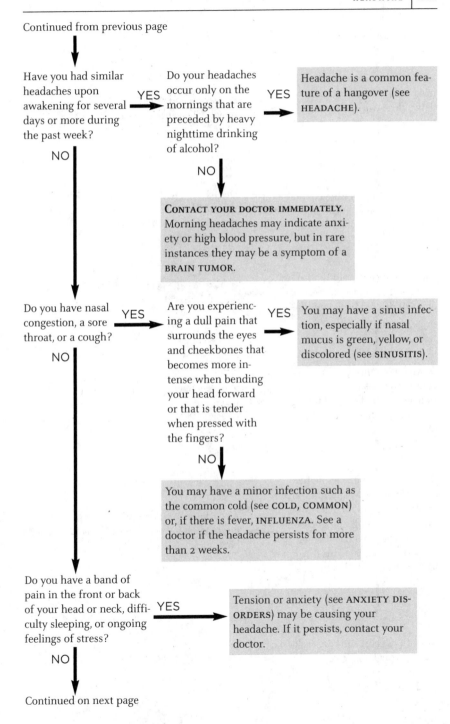

Have you had similar headaches upon awakening for several days or more during the past week?

YES →

Do your headaches occur only on the mornings that are preceded by heavy nighttime drinking of alcohol?

YES →

Headache is a common feature of a hangover (see HEADACHE).

NO ↓

CONTACT YOUR DOCTOR IMMEDIATELY. Morning headaches may indicate anxiety or high blood pressure, but in rare instances they may be a symptom of a BRAIN TUMOR.

NO ↓

Do you have nasal congestion, a sore throat, or a cough?

YES →

Are you experiencing a dull pain that surrounds the eyes and cheekbones that becomes more intense when bending your head forward or that is tender when pressed with the fingers?

YES →

You may have a sinus infection, especially if nasal mucus is green, yellow, or discolored (see SINUSITIS).

NO ↓

You may have a minor infection such as the common cold (see COLD, COMMON) or, if there is fever, INFLUENZA. See a doctor if the headache persists for more than 2 weeks.

NO ↓

Do you have a band of pain in the front or back of your head or neck, difficulty sleeping, or ongoing feelings of stress?

YES →

Tension or anxiety (see ANXIETY DISORDERS) may be causing your headache. If it persists, contact your doctor.

NO ↓

Continued on next page

Continued from previous page

Before the onset of your
headache, were you reading or
doing close work such as
sewing?

YES Eye strain and muscle strain in the neck
may be the cause (see HEADACHE).

NO

Are you taking over-the-counter
or prescription medications?

YES Discuss this with your doctor to determine
if your headache is a side effect of or a reaction to your medications.

NO

Have you recently eliminated
sources of caffeine (coffee, tea,
and soft drinks) from your diet?

YES Headaches are a common response to withdrawal from caffeine.

NO

Do you have episodes in which
your headaches recur over a period of several days and then go
away for weeks or months at a
time?

YES You may have cluster headaches (see
HEADACHE).

NO

During the 12 hours before the
onset of your headache, did you
experience any of the following:
exposure to strong sunlight, exposure to poorly ventilated or noisy
atmosphere, a missed meal, a
larger intake of alcohol than
usual?

YES All of these circumstances are apt to cause
headaches in otherwise healthy people and are
rarely a cause for concern (see HEADACHE).

NO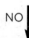

If no diagnosis can be made with the
use of this chart and your headache
lasts overnight or accompanying
symptoms develop, seek a medical
evaluation.

Nausea or vomiting

Throwing up of the contents of the stomach (vomiting), often preceded by an unpleasant sensation (nausea).

START

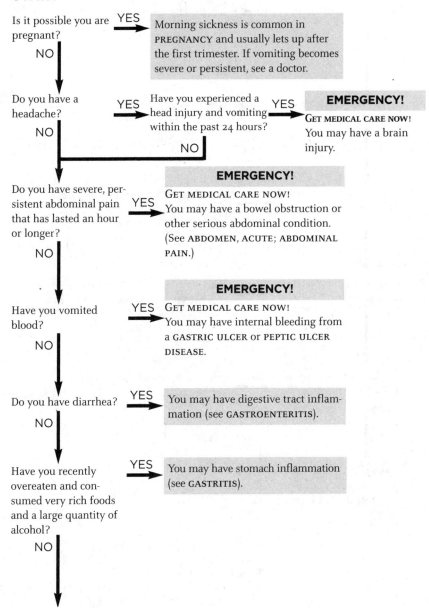

Is it possible you are pregnant?

YES → Morning sickness is common in PREGNANCY and usually lets up after the first trimester. If vomiting becomes severe or persistent, see a doctor.

NO

Do you have a headache?

YES → Have you experienced a head injury and vomiting within the past 24 hours?

NO

YES → **EMERGENCY!**
GET MEDICAL CARE NOW! You may have a brain injury.

NO

Do you have severe, persistent abdominal pain that has lasted an hour or longer?

YES → **EMERGENCY!**
GET MEDICAL CARE NOW! You may have a bowel obstruction or other serious abdominal condition. (See ABDOMEN, ACUTE; ABDOMINAL PAIN.)

NO

Have you vomited blood?

YES → **EMERGENCY!**
GET MEDICAL CARE NOW! You may have internal bleeding from a GASTRIC ULCER or PEPTIC ULCER DISEASE.

NO

Do you have diarrhea?

YES → You may have digestive tract inflammation (see GASTROENTERITIS).

NO

Have you recently overeaten and consumed very rich foods and a large quantity of alcohol?

YES → You may have stomach inflammation (see GASTRITIS).

NO

Continued on next page

Continued from previous page

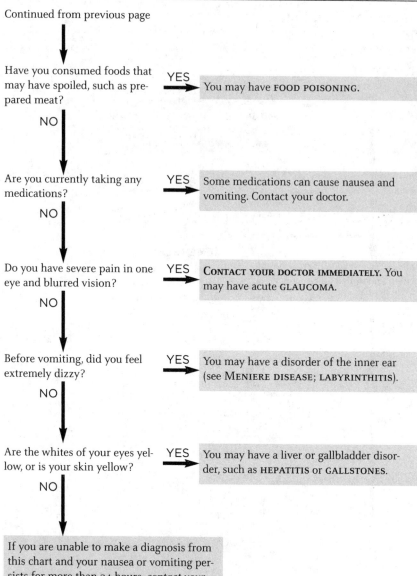

Have you consumed foods that may have spoiled, such as prepared meat?

YES → You may have FOOD POISONING.

NO

Are you currently taking any medications?

YES → Some medications can cause nausea and vomiting. Contact your doctor.

NO

Do you have severe pain in one eye and blurred vision?

YES → **CONTACT YOUR DOCTOR IMMEDIATELY.** You may have acute GLAUCOMA.

NO

Before vomiting, did you feel extremely dizzy?

YES → You may have a disorder of the inner ear (see MENIERE DISEASE; LABYRINTHITIS).

NO

Are the whites of your eyes yellow, or is your skin yellow?

YES → You may have a liver or gallbladder disorder, such as HEPATITIS or GALLSTONES.

NO

If you are unable to make a diagnosis from this chart and your nausea or vomiting persists for more than 24 hours, *contact your doctor.*

Numbness or tingling

Absence of feeling or a "pins and needles" sensation in any part of the body.

START

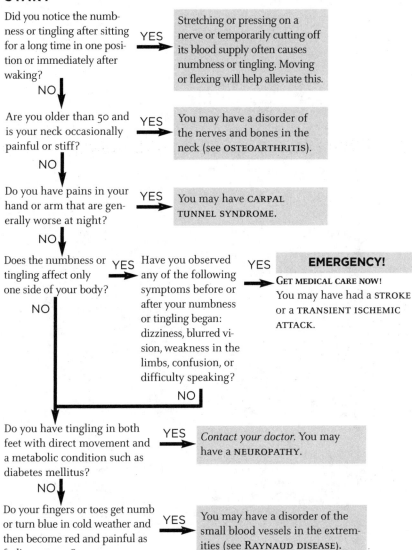

Did you notice the numbness or tingling after sitting for a long time in one position or immediately after waking?

YES → Stretching or pressing on a nerve or temporarily cutting off its blood supply often causes numbness or tingling. Moving or flexing will help alleviate this.

NO ↓

Are you older than 50 and is your neck occasionally painful or stiff?

YES → You may have a disorder of the nerves and bones in the neck (see OSTEOARTHRITIS).

NO ↓

Do you have pains in your hand or arm that are generally worse at night?

YES → You may have CARPAL TUNNEL SYNDROME.

NO ↓

Does the numbness or tingling affect only one side of your body?

YES → Have you observed any of the following symptoms before or after your numbness or tingling began: dizziness, blurred vision, weakness in the limbs, confusion, or difficulty speaking?

YES → **EMERGENCY!** GET MEDICAL CARE NOW! You may have had a STROKE or a TRANSIENT ISCHEMIC ATTACK.

NO

NO

Do you have tingling in both feet with direct movement and a metabolic condition such as diabetes mellitus?

YES → *Contact your doctor.* You may have a NEUROPATHY.

NO ↓

Do your fingers or toes get numb or turn blue in cold weather and then become red and painful as feeling returns?

YES → You may have a disorder of the small blood vessels in the extremities (see RAYNAUD DISEASE).

NO ↓

If you cannot make a diagnosis from this chart, contact your doctor if symptoms persist.

Concise
Medical
Encyclopedia

Abdomen

The region of the body that lies between the chest (thorax) and the pelvis. The abdomen encloses a cavity that houses organs of the digestive system and urinary tract, and within the bony structure of the female pelvis are the organs of the reproductive system (see REPRODUCTIVE SYSTEM, FEMALE; REPRODUCTIVE SYSTEM, MALE).

Abdomen, acute

The medical term for sudden, persistent, and severe ABDOMINAL PAIN. A person with symptoms of an acute

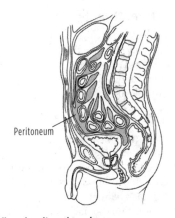

Inflamed peritoneal membrane
The most common cause of acute abdomen is inflammation of the peritoneum, the membrane that lines the abdominal cavity. It usually occurs as the result of perforation of the stomach or intestine, which allows bacteria and digestive juices to leak from the digestive tract into the abdominal cavity.

abdomen should get an immediate medical evaluation. In addition to conducting a thorough physical examination, the doctor will ask about other general symptoms such as nausea, vomiting, changes in stool, fever, fatigue, and malaise. Treatment depends on the underlying disorder.

Abdominal pain

For symptom chart, see ABDOMINAL PAIN, page viii.

Discomfort in the abdominal area or stomach region. Treatment depends on the diagnosis of the underlying disorder. Urgent medical evaluation must be sought if the abdomen is tender to the touch or rigid and board-like or if there is vomiting of blood or bloody stools.

Ablation

The destruction of a growth or harmful tissue. Ablation may refer to the use of surgical equipment, electrical current, or a laser to destroy tissue.

Ablation therapy

A procedure in which a catheter (thin tube) is used to control certain types of abnormally fast, uncoordinated heartbeats, or arrhythmias, by destroying the small areas of heart tissue that are the focus of the abnormality. Destruction of the tissue causing the heart to beat quickly and uncontrollably can prevent arrhythmias from developing and allows the heart to return to a more normal rhythm.

Abortion, elective

The voluntary termination of a pregnancy. The 1973 *Roe v. Wade* decision by the US Supreme Court ruled that American women have a constitutional right to have abortions, legalizing abortion in all 50 states. States may regulate abortions performed after 12 weeks of pregnancy. Some states have passed laws requiring a 24-hour waiting period before an abortion can be performed. Minors must obtain parental consent or approval by a court before an abortion can be performed in some states.

The earlier in pregnancy an abortion is performed, the safer the procedure is for a woman, and the less likely that complications will occur. Most abortions are performed during the first 12 weeks of pregnancy; however, sometimes a maternal illness occurs, or if the fetus dies or has a serious abnormality, an abortion is done after 12 weeks.

The choice of procedure is usually determined by the stage of the pregnancy. The most common methods of abortion are medical abortion, suction CURETTAGE, D AND E (dilation and evacuation), and labor-induced abortion. Medical abortions utilize drugs to induce the abortion and require a visit to a doctor. Suction curettage and dilation and evacuation procedures can be safely performed in a doctor's office or clinic. Labor-induced abortions are usually performed in hospitals or specialty clinics.

Immediately after an abortion, a woman's blood pressure and pulse are monitored, and she is examined for signs of excessive bleeding. After any abortion procedure, patients typically experience mild cramping and bleeding similar to that experienced during a normal period. A mild painkiller, such as ibuprofen or acetaminophen, can be taken to relieve any discomfort. Severe complications are rare.

Abortion, missed

Retention of a fetus that has died in the uterus. A missed abortion may have no signs or may be characterized by the absence of a fetal heartbeat, or a uterus that is hard, not growing, or decreasing in size. If a fetal heartbeat is not detected, an ultrasound is performed to confirm whether the fetus has died. Once the death of the fetus is confirmed, the woman and her physician will decide whether to wait and see if a spontaneous abortion (see ABORTION, SPONTANEOUS) will occur or whether to induce labor (see INDUCTION OF LABOR) or perform a dilation and evacuation (D AND E) procedure.

Abortion, spontaneous

The expulsion of a fetus by the mother's body after the fetus has died in the uterus. Also called a MISCARRIAGE.

Abortion, threatened

Any bleeding during the first half of a pregnancy, before the cervix is dilated (open). Because one in four women may have some spotting or slight bleeding, a threatened abortion is a common diagnosis. With rest, symptoms usually subside, and the pregnancy progresses normally. However, a threatened abortion may proceed to an actual MISCARRIAGE. If vaginal bleeding is accompanied by lower back pain or cramping abdominal pain, a miscarriage is more likely. Even without pain, bleeding can be a sign of a miscarriage or serious complication. A woman who is pregnant should immediately notify her doctor if she has vaginal bleeding or light spotting. A doctor may recommend a fetal ultrasound alone or in conjunction with a hormone level test, to rule out complications and assess the viability of the fetus. When a threatened abortion is diagnosed, a woman may be asked to decrease her level of activity or rest in bed until the bleeding stops.

The symptoms and the stage of the pregnancy offer clues as to the cause of the bleeding. Early in pregnancy, bleeding or light spotting may occur when a fertilized egg implants in the uterus or at the time a woman's period would have been due. However, bleeding in early pregnancy can also be due to an ECTOPIC PREGNANCY, a serious condition in which a pregnancy has developed outside the uterus. Bleeding can also result from an abnormality of the cervix or an inflammation of the vagina. Bleeding late in pregnancy can be a sign of a serious complication, such as a disorder of the placenta, or it may simply signal the beginning of labor.

Absence seizure

Also known as petit mal, a type of seizure characterized by brief episodes of loss of awareness. (See SEIZURE.) Persons having an absence seizure are described as staring or daydreaming. These seizures commonly occur during childhood and often disappear during adolescence. However, people with absence seizures are at greater risk for developing major motor or grand mal seizures during adolescence or young adulthood. Absence seizures are diagnosed by a characteristic electroencephalogram (EEG) pattern. Some children experience frequent brief seizures throughout the day that impair the ability to concentrate and learn. Treatment with appropriate medications usually allows a return to full participation in school and social activities.

Abuse, child

The physical, emotional, or sexual mistreatment or neglect of a child. National studies show that one in 20 American children are physically abused each year. The physical and psychological effects of abuse can be extensive and severe. Abuse can impair brain development and intellect, delay development of skills such as walking and speaking, and cause physical disabilities and other long-term health problems. The psychological damages of abuse continue beyond the actual episodes of mistreatment. Some abused children develop posttraumatic stress disorder, leading to symptoms such as nightmares and irritability.

Physical symptoms of abuse may include unexplained burns, bruises, or broken bones. Infants or children who have been abused or neglected often show a FAILURE TO THRIVE, a condition in which the child does not grow at the expected rate for his or her age and sex. Emotionally abused children can appear unhappy and withdrawn. A child who has been sexually abused may have recurrent infections and be overly explicit in play or conversation. There is reason to suspect abuse if the explanation a parent or caregiver gives for an injury seems inconsistent with the injury or if different caregivers' accounts contradict each other.

A child who has been abused needs treatment and protection as soon as possible. Early detection and treatment increase the likelihood of a full recovery. Whenever there is a possibility that a child is at risk, it is important to inform a doctor, social services agency, or police department. Parents who suspect their children have been abused should seek help immediately. Seeing the pediatrician or family physician is the first step. Treatment will depend on the type of abuse. The doctor can evaluate the child's condition and treat any physical problems. He or she may also refer the child to a child psychiatrist, child psychologist, clinical social worker, or rape victim advocate. Most abused children benefit from psychological counseling, especially those who have been abused by a parent or other close relative.

Doctors are required by law to report every suspected case of abuse to legal authorities, such as the state child protection agency. Once a case is reported, the agency must investigate it. For his or her own safety, a child is sometimes removed from the home while an investigation takes place. Hospital admission may be required to allow the opportunity for an in-depth medical and social evaluation. Troubled families are then given professional support and guidance. When possible, families are kept together.

Abuse, emotional

The intentional use of psychological force to hurt or destroy another person. Emotional abuse can occur between spouses and other sexual partners, between adult children and older parents, or, most commonly, between parents and children. Emotional abuse takes a number of forms, including withholding affection; using threats or terror to control the other; coercive or erratic discipline; scapegoating and rejection; failure to meet such basic physical needs as food, water, and sleep; and failure to provide love, affection, warmth, and security. Emotional abuse can occur alone or along with physical or sexual abuse (see ABUSE, SEXUAL).

Abuse of older people

Neglect or physical, psychological, or financial mistreatment of an older person. An estimated one in four older people in the United States is subjected to some form of abuse or neglect. All 50 states have passed legislation to protect older people against abuse. Abuse can occur in the home, a caregiver's home, or a long-term care facility such as a nursing home. A nearly equal number of males and females are abusers. Two-thirds are family members, most often an adult child of the abused person. Close to 70 percent of abused elders are women. The older or more disabled a person is, the more likely a caretaker will abuse her or him. The demands of caring for an infirm person, especially a person with severe mental or physical impairment, can produce stress; stress and frustration sometimes get expressed as violence. (See STRESS.)

The appearance of physical injuries, such as bruises, welts, lacerations, unhealed open wounds, broken bones, or burns, must be investigated. A caretaker's refusal to let visitors see an older person alone may signal an abusive situation. Psychological abuse and neglect can be the most difficult to detect because they do not leave obvious signs, and abused older people can be fearful and reluctant to speak up for themselves. Symptoms of psychological abuse may include agitation, withdrawal, and apathy. Unusual behavior, such as rocking or biting, or the older person's own reports of mistreatment, are strong indicators of abuse. Dehydration, malnutrition, and lack of personal hygiene are common signs of neglect.

Abuse, partner

Physical, sexual, or psychological abuse of one person in a relationship by another. Partner abuse is the most common pattern of domestic or family violence, in which one partner establishes power and control over the other through fear, domination, and intimidation. Although women are most often the victims of domestic violence, women also abuse their male partners. Partner abuse also occurs within same-sex relationships. Partner abuse generally begins with threats, name-calling, and physically destructive acts to objects or pets, escalating to violent behavior such as pushing, slapping, punching, kicking, breaking of bones, bruising, or even to the final violent act of murder. In the United States, partner abuse is considered a crime, but laws vary by state.

Abuse, sexual

Coercing another person by means of physical force, tricks, bribes, or threats into a sexual activity that gratifies the abuser. Sexual abuse can occur between adults and children or adolescents; between adolescents or older children and young children; and between adults, both heterosexual and homosexual. Sexual abuse between adults or between children or adolescents of different ages is commonly referred to as rape or sexual assault, which includes forced or coerced vaginal, oral, or anal intercourse or penetration with an object. (See also RAPE.) Under the laws of some states, it may also include fondling or erotic touching without the consent of the person being touched. Sexual abuse of children includes not only intercourse or penetration, but also fondling, looking at, or photographing a child's nude body; display of the adult's genitals to the child; and sexual activity in front of a child, including self-stimulation by an adult or intercourse between two individuals.

Children are most often sexually abused by members of their own family, which constitutes INCEST. Sexual abuse may cause physical injuries, but most of the damage is psychological and can last long after the abusive incidents. Sexual abuse of all varieties is illegal under state law.

ACE inhibitors

See ANTIHYPERTENSIVES.

Achalasia

A rare disorder in which the sphincter muscle at the lower end of the esophagus, a tube that connects the throat and stomach, fails to contract and relax properly. Achalasia causes difficulty in swallowing solids and liquids. Symptoms of achalasia include regurgitation of food eaten in the preceding day or two, chest pain, an unpleasant taste in the mouth, and bad breath.

In some cases, the symptoms of achalasia can be relieved for 6 months to several years by dilating the esophagus in a special procedure that can be repeated as necessary. In resistant cases, surgery may be required. Recently, some relief has been obtained by injection of botulinum toxin into the lower esophageal sphincter.

Achilles tendinitis

A painful inflammation of the tendon that connects the calf muscles of the legs to the heel bones. The Achilles tendon raises and flexes the foot and ankle downward during walking and running. Achilles tendinitis can cause severe pain that inhibits or prevents movement and weight-bearing function in the back of the lower legs. It is usually caused by injury or overuse.

The most important treatment for this condition is a reduction in the activity that brought on the symptoms. Gentle stretching of the calf muscles before and after an athletic activity or a workout may be helpful. Applying ice to the painful area after training may also help. The use of orthotics (special shoe inserts) in combination with a heel lift inserted in the shoes may minimize pain by reducing stress on the inflamed tendon. Physical therapy includes the use of whirlpool, electrical stimulation, and ultrasound treatment.

Achondroplasia

A common genetic disorder of bone growth that is usually evident at birth. Children with achondroplasia have short arms and legs, particularly upper arms and thighs; large heads with prominent foreheads and noses that are flat at the bridge between the eyes; curved lower spines; bowed lower legs; short stubby fingers; short, flat feet; and poor muscle tone.

Other problems include frequent ear infections that can cause hearing loss and back and leg pain and paralysis due to pressure on the spinal nerves from spinal deformities.

Achondroplasia affects one in every 10,000 births and equally affects both sexes and all races. The disorder generally does not include mental retardation, and the life span is usually normal.

Achondroplasia, a dominant genetic disorder, is caused by an abnormal gene on chromosome 4. Affected individuals have a 50 percent chance of passing it on to their children. However, in 80 to 90 percent of cases, neither of the parents is affected, and the achondroplasia is caused by a spontaneous mutation in the gene of the affected individual. Paternal age seems to be a factor in these sporadic mutations; men who become fathers when they are 40 years old or older are more likely to have children with achondroplasia than men who are younger. Maternal age is not a factor.

There is no current treatment to normalize skeletal development of children with achondroplasia. Infants and children with the disorder should be evaluated by a doctor experienced with the disorder, such as a geneticist or an orthopedist. Detection of spinal abnormalities likely to cause spinal cord compression is particularly important, since breathing difficulties and leg paralysis can result from such compression. Surgery may be necessary to prevent bowed legs or to relieve nerve or spinal cord pressure from surrounding bones. Humps may develop in the middle back that usually go away when the child begins to walk. When the humps fail to go away, surgery may be required.

Acid

A chemical compound capable of neutralizing alkalis and releasing hydrogen ions when in solution. Acids are corrosive and usually have a sour taste. An acid reacts with a base to form a salt, has a pH (a measure of the acidity of a solution) less than 7, and will turn blue litmus red.

Acid reflux

See ESOPHAGEAL REFLUX

Acid-base balance

A state of equilibrium between acidity and alkalinity of body fluids. The acid-base balance keeps body fluids at or near a neutral pH (neither acidic nor basic) for normal body function. Such a balance is necessary because most of the body's metabolic processes produce acids, while vital cellular activities require a somewhat alkaline, or basic, body fluid. Acid-base balance requires a body fluid pH of between 7.35 and 7.45 if enzyme systems and other metabolic activities are to function normally. If the body fluid pH falls below 7.30, ACIDOSIS is said to exist; if it rises above 7.50, a state of alkalosis exists. Both acidosis and alkalosis are considered serious.

Acidosis

A serious metabolic disorder that results from the accumulation of acid or a depletion of the alkaline content of the blood and tissues. The pH of the blood becomes abnormally low, indicating that the blood is excessively acidic. Acidosis occurs in cases of uncontrolled type 1 diabetes (see DIABETES MELLITUS, TYPE 1), severe kidney disorders, and some lung diseases. Respiratory acidosis can result from conditions that prevent the lungs from ventilating properly, causing carbon dioxide to accumulate. Treatment for acidosis depends on the underlying cause. For example, KETOACIDOSIS from uncontrolled diabetes requires administration of intravenous fluids and insulin. In severe cases, sodium bicarbonate to neutralize the acid may be given, or a mechanical ventilator may be used to improve respiration.

Acne

An inflammatory condition characterized by whiteheads, blackheads, and pimples. Acne lesions are seen most frequently on the face but may also develop on the back, chest, shoulders, and neck. Whiteheads—small, hard, painless, white blemishes—commonly occur in clusters on the cheeks, nose, and chin. Blackheads are composed primarily of dried body oils and shed skin cells, while pimples contain pus. While acne can occur at any age, it is most common during adolescence.

As people age, acne usually disappears on its own. However, if left untreated, it can lead to permanent scarring. Fortunately, there are many antiacne treatments. Topical medications are available both over-the-counter and by prescription. In moderate to severe cases of acne, doctors prescribe oral medications such as antibiotics and isotretinoin. Scars resulting from acne may be improved by procedures including CHEMICAL PEEL, DERMABRASION (removal of the surface layer of skin by high-speed sanding), and LASER RESURFACING.

Topical medications—lotions and creams—are good for treating acne accompanied by dry skin, while alcohol-based gels and solutions are best for treating acne-prone oily skin. These medications are designed to decrease inflammation and limit the formation of new pimples. Prescription topical drugs include benzoyl peroxide (in a more powerful concentration than the over-the-counter brands), tretinoin, and antibiotics. Tretinoin, a type of drug called a retinoid, is a derivative of vitamin A and one of the most effective topical antiacne medications.

Acoustic neuroma

A benign tumor of the eighth cranial nerve (also known as the acoustic nerve, the auditory nerve, and the vestibulocochlear nerve; it is located in the head). The cause of acoustic neuromas is believed to be a defect in a tumor suppressor gene, and bilateral acoustic tumors are associated with a genetic disorder known as NEUROFIBROMATOSIS TYPE 2 (NF2). Acoustic neuromas are almost always noncancerous and do not spread or metastasize to other parts of the body. However, they can grow quite large, causing damage to surrounding structures.

Acoustic neuromas are rarely seen in people younger than 30 years. Acoustic neuromas can press against the hearing and balance nerves, leading to symptoms of hearing loss, ringing in the ears (tinnitus), and dizziness. Other symptoms include headache, trouble understanding speech, vertigo, loss of balance, and facial numbness or pain. Larger tumors can affect the facial nerve, leading to facial paralysis. Ultimately, if untreated, a large tumor can cause increased pressure on the brain, which may result in lethargy, nausea and vomiting, and a dilated pupil in one eye. In these cases, acoustic neuromas become life-threatening.

MRI (magnetic resonance imaging) of the head is the most effective means of diagnosing an acoustic neuroma. Other helpful tests include CT (computed tomography) scans, hearing tests, caloric stimulation (a test for dizziness or vertigo), electronystagmography (a test of equilibrium and balance), and brain stem auditory evoked response (a test of hearing and brain stem function). The doctor will also take a careful history and perform a neurological examination.

Surgical removal of the tumor is the usual treatment of choice. Another treatment option is radiation therapy, which slows the growth of the tumor rather than removing it. Radiation may be recommended for older or sicker people who cannot tolerate brain surgery or following a proce-

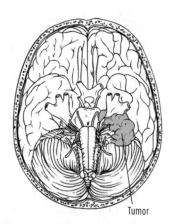

Tumor

Tumor on a cranial nerve

An acoustic neuroma forms on the eighth cranial nerve, which passes through a bony canal between the brain and the inner ear. The facial nerve passes through the same canal.

dure in which it was not possible to remove the entire tumor.

Acquired immunodeficiency syndrome

A life-threatening disorder caused by infection with HIV (human immunodeficiency virus) and characterized by a breakdown of the body's immune defenses. See AIDS.

Acromegaly

A rare, slowly progressive, chronic hormonal disorder caused by an overproduction of growth hormone by the pituitary gland. In most cases, the excess production of growth hormone is caused by an ADENOMA, a benign (not cancerous) tumor, which in acromegaly affects the pituitary gland. Treatment options include surgery to remove the adenoma, medication, and radiation of the pituitary gland.

Acrophobia

An abnormal fear of heights. If acrophobia is a symptom of DEPRESSION or if it interferes with the everyday tasks of living, psychological treatment is recommended.

ACTH

Adrenocorticotropic hormone; also known as corticotropin or adrenocorticotropin. ACTH is a hormone that controls the production and secretion of certain other hormones from the ADRENAL GLANDS.

Actinic keratosis

A red, scaly, precancerous skin lesion that is the result of years of sun exposure. Actinic keratoses usually occur on parts of the body that experience the most exposure to ultraviolet light, such as the face, ears, and backs of the hands. Most lesions develop in middle age or later; appear as small (less than $3/4$ inch), dry, scaly bumps on the skin surface; and may be tan, pink, or red. Actinic keratoses are precancerous, meaning that, if left untreated, a lesion may develop into SQUAMOUS CELL CARCINOMA, a serious type of SKIN CANCER. Squamous cell carcinoma is usually not life-threatening if detected and treated early but, if left untreated, it can spread into lymph nodes or internal organs and become incurable.

Actinic keratoses can be removed by CRYOSURGERY (freezing with liquid nitrogen), topical chemotherapy, curettage (scraping), electrodesiccation (burning with an electric current delivered through a probe), or CHEMICAL PEEL (use of a chemical agent to remove damaged skin).

Acupressure

A noninvasive method to relieve pain and manage stress using the fingertips or hands to stimulate the body's self-curative abilities. Acupressure is an ancient form of Chinese medicine that uses pressure exerted by the hands to aid healing.

Acupuncture

A technique in which extremely thin needles are inserted into specific points on the body to treat or prevent illness. Acupuncture is an ancient form of traditional Chinese medicine that has been practiced for 3,000 years.

In the United States, acupuncture has most often been used to relieve chronic pain caused by arthritis, migraine headache, premenstrual syndrome (PMS), or back pain. Another common use of acupuncture is to assist people in withdrawal from drug and alcohol dependency. Some acupuncturists use it to reduce pain during surgery.

Acute

A term that describes symptoms or disease that begins abruptly and subsides within a relatively short period. In contrast to CHRONIC health problems, the onset of abrupt or acute symptoms is characterized by sharpness, severity, or intensity.

ADA

See AMERICANS WITH DISABILITIES ACT (ADA).

ADD

The acronym for attention deficit disorder. See ATTENTION DEFICIT/HYPERACTIVITY DISORDER.

Addiction

A behavior pursued not for the pleasure or gain it provides but as a way of satisfying a physical or deep-seated psychological compulsion. Addiction often refers to the use of chemicals, such as alcohol (see ALCOHOL DEPENDENCE), tobacco (see SMOKING, TOBACCO), and illegal drugs such as cocaine, crack cocaine, heroin, amphetamines, and marijuana (see DRUG ADDICTION). Addiction can also arise with gambling (see GAMBLING, ADDICTIVE) and sexual activity (see SEXUAL ADDICTION). A person may have more than one addiction and be genetically predisposed to abusing drugs and alcohol.

Addison disease

A rare hormonal disorder that is caused by an inadequate production of cortisol, a hormone produced by the adrenal glands; also known as chronic adrenal insufficiency, hypoadrenocorticism, and hypocorticalism. Addison disease is usually the result of an autoimmune disorder. Less frequently, Addison disease can be caused by tuberculosis, fungal infections, the spread of cancer cells to the adrenal glands, AMYLOIDOSIS, surgical removal of the adrenal glands, and failure of the pituitary gland to produce enough ACTH (adrenocorticotropic hormone). Symptoms tend to begin gradually and include chronic fatigue, muscle weakness, loss of appetite, weight loss, nausea, vomiting, diarrhea, low blood pressure, a low blood sugar level, and hyperpigmentation. Untreated, this illness can lead to shock and death.

The most specific test for diagnosing Addison disease is the ACTH stimulation test, in which levels of cortisol in the blood or urine are measured before and after a synthetic form of ACTH is injected.

Treatment is aimed at replacing the missing hormones with synthetic forms, such as the oral medication hydrocortisone. Fludrocortisone acetate is a medication taken when ALDOSTERONE, a hormone also made by the adrenal glands, is deficient.

Adenitis

An inflammatory condition of a LYMPH NODE; also known as lymphadenitis. The condition may affect lymph nodes in the neck; at the back of the neck; in the mesentery, the membrane that attaches organs to the abdominal wall; or all the lymph nodes.

Treatment of localized adenitis requires the use of antimicrobial agents to treat the primary infection causing the condition. The application of warm compresses to the affected sites may help relieve discomfort. In severe forms, adenitis is treated surgically to drain the nodes.

Adenocarcinoma

A cancer derived from glandular tissue. Adenocarcinomas develop on the linings or inner surfaces of organs, such as the lung, pancreas, breast, prostate, esophagus, stomach, vagina, urethra, or small intestine. Nearly all colon cancers and about 40 percent of lung cancers are adenocarcinomas.

Adenoidectomy

The surgical removal of enlarged ADENOIDS (clusters of tissue at the back of the nose and throat), usually of a child. Adenoids are surgically removed only if they significantly interfere with a child's ability to breathe, swallow, or speak. Surgery may also be performed to treat a recurring severe sore throat caused by a "strep" infection; an abscess involving the tonsils; a suspected cancerous enlargement of the tonsil; or a middle ear infection that does not respond to other treatments, such as antibiotics or the placement of drainage tubes in the ears (see OTITIS MEDIA).

Adenoids

One of two small masses of tissue at the back of the nose above the tonsils. Also known as pharyngeal tonsils, the adenoids are part of the LYMPHATIC SYSTEM, and their function is to stop disease-causing microorganisms from entering the body through the nose or mouth. Adenoids tend to enlarge during childhood and are a frequent site of infections. But adenoids shrink in most children after age 5 and may disappear by puberty.

Adenoma

A benign (not cancerous) tumor of a glandular structure. Adenomas affect many organs such as the pituitary gland, the adrenal glands, and the thyroid glands (see THYROID NODULE).

Pituitary adenomas

A pituitary adenoma occurs in the pituitary gland, which is located at the base of the brain and produces many hormones that are involved in governing the activity of other glands. Adenomas on the pituitary gland can lead to diseases such as ACROMEGALY and CUSHING SYNDROME.

The rate of growth for a pituitary adenoma varies. It may grow gradually, causing few if any symptoms, or it may show aggressive growth and compress surrounding brain tissues as it expands. Symptoms could include headache and vision disturbances such as loss of peripheral vision, double vision, and drooping of the eyelids. Excessive thirst and urination, fatigue, light-headedness, and intolerance to cold are other symptoms of a pituitary adenoma.

Adrenal adenomas

Adrenal cortical adenomas are located on the adrenal cortex (the outer layer of the adrenal glands). These tumors are usually benign, tend to affect women more than men, and are more common in people older than 40 years. Adrenal tumors can result in Cushing syndrome or high blood pressure and low potassium levels.

Treatment

Treatment of adenomas may require surgical removal in combination with hormonal therapy to reestablish the proper balance of hormones in the body. Adenomas that do not cause symptoms may not need surgery immediately and may be monitored by your doctor.

Adenomyosis

A condition characterized by abnormal menstrual pain, typically affecting women in their 40s. As a woman ages, endometrial tissue can become embedded in the muscular wall of the uterus. As a result, a woman may experience bleeding and painful menstruation. A doctor may prescribe hormonal medication to control pain and bleeding. If hormonal medications do not alleviate the woman's symptoms, a hysterectomy may be recommended. Menopause usually brings relief.

Adenosine diphosphate

See ADP.

Adenovirus

A type of virus most commonly associated with respiratory illness. Adenoviruses can also cause gastroenteritis (particularly watery diarrhea), conjunctivitis, cystitis, and rash. When this virus causes respiratory illness, the infection may range from the level of the common cold to more serious illness including pneumonia, croup, and bronchitis. Infections caused by this virus are usually mild, and generally only the symptoms are treated. When serious illness results, it is managed by treating symptoms and complications since no virus-specific therapy is available.

ADH

Antidiuretic hormone; also known as vasopressin. A naturally occurring hormone, produced by the hypothalamus, that regulates fluid balance, blood pressure, and the volume of urine produced by the kidneys.

ADHD

The acronym for ATTENTION DEFICIT/ HYPERACTIVITY DISORDER.

Adhesions

Bands of scar tissue that form between the loops of the intestines or between the intestines and the abdominal wall. Adhesions develop as tissues heal after abdominal surgery or when there is inflammation of the membrane lining the abdominal wall. Adhesions may cause pain in the abdomen when they are pulled or stretched because scar tissue is not elastic.

Abdominal adhesions can occasionally lead to an obstruction of the intestine (see INTESTINE, OBSTRUCTION OF). Gangrene, the death of tissue, can develop if the blood supply to part of the intestine is interrupted. If the problem is not resolved, either spontaneously or by using techniques such as decompressing the intestine with suction, surgery may be necessary.

Adhesive otitis media, chronic

The end stage of middle ear effusion (accumulation of fluid) that leads to EUSTACHIAN TUBE dysfunction. The eardrum becomes thinner and retracts toward the inner wall of the middle ear. In time, the drum may contact the incus and stapes (small middle ear bones) and even drape over them or touch the inner wall of the middle ear. Early on, this process can be reversed by placement of a drainage tube. In time, the drum may become scarred at the areas of contact, and the volume of air or fluid in the middle ear will shrink—sometimes down to nothing. The middle ear bones may erode, and sometimes tissue with a grainy texture (granulation tissue) grows from poorly covered bone. The ear may drain, and the tissue growth may resemble a tumor.

Fortunately, hearing loss is usually mild with this condition and usually does not progress. In cases of more severe hearing loss, a hearing aid or surgery is an option, but surgery is difficult and requires a lifetime of tubes to maintain any gain. Examination once or twice a year for a few years by a doctor is needed once this diagnosis is made. See also OTITIS MEDIA.

Adipose tissue

Animal tissue containing fat. Adipose means "fat," and adipose tissue refers specifically to tissue found under the skin or around internal organs that is chiefly made up of fat cells.

Adjustment disorder

A mental illness characterized by a disturbing emotional or behavioral reaction to stress that affects the individual's ability to function, or that greatly exceeds the normal reaction to stress. If adjustment disorder begins in response to a single event, it arises within 3 months of the event and usually improves within 6 months. If the source of stress is ongoing, the disorder may persist for longer than 6 months.

In most cases, some form of therapy is recommended. Medication may be used with therapy.

Adolescence

A period of rapid physical, emotional, social, and intellectual growth from ages 10 through 21. Adolescence begins at PUBERTY with the onset of physical and sexual developments that enable reproduction and ends with the transition into adulthood. Developmentally, adolescence is viewed as beginning at age 10 and proceeding in three stages: early (ages 10 to 13); middle (ages 14 to 17); and late (ages 18 to 21).

The early stage is characterized by the start of puberty (sexual maturation) and a major growth spurt. Girls usually experience puberty a year or two before boys. With the middle stage come intensified sexual desires, increased sociability, and experiments with risky behavior such as smoking, trying alcohol and drugs, and having unprotected sex. Peer pressure becomes a strong influence. In the late stage, the adolescent begins to settle down and focus energies on plans for the future. The psychosocial development of adolescence involves several tasks concerned with transforming the child into an adult. They include establishing independence, achieving a realistic and satisfying self-image, exploring sexuality, and choosing life roles (for example, a career). As the child tries to accomplish these tasks, conflicts often arise.

Because of the tremendous growth spurt that takes place during puberty, teenagers require extra calories and good nutrition. Calcium is essential, because half the body's total bone mass is formed during these years.

ADP

Adenosine diphosphate. An organic compound that consists of adenine, ribose, and two phosphate units. ADP is formed when adenosine triphosphate (ATP) is broken down by its re-action with water so one phosphate unit and one hydrogen ion are removed from the ATP molecule. Most of the reactions that consume energy in the cells are driven by the conversion of ATP to ADP. These reactions include transmitting nerve signals, moving muscles, synthesizing protein, and dividing cells.

Adrenal failure

A sudden, potentially fatal condition that occurs when the adrenal glands do not produce and release a sufficient amount of cortisol; also known as adrenal crisis, addisonian crisis, or acute adrenal insufficiency. Cortisol is a hormone that enables the body to use nutrients, cope with stress, and regulate the immune system. Symptoms include headache, profound weakness, fatigue, nausea, decreased blood pressure, dehydration, and high fever. Adrenal failure can be diagnosed by the ACTH (adrenocorticotropic hormone) stimulation test, other blood tests, and urine analysis.

Adrenal failure is a medical emergency that requires immediate treatment to avoid shock or even death. Emergency treatment for adrenal failure includes an injection of the corticosteroid hydrocortisone and hospitalization for general observation and for treatment of low blood pressure with intravenous fluids. Antibiotics may be given if infection is involved.

Adrenal glands

The two vital organs that produce and secrete hormones into the bloodstream via veins that drain them; also known as suprarenal glands. The triangular-shaped adrenal glands are located on top of the two kidneys. The adrenal glands have two different kinds of cellular tissue that each have their own unique cellular function. The inner portion of an adrenal gland is called the adrenal medulla and secretes the hormone EPINEPHRINE, which is produced by the sympathetic nervous system at times of stress, regulates blood pressure, increases heart rate, and raises the blood sugar level. The adrenal medulla also secretes NOREPINEPHRINE, a hormone that helps maintain normal blood pressure.

The outer layer of the adrenal glands, called the adrenal cortex, secretes as many as 30 different steroid hormones including ALDOSTERONE, which is important for regulating salt and water in the body, and CORTISOL, which is essential for regulating the response to stress, as well as for regulating the metabolism of fat, carbohydrate, and protein. Adrenal sex steroids are usually the major source of testosterone in women. However, adrenal testosterone is of little importance in men because the testicles make larger amounts of testosterone.

Adrenal hyperplasia, congenital

A group of disorders caused by a deficiency of the enzyme that is essential to the production, by the adrenal cortex (the outer layer of the adrenal glands), of steroid hormones called corticosteroids. The enzyme deficiency in a fetus is the result of inheriting two defective genes, one from the father and one from the mother.

When severe, congenital adrenal hyperplasia produces an inability to respond to stress and properly maintain the balance of salt and water in the body. An affected fetus may become extremely dehydrated, and AD-RENAL FALURE may occur. Less severe forms may result in early sexual development and rapid growth in childhood. Adolescent girls may experience growth of unwanted facial and body hair and irregular menstrual periods. Male and female adolescents may have severe acne. Women who have difficulty getting pregnant because of congenital adrenal hyperplasia may undergo treatment with hormone replacement therapy.

Congenital adrenal hyperplasia is diagnosed by analysis of blood and urine. The condition is generally treated in children by administering hydrocortisone medication, orally or by injection. In adolescents and adults, a more potent, longer-acting corticosteroid may be given. There is also medication to correct salt imbalance. Genital surgery may be necessary for affected females. Psychological counseling is often recommended before puberty, especially for girls.

Adrenaline

See EPINEPHRINE.

Adrenocorticotropic hormone

See ACTH.

Adrenogenital syndrome

A condition, affecting both men and women, caused by the secretion of excess adrenal SEX HORMONES, typically male sex hormones. Adrenogenital syndrome is generally caused by a tumor on the adrenal cortex (the outer layer of the adrenal glands). An affected woman will have masculine hair growth patterns (includ-

ing excess facial hair and sometimes male-pattern hair loss), deepening of the voice, an enlarged clitoris, and a masculine appearance of the skin and muscles. When adrenogenital syndrome occurs in boys before puberty, rapid sexual development may occur at an abnormally young age. In adult males, testosterone may obscure the signs. In rare cases, the adrenal tumor may secrete female hormones, producing enlarged breasts in men.

Advance directives

Legal documents that state how a person's health care should proceed if he or she becomes physically or mentally unable to communicate his or her wishes. Advance directives specify the type of care and who makes the care decisions and may provide instructions on other matters such as ORGAN DONATION. Their primary function is to give a person the option of avoiding aggressive treatments that may cause pain or incur great expense but offer little benefit. Commonly prepared for older people, advance directives are also used by people with terminal illnesses, those with a condition that has a poor outlook, those who have a strong point of view concerning their care, and parents who do not want to spend their resources on their own terminal care.

Types of directives include: a living will, which specifies which medical treatments an individual wants or does not want, in the event that he or she becomes unable to make decisions or communicate them; a durable power of attorney for health care, which, when signed, dated, and witnessed, designates a surrogate decision maker to make critical health care decisions after an individual becomes incapacitated; and a do-not-resuscitate order (DNR order), which designates that cardiopulmonary resuscitation (CPR) will not be administered if an individual's heart stops.

Legal Aspects

Laws concerning advance directives differ from state to state. Most states recognize the validity of advance directives written in another state. To ensure that advance directives are followed, one copy is usually given to the doctor and another to a family member, friend, or lawyer. All advance directives can be changed or cancelled at any time.

Adverse drug reaction

An unexpected and potentially harmful response to a drug that is unrelated to its intended effect. Adverse drug reactions can occur because of the nature of the drug taken or because the person taking it is allergic to the drug. Adverse drug reactions can be mild, moderate, or severe and life-threatening. Because most drugs are taken orally, either as pills or capsules, and are digested in the gastrointestinal tract, the most common reactions are nausea, loss of appetite, and diarrhea. Rashes are also a common adverse drug reaction.

Aerobic

Requiring oxygen. Aerobic is an adjective used to describe activities, life forms, or events that depend on the presence of oxygen.

Affective disorders

Another term for mood disorders, which are characterized by a distur-

bance in emotions and feelings. The disturbance may be expressed as either elation or unhappiness. There are various types of mood disorders, including DYSTHMIA (a low-grade depression), major DEPRESSION, and BIPOLAR DISORDER.

AFP test

Alpha-fetoprotein test. A measurement of the level of alpha-fetoprotein (AFP) in a pregnant woman's blood; it reflects the amount of AFP produced by a developing fetus. The test is used to detect birth defects. A high level of AFP in a woman's blood sometimes indicates that the fetus has a neural tube defect, a birth defect in which the skull, brain, or spinal cord does not develop properly. AFP testing combined with other biochemical and hormonal measurements can also screen for other fetal abnormalities, including Down syndrome.

Afterbirth

The PLACENTA and membranes that are expelled from the mother's body shortly after the birth of the baby. Delivery of the afterbirth commonly occurs within 30 minutes after delivery of the baby and is the final stage of LABOR.

Afterpains

Abdominal cramps a woman feels after childbirth. After delivery, hormones stimulate contractions that help shrink the uterus to its prepregnancy size. Contractions may last for several days after the birth.

Agar

A gelatinlike substance made from red seaweed. Agar is best known as a solidifying component used to culture bacteria for laboratory analysis.

Agenesis

Absence or lack of development of an organ in an embryo. Examples of agenesis include the absence of ovaries (ovarian agenesis), a defective development of part of the brain (callosal agenesis), or absence of kidneys (renal agenesis).

Agent

Any physical substance capable of producing an effect. A pharmacological agent, for example, is one capable of causing a biological response, while a pathological agent is one capable of causing disease.

Agent Orange

An herbicide and a defoliant used by the United States military during the Vietnam War to kill vegetation in forested areas so enemy guerrilla soldiers would be visible. Agent Orange was a mix of two weed killers developed in the 1940s containing dioxin.

Exposure to Agent Orange has been linked to certain chemical acne, non-Hodgkin lymphoma, HODGKIN DISEASE, and soft-tissue SARCOMA.

Aging

The decline, over time, of the body's organ systems. Far-ranging physiological changes are a part of aging. Homeostasis, the process through which the body adjusts to external change, becomes impaired. The reserve, or capacity, of many body functions is decreased. However, life expectancy in the United States nearly doubled in the 20th century. Today Americans who reach age 60 can expect to live beyond 80.

The reasons people change as they grow older are not completely understood. In gerontology, the scientific study of the aging process, theories of aging fall into two major overlapping groups. Programmed theories of aging emphasize the notion of internal biological clocks. Meanwhile, damage—or error—theories stress the environmental factors that damage cells and gradually impair organ function.

People age at different rates. While innate genetic makeup cannot change, lifestyle choices, such as diet, exercise, smoking, and drinking, can modify the aging process.

Agonist

A substance responsible for triggering a response in a cell. Agonist drugs are sometimes called mimics because they mimic part of the normal activity within a cell. Agonist drugs work by enhancing or restoring a cell's normal activity.

Agoraphobia

An intense, debilitating fear of open public spaces. The disease impairs the ability of the person to work and have a social life.

Symptoms include fear of being alone, remaining intentionally housebound for long periods, fear of losing control in public places, feelings of helplessness and dependence, fear of being crazy or dying, feelings that the body or the environment is unreal, and unusual outbursts of anger with twitching. The extreme anxiety or panic is experienced as light-headedness, excessive sweating, heart palpitations, chest pain, difficulty breathing, nausea and vomiting, numbness and tingling, stomach pain or distress, chills or hot flashes, and choking. Agoraphobia may occur alone or with PANIC DISORDER. Untreated, the disease can lead to major depression.

Agoraphobia may be biologically based, but the exact cause remains unknown. Treatment works best when begun early. It consists of medication to alleviate the anxiety along with psychotherapy to teach the person techniques for reducing anxiety. People with agoraphobia should avoid caffeine and other stimulants.

Agraphia

A loss of the ability to write as a result of brain damage. (See DYSLEXIA.) Damage is commonly localized to the posterior part of the brain, although lesions elsewhere have also been associated with difficulty writing. Agraphia can be divided into the following categories: aphasic agraphia (inability to spell or use correct grammar), constructional agraphia (difficulty spacing or organizing letters correctly), and apraxic agraphia (difficulty coordinating hand movements to write).

AIDS

Acquired immunodeficiency syndrome caused by the human immunodeficiency virus, or HIV. AIDS results when a person's immune system is damaged by HIV infection; this allows other organisms to infect the body, which has become ill equipped to resist them.

A person is diagnosed as having AIDS after developing one of the opportunistic infections or conditions that are defined as AIDS-related illnesses. A person who is HIV-positive but has not had an AIDS-related ill-

ness such as recurring pneumonia or Kaposi sarcoma, for example, may also be diagnosed with AIDS based on blood tests that indicate a severely damaged immune system.

The symptoms of AIDS are similar to those of many different illnesses and infections. These symptoms include rapid weight loss; dry cough; recurring fever; profuse night sweats; severe fatigue; swollen lymph glands (located in the armpits, groin, or neck); persistent diarrhea; and memory loss, depression, dementia, and other psychological problems. Certain types of pneumonia or tuberculosis may indicate AIDS. White spots or other lesions in the mouth or on the tongue and in the throat may be symptomatic of AIDS, as are red, brown, pink, or purplish patches under the skin or inside the mouth, nose, or eyelids.

Testing options and results

It should not be assumed that symptoms alone indicate a diagnosis of AIDS. The medical diagnosis must be made by a doctor based on specific criteria, including a positive result for HIV infection, which is detected by tests for the presence of antibodies that combat HIV. These antibodies generally develop within 25 days to 3 months following infection, but may not be detectable for up to 6 months. Blood test results for HIV are typically available within 1 to 2 weeks.

Positive test results indicate an infection with HIV, but may or may not indicate that a person will develop AIDS or HIV-related symptoms and illness. Further evaluation may be necessary to discover if there is damage to the immune system or if conditions indicating AIDS are present. A person with a positive test result is infectious and capable of spreading the HIV virus to others, even if there are no symptoms.

Negative test results are not always conclusive; they may indicate that the person is not infected with HIV or that the infection has not yet produced enough antibodies to be detected; this only occurs very early in the course of infection with HIV.

Treatment

While there is no medically recognized cure for AIDS at this time, treatments are now available to help strengthen the immune system and decrease the usual speed at which HIV weakens it. Antiretroviral therapy (especially combination therapy) is able to slow the progression of the virus, and there are several treatments to prevent or cure some of the opportunistic infections associated with AIDS. Fifteen different antiviral medications are available, which when used in combination, successfully slow the progression of disease, decrease the risk of death, and improve the quality of life for people with AIDS.

Risks and prevention

Avoiding the known circumstances that result in HIV infection is the best approach to avoiding AIDS. Unprotected sexual contact or sharing needles with an HIV-infected person or with a person whose health status is uncertain or unknown carries a strong risk of contracting the HIV virus.

AIDS-related cancers

Cancers associated with AIDS (acquired immunodeficiency syndrome).

Although AIDS itself is not a cancer, it has been associated with several different cancers, including KAPOSI SARCOMA, a form of skin cancer. Kaposi sarcoma is triggered by a virus called Kaposi sarcoma–associated herpesvirus (KSHV), also known as human herpesvirus 8 (HHV-8). Other AIDS-related cancers include cancer of the cervix and various lymphomas (cancers of the lymphatic system), such as BURKITT LYMPHOMA and non-Hodgkin lymphoma (see LYMPHOMA, NON-HODGKIN).

Airway

The tubular structure in the respiratory system that carries inhaled air through the nose and mouth to the lungs. The largest airway is the windpipe, or trachea. This structure branches into two smaller airways called the bronchi, which are connected to and supply the lungs. The bronchi repeatedly divide into tiny airways called bronchioles. This system of airways is often referred to as the bronchial tree.

Al-Anon

A self-help support group that serves the needs of the families, friends, and partners of people addicted to alcohol. Al-Anon is associated with ALCOHOLICS ANONYMOUS (AA), a self-help group for people recovering from alcoholism who are committed to living sober lives. Al-Anon stresses the importance of forgiveness and detachment for people whose lives have been affected by alcoholism in family or friends.

Albinism

A group of inherited conditions in which no or little pigment—or coloring agent, called melanin—is present in eyes, skin, and hair. There are about ten different types of albinism, based on the amount of pigment, that can vary considerably from person to person. Most people with albinism have very light eyes, skin, and hair. All types of albinism lead to problems with vision, usually decreased visual acuity, involuntary eye movements (nystagmus), and increased sensitivity to light. Some people are legally blind, while others have "crossed eyes" or "lazy eye" (STRABISMUS). Some types of albinism involve reduced pigment only in the eyes (ocular albinism). People with albinism live normal life spans.

The diagnosis of albinism is usually made through observation of the skin, hair, and eyes. Definitive diagnosis is based on an eye examination, because it is the presence of eye problems that defines the condition. Treatment is intended to reduce symptoms and depends on the extent of the disorder. Skin and eyes must be protected from the sun: sunglasses with UV (ultraviolet) protection should be worn; and skin must always be shielded from the sun by sunscreens with a high SPF (sun protection factor) and by complete coverage with clothing.

Albumin

A simple protein found in plant and animal tissues. Albumins are water soluble and can be coagulated or made semisolid with the application of heat. In the blood, albumins have an important role in regulating the distribution of water throughout the body and may bind to certain drugs, making them less active. Albumin infusions are often used therapeutically to treat shock, burns, liver failure, and kidney disease.

Albuminuria

Abnormally high amounts of the protein albumin in the urine. Excessive levels of protein in the urine usually result from damage to the glomeruli (the filtering units of the kidneys). Albuminuria may have a number of different causes but is a common problem in people with kidney disease that stems from having diabetes mellitus for an extended period of time. See also MICROALBUMINURIA.

Alcohol dependence

A disorder involving addiction to alcohol and characterized by tolerance (the need to consume increasingly larger amounts of alcohol to feel its effects), physical symptoms if alcohol is withdrawn, or both. Alcohol dependence is also known as alcoholism, and alcohol-dependent people are known as alcoholics. Untreated, the disease has severe physical, social, and personal consequences.

Symptoms

Alcohol dependence is characterized by constant or periodic preoccupation with alcohol, distorted thinking (particularly denial that alcohol poses a problem), lack of control regarding alcohol use, and continued drinking despite obvious adverse results, such as legal problems, family breakup, health problems, or job loss. Denial is one of the key signs of alcohol dependence. Alcohol-dependent people typically use alcohol to relieve symptoms such as pain or anxiety.

The majority of alcohol-dependent people who stop drinking experience some anxiety, insomnia, and tremors for a few days; some have few or no symptoms; and a minority have more severe symptoms requiring medical detoxification. Symptoms, if they appear, may include hand tremors; increased blood pressure, pulse, and body temperature; nausea or vomiting; and an inability to sleep (insomnia). In some cases, withdrawal causes delirium tremens (DTs), which can involve confusion and altered mental state (delirium), agitation, hallucination, feelings of persecution, seizures, and severe tremors. DTs can be dangerous; medical intervention is required.

Consequences

Excessive alcohol consumption over a period of years has serious consequences, causing impaired health and premature death. Common alcohol-induced impairments include brain

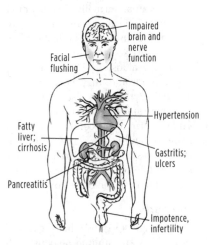

Impaired brain and nerve function

Facial flushing

Hypertension

Fatty liver; cirrhosis

Gastritis; ulcers

Pancreatitis

Impotence, infertility

Physical effects of abusing alcohol
Long-term heavy drinking causes damage throughout the body and is a leading cause of death in the United States. A variety of serious health problems arise from drinking more than one drink a day for women or two drinks a day for men.

damage; short-term memory damage; wernicke-korsakoff syndrome; ulcers and other gastrointestinal problems; damage to the liver and pancreas; an increase in blood pressure and damage to the heart muscle; sexual dysfunction in both men and women; and an increased risk of cancer.

Since depression often accompanies alcohol dependence, suicide is possible. Women who drink while pregnant may give birth to a baby with FETAL ALCOHOL SYNDROME.

Treatment

The first step in treatment is getting the person to recognize the problem. Once the problem is recognized, treatment begins with detoxification, which involves the person's withdrawal from alcohol in a supervised setting that lasts from 4 to 7 days.

The next step involves providing emotional and physical support to help the person remain abstinent from alcohol. Drugs may also be prescribed. Many people recovering from alcohol dependence rely on self-help peer groups, such as ALCOHOLICS ANONYMOUS (AA).

Alcohol intoxication

The impaired mental or physical functioning that comes from the consumption of alcohol; also known as inebriation or drunkenness. Alcohol (known medically as ethanol, or EtOH) is a central nervous system depressant drug, one that slows the activity of the central nervous system, particularly the brain. Alcohol requires no digestion and is absorbed directly into the bloodstream.

The level of alcohol in the blood after drinking depends primarily on the amount consumed. Alcohol is metabolized largely in the liver, with some also expelled through the kidneys and lungs. Typically, an adult can metabolize approximately 1 ounce of alcohol per hour.

As the blood alcohol level rises, several stages of intoxication may occur: at a blood alcohol level of approximately 0.02 percent, the person is talkative and sociable. At a blood alcohol level of 0.08 a person is above the legal limit for driving a car in most states; at a blood alcohol level of approximately 0.20 percent, the person experiences some loss of control over talking and walking, with slurred speech, staggering, disorientation, double vision, and exaggerated mood.

Alcoholics Anonymous (AA)

A self-help group for men and women recovering from alcohol dependency that provides an effective model of total abstinence; commonly abbreviated to AA. Founded in 1935 on the principle that alcohol dependency is a disease and that each person's experience is unique, Alcoholics Anonymous follows the Twelve Steps (see TWELVE-STEP PROGRAM), which serve as practical suggestions to help people lead sober lives by accepting their powerlessness around alcohol and being honest about their past and present lives.

Alcoholism

A disorder involving addiction to alcohol and characterized by tolerance (the need to consume increasingly larger amounts of alcohol to feel its effects) to increasing amounts of alcohol, or by physical symptoms if alcohol is withdrawn, or both. See ALCOHOL DEPENDENCE.

Aldosterone

A hormone produced by the adrenal cortex (the outer layer of the adrenal glands). Aldosterone controls the levels of sodium and potassium in the blood to help regulate water balance, blood volume, and blood pressure. The production of aldosterone is stimulated by the hormone RENIN, which is produced by the kidneys.

Aldosteronism

A condition in which the adrenal cortex (the outer layer of the adrenal glands) secretes abnormally high levels of ALDOSTERONE, a hormone that regulates blood volume and the balance of sodium and potassium in the blood; also known as hyperaldosteronism. If aldosteronism results in a severe depletion of potassium, muscle weakness and even paralysis can result. Excessive water and sodium retention can abnormally elevate blood pressure. Aldosteronism can also result in arrhythmias and other cardiac abnormalities.

Primary aldosteronism, also called Conn syndrome, may be caused by adrenal hyperplasia (see ADRENAL HYPERPLASIA, CONGENITAL). The secondary form of the condition is more common and is associated with congestive heart failure, cirrhosis, and kidney failure. Surgery may be considered to treat the condition.

Allergen

Any foreign substance that is capable of causing an immune response. Allergens produce what is called an allergic reaction. This occurs when the immune system mistakes allergens, which are normally nonharmful substances, for substances that are potentially harmful. The most common allergens are plant pollens, house dust mites, fungi spores, certain food items, medications such as penicillin, and the dander of domestic animals such as cats and dogs.

Allergic reaction

A disorder caused by hypersensitivity to a substance, such as a medication. An allergic reaction occurs when the immune system attacks a substance that is normally harmless as if it were a disease-causing organism. Allergic reactions to medication can include hives, itching, wheezing, throat tightening, and rarely, shock, an intense reaction quickly leading to difficulty in breathing, low blood pressure, rapid pulse, sweating, and collapse.

Allergic reactions to medication are difficult to prevent, but symptoms can be treated with antihistamines, corticosteroids, or epinephrine.

Allergies

Abnormal responses of the immune system that produce physical symptoms caused by contact with a substance that is normally harmless. Allergies occur when an ANTIBODY responds to a specific ANTIGEN. The substance producing the response is called an ALLERGEN. These antigens or allergens typically do not produce a strong immune response in most people but can cause an immune response in those who are allergic to the antigen.

How allergies occur

Allergic reactions occur when the immune system attacks what is perceived to be a hostile invader by producing antibodies to defend the body against the invader. HISTAMINE, the best known of the many chemicals released during an allergic reaction, may trigger an inflammatory response ranging from a mild runny nose and itchy, watery eyes to a severe life-threatening reaction called ANAPHYLAXIS.

If an allergen gets into the bloodstream, the effects may be more far-reaching. When this occurs, the allergen may cause symptoms in addition to those occurring at the site of the reaction. For example, a food allergen that is ingested may cause hives as well as gastrointestinal symptoms.

Symptoms, diagnosis, and treatment

Symptoms depend on the part of the body affected. If the allergic reaction occurs in the ears, nose, throat, or sinuses, the membranes lining these cavities become swollen as a result of the immune system's inflammatory response to the allergen. The person may have a stuffy or runny nose with frequent sneezing, coughing, and wheezing and an itchy sensation in the eyes, nose, throat, or roof of the mouth. If NASAL POLYPS have developed, the person may have difficulty breathing and a loss of the sense of smell. One of the most common allergies is medically known as seasonal allergic rhinitis, which is also called HAY FEVER. This is usually caused by a reaction to airborne allergens, such as pollen, and occurs on a seasonal basis when the pollens are abundant in the outdoor environment. The allergy may be diagnosed after a doctor's evaluation of a complete history including the time of day and the season in which the allergies occur. A skin SCRATCH TEST may be performed to determine the allergen responsible. Treatment is generally based on avoidance of the known allergen and on medications such as antihistamines and decongestants. A medical procedure known as immunotherapy, which is a series of injections to desensitize the system to specific allergens, may be tried in severe cases.

Food allergies can produce symptoms including abdominal pain, diarrhea, nausea, and vomiting. Nasal congestion may also occur, and the lips, eyes, face, tongue, and throat may become swollen. Hives and asthma may also develop from food allergies. The affected person may be required to follow a strict program, called an elimination diet, to determine the allergen causing the reaction. Skin scratch tests and specific blood tests may also be used in the diagnosis. The only treatment for food allergies is complete avoidance of the food. For some people, physical contact with the food allergen is to be avoided as strictly as ingestion of the allergens. People with serious food allergies must carry an emergency kit containing epinephrine at all times.

Allergies to medications can cause symptoms including wheezing and difficulty breathing, rash or hives, overall itching, and, in severe cases, shock or anaphylaxis. These allergies may be treated with adrenaline (epinephrine), antihistamines, or corticosteroid medications.

Allergies to insect stings may involve symptoms such as pain and severe itching at the site of the sting, hives, itchy eyes, and a constricted feeling in the throat and chest. Anaphylaxis can occur, causing severe swelling of the eyes, lips, or tongue and a swelling of the throat that makes it difficult to breathe. Anaphy-

laxis can involve obstruction of the airways and lungs and can even cause shock. Severe reactions can occur within 10 to 20 minutes of the insect bite and require emergency medical attention, often an injection of epinephrine.

Allograft

A surgical procedure in which tissue or an organ is taken from one person and transplanted into or implanted onto another individual. See TRANSPLANT SURGERY.

Aloe

Dried juice of the leaves from various species of lilac plants. Aloe, or aloe vera, is chiefly used to ease the pain of sunburn, frostbite, and other skin irritations, but the natural medicine is not regulated by the Food and Drug Administration.

Alopecia

Baldness; absence of hair from areas where it normally is present. Alopecia can stem from genetic causes and is also associated with radiation therapy, chemotherapy, scarring, stress, endocrine disorders, certain drugs, and other factors. Male pattern baldness (androgenic alopecia), the most common type of baldness, is characterized by a progressive symmetrical loss of scalp hair in men in their 20s and 30s, starting at the front, eventually leaving only a peripheral ring of hair. It is an inherited condition that can also affect women.

Alopecia areata is a loss of scalp and beard hair in patches, due to an immune response. It is usually reversible. Alopecia totalis is the entire loss of hair from the scalp due to alopecia areata. In scarring alopecia, the hair loss is associated with inflammation and scarring of the hair follicles. Scarring alopecia is usually the result of a skin disorder.

Alpha 1-antitrypsin deficiency

A common hereditary disorder characterized by a deficiency in levels of the blood protein alpha 1-antitrypsin (AAT). AAT is produced in the liver and inhibits the inflammatory response of the body. When AAT is deficient or absent, infection or uncontrolled inflammation can destroy tissue cells, which is seen most often in the lungs, particularly when they are exposed to cigarette smoke. Approximately 75 percent of adults with AAT deficiency who smoke will develop EMPHYSEMA, a serious respiratory disease, usually before age 40.

Symptoms and treatment

Signs associated with AAT deficiency may include shortness of breath, unintended weight loss, wheezing, chronic cough, yellow skin (jaundice), barrel-shaped chest, accumulation of fluid in the tissues (edema), and abnormal liver test results.

Diagnosis is made on the basis of physical examination, chest X ray, and various tests, including tests of pulmonary function and arterial blood gases. A test to measure the AAT levels in the blood may also be done.

There is no proven treatment to reverse the deficiency itself. However, the disorders associated with it, such as emphysema, asthma, chronic bronchitis, and cirrhosis, can be treated. When the deficiency is detected before symptoms are present, treatment focuses on prevention.

Alpha blockers

Drugs that help lower blood pressure by preventing blood vessels from constricting. Alpha blockers work by preventing stress hormones from stimulating receptors in the blood vessels, thereby preventing arteries and veins from constricting, which is what raises blood pressure.

Side effects of alpha blockers include dizziness, headaches, heart palpitations, nausea, and mild fluid retention.

Alpha-fetoprotein (AFP) test

See AFP TEST.

Alpha-tocopherol

Another name for VITAMIN E. Alpha-tocopherol may protect cells from some kinds of damage and helps slow the cell damage that happens naturally as a person ages. Vitamin E is thought to interfere with the oxygen-controlled signals that make cancer cells grow. Vitamin E is found naturally in nuts, sunflower seeds, mayonnaise, cold-pressed vegetable oils, spinach, sweet potatoes, and yams. There is no evidence that vitamin E supplements reduce the risk of heart disease or of cancer, but they are widely used on that assumption.

ALS

Amyotrophic lateral sclerosis, the most common form of MOTOR NEURON DISEASE, characterized by progressive muscle atrophy (shrinking) and the loss of muscle function. ALS is commonly referred to as Lou Gehrig disease (the only disease to be named after a patient), after the baseball player who died of the disease in 1939. In ALS, the nerves that control muscle activity progressively degenerate within the brain and spinal cord, resulting in the characteristic muscle wasting and weakness. ALS is rare and the cause is unknown. About one in ten people with ALS have a family history of the disorder.

Symptoms

The onset of ALS generally occurs after age 50 years. In limb-onset ALS, weakness is first experienced in the arms or legs, making it difficult to walk or perform tasks that require manual dexterity. Bulbar-onset ALS first involves problems with speaking or swallowing.

In ALS, muscle strength and coordination gradually decrease, while mental functioning remains unaffected.

As the loss of muscle control continues to progress, and more muscle groups become involved, the person becomes more disabled. Eventually all four limbs become involved. Deterioration finally results in speech impairment, difficulty swallowing, and trouble breathing. Death results from paralysis of the respiratory muscles. This typically occurs in 3 to 5 years. However, exceptions occur, and some people have lived 20 years or more following diagnosis.

Diagnosis

Accurate diagnosis of ALS can be difficult because it can be confused with a number of other neurological disorders that require different treatment. Diagnosis of ALS is made through neuromuscular examination that indicates muscle weakness without loss of sensation. Weakness often begins in a single limb or in the shoulders or hips. Examination may also reveal tremors, spasms, contractions, atrophy, abnormal reflexes, and a clumsy gait (walk). Tests to confirm diagnosis and rule out other causes include electromyography (measurement of muscle electrical activity), blood studies, CT (computed tomography) scanning, and MRI (magnetic resonance imaging). At times, a muscle biopsy is necessary. Genetic testing may be recommended if there is a family history of ALS.

Treatment

Because there is no cure for ALS, the goal of treatment is to control symptoms. Medication may be prescribed to manage spasms and the ability to swallow. Since there is a progressive loss of the ability to care for oneself, helpful measures include physical therapy, rehabilitation, and orthopedic appliances (such as a wheelchair). To prevent choking, a tube may need to be placed into the person's stomach for feeding. Because mental functioning remains intact, emotional support is vital for coping with this disorder.

Alternative medicine

Techniques, methods, and practices of health care used as alternatives to conventional medicine. Examples of alternative medicine include ancient healing traditions such as ACUPUNCTURE, HERBAL MEDICINE, to newer methods, such as CHIROPRACTIC and megavitamin therapy.

An idea key to all forms of alternative medicine is that health is more than simply the absence of disease. Most forms of alternative medicine assume that health care involves more than just the physical body. Alternative medicine generally focuses on the whole person and takes into account his or her physical, emotional, spiritual, nutritional, and social needs.

Complementary medicine combines alternative therapies with techniques used by conventional medical practitioners. Massage therapy, bodywork, and MEDITATION are examples of techniques that may be used to complement traditional therapies.

Altitude sickness

A disorder caused by a lack of oxygen at altitudes above 8,000 feet. The disorder occurs because as altitude increases, both atmospheric pressure and the amount of oxygen available in the atmosphere decrease. Initial symptoms, often referred to as acute mountain sickness, include headache, sleep disturbance, fatigue, shortness of breath, dizziness, and nausea. Symptoms of altitude sickness usually wear off within 24 to 48 hours, as the body adapts to the altitude.

More serious symptoms can develop above 9,000 feet, causing high-altitude pulmonary edema and high-altitude cerebral edema, both of which can be fatal. High-altitude pulmonary edema is characterized by strong coughing that produces frothy, blood-tinged sputum, while high-altitude cerebral edema is associated with staggering, hallucinations, confusion, and coma.

Altitude sickness can usually be prevented by a slow ascent.

Alveolectomy

Dental surgery to trim or remove the bone or gum tissue in the jawbone that holds the roots of the teeth. The procedure is usually performed along with tooth extractions.

Alveoli

Microscopic air sacs within the lungs and the site of gas exchange. The alveoli are clustered together like grapes at the end of a bronchiole (small air tube). Each alveolus is made of connective tissue surrounded by very small blood vessels called capillaries. Air that is inhaled travels through the successively finer air passageways of the RESPIRATORY SYSTEM to the alveoli.

Alveolitis

A lung disease that results from an inflammation of the alveoli, which are the tiny round air sacs found at the ends of the bronchioles in the lungs.

Allergic alveolitis (also called hypersensitivity pneumonitis) is caused by an allergic response in those who are sensitive to organic dusts. Contact with organic dusts often occurs in the workplace, and the different forms of alveolitis are often named according to the manner in which they were acquired. The two most common of these are FARMER'S LUNG, which is generally caused by continual inhalation of spores from moldy hay, and byssinosis, which occurs in workers who produce cotton, flax, jute, and hemp for yarn or rope.

In people who are sensitive to these specific dusts, exposure can cause symptoms, generally from 6 hours to days after exposure. The symptoms include a persistent cough, a sensation of tightness in the chest, wheezing, shortness of breath, and decreased lung function. There may also be recurrent episodes of fever, chills, dry coughing, and very labored breathing.

Diagnosis is based on characteristic symptoms and a history of environmental exposure and may be confirmed with the results of PUL-

MONARY FUNCTION TESTS, X rays, and blood tests. Avoiding exposure to the dust that irritates the alveoli generally relieves symptoms. In some cases, a corticosteroid may be prescribed to open airways and ease breathing.

Alzheimer's disease

An irreversible brain disease, usually found in older people, that causes a progressive decline in mental function. Alzheimer's disease (AD) is the most common cause of dementia, a syndrome characterized by a gradual loss of memory and other intellectual functions. Typically in Alzheimer's disease (AD), brain cells die and the connections between them deteriorate. Researchers suspect AD may be caused either by a deficiency in a brain chemical or a genetic defect.

Early on, AD affects cells in the hippocampus, a brain area related to memory. Early signs of AD, such as forgetfulness and a loss of concentration, are subtle. Ordinary forgetfulness is not a sign of the disorder, but memory loss that interferes with function is. Later stages of the disease target the cerebral cortex, where language and reasoning originate. In addition to memory loss, a person with AD eventually loses the abilities to reason and communicate. An affected person gradually worsens and at last becomes incapacitated. The course of the disease varies greatly among individuals. On average, people live from 8 to 10 years after diagnosis but can live as long as 20 years.

Anatomic hallmarks of the disease are the distinct pathologic abnormalities called plaques and tangles, which have been detected in the brain tissue of people who have AD. Plaques are dense protein deposits found around the brain's nerve cells. Tangles are twisted protein fibers that appear inside the nerve cells. Both are associated with AD, but their precise role in the disease is not clear.

Other than a brain biopsy demonstrating the characteristic changes in brain tissue, no physical, psychological, or laboratory test provides a definitive diagnosis of AD. However, based on medical observation, the accuracy rate of AD diagnosis by experienced clinicians is high; autopsies confirm clinical AD diagnoses from 85 to 95 percent of the time.

Diagnosis is made by a complete physical examination, personal and family medical histories, and tests. An important part of evaluating people for AD is ruling out possible causes of symptoms that may be reversible.

Tests may include basic analyses of blood and urine; a mental status examination; and neuropsychological tests of memory, problem solving, and language. Imaging studies of the brain, such as CT (computed tomography) scanning or MRI (magnetic resonance imaging) frequently are used to rule out other causes of dementia.

Medications called cholinesterase inhibitors can be taken to slow the progression of cognitive symptoms in the early to middle stages of the disease.

Behavioral approaches sometimes improve the control of symptoms such as depression, frustration, agitation, and anger. Community resources are useful for dealing with the behavior of people with AD. Most people with AD will eventually require the skilled and constant care of a LONG-TERM CARE FACILITY.

Being genetically linked to a relative who has or had the disease is a risk factor for AD, as is being older than 65.

Amaurosis fugax

Loss of vision in one eye that lasts for seconds to minutes for up to 24 hours. The visual loss from amaurosis fugax is often described as if a curtain is coming down from above or across the field of vision. The usual cause is a spasm or blockage in a small blood vessel leading to a lack of blood in the retina (the light-sensitive layer in the back of the eye). The condition can be a sign that a person is at increased risk for stroke.

Amblyopia

Poor vision in one eye resulting from a failure to develop normal sight during childhood; commonly known as "lazy eye." The brain's center of vision usually develops from birth to age 6 or 7 years. If the brain's visual center has not developed by then, vision may be permanently impaired.

Amblyopia can be caused by any disease that prevents clear focusing. The most common cause is STRABISMUS, known commonly as "crossed eyes." Other causes include farsightedness, nearsightedness, or astigmatism that is more severe in one eye than the other. In rare instances, amblyopia is caused by a cataract (clouding of the lens of the eye).

Except in obvious cases of strabismus, amblyopia can be difficult to detect. Physicians check for the condition by watching how well a child can follow objects with one eye covered.

Amblyopia does not usually improve after the age of 9 years, making it very important to detect and treat it before then to ensure the development of normal vision.

Treatment is usually successful, particularly in younger children. Treatment relies on inducing the child to use the weak eye. Often this is accomplished by placing a patch over the good eye, requiring the child to rely on vision from the amblyopic eye for an extended period. In some cases, drops that blur vision in the good eye are used instead of a patch, but this approach is usually less effective.

Amebiasis

An infectious intestinal disease caused by a microscopic, one-celled parasite. Symptoms, which are rare and often mild, include diarrhea, abdominal pain and cramping, nausea, weight loss, and sometimes fever. Amebiasis in its most severe form is called AMEBIC DYSENTERY. Symptoms of amebic dysentery include stomach pain, bloody mucous stools, and fever. In rare cases, the parasite may spread to the liver and form an abscess, and in even rarer cases, the parasite may invade other parts of the body, including the lungs or brain.

Infected people are the only source of the parasite that causes amebiasis, and it is spread by contact with fecal material from people who carry the parasite. Symptoms usually occur within 2 to 4 weeks of exposure, but may appear within a few days to a few months. A person with amebiasis can carry the parasite for several weeks to several years, often with no symptoms.

Amebiasis is diagnosed by examining a person's stool sample under a microscope. A blood test may be recommended if there is the suspicion that the infection has spread to the wall of the intestines or to the liver.

The infection is treated with specific antibiotics. Once treated, a person will no longer carry the parasite in the intestinal tract and in most cases is unlikely to become reinfected.

Amebic dysentery

Inflammation of the colon caused by infection with an ameba (a single-celled parasite), causing bloody DIAR-RHEA, excess mucus secretion, and abdominal cramps. Amebic dysentery is most common in countries with poor sanitation and is caused by consuming water or food that is contaminated with particles of feces that contain amebae.

Diagnosis of amebic dysentery can be made by analyzing stool samples, by blood tests, or by SIGMOIDOSCOPY. Antiamebic drugs are usually effective in treating the disease. Untreated amebic dysentery can cause an abscess in the liver (see LIVER ABSCESS) to develop.

Amenorrhea

The absence of menstruation either in a woman who has never menstruated or in a woman whose regular menstrual cycle has ceased temporarily or permanently. See MENSTRUA-TION, DISORDERS OF.

American Medical Association (AMA)

The largest physician organization in the United States. Founded more than 150 years ago, the AMA is committed to education, research, and service. It develops and promotes standards in medical practice, ethics, and research and promotes excellence in medical education and practice. In addition, the AMA serves as an advocate on behalf of physicians and patients in the legislative and judicial arenas, and it provides timely information on health matters through a wide range of sources, including accreditation and education activities, scientific journals, the AMA Web site (http://www.ama-assn.org), and physician and consumer book publishing divisions.

Americans with Disabilities Act (ADA)

A civil rights law enacted in 1990 to eliminate discrimination against individuals with disabilities and to provide disabled Americans with a system of legal redress. The Americans with Disabilities Act (ADA) prohibits discrimination by private and public services in many areas, including employment, housing, public accommodations, education, transportation, communications, and health services, on the basis of disabilities.

The term "disability" is defined by the ADA to include a functional physical or mental impairment that substantially limits one or more major life activities. Physical impairment generally refers to a physiological disorder or condition, a disfigurement, or an anatomical loss. Mental impairment refers to mental or psychological disorders such as mental retardation, emotional illness including alcoholism, and learning disabilities.

Amino acids

Organic compounds are the building blocks of all proteins. Amino acids are found in both plants and animals. The human body can synthesize some amino acids, while essential amino acids must be obtained from protein consumed in the diet. When a person ingests protein, the body breaks it down into amino acids. Then the amino acids are transported through the bloodstream to various cells of the body, where they are used for growth, maintenance, and repair.

Aminoglycosides

A type or class of antibiotics used to treat infections caused by aerobic, gram-negative bacteria. Aminoglycosides work by preventing proper protein synthesis in disease-causing bacteria. Among the bacteria that are vulnerable to aminoglycosides are Pseudomonas, Klebsiella, Escherichia coli (see E. COLI), Staphylococcus aureus, and Mycobacterium tuberculosis.

Aminoglycosides are used to treat bacterial "blood poisoning" (septicemia), urinary tract infections, and treat active tuberculosis.

Amnesia

The loss of memory. (See also MEMORY, LOSS OF.) Amnesia can be the result of brain damage or severe emotional trauma. Depending on its cause, memory loss may be temporary or permanent and may come on slowly or suddenly. Common causes of amnesia include alcoholism, general anesthetics, brain surgery, drug reactions, ECT (electroconvulsive therapy), head trauma or injury, hysteria, and migraine.

There are three major forms of amnesia: anterograde, retrograde, and transient global amnesia. Anterograde amnesia is caused by brain trauma and is characterized by an inability to form new memories or remember newly learned material.

In retrograde amnesia, also the result of trauma, the affected person can recall only the events that occurred after the trauma.

In transient global amnesia, there is a sudden loss of memory and a transient inability to recall new information.

To diagnose the underlying cause of memory loss, doctors usually conduct thorough physical and neurological examinations and take a detailed medical history. Tests that may be used include cerebral angiography, MRI (magnetic resonance imaging) or CT (computed tomography) scanning of the head, electroencephalogram (EEG), blood tests, and psychometric or cognitive tests. Treatment of amnesia depends on its underlying cause.

Amnio infusion

A procedure used during labor in which saline (a salt solution that has the same concentration as body fluids) is instilled into the uterus at a constant rate. The objectives of this treatment include flushing out thick waste-stained fluid and reversal of abnormal fetal heart rate patterns, which may be related to umbilical cord compression.

Amniocentesis

A test commonly performed between weeks 14 and 16 of pregnancy to diagnose hereditary diseases and congenital defects in a fetus. Amniocentesis involves removing some of the amniotic fluid that surrounds a fetus in the uterus. The test is performed in women thought to have an increased risk of bearing a child with a genetic

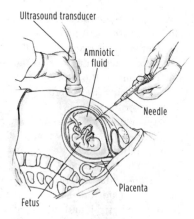

How amniocentesis is performed

The woman is given a local anesthetic. Then a needle will be inserted into the uterus to withdraw amniotic fluid (the liquid that surrounds the fetus). The position of the fetus, placenta, and umbilical cord are monitored using ultrasound imaging.

disorder or other detectable birth defects.

During the procedure, a very fine needle is passed through the abdominal wall into the uterine cavity to withdraw about an ounce of amniotic fluid for analysis. Fetal cells obtained from the amniotic fluid are tested for levels of various substances. Also, the amniotic fluid is analyzed to detect abnormalities in chromosomes or genes or birth defects. Disorders that can be detected through amniocentesis include Down syndrome and spina bifida (a neural tube defect).

Amniotic fluid

The clear, watery fluid that surrounds and protects a fetus in the uterus (the organ in which the baby grows). The amniotic fluid is contained in a membrane called the amniotic sac. The fluid cushions the fetus from the pressure of the woman's internal or-gans and protects the fetus from injury. Maintaining the proper amount of fluid is important to the health of the fetus. POLYHYDRAMNIOS is a condition in which excess amniotic fluid is detected; it occurs once in about 250 pregnancies. OLIGOHYDRAMNIOS is an extremely rare condition in which an abnormally small amount of amniotic fluid is produced.

Amniotomy

A procedure used to start or speed up labor. The membranes of the amniotic sac surrounding the baby are broken and the AMNIOTIC FLUID is released, leading to stronger and more frequent contractions of the uterus. See LABOR.

Amsler grid

A chart used to detect a type of age-related change in central vision known as MACULAR DEGENERATION. The chart looks like a piece of paper with dark lines forming a square grid around a dot in the center. The grid is held at a comfortable reading distance with one eye covered while the person focuses on the center dot; the test is then repeated with the other eye covered. Blurring of the grid or distortion of its lines into wavy, fuzzy, or missing areas of vision can indicate damage to the macula, most commonly from macular degeneration. See also VISION TESTS.

Amyloidosis

An uncommon disease caused by the abnormal protein amyloid being deposited in tissues or organs of the body, most frequently in the heart, kidneys, nervous system, or gastrointestinal tract. Amyloidosis may be associated with an underlying inflammatory disease or cancer.

Amyotrophic lateral sclerosis

See ALS.

Amyotrophy

ATROPHY or wasting of the muscles. Amyotrophy is a common symptom of motor neuron diseases, such as ALS, but it is also seen in many other conditions, including diabetes, syphilis, and cancer.

Anabolic steroids

Synthetic male sex hormones (androgens). Anabolic steroids promote the growth of skeletal muscle (anabolic effects) and the development of male sexual characteristics (androgenic effects). They were originally developed to treat a condition called hypogonadism, in which the testes do not produce enough testosterone for normal growth and sexual functioning. Some athletes, especially bodybuilders, abuse steroids to increase muscle size and to decrease body fat. Anabolic steroids can cause liver failure, abnormal hair distribution, oily skin, and, in women, masculine characteristics.

Anal dilation

The widening of the anal sphincter muscle to treat hemorrhoids or to repair an ANAL FISSURE, a tear or ulcer in the lining of the anal canal. It is also performed if there is a narrowing of the anal canal that interferes with the normal passage of stools. The procedure can stop the pain, spasms, and bleeding associated with anal fissures, and healing is relatively quick.

Anal discharge

Secretion of substances, such as blood, mucus, or pus, from the anus. Anal discharge is often the result of a relatively minor problem, such as hemorrhoids or an anal fissure (a tear or ulcer in the lining of the anal canal). However, in some cases, a discharge may be the sign of a more serious disorder, such as CROHN DISEASE, COLITIS, or colon cancer (see COLON, CANCER OF THE). For this reason, doctors recommend that individuals who experience an anal discharge seek medical attention as soon as possible. This is critically important in cases of a bloody discharge.

Anal fissure

A tear or ulcer in the lining of the anal canal that extends inside the canal from the anal opening. Fairly common, anal fissures may be linked to constipation and diarrhea, although their exact cause remains unknown. The first symptom of an anal fissure is usually rectal pain and occasional bleeding. The pain may be sharp and burning and increases during defecation. Pain may cause people to avoid defecation, which worsens the situation. Other symptoms include spasm of the anal muscles and anal discharge.

An anal fissure is usually diagnosed by physical examination. In most cases, topical ointments and stool softeners are prescribed. Doctors also recommend a high-fiber diet, adequate fluids, and warm baths after painful bowel movements to reduce spasms. With these measures, many anal fissures resolve spontaneously. In other cases, minor surgery is necessary. See ANAL DILATION and SPHINCTEROTOMY.

Anal fistula

Formation of an abnormal channel between the anal canal and the skin surrounding the anus. The continual discharge of watery pus from the fistula can irritate the skin and result in itching, discomfort, and pain. Most anal fistulas are caused by abscesses (pus-filled sacs) that spread from inside of the anus to the outer surface of the skin. Sometimes, a fistula may result from CROHN DISEASE, COLITIS, or colon cancer (see COLON, CANCER OF THE). The doctor will perform tests, such as X rays and a SIGMOI-DOSCOPY.

When an abscess is present, minor surgery is performed to remove the fistula and drain the abscess. Most fistulas persist until they are surgically removed. Afterward, stool softeners, antibiotics, and rest are usually prescribed.

Anal stenosis

Narrowing of the anus, which is also known as anal stricture. In this condition, the anal opening is too small to permit the normal passage of feces. Symptoms of anal stenosis include constipation and pain during defecation. In many cases, anal stenosis is present from birth. Sometimes, it is the result of INFLAMMATORY BOWEL DISEASE (IBD). The chronic inflammation characteristic of IBD causes scarring in the anus that can eventually lead to stenosis.

Diagnosis of anal stenosis is made by physical examination, X rays, and SIGMOIDOSCOPY (visual examination of the rectum and sigmoid colon using a lighted tube called a sigmoidoscope). Treatment with daily digital dilation may successfully widen the anal opening in infants. Sometimes, surgery is necessary to correct the condition.

Analgesia, patient-controlled

A method of diminishing pain, most commonly after surgery, in which the patient chooses, within limits set by the physician, how often to receive medication needed to overcome discomfort. Patient-controlled analgesia or PCA (pain control without loss of consciousness), is often used to replace periodic painkiller (analgesic) injections after surgery. PCA allows for a more even administration of medication, generally resulting in improved pain control, in contrast to injections that may produce variable levels of pain control.

Analgesics

Painkillers. An analgesic is any drug used to relieve pain without loss of consciousness. Painkillers usually have only a temporary effect. There are more than 100 different analgesics on the U.S. market. They are divided into two main classes: nonnarcotics and narcotics.

Nonnarcotics include acetaminophen and nonsteroidal anti-inflammatory drugs (NSAIDs), such as aspirin and ibuprofen. NSAIDs work by blocking the production of prostaglandins, naturally occurring substances present in many tissues that stimulate nerve endings, which are sensitive to pain.

Acetaminophen works by blocking the production of prostaglandins in the brain, but the drug has no ability to block production in the rest of the body so it does not reduce inflammation.

Narcotic analgesics combine with pain receptors in brain cells to block the transmission of pain signals within the brain and spinal cord. The most effective narcotic analgesics are the opioids, such as morphine. Codeine is a milder narcotic analgesic. Any narcotic painkiller can impair a person's ability to drive or operate dangerous machinery and must be used with care. Overdose can cause breathing distress, coma, and death.

Anaphylactic reaction

A rapid allergic reaction that can be life-threatening. Anaphylaxis is an acute systemic type of allergic reaction that affects the entire body. During an anaphylactic reaction, the immune system releases antibodies and the tissues release substances such as histamine, which causes the airways to narrow, resulting in wheezing and labored breathing. Histamine also causes the blood vessels to dilate, or widen, which leads to a drop in blood pressure, resulting in shock. Hives often occur, and irregular heartbeats (arrhythmias) can occur during prolonged reactions.

Anaphylactic reactions can occur in response to any allergen, or allergy-producing substance, but are commonly associated with insect bites or stings, horse serum used in certain vaccines, food allergies, and drug allergies. Pollen and other inhaled environmental allergens rarely cause anaphylactic reactions.

Anaphylactoid purpura

An allergic reaction of unknown origin that causes a skin rash and other potentially serious symptoms.

Anaphylaxis

A severe, potentially life-threatening allergic reaction that is characterized by swelling of the throat, difficulty breathing, and a sudden fall in blood pressure. Anaphylaxis, which is also called anaphylactic shock, is an infrequent but very serious allergic reaction and an example of immediate HYPERSENSITIVITY. It usually occurs within seconds or minutes of exposure to minute amounts of an ALLERGEN (allergy-causing substance) to which a person is highly sensitized. The body's immune response to the allergen involves the release of histamine and other body chemicals. These immune chemicals produce hives, swelling of the skin, and severe breathing problems caused by swelling tissues in the throat and a narrowing of the airways. The blood vessels swell and become wider, which results in a dramatic drop in blood pressure. These symptoms are a medical emergency, and immediate medical attention can be lifesaving.

Causes and symptoms

There are many substances that tend to be more commonly associated with this severe allergic reaction, including eggs, seafood, nuts, grains, milk, or peanuts; antibiotics from the penicillin and cephalosporin groups; vaccinations; and insect stings. This severe allergic reaction may occur when analgesics, such as aspirin or nonsteroidal anti-inflammatory drugs, are injected intravenously. Latex and rubber products, including the latex gloves worn by health care workers, can cause allergic reactions that may escalate to anaphylaxis. Sometimes the cause of anaphylaxis may not be determined.

Symptoms appear immediately after the offending allergen has been ingested or physically contacted. Milder episodes can involve skin symptoms primarily, while more severe anaphylaxis causes severe breathing difficulties. The drop in blood pressure causes symptoms such as a rapid pulse, dizziness, wheezing, sweating, weakness, coughing, a sensation of tightness in the chest, and fainting or unconsciousness. The skin may turn a pale or bluish color. Intensely itching hives may affect large areas of swollen skin, and the lips, tongue, or eyes may become very swollen. Gastrointestinal symptoms may include nausea, abdominal cramps, vomiting, and diarrhea. Cardiac collapse may occur.

The throat may feel constricted and swollen, and there may be hoarseness. An obstructed airflow makes it difficult to breathe. Once these symptoms have started, a person may die within minutes to hours if treatment is not started.

Diagnosis, treatment, and prevention

Anaphylaxis is recognized immediately by the characteristic symptoms. Treatment consists of an immediate injection of adrenaline (epinephrine) to open airways and reduce swelling, as well as rapid injection of intravenous fluids. CARDIOPULMONARY RESUSCITATION (CPR) to assist in breathing and to restore the person's heartbeat may be necessary. Sometimes an emergency tracheotomy to open the main airway and restart breathing may need to be performed. Subsequently, oxygen therapy and mechanical VENTILATION may be required to help the person breathe. With proper medical treatment, a person who has undergone anaphylaxis can recover completely. How-

ever, a person who has had this reaction remains at risk for future episodes following ingestion of or contact with the causative allergen.

It is a good idea for a person who has experienced anaphylactic shock and determined the cause to wear a medical-alert bracelet or necklace that identifies the problem and its source. Allergens that trigger the symptoms must be strictly avoided.

Doctors may also recommend that a person have available a preloaded syringe of epinephrine to be injected at the first sign of symptoms. These injections should be considered only as interim measures when anaphylactic shock occurs, and emergency medical attention should always be sought.

Androgens

Male sex hormones. Testosterone is the principal male steroid hormone, produced in the testes in men and in small amounts in the ovaries and adrenal glands in women. Testosterone is responsible for the growth and development of male sex organs as well as for some physical characteristics in men, such as beard, body hair, and a lowered voice. Androgen hormone replacement is prescribed to replace testosterone in men who have low levels of it in their blood or who have lost testicular function. Women may receive testosterone to treat metastatic cancer (cancer that has spread from one area of the body to another).

Anemia

A condition marked by the presence of an abnormally low number of red blood cells or hemoglobin molecules, the iron-containing compound in red blood cells that transports oxygen.

There are many different types of anemia, each one with its own cause. As a group, anemias are the most common diseases affecting the blood.

In a healthy person, red blood cells are produced in the bone marrow and have a life span of approximately 120 days, at which point new red blood cells replace them. In healthy individuals, the formation of new red blood cells balances the destruction of old cells, and the amount of hemoglobin remains steady within the normal range. Anemia can result if red blood cells are destroyed prematurely, if the bone marrow loses the ability to make a sufficient number of new red blood cells, or if a person experiences blood loss from bleeding. The net result is a deficiency in red blood cells or hemoglobin. This loss in the body's ability to transport oxygen produces the symptoms of anemia.

Symptoms

Most anemias start with mild symptoms that may hardly be noticed. Symptoms worsen as the disease progresses. A person with anemia may feel fatigued and appear paler than usual. The pallor is more apparent in the nail beds of the fingers and toes, the insides of the eyelids, and the palms, where the creases may become as pale as the skin surrounding them. The heart rate often increases as the heart works harder to pump blood throughout the body in an effort to compensate for the oxygen deficit. Shortness of breath when exercising may also occur.

Anemias may be caused by iron deficiency (see ANEMIA, IRON-DEFICIENCY); insufficient vitamin B12 (see ANEMIA, PERNICIOUS) and folic acid deficiency; disease processes in which red blood cells break down faster than bone marrow can produce them (see ANEMIA, HEMOLYTIC); the failure of bone marrow to properly develop all types of blood cells, including red blood cells (see ANEMIA, APLASTIC); or genetic abnormalities that cause the body to manufacture defective hemoglobin (see SICKLE CELL ANEMIA and THALASSEMIA).

Anemia, aplastic

A disease in which the bone marrow fails to produce all types of mature blood cells in sufficient numbers. In addition to the symptoms commonly associated with anemia, aplastic anemia can lead to leukopenia (low white blood cell count), which increases the risk of infection, and thrombocytopenia (low platelet count), which results in bleeding from the skin and the mucous membranes, such as those of the nose and gums, and causes easy bruising. Aplastic anemia may be acute or chronic, and it is always progressive, becoming worse over time. Left untreated, the disease leads to death.

The bone marrow in a person with aplastic anemia contains very few stem cells, the cells from which mature bone marrow cells are derived. In some cases, aplastic anemia is thought to develop from an autoimmune disorder, in which a person develops antibodies against his or her own cells. Aplastic anemia can also be caused by exposure to toxins (such as organic solvents, cleaners, and paint removers), chemotherapy, radiation therapy, certain medications and illegal drugs, pregnancy, infections, and systemic lupus erythematosus.

Mild cases of aplastic anemia are

treated with supportive care, such as blood transfusions and platelet transfusions to raise the number of blood cells to normal and antibiotics to fight infections. If the disease is severe and life-threatening, bone marrow transplant (see BONE MARROW TRANSPLANT, ALLOGENEIC) is the most effective treatment for people younger than 30. People who are older than 40 or who lack a matching bone marrow donor are treated with antithymocyte globulin, a serum that suppresses the immune system.

Anemia, hemolytic

A group of diseases in which red blood cells are destroyed faster than they are produced, resulting in anemia. Symptoms include fatigue, pallid skin, breathlessness, rapid heartbeat (particularly on exertion), jaundice, dark urine, and enlarged spleen. Hemolytic anemias are sometimes difficult to treat, but they are rarely fatal.

Some hemolytic anemias are inherited; others are acquired. The hemolysis, or breakdown of cells, may develop during an infection or after exposure to certain chemicals, such as mothballs, and specific drugs, such as antimalarial agents, sulfonamide antibiotics, nonsteroidal anti-inflammatory drugs (NSAIDs, such as aspirin and ibuprofen), and quinine. This type of hemolytic anemia can be prevented by avoiding medications that may bring on a crisis.

An acquired form of the disease is idiopathic autoimmune hemolytic anemia. For unknown reasons, a person forms antibodies against his or her own red blood cells. The disease may begin very suddenly and severely. This hemolytic anemia is treated with prednisone, which slows the immune response. Since the spleen is the organ that removes red blood cells from the bloodstream, it is sometimes surgically removed. Drugs that suppress the immune system may also be prescribed.

Anemia, iron-deficiency

A decrease in the number of red blood cells caused by inadequate stores of iron in the body. Iron is the central component of hemoglobin, the pigment in red blood cells that transports oxygen through the body. When the iron supply in the body is inadequate, hemoglobin production falls and anemia results.

Iron deficiency is the most common cause of anemia. The principal causes of the disease are inadequate iron in the diet, insufficient iron absorption during digestion, and abnormal blood loss. In children, lead poisoning can interfere with iron utilization and cause anemia.

Mild iron-deficiency anemia often produces no symptoms. If the disease progresses, symptoms appear, which include pallid skin, fatigue, irritability, weakness, shortness of breath, postural hypotension (low blood pressure on standing up), brittle nails, headache, and sore tongue.

Iron-deficiency anemia is diagnosed by blood tests that measure the amount of hemoglobin and iron in the blood. If the iron deficiency is thought to be the result of digestive tract bleeding, other tests may be performed to identify the bleeding site. A colonoscopy is often recommended to rule out colon cancer.

Iron-deficiency anemia is treated by increasing dietary iron intake and by taking supplemental iron, typically in the form of ferrous sulfate. Iron-rich foods include red meat, raisins, fish, egg yolks, liver, poultry, legumes (peas and beans), potatoes, and whole grains. Occasionally people with iron-deficiency anemia are given supplemental iron by injection; in severe cases, blood transfusions may be given until the bone marrow can replace the blood that has been lost.

Anemia, megaloblastic

A blood disorder characterized by larger than normal red blood cells. Abnormal precursors of red blood cells called megaloblasts (from Greek roots meaning "big cell buds") occur in the bone marrow and give this anemia its name. Megaloblastic anemia commonly results from deficiency in vitamin B12 or folic acid (also known as folate). It can also be caused by leukemia, multiple myeloma, certain hereditary disorders, and some chemotherapy agents. The most common type of megaloblastic anemia is pernicious anemia (see ANEMIA and ANEMIA, PERNICIOUS).

Anemia, pernicious

A blood disorder characterized by abnormally low numbers of red blood cells and caused by an inability to absorb vitamin B12, which is needed for red blood cell production.

Pernicious anemia gets its name from the fact that, in the days before its cause was understood and effective treatment developed, it led to gradual, progressive deterioration and eventual death. Early symptoms include a sore tongue, a rapid heartbeat, limited endurance, weakness, abdominal discomfort, and weight loss due to poor appetite. The disease also affects the nerves, causing paresthesia (tingling or numbness) in the hands or feet, difficulty walking, clumsiness, slow thought processes, and impaired memory. Rarely there are psychiatric symptoms such as hallucinations or paranoia.

Pernicious anemia is usually diagnosed with blood tests that measure the level of vitamin B12 in the bloodstream. In some cases a biopsy sample of bone marrow is taken. Pernicious anemia is a megaloblastic anemia, which is characterized by the presence of abnormal red blood cell precursors (megaloblasts) in the bone marrow.

Once pernicious anemia is diagnosed, it is treated with regular injections of vitamin B12. Treatment usually reduces symptoms in 48 to 72 hours. People with pernicious anemia require injections every month or two for the remainder of their lives.

Anemia, sickle cell

See SICKLE CELL ANEMIA.

Anemia, sideroblastic

A group of blood diseases in which the red blood cells contain too much iron and hemoglobin production is defective. Sideroblastic anemia can be inherited. Other forms of the disease are acquired as a result of exposure to toxins (such as alcohol or lead), certain cancers (such as leukemia, lymphoma, or myeloma), or inflammatory disease (such as rheumatoid arthritis). In some cases, no cause can be identified. Symptoms include fatigue, shortness of breath, weakness, pallid skin, and an enlarged liver and spleen. Removing the toxin or treating the underlying disease often reverses the anemia.

Some people with sideroblastic anemia respond to high doses of vitamin B6 (pyridoxine) or androgens to stimulate the bone marrow. In addition, blood transfusions may be required, and medication may be needed to rid the body of excess iron from multiple transfusions.

Anencephaly

A severe NEURAL TUBE DEFECT in which an infant's brain and spinal cord fail to develop in utero (within the uterus). Anencephaly occurs when the top portion of an embryo's neural tube fails to close in the early stage of pregnancy. As a result, the infant is born without a forebrain (the part of the brain responsible for thinking and coordination). Remaining brain tissue is often left exposed, uncovered by skin or bone. Although reflex actions such as breathing may occur, an affected infant is usually blind, deaf, unconscious, and unable to experience sensations, such as pain. The lack of a functioning cerebrum means that the infant cannot gain consciousness. When the infant is not stillborn, death usually occurs within hours or days after birth.

Some cases of anencephaly may be detected by checking the mother's alpha-fetoprotein level early in the pregnancy. The abnormality can often be confirmed on ultrasound examination before delivery. The risk for anencephaly and other neural tube defects can be decreased if the mother takes a daily multivitamin containing 400 micrograms of folic acid as a part of regular prenatal care.

Anesthesia

A method, including medication, to cause the temporary absence of all sensation. Anesthesia makes surgery possible by eliminating the pain that a procedure would otherwise cause. Various forms and routes of pain suppression are available, depending on the person's medical history, preferences, age, and emotional makeup and on the type and duration of surgery performed. See also the following ANESTHESIA entries.

Anesthesia, epidural

A method of anesthetizing the lower half of the body by administering medication into the epidural space (a narrow area around the spinal cord) in the lower back. Typically used in labor or surgery, the procedure is also called an epidural block or a lumbar epidural block.

Often, epidural anesthesia affects the ability to urinate, and a catheter must be inserted into the bladder to drain it.

Anesthesia, general

A method of preventing pain and discomfort during surgery that makes the patient temporarily unconscious. Under general anesthesia, patients respond minimally, if at all, to intense stimulation, including pain. Breathing, heart function, and protective reflexes, such as coughing, continue but are slowed.

General anesthesia is used for surgery in the chest, abdomen, limbs, neck, and head and for almost all types of laparoscopic surgery, in which the abdomen is inflated with gas to allow the insertion of instruments through small incisions. For general anesthesia, the person inhales anesthetic gases, and intravenous medication is given.

Possible complications that can

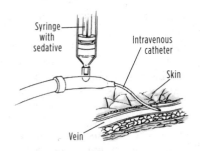

Inducing unconsciousness

To give a general anesthetic, a sedative is first administered to cause the person to lose consciousness immediately. This medication is usually injected through a catheter inserted into a vein in the hand or arm.

arise during general anesthesia include breathing difficulties, a drop in blood pressure, and irregular heartbeat.

Anesthesia, inhalation

A method of giving medication that is inhaled into the lungs as an anesthetic gas to suppress pain. Nitrous oxide, known as "laughing gas," is an odorless, colorless gas that was one of the first effective anesthetics discovered and is still the most widely used inhaled anesthetic agent, especially for dental procedures. Nitrous oxide is commonly administered with other intravenous anesthetics or other medications to decrease anxiety, relax the patient, and enhance the effectiveness of the other intravenous medications.

Another inhalation agent and a powerful anesthetic that suppresses pain very effectively is halothane. Combining halothane with nitrous oxide enhances the anesthetic effect, reduces the amount of halothane needed, and lowers the risk of circulatory complications that can be a side effect of this anesthetic.

Anesthesia, intravenous

A method that provides pain-suppressing medication through a small, flexible tube (intravenous catheter) inserted into a vein, usually in the hand or lower arm. Intravenous anesthesia can be used for general anesthesia (see ANESTHESIA, GENERAL), CONSCIOUS SEDATION, or regional anesthesia (see ANESTHESIA, REGIONAL).

Anesthesia, local

A method used to give medication to induce loss of sensation to prevent pain in a surgical site. Most local anesthetics are given as injections, but ointments or sprays containing an anesthetic agent can also be used. Local anesthetics block the nerve impulses that would otherwise communicate pain signals to the brain during diagnostic procedures, treatments, and surgery. They do not block all sensation; patients may still feel touch or pressure in the anesthetized area. Local anesthetics can be used alone or combined with CONSCIOUS SEDATION to keep the patient awake but relaxed, drowsy, and insensitive to pain.

Local anesthetics generally have little or no effect on the respiratory or circulatory systems. Nausea and vomiting, which follow general anesthesia in some patients, are very rare with local anesthesia.

The most serious possible complication to local anesthesia is accidental injection of a large volume of medication into a vein. This can lead to seizures, an abnormal heart rhythm, and even cardiac arrest, which may prove fatal. As a safeguard during the injection of local anesthetic, the physician or nurse always injects slowly and pulls back on the syringe to look for blood to ensure that the medication is not being placed in a vein. See also ANESTHESIA, REGIONAL.

Anesthesia, pediatric

A method used to suppress pain in children undergoing a surgical operation. Anesthesia in children carries a greater risk than it does in adults. Since children have a higher metabolism than adults and require more oxygen, they suffer brain damage more quickly if a complication during anesthesia stops their breathing.

Sedation, which makes the child relaxed and less anxious, is often used even before the child is taken to the operating room. Children receiving general anesthesia are often put to sleep by breathing anesthetic gases before an intravenous catheter is placed in a vein. Pleasant smells, like bubble gum or strawberry, may be added to the mask to cover the smell of the gas, which some children find unpleasant.

Regional anesthesia can be used during surgery in combination with CONSCIOUS SEDATION, which leaves the child awake, drowsy, and pain-free. This combination, with a spinal block as the regional anesthesia, is common for routine removal of the appendix.

Anesthesia, regional

The use of medication to make a portion of the body unable to feel pain. Regional anesthesia works by blocking pain impulses from nerves located in the part of the body that is anesthetized. In some cases, regional anesthesia is combined with CONSCIOUS SEDATION, leaving the person awake, relaxed, and insensitive to pain. For many types of surgery, regional anesthesia is preferred to general anesthesia because it has no effect on the respiratory system and may be safer for the patient.

Regional anesthesia in the lower part of the body is commonly produced by injecting anesthetics into the spinal column; this procedure blocks pain impulses from nerves in the legs, groin, buttocks, and lower portion of the abdomen. See also ANESTHESIA, SPINAL and ANESTHESIA, EPIDURAL.

Anesthesia, spinal

Making the lower part of the body insensitive to pain by injecting medications into the spinal column to block the nerves that lead to and from the legs, groin, buttocks, and lower region of the abdomen. Spinal anesthesia is also called a saddle block. Spinal anesthesia is used for repairing fractures in the legs and feet, hernia repair, removal of the appendix or uterus, surgery on blood vessels in the legs and lower part of the abdomen, lower back surgery, childbirth, and operations on the male and female urinary and reproductive systems. It produces excellent pain control without affecting the respiratory system.

Spinal anesthesia begins as a tingling sensation in the toes or the buttocks; then, it spreads across the entire lower part of the body. The medication blocks the nerves that control the muscles as well as the ones that convey pain, so the patient cannot move the anesthetized area. The anesthesia may last from as little as an hour to as long as several hours. When it wears off, muscle control returns first and then feeling reappears. The possible complications of spinal anesthesia include abnormally low blood pressure (HY-POTENSION), severe headache during recovery from surgery, PARALYSIS, and MENINGITIS, an inflammation of the lining of the spinal cord that usually is due to infection.

Anesthesiology

The medical specialty that focuses on relieving pain and providing medical care to surgical patients before, during, and after surgery. An anesthesiologist is a physician who specializes in anesthesiology.

Anesthetics

Drugs that cause a loss of sensation, including pain. Anesthetics may be general, which is when a temporary loss of consciousness is induced in a patient, or local, when specific nerves are targeted to produce numbness (and a loss of sensation) in only that part of the body.

Aneurysm

An abnormal widening or ballooning of a portion of a blood vessel. Common risk factors for aneurysms include HYPERTENSION (high blood pressure), ATHEROSCLEROSIS (narrowing of the arteries), and smoking. Two of the most common and serious types are cerebral aneurysms and aortic aneurysms.

Cerebral aneurysm

Aneurysms in the brain occur when there is a weakened wall in a blood vessel. They may be congenital or develop later in life. An aneurysm generally does not cause symptoms until it either ruptures or leaks blood. A cerebral aneurysm is a life-threatening condition that can lead to STROKE, SEIZURE, BRAIN DAMAGE, or death. Permanent brain damage is a result of ischemia (loss of blood flow) or of bleeding into the brain tissue.

The primary symptom of a ruptured cerebral aneurysm is the sudden onset of a severe headache and a stiff neck. This may be accompanied by nausea, vomiting, fainting, an altered level of consciousness, breathing problems, difficulty with speaking, trouble swallowing, confusion, irritability, vision problems, loss of movement or sensation, muscle aches, or seizure.

A suspected cerebral aneurysm requires immediate medical attention. Diagnostic evaluation includes a neuromuscular examination, CT (computed tomography) scanning, MRI (magnetic resonance imaging), and angiography. (See BRAIN IMAGING.) A spinal tap will reveal the presence of blood in cerebrospinal fluid. Treatment varies but usually includes life-saving interventions and supportive measures. Surgery is usually required to remove large hematomas (collections of blood) and repair the damaged blood vessel. Even with prompt treatment, the death rate approaches 50 percent.

Aortic aneurysm

An abdominal aortic aneurysm is an abnormal widening of the abdominal part of the aorta (the major artery of the body). A common complication is rupture. This is a life-threatening medical emergency that can cause profuse internal bleeding.

Symptoms of an aortic aneurysm include a pulsating abdominal mass, abdominal pain and tenderness, rigidity, lower back pain, rapid pulse, paleness, nausea, vomiting, anxiety, fatigue, clammy skin, thirst, sweating, and fainting. Diagnosis is based on physical examination of the abdomen, blood tests, and radiographic tests such as X rays, ultrasound, MRI, CT scanning, and angiography.

If the aneurysm is unruptured, treatment depends on the size of the aneurysm and the general health of the person. Smaller aneurysms are periodically monitored for changes in size. Larger aneurysms are at greater risk for rupture, and surgical repair is often recommended. Once an aneurysm ruptures, it is a life-threatening event, and fewer than half of those who experience a ruptured abdominal aortic aneurysm survive. Emergency treatment includes supportive care and surgery to repair the damaged blood vessel.

Angina

A diffuse pain or discomfort in the chest that is often described as a tightness or heaviness; the cause is insufficient blood flow to the heart. Angina is also known as angina pectoris, which is Latin for "choking pain of the chest." In most cases, attacks of angina last only a few minutes and are brought on by physical exertion or emotional stress. Angina itself is not a disease, but a symptom of heart disease.

The discomfort of angina is often felt under the breastbone (sternum) but may radiate to the back, neck, shoulder, and arm, particularly on the left side. In some cases, pain occurs only in the arm or jaw. Pain and discomfort may be accompanied by nausea, sweating, shortness of breath, and light-headedness.

Types

Stable angina arises during or just after situations in which the heart must work harder and needs increased oxygen. An attack of stable angina usually lasts from 1 to 15 minutes, subsides with rest, and tends to occur more commonly between 6 A.M. and noon. Angina attacks lasting longer than 30 minutes are rare and merit emergency evaluation.

If angina worsens in frequency or severity of attacks or occurs at rest, it is called unstable angina. Unstable angina may occur at any time, whether the person is moving or at rest, including during sleep. Unstable angina is a serious condition that indicates an increased risk for a myocardial infarction (heart attack). It is less common than stable angina and may require hospitalization.

Variant, or Prinzmetal, angina is also distinguished by attacks that occur when the person is at rest. Variant angina is often accompanied by abnormal heart rhythms, such as VENTRICULAR FIBRILLATION or ventricular tachycardia (see TACHYCARDIA, VENTRICULAR), which increase the risk of sudden death.

Diagnosis, treatment, and prevention

In many cases, a doctor can decide whether angina is present from the way a person describes an attack. A variety of tests may include exercise stress testing (monitoring the heart while exercising on a treadmill or a stationary bicycle), nuclear imaging (injecting a radioactive substance into the blood to produce images of the heart), echocardiogram (an ultrasound image of the heart), cardiac catheterization (inserting a thin tube through a blood vessel into the heart to locate artery blockages), and CT (computed tomography) scanning.

Once the severity and extent of the underlying condition have been determined, the best course of treatment can be chosen. Most people with mild stable angina are treated with a combination of lifestyle changes and medication.

Persons with unstable or severe stable angina are often treated with an invasive catheter or surgical procedure. Procedures include BALLOON ANGIOPLASTY; keyhole surgery, which can be used in some people with fewer than three blockages; or BYPASS SURGERY.

Angioedema

An allergic reaction in the skin and underlying tissue marked by swelling and red blotches. Angioedema is characterized by large welts below the surface of the skin, especially around the eyes and lips, and less frequently on the hands and feet and in the throat. It is caused by the release into the bloodstream of HISTAMINE and other chemicals related to the immune system.

There is a known hereditary component to the development of angioedema, but the specific cause of the reaction is often unknown. Foods, pollen, animal dander, medications, latex, insect stings, infections, illness, cold, heat, light, and emotional distress are common culprits.

Diagnosis of angioedema is sometimes difficult because of the wide range of possible allergens or irritants that may cause it. A detailed history of exposure to possible irritants recently may help a doctor determine a possible cause.

Treatment is generally centered on avoidance of the causative agent and may sometimes include medications

such as adrenaline (epinephrine), antihistamines, and, occasionally, an oral corticosteroid.

Hereditary or recurrent angioedema is a rare form of the disorder that can be dangerous. It involves an abnormality in a blood protein in the immune system and may require specialized treatment. This form of angioedema usually includes swelling that does not itch and is sometimes accompanied by abdominal cramps and diarrhea. If hereditary angioedema affects the throat or tongue, the swelling can obstruct the air passage and be life-threatening.

Angiogram

An X-ray film of blood vessels (either arteries or veins) after they have been filled with a CONTRAST MEDIUM. See also ANGIOGRAPHY.

Angiography

An X-ray procedure used to visualize blood vessels (both arteries and veins) after they have been injected with a CONTRAST MEDIUM. When an angiogram is used to examine arteries, it is known as an arteriogram. When an angiogram is used to examine the veins, it is called a venogram.

Angiography is generally used to detect abnormalities of the blood vessels or to evaluate the blood supply to various organs. The procedure may yield information about blood flow, the formation of an aneurysm (an abnormal ballooning of a weakened area in a wall of an artery), vascular anomalies, tumors, and hemorrhage. Deep leg veins may be examined by angiography to confirm the presence of deep-vein thrombosis, identify causes of edema, and assess vascular health after surgery.

Because angiography is an invasive procedure, there are risks involved. The risks include bleeding at the puncture site, injury to a blood vessel, allergy or other reaction to the contrast medium or other medications, and infection. Very rarely, a heart attack or stroke may occur during or after angiography. See also DIGITAL SUBTRACTION ANGIOGRAPHY.

Angioma

A benign (not cancerous) growth on the skin consisting of blood vessels. Some examples include cherry angiomas (small, bright red, domelike spots on the skin caused by dilated blood vessels) and capillary hemangioma (a reddish purple birthmark caused by an abnormal distribution of blood vessels).

Angioplasty, balloon

See BALLOON ANGIOPLASTY.

Angiotensin

A hormone that causes blood vessels to constrict and raises blood pressure. Medications that prevent the formation of angiotensin, known as angiotensin-converting enzyme (ACE) inhibitors, lower blood pressure and reduce the workload on the heart. They are commonly used in the treatment of congestive heart failure (see HEART FAILURE, CONGESTIVE) and high blood pressure (see HYPERTENSION). Another class of medications, the angiotensin-receptor blocking agents, block the effect of angiotensin and have effects similar to those of ACE inhibitors.

Angiotensin-converting enzyme inhibitors

See ANTIHYPERTENSIVES.

Ankylosing spondylitis

An inflammatory disease of the joints in the spinal column and back of the pelvis that may also involve the shoulder, hip, and knee joints. Ankylosing spondylitis generally develops in late adolescence or early adulthood and can lead to extreme rigidity, deformity, and a fusion of the bones involved.

Symptoms include morning back pain with aching and stiffness that tends to improve in 1 or 2 hours. Movement tends to lessen this pain, which often returns when the body is stationary for long periods. Over a period of several months, the pain and inflexibility tend to become more severe, moving up the spine. Other spinal components, such as ligaments and muscles, become affected, causing severe muscle spasms. These spasms produce a forward flexing of the spinal column, which causes a rounded curvature of the back. The disks, joints, and ligaments of the spinal column and eventually the hip, knee, and shoulder joints become inflamed and hardened. In severe cases, the neck may be stiff, preventing the person from being able to lift his or her head. Sites other than the spinal column can be involved, such as the eyes, heart, aorta, and lungs.

The diagnosis of ankylosing spondylitis is based on a clinical history, an evaluation of lower back stiffness and joint and tissue inflammation, and the results of laboratory tests and procedures, such as X rays and other imaging techniques. A person with this condition should sleep on a firm mattress with thin pillows to prevent muscle spasms of the back. Treatment may include physical and occupational therapy, nonsteroidal anti-inflammatory drugs (NSAIDs), and in rare severe cases, surgery to realign the spine and to replace destroyed joints in order to restore function and eliminate debilitating pain. See also SPONDYLITIS.

Ankylosis

Immobility and consolidation of a joint or joints caused by disease or injury. Ankylosis refers to the condition in which bones and other components of a joint are stiff or fixated, causing severe or complete loss of the joint's movement. It is also the term for a surgical procedure known as cervical spine fusion, which is performed to stabilize a joint, commonly in the neck or back.

Anorexia nervosa

A mental illness in which a person refuses to maintain normal body weight, is extremely afraid of gaining weight, and has a distorted image of his or her body, such as describing it as obese even when it is extremely thin. People with anorexia usually lose weight by restricting the amount and type of food they eat. In one type of anorexia similar to BULIMIA, some people engage in binge eating, or they purge themselves with self-induced vomiting, laxatives, diuretics, or enemas. People with anorexia may also exercise excessively. The disease primarily affects females, particularly during adolescence, but it also affects women at other ages, and, rarely, men.

Anorexia nervosa is often accompanied by other mental diseases, such as depression, manic-depressive illness, self-mutilation, and obsessive-compulsive disorder. As their weight drops below normal, those with anorexia often experience low moods, withdraw from social contact, have trouble sleeping, exhibit irritability, and lose interest in sex. Physical symptoms include sensitivity to cold, yellowing skin, brittle nails, low blood pressure, lack of menstrual periods, slow heartbeat (bradycardia), and, if the person is inducing vomiting, damage to tooth enamel from stomach acid. Long, fine hair may develop on the body as a way of conserving heat. Anorexia nervosa can have serious medical consequences, including heart disease, anemia, kidney disease, dental problems, and brittle bones (osteoporosis). Death from heart failure is a major risk. In severe cases, hospitalization may be necessary.

Treatment consists of increasing the person's weight into the normal range by stabilizing eating patterns coupled with psychotherapy, especially family group therapy, aimed at understanding the emotional conflicts that underlie the disorder. In some cases, medication may be used to treat accompanying depression or anxiety. In extreme cases, the person will need nutrition through intravenous therapy. Prognosis is generally good, although relapses are common.

Anorgasmia

See ORGASM, LACK OF.

Anovulation

See OVULATION, LACK OF.

Antacids

Drugs used to relieve the symptoms of indigestion and heartburn. Antacids, which are available in over-the-counter preparations, neutralize stomach acid and effectively relieve symptoms.

The use of antacids can mask the symptoms of more serious disorders, and the excessive or prolonged use of antacids can cause bloating or serious disorders of the kidneys or bones. A person who experiences indigestion, heartburn, or stomach pain for longer than 2 weeks, or pain that is not relieved by antacids, should seek medical attention.

Antagonist

A drug that binds to a cell receptor without eliciting a biological response. Antagonist drugs are substances that tend to cancel out the action of active substances.

Antepartum hemorrhage

Any vaginal bleeding after the 20th week of pregnancy. Antepartum hemorrhage may have several causes, including damage to the cervix, separation of the placenta from the uterine wall, or PLACENTA PREVIA, in which the placenta lies over the cervix. Most antepartum bleeding is mild and harmless. However, hemorrhage caused by placental separation, placental bleeding, and placenta previa can threaten both the mother and baby. Any bleeding during pregnancy should be reported to the doctor as soon as possible. Blood tests and ultrasound scanning can help identify the source of the hemorrhage. In the case of severe antepartum hemorrhage, hospitalization may be required. A blood transfusion may be needed, and the baby may need to be delivered as soon as possible, either by cesarean section or by induction of labor.

Antepartum testing

See PRENATAL TESTING.

Anthrax

An infectious disease of animals that occasionally infects people. Anthrax is found in goats, cattle, sheep, horses, and exotic wildlife such as hippos, elephants, and the Cape buffalo. The disease is unusual in humans and generally occurs in developing countries in which exposure to infected animals and their products is not adequately prevented.

Anthrax is caused by a bacterial spore that is highly resistant and can remain viable in soil and in animals for decades. People may become infected with cutaneous anthrax by handling materials from animals that have died of anthrax (the bacteria enter via a scratch or sore when contaminated animal material is handled) or from eating contaminated meat. Pulmonary anthrax (sometimes called inhalation anthrax) may occur if a person with an acute respiratory infection inhales spores of the organism that causes anthrax. Anthrax has been used in BIOTERRORISM.

Symptoms of cutaneous anthrax include an enlarging skin eruption, malaise, body aches, headache, fever, nausea, and vomiting. Pulmonary anthrax symptoms resemble those of the flu and may progress rapidly to severe respiratory distress, shock, coma, or even death.

Anthrax is suspected when there is a history detailing exposure to animals or their products, which may have transmitted the disease. Cultures of skin lesions may be taken to identify the bacteria in cutaneous anthrax, and throat swabs and sputum samples may be evaluated if pulmonary anthrax is suspected.

The cutaneous form is treated with penicillin, tetracycline, or another antibiotic to prevent the bacteria from spreading through the body and to heal the open sore on the skin. Anthrax is not contagious from person to person. Pulmonary anthrax is usually fatal if not treated early with continuous intravenous penicillin, fluoroquinolones, and, possibly, corticosteroids. A vaccine that provides some protection against anthrax infections is given mainly to military personnel and veterinarians and others who work closely with animals.

Antiaging therapies

Treatments claimed to improve and maintain optimal health for people as they age. Antiaging therapies include the use of vitamins, minerals, hormones, and some drugs of unproven benefit. There is no evidence, however, that external therapies can reverse or retard the aging process.

Some antiaging therapies recommend large doses of hormones, such as estrogen and testosterone, to reverse the aging process, although no evidence exists to demonstrate that this remedy is effective.

Antianxiety drugs

Antianxiety drugs, also known as anxiolytics, do not cure anxiety disorders but can effectively relieve unpleasant symptoms. A common class of antianxiety drugs are the BENZODIAZE-PINES, which work by enhancing the function of a neurochemical called GABA (gamma-aminobutyric acid). Benzodiazepines are fast-acting but can be associated with addiction,

abuse, and the impaired ability to drive.

Some antianxiety drugs are BETA BLOCKERS, which reduce the effects of adrenaline. Also fast-acting, these drugs are not habit-forming. Other drugs used to treat the symptoms of anxiety include ANTIDEPRESSANTS, many of which work by enhancing or regulating the activity of serotonin, a chemical in the brain known to affect a person's mood.

Antiarrhythmics

Drugs that correct an irregular heartbeat by restoring normal rhythm. Antiarrhythmics can also help the heart work more efficiently by slowing it down when it beats too fast or by helping it beat more regularly. The pace at which the heart beats is controlled by electrical signals that start in one part of the heart and spread throughout the entire organ. Arrhythmias develop when this control mechanism is disrupted.

Antibiotics

Among the first antibiotic to be used to treat disease was penicillin (see PENICILLINS).

Antibiotics can kill harmful bacteria that cause infection and disease. When a person takes an antibiotic, it overpowers and kills the bacteria causing the infection, or it prevents the bacteria from multiplying. Doctors always recommend that a person finish the entire course of antibiotics.

When organisms invade the body, they reproduce and multiply rapidly. At the same time, they compete with the body's natural metabolism, in some cases by producing poisons that injure cells. Bacterial infections can be extremely serious and even fatal. The extent to which an infected person is ill depends on the type and number of the invading organisms, as well as on the person's general health. There are several types of bacterial infection for which antibiotics are prescribed—including infections caused by staphylococcus, streptococcus, and E. coli bacteria.

Antibiotics generally are only useful in the treatment of bacterial infection. Not all fevers are caused by infection, and not all infections are caused by bacteria. Many infections are caused by viruses, and antibiotics cannot treat viral infections. Colds and flu, for example, are respiratory infections caused by viruses and do not respond to antibiotics.

Sometimes viral infections such as colds and flu can lead to secondary infections that are caused by bacteria. Secondary bacterial infections, such as ear or sinus infections, can be treated with antibiotics. However, not all bacterial infections need to be treated with antibiotics.

Because over time antibiotics have been overused and used inappropriately, tough new strains of bacteria have developed that are resistant to antibiotics. As bacteria reproduce, they change their cellular makeup to protect themselves from future attack, including the attacks made on them by drugs.

Many bacteria have adapted and become invulnerable to antibiotics. As a result, the number of deaths from infectious diseases has risen, in part because many bacteria have acquired resistance against antibiotics.

Antibody

A mechanism used by the body for fighting infection. Antibodies are protein that react to antigens (foreign substances in the body) in a number of ways. An antibody recognizes a specific ANTIGEN and binds to it or coats it to inactivate or destroy the antigen. Antibodies are secreted into the body's fluids by B cells, which are a type of white blood cell called a lymphocyte.

Each B cell makes a specific antibody to combat a specific antigen. For example, one B cell is programmed to make an antibody to block the virus that causes the common cold, while another B cell can make antibodies to stave off the Streptococcus bacteria that result in strep throat.

Antibodies are large protein molecules that belong to the group of proteins known as immunoglobulins. The action of antibodies varies with the nature of the antigen with which they are interacting. Most commonly, after the antibody bonds to the antigen, it forms a complex protein which trigger a set of reactions that are lethal to the antigen.

Antibody, monoclonal

An ANTIBODY produced in large quantities by a single cell directed for use against a specific antigen. If the body produces an excess of a monoclonal antibody, this may be a sign of a plasma cell disorder such as multiple myeloma, a type of cancer.

Monoclonal antibodies are currently used clinically as a method for identifying the myriad cells involved in the immune response and as diagnostic tools for cancer and other diseases and for treatment of several autoimmune disorders. Doctors are also researching the use of monoclonal antibodies in a technique to target cancer cells for treatment and as an agent to target tissues for treatment in nuclear medicine.

Preparations of monoclonal antibodies can be used diagnostically to measure proteins, medications, and other substances in the blood. They may be useful for typing tissue and blood and for identifying infectious agents. They are also used to treat allograft rejection in organ transplant recipients. In the diagnosis and treatment of leukemias and lymphomas, monoclonal antibodies are used to identify cluster designations (abbreviated CD and used with a number, such as CD3) for classification of and follow-up on tumors. Monoclonal antibodies are useful for identifying tumor antibodies and autoantibodies in a variety of other diseases, too. For example, monoclonal antibodies are used in organ transplant patients to help stop rejection of the transplanted organ.

Anticholinergic agents

Drugs that block the action of acetylcholine (a chemical messenger in the nervous system) in the body. Anticholinergics are used to treat Parkinson disease, muscle rigidity, and muscle spasms caused by psychoactive medications. Anticholinergics work by blocking acetylcholine receptors in the brain and other tissues, reducing the effects of acetylcholine and restoring balance with dopamine. Some anticholinergics are also used to prevent nausea and vomiting caused by motion sickness and to treat asthma.

Examples of anticholinergics include belladonna alkaloids, which contain naturally occurring anticholinergics that have been used for centuries, and benztropine.

Anticoagulants

Drugs that prevent clotting of blood; also called "blood thinners." Anticoagulants are used to maintain normal blood flow in people who are at risk for excessive clot formation, such as people who are immobile. Anticoagulants prevent new clots or the enlargement of existing clots; they do not dissolve existing clots.

Anticoagulants are prescribed for people who have had recurrent heart attacks or stroke. They are also given to people who have transient ischemic attacks (TIAs), an arterial embolism, or a pulmonary embolism and to people at risk for developing blood clots, such as those with irregular heart rates.

Anticonvulsants

Drugs used to control seizures. Anticonvulsants are used to treat EPILEPSY and other SEIZURE disorders, such as a seizure following neurosurgery and a seizure associated with brain tumors. Anticonvulsants act on the central nervous system by inhibiting activity in the part of the brain responsible for grand mal or generalized seizures in which the entire body shakes uncontrollably.

Antidepressants

Drugs used to treat DEPRESSION and other conditions associated with reduced levels of two neurotransmitters: norepinephrine and serotonin. Most antidepressants work by raising the levels of norepinephrine and serotonin in the brain or by preventing their inactivation in the brain. Under normal circumstances, the neurotransmitters stimulate the brain when they are released and are reabsorbed by brain cells, then broken down by an enzyme called mono-amine oxidase (MAO). When levels of these neurotransmitters are low, the brain is understimulated.

Tricyclic antidepressants

This class of antidepressants is named for its chemical structure. Tricyclics increase the levels of both serotonin and norepinephrine by blocking their reabsorption into nerve cell endings. Tricyclics are very effective at treating symptoms of depression, but they are associated with many troublesome side effects, such as drowsiness, dry mouth, and constipation. In overdose, they can be deadly.

MAO inhibitors

This class of antidepressants is named for its action. By inhibiting monoamine oxidase, the levels of neurotransmitters in the brain are increased. MAO inhibitors are very effective at reducing symptoms of depression, but MAO is also involved in the metabolism of tyramine, an amino acid. People who take MAO inhibitors must be very careful not to eat or drink certain foods or beverages that contain large amounts of tyramine. The combination of tyramine and an MAO inhibitor can cause the person to have a dangerous increase in blood pressure.

SSRIs

Selective serotonin reuptake inhibitors (SSRIs) make up the newest class of antidepressants. They are less likely to cause side effects than either tricyclics or MAO inhibitors. They work by blocking the reabsorption of serotonin in the brain, thereby increasing the available supply and enhancing a person's mood. SSRIs are associated with some side effects, but they are usually mild. Some people taking SSRIs experience sexual difficulties.

Antidiuretic hormone

See ADH.

Antiemetics

Drugs used to prevent or relieve nausea and vomiting, usually from motion sickness, gastroenteritis, morning sickness, and cancer. Four kinds of drugs are prescribed for nausea and vomiting: phenothiazines, antihistamines, anticholinergics, and selective serotonin antagonists. Phenothiazines work by depressing the central nervous system; antihistamines have a depressant effect on nerve pathways; anticholinergics inhibit nerve impulse transmissions; and serotonin antagonists block the stimulation that causes vomiting. The latter type of drug is often used to treat nausea and vomiting due to cancer chemotherapy. All are powerful drugs that act at one or more of the places in the body responsible for causing nausea and vomiting, and they must be taken with care.

The herbal agent ginger may also be useful as a mild antiemetic; it is sometimes used to treat motion sickness and morning sickness in pregnancy.

Antiepileptic agents

See ANTICONVULSANTS.

Antifungal drugs

Drugs used to treat infections caused by fungi. Fungi are single-cell life forms that survive by invading and living off other living things. They thrive in moist, dark places, including some parts of the human body. Examples of fungal infections that affect the skin include candidiasis (also known as thrush or yeast infection), histoplasmosis, and aspergillosis.

Antigen

A substance that, on entering the body, is recognized as foreign and responded to by the person's immune system. An antigen is a molecule that can produce a specific immune response when it is introduced into the bloodstream. A specific configuration on the surface of certain large molecules makes a particular molecule an antigen that attracts a specific ANTI-BODY. Different types of antibodies recognize the different configurations as sites that they can combine with. The combining sites of the antibody and antigen form a bond that locks them tightly at surface sites that complement each other like pieces of a jigsaw puzzle.

Antihistamines

Any drug that counteracts histamine, a chemical released within the body during an allergic reaction. Antihistamines do not alter the cause of the reaction but suppress the symptoms associated with the release of histamine, such as swelling, irritation, and watery discharge from the eyes and nose. Antihistamines work by blocking histamine receptors.

Antihistamines are most often used to suppress the symptoms of hay fever and related allergies. They are also available in topical form as creams and ointments to reduce skin inflammation and itching caused by allergic reactions.

Antihypertensives

Drugs that help lower blood pressure. Blood pressure measures the force with which blood moves through the blood vessels. While blood pressure normally varies throughout the day, rising during exercise and falling during sleep, in some people the blood pressure stays high all the time. There are five major classes of medication used to treat hypertension.

- *DIURETICS* work by preventing the kidneys from retaining water and salt. By increasing the amount of fluids and salt excreted by the kidneys, the amount of fluid in the bloodstream is reduced, which reduces pressure on the artery walls of the blood vessels.

- *BETA BLOCKERS* reduce high blood pressure by slowing the force and speed of the action of the heart, including the rate at which it contracts. The medication may also reduce blood pressure by directly affecting the central nervous system, altering the body's response to certain nerve impulses.

- *ANGIOTENSIN-CONVERTING ENZYME (ACE)* inhibitors lower blood pressure by blocking production of angiotensin II, a chemical the body produces to raise blood pressure. Normally, angiotensin maintains blood pressure by tightening the arteries and causing the retention of sodium (salt) and water.

- *ANGIOTENSIN II RECEPTOR ANTAGONISTS* lower blood pressure by blocking angiotensin from binding to receptor sites in the smooth muscles of the blood vessels. This stops the angiotensin from tightening the arteries and raising the blood pressure.

- *CALCIUM CHANNEL BLOCKERS* reduce blood pressure by dilating the arteries, thereby reducing resistance to blood flow.

There are also other drugs that can lower blood pressure by relaxing the muscles in the walls of the arteries or veins, thereby reducing blood pressure. These drugs are sometimes considered vasodilators. They include clonidine, guanfacine, and hydralazine.

Antimicrobial agents

A general term referring to several categories of drugs, including antibiotics, antifungals, antiprotozoals, and antivirals. The most important characteristic of an antimicrobial agent is that it acts to inhibit or kill a target pathogen, or disease-causing entity, but has no toxic effect on the host. Antimicrobials affect the biochemical processes of microbes, but not those of humans or other animals.

Antioxidants

Substances able to neutralize OXYGEN FREE RADICALS produced in the body during metabolism. Antioxidants act by interrupting a process called oxidation, in which free radicals (molecules with unpaired electrons) react with other molecules in a series of chain reactions. Free radicals are produced normally by the body, as are antioxidants, to help body systems maintain a healthy balance. Stress, aging, and pollution can add to the number of free radicals in the body, thereby disrupting the delicate balance by damaging DNA in cells.

Because antioxidants prevent or slow oxidation by free radicals, they are assumed to provide a protective effect and are thought to be able to reduce the risk of cancer, heart disease, and stroke, among other diseases associated with aging. Although some people believe that adding antioxidants to the diet by consuming dietary supplements is desirable, this view is not medically proven.

Anti-Parkinson drugs

Drugs that address an imbalance between the primary neurotransmitters dopamine and acetylcholine. Parkinson disease is caused by an imbalance of the two neurotransmitters responsible for transmitting nerve impulses from the brain to the muscles. One group of anti-Parkinson drugs works by stimulating production of dopamine in the brain, supplying the substance from which it is formed (levodopa) to be converted to dopamine in the brain. Dopamine levels can also be increased by reducing the breakdown of dopamine in the brain or by stimulating its release.

Another group of drugs, called anticholinergic drugs, restores the balance between the two neurotransmitters by blocking the action of acetylcholine.

Antipsychotic drugs

Drugs that reduce psychotic symptoms. Antipsychotic drugs do not cure schizophrenia or other psychotic disorders, but help make it possible for people with those diseases to function more effectively.

It is thought that in psychotic disorders, the brain cells release too much dopamine, which causes overstimulation of brain activity. Antipsychotic drugs block the stimulatory actions of dopamine. They are chiefly used to treat the hallucinations and delusions associated with schizophrenia and other psychotic disorders. Antipsychotic drugs are less able to modify symptoms such as reduced motivation or the absence of emotion.

Antipyretic drugs

Drugs that reduce FEVER. Fever can be reduced by drugs representing three different classes. Many of them are available without a prescription. The three types of antipyretics are salicylates, including aspirin; acetaminophen, sometimes called nonaspirin pain relievers; and nonsteroidal anti-inflammatory drugs (NSAIDs), such as ibuprofen, naproxen, and ketoprofen. Aspirin should not be taken by children to reduce fever because of its association with Reye syndrome, a rare disorder that can cause brain and liver damage. In children, the most commonly used antipyretic drugs are acetaminophen and ibuprofen.

Antiseptics

Substances that destroy or inhibit the growth of bacteria and other microorganisms. Antiseptics are used topically to treat wounds and infections, to sterilize surfaces and medical instruments, to promote general hygiene, to preserve foods, and to purify sewage. Common antiseptic chemicals include iodine, alcohol, hydrogen peroxide, and boric acid, each of which works differently. Iodine, for instance, can kill bacteria within 30 seconds, while other antiseptics work more slowly.

Antisocial personality disorder

See PERSONALITY DISORDERS.

Antitoxin

A specific type of ANTIBODY that combines with and inactivates the toxins produced by certain bacterial microorganisms that cause infections. Antitoxins are proteins that exist naturally in the body or develop in response to the presence of toxins in the bloodstream. Toxins known as exotoxins are produced by the bacteria that cause botulism, diphtheria, and tetanus and are among those that are inactivated by antitoxins.

Antituberculosis drugs

Drugs used to cure tuberculosis infection. Pulmonary tuberculosis is caused by a bacterium called Mycobacterium tuberculosis and is treated with daily oral doses of antibiotics for at least 9 months. In some cases, the bacteria that cause tuberculosis have developed immunity to specific antituberculosis drugs, so most people with the disease take three or four drugs. Antituberculosis drugs are available by prescription only. They are all associated with some side effects.

Antivenin

A substance containing purified antibodies used to neutralize the venom of a poisonous animal. Antivenin is a type of antiserum that comes from the serum of an animal that has been deliberately immunized against a particular venom. Antivenin is available to counteract animal bites from poisonous snakes, spiders, and scorpions.

Anuria

Serious kidney malfunction that results in little or no urine production. Failure to pass urine is an indication of a serious problem in the urinary tract. In patients with only one kidney, anuria is often caused by a stone. In patients with both kidneys, the condition may be caused by a tumor blocking the kidneys, kidney disease, or abnormally low blood pressure caused by shock. Treatment is urgent and depends on the cause of the condition. Dialysis may be used to rid the body of wastes temporarily.

Anus

The opening at the lower end of the DIGESTIVE SYSTEM through which the feces, or stool, passes out of the body. About 1 to 2 inches long, the anus comprises two circular muscles. The internal anal sphincter muscle is a smooth, involuntary muscle; the external anal sphincter is a voluntary, striated muscle that can be relaxed at will to allow a bowel movement. The two muscles work together to open and close the anus.

Anus, cancer of

An uncommon cancer that develops in the inch-long muscular tube where the rectum opens. Anal cancer is a form of colon cancer (see COLON, CANCER OF THE) that is highly treatable and potentially curable. The earliest sign of anal cancer usually is bleeding and is often mistaken as a sign of hemorrhoids. Other common symptoms include pain or itching in the anal area, straining during bowel movements, or a discharge from the anus. Less common symptoms may include swollen lymph nodes in the groin or anal area and changes either in bowel habits or in the size of the stool.

Treatment usually consists of radiation and chemotherapy. If the tumor is not eradicated, surgery may be needed.

Anus, imperforate

A birth defect in which an infant is born without a fully developed anus. (See also BIRTH DEFECTS.) The anus is the external opening of the rectum through which stools pass. When a baby is born with an imperforate, or closed, anus, there are two possible causes. The anus may be covered with skin, or, more rarely and seriously, the anal canal fails to develop before birth.

Surgery is necessary to correct an imperforate anus. If the anus is simply covered, the surgeon will remove the skin. If the anal canal did not develop, more complicated reconstructive surgery is required. Most children recover completely. Eight of ten children born with an imperforate anus are toilet-trained by age 4.

Anxiety disorders

A group of mental illnesses characterized by overpowering and long-lasting fear, dread, unease, apprehension, obsessions, compulsions, and unpleasant physical symptoms, such as sweating, elevated heartbeat, shaking, or trembling. Anxiety disorders interfere with day-to-day functioning and may make it difficult or impossible for an individual to hold a job or enjoy a family or social life. They are the most common mental illnesses in the United States.

Types of anxiety disorders

- *GENERALIZED ANXIETY DISORDER (GAD)* is characterized by excessive, constant anxiety and worry about a number of life problems, such as marriage and money, for a period of 6 or more months.

- *PANIC DISORDER* is distinguished by unpredictable bouts of extreme anxiety that seem to start suddenly and peak quickly, usually within 10 minutes. Unpleasant physical symptoms can include elevated blood pressure and heartbeat, disorientation, dizziness, numbness, a looming sense of danger, choking sensations, and a strong desire to escape. (See PANIC DISORDER.)

• *PHOBIA.* People with phobias have an exaggerated, extreme, and irrational fear of specific situations or objects. The feared situation or object varies with the individual. Common phobias include objects such as needles, knives, or animals, particularly snakes, dogs, or spiders (simple phobia); social situations (social phobia); and public spaces such as churches and stadiums (agoraphobia). These fears are common in children and are not a sign of a psychiatric disorder. See PHOBIA.

• *OBSESSIVE-COMPULSIVE DISORDER (OCD)* is distinguished by persistent, intrusive, and distressing thoughts, images, or impulses that occupy the mind (obsessions) and by repetitive actions the individual thinks he or she must perform (compulsions). Typical obsessions include fear of contamination by dirt, germs, or viruses; extreme need for objects to be in an exact order; heightened vigilance, such as keeping all windows and doors locked at all times; and fear of unlucky numbers. Typical compulsions include washing the hands repeatedly, checking door and window locks again and again, and hoarding supplies against unlikely disasters. OCD is equally common in males and females. See OBSESSIVE-COMPULSIVE DISORDER.

• *POSTTRAUMATIC STRESS DISORDER (PTSD)* represents an immediate or delayed response to a traumatic event that evokes intense fear, helplessness, and horror through flashbacks, or nightmares coupled with avoidance of all things associated with the event and increased vigilance and arousal, such as extreme alertness and difficulty sleeping. PTSD can arise after accidents involving maiming or death, natural disasters, war, physical abuse, assault, rape, and torture. It usually develops within 3 months of the trauma but can begin years later. See POSTTRAUMATIC STRESS DISORDER.

Treatment and outcome

Anxiety disorders are typically treated with a combination of medications to improve the person's physical and emotional symptoms and psychotherapy aimed at teaching the individual how to handle anxiety-provoking situations. A number of medications are available, including sedatives, antihistamines, tranquilizers, benzodiazepines, and antidepressants. People with anxiety disorders should avoid alcohol and stimulants, including caffeine.

Anxiolytics

See ANTIANXIETY DRUGS.

Aorta

The largest artery in the body. All other arteries branch out from the aorta to carry oxygen-rich blood from the heart to the rest of the body tissues. The aorta, which is about an inch wide, begins in the left ventricle, one of the four chambers of the heart. When the heart beats, the aortic valve opens to allow oxygen-rich blood to flow from the ventricle into the aorta. See CARDIOVASCULAR SYSTEM; HEART.

Aortic insufficiency

Leakage in the valve between the heart and the aorta (main artery of the body); also known as aortic regurgitation. Aortic insufficiency occurs when blood leaks back from the aorta into the heart, decreasing blood flow into the body and forcing the heart to pump harder to compensate. Over time, the heart chamber known as the left ventricle, where the aortic valve is located, may enlarge and weaken, causing congestive heart failure (see HEART FAILURE, CONGESTIVE).

The symptoms of aortic insufficiency include shortness of breath during exercise, difficulty breathing when lying down at night, weakness on exertion, swelling in the ankles, angina (chest pain), night sweats, fainting spells, and irregular heartbeat. The disease can be caused by degeneration of the aortic valve with aging, damage from infection (associated with endocarditis or rheumatic fever), or congenital abnormality. Severity of the disease varies from mild to life-threatening.

Aortic insufficiency is diagnosed in a variety of ways. A doctor listening to the heart through a stethoscope may detect the characteristic sounds of a valve defect even before symptoms appear. Abnormalities may also be detected by an electrocardiogram, a chest X ray, or an echocardiogram.

A person with aortic insufficiency needs to take antibiotics before dental or invasive surgical procedures to prevent infection of the valve. A valve infection (such as that associated with ENDOCARDITIS, inflammation of the lining of the heart that usually affects the valves) is a life-threatening condition that worsens the disease. Other medications may be used to treat the symptoms of aortic insufficiency, such as angiotensin-converting enzyme (ACE) inhibitors, calcium channel blockers, anticoagulants, and diuretics.

Aortic stenosis

Narrowing of the valve connecting the heart to the body's main artery (aorta). Because the narrowing partially blocks the outflow of blood from the heart to the aorta, blood flow to the body is reduced, and the heart must work harder to compensate. The greater workload can enlarge the heart chamber known as the left ventricle, where the aortic valve is located. Congestive heart failure (see HEART FAILURE, CONGESTIVE), which

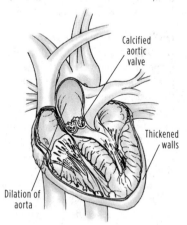

Calcified aortic valve

Thickened walls

Dilation of aorta

Damage from aortic stenosis
A calcium buildup on the aortic valve, usually the result of aging, obstructs blood flow from the left ventricle into the aorta. Pressure builds in the ventricle (the heart's main pumping chamber) and, over time, its walls thicken. The aorta dilates (widens) in an effort to keep blood pumping adequately to the rest of the body.

is life-threatening, can result. Aortic stenosis is more severe if the coronary arteries are narrowed by fat deposits because the enlarged heart is deprived of the blood supply it needs.

Aortic stenosis may exist in a mild form for years before symptoms appear. Symptoms include fatigue, fainting spells, shortness of breath with exercise, difficulty breathing while lying down at night, angina (chest pain), and swelling in the ankles. The disease may be caused by damage to the heart from rheumatic fever, valve defects present at birth (congenital), or the buildup of calcium deposits on the aortic valve because of aging.

Aortic stenosis is diagnosed by a doctor listening to the heart through a stethoscope, an electrocardiogram, chest X rays and echocardiograms. Cardiac catheterization, a procedure in which a catheter (thin tube) is threaded from a vein into the heart, is sometimes needed to confirm the diagnosis and to establish the severity of the disease.

A person with aortic stenosis needs to take antibiotics before dental, medical, or surgical procedures to prevent infection of the valve, which worsens the disease. Other medications may be used to treat the symptoms of aortic stenosis, such as angiotensin-converting enzyme (ACE) inhibitors; anticoagulants, which inhibit the formation of blood clots; and diuretics, which help remove excess body fluid. Once symptoms of aortic stenosis become severe, surgery to repair or replace the valve is the preferred treatment. The long-term prognosis is poor for those with symptoms who do not undergo surgery.

Aortitis

Inflammation of the aorta, the main artery leading from the heart into the body. Aortitis is commonly caused by advanced syphilis or an autoimmune disorder such as rheumatoid arthritis.

Apgar score

A scoring system used by doctors to assess the need for resuscitation and care of a baby at 1 minute after birth and again at 5 minutes after birth. To arrive at the Apgar score, the doctor evaluates five signs of the baby's condition: heart rate, breathing and crying, skin color, muscle tone, and reflexes. The total score ranges from 0 to 10. Babies who have endured a long or difficult delivery may have low Apgar scores and may require medical attention right after birth. Apgar scores alone are of limited value in predicting long-term outcomes.

Aphakia

Absence of the natural lens of the eye. In the normal eye, the lens is a clear, crystalline structure located behind the iris (the colored part of the eye) that focuses light coming into the eye. The cause of aphakia can be a congenital abnormality (lacking lenses at birth), an injury that destroys the lens, or surgical removal. Surgical removal of the lens is standard treatment for cataract, a disease in which the lens becomes cloudy or opaque. Aphakia causes extreme farsightedness, which can be treated with glasses or contact lenses or by surgery to insert a plastic lens implant in the eye.

Aphasia

Language problems caused by injury to the brain. People with aphasia have problems with speaking, understanding, reading, or writing. Aphasia is sometimes confused with DYSARTHRIA, which is trouble speaking or forming words because of an impairment in the function of the muscles required for speech.

Depending on the location and extent of brain damage, the resulting difficulties can range from mild to severe. Other causes of aphasia include brain trauma and BRAIN TUMOR. Lesions in the front part of the brain lead to problems with expression (Broca aphasia), while problems in the back of the brain lead to comprehension problems (Wernicke aphasia).

A person who has experienced a brain injury is usually hospitalized under the care of a neurologist. After his or her condition has stabilized, most doctors recommend a thorough speech and language evaluation by a speech-language pathologist (or speech therapist).

People who experience speech problems at any age can benefit from SPEECH THERAPY.

Aplasia

The absence of an organ or tissue due to developmental failure. In aplastic anemia (see ANEMIA, APLASTIC), there is a failure in the normal generation and development of blood cells.

Apnea

A total cessation of breathing, either momentarily or for a prolonged period. Prolonged apnea, which can be life-threatening, may occur as a result of a stroke or transient ischemic attack (a brief interruption in blood supply to the brain, resulting in temporarily impaired sensation, movement, vision, or speech); as an effect of certain drugs; or as a result of airway obstruction. Loud snoring accompanied by pauses in breathing while sleeping is a symptom of potentially life-threatening SLEEP APNEA SYNDROME. Other symptoms of sleep apnea include daytime sleepiness, fatigue, and headache. Sleep apnea is most common in overweight people, as excessive body fat puts pressure on breathing passages. In CHEYNE-STOKES respiration, alternating periods of apnea and deep, rapid breathing occur.

Treatment of apnea depends on its severity and underlying cause. Remedies for mild sleep apnea include weight reduction; exercise; avoidance of alcohol, tranquilizers, and sleeping pills; sleeping on the side or abdomen rather than the back; and the use of medications prescribed or recommended by the physician. More serious cases can require medication, the administration of oxygen using a mask during sleep, or surgery. Untreated sleep apnea can lead to hypertension, heart disease, and stroke.

Apolipoprotein

The protein component of lipoprotein complexes.

Appendectomy

Surgical removal of the appendix, which is a small finger-shaped pouch that branches off from the large intestine. An appendectomy is performed to treat APPENDICITIS (an acute inflammation of the appendix) and is a simple operation associated with few risks.

Appendicitis

Acute inflammation of the appendix (a small finger-shaped pouch that branches off from the large intestine in the lower right part of the abdomen). The appendix can become inflamed and fill with pus when a small piece of stool or debris blocks its opening. To avoid serious complications, an APPENDECTOMY (surgical removal of the appendix) is usually required.

The first symptom of appendicitis is usually vague pain and discomfort around the navel. Within a few hours, the pain moves to the lower right part of the abdomen and becomes more intense.

Diagnosis is based on a physical examination of the abdomen by a doctor. Applying pressure to the spot where an inflamed appendix is located causes increased pain. If the diagnosis is uncertain, the doctor may order blood and imaging tests, such as abdominal X rays, a CT (computed tomography) scan, or ultrasound scanning.

An inflamed appendix must be removed as early as possible to prevent serious complications. Possible complications include GANGRENE, an abscess, or rupture of the appendix that can lead to PERITONITIS (a life-threatening inflammation of the peritoneum, the membrane that lines the abdominal cavity). Although removing an appendix is a simple operation, the risk of complications increases greatly if the appendix ruptures.

Appendix

A small organ hanging down from the upper part of the large intestine (cecum) into the abdomen. Medically known as the vermiform, the appendix is an organ of the IMMUNE SYSTEM. The appendix contains abundant lymphatic tissue and apparently serves to destroy disease-causing microorgan-

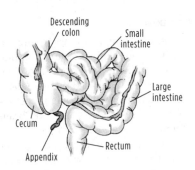

Location of appendix
The appendix is a narrow tube, closed at one end, that extends down from the front portion (cecum) of the large intestine into the lower abdomen. It secretes mucus that flows into the cecum.

isms that might enter the body or multiply rapidly through the digestive system (although its role is not entirely clear). The most common disorder is APPENDICITIS, an inflammation of the appendix, which is treated by surgical removal of the appendix.

Appetite stimulants

Drugs used to stimulate feelings of hunger. These drugs are often used to help in the treatment of people with cancer and AIDS (acquired immunodeficiency syndrome). Appetite stimulants seem to be most effective if they are introduced during the early stages of weight loss.

Appetite suppressants

Drugs that are intended to reduce feelings of hunger. No convincing evidence is available showing that any product available over-the-counter can help people lose weight. Appetite suppressants can be dangerous if they are taken by people with high blood pressure, heart disease, glaucoma, diabetes, thyroid disease, or kidney problems.

Apraxia

A loss of the ability to carry out previously learned skills or gestures despite normal muscle power and coordination. Apraxia is caused by brain damage associated with problems such as ALZHEIMER'S DISEASE, STROKE, brain tumor, or head injury. Symptoms can include difficulty using an arm or leg or even making purposeful facial movements on command.

Arm, fractured

A break in one or several of the bones in the arm, generally caused by physical trauma, undue pressure, or other injury to the arm. Immediately following the event that produces the fracture, there may be acute pain, localized tenderness to the touch, muscle spasms, and greater pain or numbness with movement or use of the arm, followed by numbness, tingling, weakness, or paralysis. A fractured arm is generally diagnosed by the presence of deformity and an evaluation of X rays. Generally, treatment is that the broken bones are aligned into an immobile position, usually with a cast or splint for a specified time. During the healing period, a sling may be used to support the arm and hold it stationary against the body. In more complex fractures, traction and surgical repair may become necessary. See also FRACTURE.

Aromatherapy

The use of fragrant plant oils for psychological and physical well-being. The plant oils are inhaled, rubbed onto the skin, or swallowed. Aromatherapy is said to help relieve stress, enhance the immune system, and unlock buried emotions.

Arrhythmia, cardiac

A disturbance or abnormality in the rhythm of the heartbeat. Cardiac arrhythmias vary in severity from annoying to life-threatening.

Types and symptoms

The least serious and most common cardiac arrhythmia is the ectopic heartbeat, or extrasystole. This is a simple variation in a normal heartbeat, possibly the source of the phrase "my heart skipped a beat." An occasional extra systole is harmless and requires no treatment.

An arrhythmia that causes the heart to beat too slowly is called BRADYCARDIA. In some situations, the heart may not pump fast enough to keep the body supplied with the oxygen-rich blood it needs, and symptoms such as fatigue, dizziness, lightheadedness, or fainting can occur.

An arrhythmia that causes the heart to beat too rapidly is known as TACHYCARDIA or tachyarrhythmia. Symptoms can include palpitations (the sensation of an unusually fast or irregular heartbeat), chest pain, dizziness, light-headedness, or fainting. If the atria are beating too rapidly, the condition is known as supraventricular tachycardia (SVT); if the beat of the atria is irregular, it is known as ATRIAL FIBRILLATION. Both SVT and atrial fibrillation tend to occur in episodes, with periodic attacks separated by periods of normal heart rhythm.

Paroxysmal supraventricular tachycardia (PSVT) (see TACHYCARDIA, PAROXYSMAL SUPRAVENTRICULAR) causes sudden attacks in which the heart races suddenly at between 140 and 240 beats a minute (versus the normal 60 to 100). PSVT is not usually life-threatening, but repeated attacks increase the risk of developing congestive heart failure.

In ventricular tachycardia (see TACHYCARDIA, VENTRICULAR), the ventricles contract too rapidly. Ventricular tachycardia, usually associated with heart disease, is a common complication during the first several days after a heart attack. In the more serious condition known as VENTRICULAR FIBRILLATION, the ventricles contract in such a weak, rapid, and uncontrolled way that the heart essentially ceases to pump. If a normal rhythm cannot be reestablished within a few minutes, death can result.

Diagnosis and treatment

Accurate, early diagnosis of a cardiac arrhythmia is important in order to begin treatment. As part of evaluation by a physician, persons with symptoms suggesting arrhythmia may need to wear a HOLTER MONITOR, which is a portable device that records and analyzes the electrical activity of the heart, for one to two days. Or an event monitor may be worn for a longer period.

Treatment depends on the type of arrhythmia and its severity. Some arrhythmias can be controlled with lifestyle changes. Medications that control or change heartbeat may also be prescribed.

For people with bradycardia, a PACE-MAKER can be surgically implanted in the chest to accelerate the heart via electrical impulses whenever it beats too slowly. For people with ventricular tachycardia, a device called an implantable cardioverter DEFIBRILLATOR can be placed surgically in the chest to monitor and correct heartbeat if it becomes abnormally fast.

Arteries

Vessels that carry blood away from the heart to the rest of the body.

Arteriosclerosis

Thickening and loss of elasticity in the walls of the arteries; also known as hardening of the arteries. The most common type of arteriosclerosis is ATHEROSCLEROSIS, in which fat deposits build up in the arteries.

Arteriovenous malformation

A tangled mass of small arteries intertwined with small veins that is present at birth; commonly abbreviated as AVM. Blood flows directly from the arteries into the veins, not through the bed of capillaries (very small blood vessels) that normally lie between them. An AVM is most serious when it occurs in the brain; this condition is called cerebral AVM.

Symptoms of a ruptured or leaky cerebral AVM include headache, blurred vision, slurred speech, vomiting, stiff neck, muscle weakness and loss of sensation in a part of the body, fainting, drooping eyelid, altered vision, facial paralysis, or change in mood. A ruptured cerebral AVM can be fatal. Treatment usually consists of surgery to remove the malformation.

Arteritis

Inflammation of an artery or arteries. The inflammation can block the artery, reducing blood flow to the affected area and possibly weakening the artery wall, which in turn leads to swelling of the artery into a balloonlike form called an aneurysm. Arteritis is usually treated with anti-inflammatory medications, such as corticosteroids. In some cases, surgery is needed to remove the blockage and restore normal blood flow.

Arteritis, giant cell

Chronic inflammation of large and medium arteries, usually in the head and neck, less commonly throughout the body; also known as temporal or cranial arteritis. The disease takes its name from the extremely large cells that develop in the inflamed blood vessels. Symptoms resulting from the inflammation include fever, headache, scalp tenderness, jaw pain, double vision or blindness, weakness, loss of appetite and weight, muscle aches, and excessive sweating. The cause of giant cell arteritis is unknown, but it is thought to result from a disorder of the immune system. Treatment consists of anti-inflammatory medications, such as aspirin and corticosteroids.

Arthritis

The inflammation of a joint, which causes localized pain, swelling, and stiffness. There are several different types of arthritis. The most common type is OSTEOARTHRITIS, or degenerative arthritis, which involves changes in the joint cartilage as a result of aging and use. The affected joint may become swollen. Because movement of the joint is restricted and painful, the associated muscles begin to shrink from lack of use.

The pain and discomfort of osteoarthritis may be treated with aspirin, ibuprofen, or other nonsteroidal anti-inflammatory drugs (NSAIDs); injections of corticosteroid drugs; or PHYSICAL THERAPY. When joints are severely damaged by osteoarthritis, producing chronic pain and preventing normal movement of limbs, they

may be surgically replaced with artificial joints. Hip and knee joints are often successfully replaced. (See also JOINT REPLACEMENT, HIP; JOINT REPLACEMENT, KNEE.)

Other types of arthritis include gouty arthritis, which is caused by urate crystals forming in the joints (see GOUT), and a temporary form of arthritis that may accompany acute rheumatic fever.

Rheumatoid arthritis, an autoimmune disease, is a more serious, systemic form of arthritis, which may affect the heart, lungs, and eyes, as well as multiple joints. See also RHEUMATOID ARTHRITIS.

Arthrodesis

The surgical fusion or immobilization of the bones in a damaged joint for the purpose of supporting the joint and relieving pain. The procedure, often performed on the foot or ankle, involves removing the weight-bearing surfaces of the joint. A fixation device is then implanted to hold the bones together during the healing process. As they heal, the bones grow together until they are united.

Arthroplasty

See JOINT REPLACEMENT.

Arthroscopic surgery

Joint surgery performed using a technique called arthroscopy, which involves the use of a specialized viewing instrument to observe the interior of a joint. Arthroscopic surgery is performed to remove unattached pieces of cartilage, repair or remove torn knee cartilage, and obtain a biopsy specimen to diagnose infections, rheumatoid arthritis, gout, or disorders of the connective tissue.

Arthroscopy

See ARTHROSCOPIC SURGERY.

Artificial insemination

The placement of sperm inside the female reproductive tract by artificial means rather than sexual intercourse.

Artificial insemination is used when the man has difficulty having natural intercourse or has a very low sperm count or semen volume. It is also often used when the woman's ovulation is being controlled with fertility drugs and timed so the maximum number of sperm will reach the egg when it is released. (See also ASSISTED REPRODUCTIVE TECHNOLOGY; INFERTILITY.)

Artificial kidney

Popular name for the machine that cleans and filters the blood by removing waste products and fluid. See DIALYSIS MACHINE.

Artificial respiration

The forcing of air into and out of the lungs of one person by another or by mechanical means. Artificial respiration, also called rescue breathing, is usually performed when natural breathing stops because of disease, trauma, overdose of drugs, or by suffocation caused by drowning or other means. If the brain is deprived of oxygen for even 5 minutes, permanent damage can result, and after a few more minutes, death is likely to occur.

Asbestosis

A form of the lung disease PULMONARY FIBROSIS that is caused by breathing asbestos dust particles and results in extensive scarring of the lung tissue. Asbestos is a tough, nearly indestructible fiber composed of mineral silicates. Asbestosis can also cause thickening of the membrane layer, called the pleura, that covers the lungs. The risk of developing asbestosis is greater among people who have ongoing exposure to asbestos, such as demolition workers who work on old buildings that are insulated with material containing asbestos. The greater and longer the exposure to asbestos-containing materials, the higher the risk becomes.

Initial symptoms include mild shortness of breath and a reduced capacity for strenuous activity. Coughing and wheezing are common among people who smoke heavily or have chronic bronchitis in addition to asbestosis. Over time, breathing becomes increasingly difficult. In severe cases, people with asbestosis develop severe shortness of breath and respiratory failure.

Diagnosis of asbestosis is based on a clinical history that includes prolonged exposure to asbestos combined with characteristic chest X-ray findings and the detection with a stethoscope of abnormal lung sounds.

Treatment (oxygen therapy, eliminating future asbestos exposure, and a procedure to drain fluid from around the lungs if present) is aimed at easing symptoms. In severe cases, lung transplantation may be the only effective treatment.

Prevention of asbestosis focuses on minimizing or eliminating asbestos dust and fibers in the workplace.

Ascariasis

An infection caused by a parasitic roundworm. Ascariasis occurs when food or drink contaminated with roundworm eggs is ingested. When the eggs hatch, the roundworm's larvae are released into the intestine. These larvae migrate through the intestinal wall into the bloodstream to the lungs, where they travel up the respiratory system and are swallowed. This returns the larvae to the intestines where they mature into adult roundworms. The mature roundworms live in the intestine and lay eggs that are expelled with the stool.

Symptoms of ascariasis may include the passing of roundworms in the stool, in vomiting, or through the nose or mouth.

Ascariasis is diagnosed by an examination of stool samples for parasites and eggs and by abdominal X ray. The infection is treated with medication that destroys intestinal parasitic worms. The condition is usually cured with prescribed medication or may improve without treatment.

Ascites

A swollen abdomen that results from an abnormal collection of fluid inside the abdominal cavity. Ascites can be a symptom of cancer, infection, cirrhosis (a type of severe liver disease), portal hypertension (increased blood pressure in the portal vein, which carries blood from the intestines to the liver), or heart or kidney disease. Ascites itself can be treated with diuretic drugs and by restricting sodium intake. If this fails to reduce the amount of fluid, or if breathing becomes impaired, draining the ascitic fluid is required.

Ascorbic acid

See VITAMIN C.

Aseptic technique

Any health care procedure in which strict precautions are observed to avoid contamination by microorganisms.

Aspartame

One of the nonnutritive artificial sweeteners. A combination of the amino acids aspartic acid and phenylalanine, aspartame also contains a small amount of methanol.

Asperger disorder

A pervasive developmental disorder (see DEVELOPMENTAL DISORDER, PERVASIVE) that is probably related to autism but is not associated with delays in language development. Treatment is generally directed at symptoms, such as poor relationships with peers or family members or the inability to adapt to school or work. Methods of treatment may include family therapy, group social skills training, and individual coaching. Medication may be necessary to treat coexisting psychiatric disorders, such as depression, anxiety disorders, and obsessive compulsive disorder.

Asphyxia

Suffocation; interruption of breathing. Asphyxia is suffocation caused by a blocked airway or the breathing in of toxic gases. Asphyxia is the direct result of a lack of oxygen and an excess of carbon dioxide in the body, which leads to unconsciousness; if untreated, asphyxia may lead to death.

Aspiration

Drawing in or out with suction. Aspiration can also refer to the accidental inhalation of a foreign object or body fluids, the removal of harmful substances (such as bone fragments or body fluids), and the extraction of tissue samples for testing (as in a fine-needle aspiration of the breast).

Aspirin

Acetosalicylic salicylate; a drug used to reduce pain, fever, and inflammation. Aspirin reduces pain by acting on the hypothalamus and by blocking pain impulses in muscles. The fever-reducing activity in aspirin involves the heat-regulating center in the hypothalamus: aspirin increases sweating, which leads to cooling of the body by evaporation.

At low doses, aspirin reduces blood clotting by preventing formation of a substance needed for clotting of platelets. Aspirin is used by doctors to treat people who have transient ischemic attacks (TIAs), thromboembolic disorders, and unstable angina, as well as to prevent heart attack. But a person should not use aspirin for more than 3 days without consulting a doctor.

Assault

In law, the attempt or threat to use violence to harm another person; if actual violent contact is made with the other person's body, BATTERY has been committed in addition to assault. See also ABUSE, PARTNER.

Assault, sexual

Forced sexual activity or contact without consent; also called rape. Sexual assault is a gender-neutral term currently in use in many states instead of "rape," which has traditionally been defined as forced vaginal penetration of women by men. Sexual assault is the most rapidly growing violent crime in the United States. See also ABUSE, SEXUAL; RAPE.

Assisted reproductive technology

Generally, infertility treatments using advanced technology to treat a variety of conditions associated with infertility. The most common form of assisted reproductive technology (ART) is IN VITRO FERTILIZATION (IVF) for treating female infertility. Other ART techniques include gamete (the female egg and male sperm) intrafallopian transfer (GIFT), zygote intrafallopian transfer (ZIFT), and INTRACYTOPLASMIC SPERM INJECTION (ICSI). See also INFERTILITY.

Asthma

A condition that causes inflammation, excessive mucus secretion, and reversible constriction of the smooth muscle in the lung's airway. Asthma can produce wheezing, coughing, and shortness of breath; these symptoms may vary in severity. If a person's air supply becomes seriously restricted, confusion and lethargy can occur, and the skin may turn blue. Emergency medical treatment is essential if these symptoms are present. An asthma attack may be triggered by a

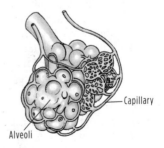

Alveoli

In healthy alveoli, oxygen passes through the walls and into the blood, which carries it to tissue throughout the body. During bronchial spasms, however, air is trapped in the alveoli.

person's sensitivity to certain substances, exercise, dusts, viral infections, smoke, cold air, stress, anxiety, and other conditions that produce inflammation of the airways.

Patients rarely die, even in cases of severe asthma attacks, if proper treatment is obtained early in the course of the attack. However, delaying treatment can cause a life-threatening attack.

Asthma is suspected on the basis of a description of characteristic symptoms. If a person has narrowed airways at the time he or she visits a doctor, the doctor may hear wheezing, in which case SPIROMETRY, a test that measures air movement, may confirm bronchoconstriction.

The most commonly used medications to relieve asthma symptoms are BRONCHODILATORS, which stimulate certain receptors in the airway to relax the smooth muscle and dilate (widen) the airways. Bronchodilators may be taken by mouth, by injection, or by inhalation. Inhaler devices deposit the medication directly into the airways during an attack and immediately dilate the airways, but in cases of severe bronchoconstriction the airways may be so narrow that the inhaled medication has difficulty reaching all the affected airways. Oral bronchodilators can reach all the obstructed airways but act more slowly than inhaled forms and usually have more side effects.

Inhaled, oral, or injected CORTICO-STEROIDS can counteract the inflammatory response and are very effective at controlling symptoms. When taken over time, these medications gradually act to prevent attacks by reducing inflammation and blocking the sensi-tivity of the airways to allergens and other stimuli.

An acute asthma attack should be treated immediately using additional medications or higher doses or different forms of the medications used on an ongoing basis to control or prevent asthma. Oxygen and intravenous fluids may also need to be given, and antibiotics may be necessary if an underlying infection is present.

Asthma, cardiac

Wheezing that results from the pooling of fluid in the lungs because of heart failure (see HEART FAILURE, CONGESTIVE). Similar symptoms can arise from other diseases, including PANIC DISORDER, COR PULMONALE, and SLEEP APNEA SYNDROME. To get relief, the person must sit upright and sometimes must resort to sleeping in a chair.

Astigmatism

A defect in vision caused by uneven curvature of the eye's clear outer covering (cornea). The normal cornea is round, curving equally from top to bottom and side to side. In astigmatism, the cornea curves more in one direction than the other, making it asymmetrical.

Astringents

Agents that cause contraction after they are applied to the skin. Examples include calamine lotion and witch hazel.

Asymptomatic

A term that describes a person who does not have symptoms or any indications of sickness or disease. When a person has a condition but exhibits no recognizable signs of it, he or she is said to be asymptomatic. See also SYMPTOM.

Asystole

The absence of a heartbeat. See also CARDIAC ARREST.

Ataxia

Lack of coordination caused by nerve or brain damage. Ataxia may impair balance, gait, movement, or speech. Ataxia can also be caused by intoxication with medications or alcohol, infections, strokes, tumors, or chronic hereditary degenerative syndromes, such as FRIEDREICH ATAXIA or olivopontocerebellar atrophy. Slow or clumsy movement in the early stages of these diseases can eventually become so pronounced that a person requires a wheelchair. Hereditary ataxias may also affect speech and swallowing. These progressive diseases may shorten a person's life span as a result of complications such as heart disease and respiratory difficulties. The treatment of ataxia is based on the cause.

Atelectasis

A chronic or acute condition that arises when a small portion of the lung tissue collapses, usually caused by obstruction of a bronchial tube. As a result, the collapsed tissue is unable to properly exchange oxygen. The condition may be caused by obstruction of the airway by a tumor, mucous plugs, or foreign bodies lodged in the bronchi; abnormalities in the bronchial structures; external compression of an airway from an enlarged lymph node; or compression of the lungs caused by the abnormal presence of fluids or gases. Atelecta-

sis is a common postoperative complication of surgery performed in the upper abdomen, on the lungs, or on the heart.

Atelectasis may cause few symptoms or may cause chest pain, cough, and shortness of breath. If a person's oxygen supply is affected, there may be a blue discoloration of the skin, a drop in blood pressure, an irregular heartbeat, and an elevated temperature. Chronic atelectasis may have no symptoms or may result in severe, dry coughing. Acute pneumonia may develop from the chronic form.

Atelectasis is diagnosed on the basis of a physical examination and X-ray findings that reveal a decrease in lung size and an opaque, airless area within the lung. A CT (computed tomography) scan may be used to detect any underlying lung disease, and a fiberoptic bronchoscope may be used to detect the cause of obstruction.

Treatment is generally aimed at the cause of the condition. In many cases, suctioning or respiratory and physical therapy can treat the problem. Antibiotics are used to treat underlying infections. In some chronic cases, or if a mass is compressing the airway, surgery may be recommended.

Atenolol

See BETA BLOCKERS.

Atherectomy

See BALLOON ANGIOPLASTY.

Atheroma

An abnormal growth of fatty tissue in or on the walls of a major artery. Atheromas have a central role in the disease ATHEROSCLEROSIS.

Atherosclerosis

A disease in which deposits of fat and other materials accumulate in and on the inner walls of the arteries, narrowing them and causing them to lose their elasticity, strength, and flexibility. The fatty deposits are often called atheromas or plaques. Atherosclerosis is often referred to popularly as hardening of the arteries.

The coronary arteries, which surround the heart and supply it with blood, are a common site of atherosclerosis. If the blood flow is restricted to the extent that there is an imbalance of oxygen supply to oxygen demand, the chest pain known as ANGINA often results. Complete blockage of one of the coronary arteries by atherosclerotic plaque is a principal cause of heart attack, and it can lead to sudden death.

Atherosclerosis in the arteries that supply blood to the brain (the carotid and cerebral arteries) is one cause of STROKE. Severe plaque in the arteries providing blood to the lower limbs (see CLAUDICATION) may cause poor circulation, sores, and gangrene, and amputation may be necessary.

Sometimes a doctor suspects atherosclerosis during a routine physical examination. Through a stethoscope applied to the neck, groin, or abdomen, the doctor may be able to hear the characteristic bruit (blowing sound) caused by turbulent blood flow that results from atherosclerotic narrowing. Also, a weak pulse in the wrists, legs, or feet may indicate partially obstructed blood flow.

When atherosclerosis is suspected, a number of noninvasive tests can be used to identify and assess the disease. One is the electrocardiogram (ECG). Ultrafast CT (computed tomography) scanning takes multiple views of the heart and is useful in determining the amount of calcification in the artery.

When atherosclerosis is advanced, an invasive test called an angiogram is often performed to confirm the presence of the disease and determine how severe it is.

Controllable risk factors for atherosclerosis are smoking, hypertension, obesity, diabetes mellitus, and high blood cholesterol.

The best treatment for atherosclerosis is preventing the disease in the first place, by eliminating or reducing the controllable risk factors for the disease.

A number of medications are useful in treating atherosclerosis. Aspirin inhibits the formation of blood clots and may help prevent a damaged blood vessel from becoming blocked. ANTIHYPERTENSIVES such as beta blockers reduce the workload on the heart. Drugs to lower blood cholesterol levels may be prescribed for people with elevated blood fat levels. Certain vitamins may also be helpful, particularly folic acid, one of the B vitamins.

Invasive procedures are used for advanced disease, particularly when an artery has been blocked. BALLOON ANGIOPLASTY and CAROTID ENDARTERECTOMY correct narrowed or blocked arteries. In coronary artery bypass surgery, veins harvested from the legs are grafted to the coronary arteries to bypass blockage.

Athlete's foot

A common infection of the skin between the toes, which leads to itching and soreness; also known as tinea pedis. Athlete's foot is a form of TINEA (a group of related skin infections caused by different species of fungi).

The rash may spread to other parts of the foot; in some people, it may manifest as redness and scaling on the soles and sides of the feet. Infection may spread to the toenails (onychomycosis).

Athlete's foot is diagnosed by the characteristic appearance of the skin and by examining pieces of skin, obtained through scraping, under a microscope, to detect fungus growth.

Simple cases of athlete's foot respond well to treatment with antifungal creams. The skin should be kept clean and dry. Severe infections require stronger oral antifungal medications that may cause side effects.

Atony

A loss of muscle tone (the normal degree of resistance a relaxed muscle gives to passive movement) resulting in weakness of the body or of a muscle or organ. Atony is a symptom of many diseases, including MULTIPLE SCLEROSIS, MUSCULAR DYSTROPHY, MYASTHENIA GRAVIS, and STROKE.

Atresia

From birth, the absence of a normal body opening or the abnormal closure of an opening. Examples of atresia include a closed anus, the absence or closure of the outer ear canal, and narrowing of certain blood vessels.

Atrial fibrillation

A rapid, highly irregular heartbeat caused by abnormalities in the electrical signals generated by the atria (upper chambers) of the heart.

At first, atrial fibrillation tends to occur in episodes lasting minutes or hours, with long periods of normal heart rhythm separating the attacks. If the attack is severe, chest pain, shortness of breath, light-headedness, fainting, or fatigue can also result. Over time, atrial fibrillation can become chronic. The principal risk posed by atrial fibrillation is stroke. Atrial fibrillation also increases the risk of heart failure (see HEART FAILURE, CONGESTIVE), CARDIOMYOPATHY (impaired heart muscle function), and HEART ATTACK.

Atrial fibrillation is the most common type of sustained abnormal heart rhythm (see ARRHYTHMIA, CARDIAC, for information on how atrial fibrillation compares with other heartbeat disorders). The disease is estimated to affect 2 million Americans. It is more common in older people and affects 5 percent of those over 65 in the US.

The episodic nature of atrial fibrillation makes diagnosis difficult in some cases. A doctor using a stethoscope can listen for heart rhythms that indicate atrial fibrillation. Irregularities in heart rhythm may also be captured by an electrocardiogram (ECG), a Holter monitor, an event recorder, a stress test, echocardiography, or transesophageal echocardiography.

Treatment depends on the severity of the atrial fibrillation. Any underlying condition, such as hypertension or coronary artery disease, must be treated as well. A number of medications are useful in the treatment of atrial fibrillation. Beta blockers, calcium channel blockers, and digoxin slow the ventricular heart rate, reduce the work load on the heart, and lower blood pressure. The risk of stroke in people with atrial fibrillation is about 5 percent per year, so anticoagulants are used to prevent clots.

More invasive treatments are available if needed. CARDIOVERSION uses drugs or electrical shock to return the heart to a normal rhythm. An implantable cardioverter DEFIBRILLATOR (ICD) can be placed surgically in the chest to monitor heartbeat and correct it if it becomes abnormally fast. Radiofrequency ablation (see ABLATION THERAPY) or the Maze procedure may be needed.

Atrial flutter

A rapid but relatively regular heartbeat caused by abnormalities in the electrical signals generated by the atria (upper chambers) of the heart. Atrial flutter is a common type of cardiac arrhythmia, or abnormal heartbeat. Atrial flutter causes the heart to pump less effectively, reducing the amount of blood being pumped throughout the body. The condition is often associated with heart attack or surgery on the heart or lungs.

Atrial flutter tends to occur in episodes lasting minutes or hours, with periods of normal heart rhythm separating the attacks. When an attack occurs, it is likely to cause palpitations (the physical sensation of rapid heartbeat). If the attack is severe, chest pain, shortness of breath, light-headedness, fainting, or fatigue can result.

The episodic nature of atrial flutter makes diagnosis difficult in some cases. A doctor using a stethoscope can listen for heart rhythms that indicate atrial flutter. Abnormal rhythm can also be detected by an electrocardiogram (ECG), a Holter monitor, an event recorder, a stress test, or echocardiography.

A number of medications are useful for treating atrial flutter. Beta blockers, calcium channel blockers, and digoxin slow the overall heart rate, reduce the workload on the heart, and lower blood pressure. CARDIOVERSION

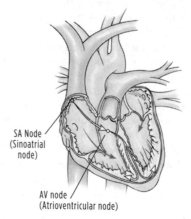

SA Node
(Sinoatrial
node)

AV node
(Atrioventricular node)

Electrical signals in the heart

In the healthy heart, electrical signals originate in the sinoatrial (SA) node, and the atrioventricular (AV) node conducts the electrical signals throughout the heart.

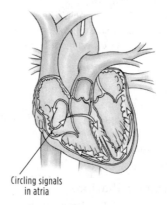

Circling signals
in atria

Quickened heartbeat

If electrical problems in the heart cause the atria to beat too quickly, but evenly, the result is atrial flutter. Impulses travel in circles in the atria, causing the atria to beat far too rapidly.

uses drugs or electrical shock to return the heart to a normal rhythm.

Atrial septal defect

See SEPTAL DEFECT, ATRIAL.

Atrium

Either of the two upper chambers of the heart. The right atrium receives oxygen-depleted blood from the body and moves it into the right ventricle, where the blood is pumped into the lungs to dispose of waste products (carbon dioxide) and receive oxygen. The oxygen-rich blood then returns to the left atrium, passes into the left ventricle, and is pumped through the aorta into the rest of the body. The tricuspid valve divides the right atrium from the right ventricle, letting blood flow from the one into the other and preventing backwash. The mitral valve performs the same function between the left atrium and the left ventricle. See HEART.

Atrophy

Wasting or diminution in size or activity of a part of the body. Atrophy is caused by factors such as disease, aging, nutrition, immobility, and lack of exercise.

Attending physician

The physician in charge of a person's overall care in the hospital. The term is also used to refer to full-fledged members of a hospital medical staff. An attending physician may be a primary care doctor, a doctor on the hospital staff, or a specialist.

Attention deficit/ hyperactivity disorder

A mental illness characterized by difficulty paying attention and a high degree of restlessness and impulsive behavior; the name of the disorder is commonly abbreviated as ADHD. Symptoms begin before age 7, last for at least 6 months, and cause the child substantial difficulty in at least two settings, usually family and school.

In some cases, the disorder resolves during adolescence. More often, it lasts into adulthood and becomes a lifelong condition, although the symptoms may be less pronounced than they were in childhood. ADHD is more common in males than in females.

ADHD is often accompanied by other disorders. Approximately half of the children with the disorder are hostile and negative in their behavior, and a smaller number engage in aggressive behavior toward people or animals, vandalism, or breaking important rules. Anxiety and depression may also affect children and adults with ADHD. Untreated ADHD increases the risk of substance abuse, academic and vocational problems, marital discord, and emotional distress. There is also a connection between ADHD and TOURETTE SYNDROME, a disease of the nervous system that causes repeated involuntary movements called tics.

ADHD is usually treated with a combination of medications to stabilize brain activity and counseling or therapy to help the individual learn how to cope with the disorder. The most commonly used medications are stimulants to increase the activity of dopamine and thus may help raise the level of activity in areas of the brain that control attention and impulse control. Antidepressants and tranquilizers have also proved useful.

Audiology

The study of hearing. This branch of scientific study deals with the identification, assessment, and nonmedical management of auditory (hearing-related) and balance disorders. An audiologist is a specialized health care professional who holds a master's or doctoral degree from an accredited university graduate program.

Audiometry

Measurement of hearing ability using specific tests. The purpose of the tests is to diagnose hearing problems, including HEARING LOSS from any cause.

Aura

An unusual sensation that is often a warning of an impending MIGRAINE headache or a SEIZURE, a sudden episode of uncontrolled electrical activity in the brain, causing a series of involuntary muscle transactions or a temporary lapse in consciousness. An aura may consist of a strange feeling, abnormal perceptions, or visual disturbances such as seeing stars or flashes.

Autism

A nervous system disorder beginning in early childhood and characterized by impaired social interaction, problems with communication and imagination, and unusual or limited activities or interests. Doctors classify autism as one of the pervasive developmental disorders (see DEVELOPMENTAL DISORDER, PERVASIVE). Some individuals are only mildly affected, while others exhibit extremely repetitive, unusual, aggressive, or self-injurious behavior. Some degree of mental retardation occurs in 75 percent of those affected. However, in some people, an inability to communicate and other symptoms conceal a considerable intelligence. Some individuals who have autism possess unique aptitudes that are often quite remarkable, such as musical ability. The term autism spectrum disorder is increasingly used to describe a wide range of symptoms and outcomes.

The exact cause of autism remains unknown. Researchers believe that a combination of genetic and environmental factors contribute to its development. There is no specific medical test to diagnose autism. Children are diagnosed according to their symptoms and results of psychological testing.

Treatment is designed to meet the individual needs of each child. Educational and behavioral interventions can help children to develop social and language skills. Child and adolescent psychiatrists or other physicians with special training in autism may prescribe medication to ameliorate symptoms, such as aggressive behavior.

Outlook is often related to intellectual ability. Symptoms change over time, requiring different needs to be met. Only one of six children with autism grow up to be functionally independent adults. See also ASPERGER DISORDER.

Autoimmune disorders

Disorders that occur as a result of a mistaken immune response to the body's own tissues. Autoimmune disorders develop when a HYPERSENSITIVITY reaction causes the immune system to respond inappropriately, excessively, or inadequately.

Autoimmune disorders can destroy

one or more organs or types of body tissues. The resulting destruction of tissue can cause abnormal growth of an organ or changes in the organ's function. Tissues of the muscles, joints, and skin are commonly affected. Blood components, including red blood cells and blood vessels, can also be destroyed by autoimmune disorders, as can connective tissues and endocrine glands, including the thyroid and the pancreas. Kidney disease can also occur.

Signs and symptoms of autoimmune disorders are related to the specific disease or condition that results and the tissues or organs affected. These include RHEUMATOID ARTHRITIS, systemic lupus erythematosus (see LUPUS ERYTHEMATOSUS, SYSTEMIC), ADDISON DISEASE, diabetes mellitus (see DIABETES MELLITUS, TYPE 1; DIABETES MELLITUS, TYPE 2), HASHIMOTO THYROIDITIS, MULTIPLE SCLEROSIS, REITER SYNDROME, SJÖGREN SYNDROME, and GRAVES DISEASE.

Nonspecific symptoms are frequently associated with all disorders related to autoimmunity. These include a tendency to tire quickly or be easily fatigued, dizziness, general malaise, weight loss, and a low-grade fever. Autoimmune disorders may be diagnosed with specialized blood tests.

Symptoms and deficiencies related to specific disorders are treated accordingly. If the disorder results in insufficient hormones or other substances essential to normal body functions, vitamins, thyroid supplements, insulin, or other medications can be taken or administered to compensate for the deficiency. If components of the blood are affected, blood transfusions may become necessary. If the bones, joints, or muscles are affected, physical therapy may be needed.

Most autoimmune disorders are chronic, but they can be managed with proper medical treatment of specific symptoms and of the underlying disorder. Medications such as corticosteroids or immunosuppressive drugs may be used to blunt the body's immune response and thereby help control the disease.

Autologous blood donation

Donation of one's own blood to oneself. Autologous blood donation may be used by people with a scheduled surgical procedure to ensure that any blood they may require during the surgery will be their own. The advantage of autologous blood donation is that it is the safest blood available.

Autologous bone marrow transplant

See BONE MARROW TRANSPLANT, AUTOLOGOUS.

Autonomic nervous system

The part of the NERVOUS SYSTEM that controls involuntary activities, such as blood pressure and heartbeat. The autonomic nervous system consists of a network of nerves divided into two parts: the parasympathetic nervous system and the sympathetic nervous system. The two systems act together and normally balance each other. The parasympathetic nervous system predominates during times of relaxation, acting to conserve and restore energy. The sympathetic nervous system prepares the body to cope during times of stress.

Autopsy

Examination of a body after death. An autopsy, a legal and medical procedure also called a postmortem examination, is performed by a medical examiner or by a pathologist to establish the cause of a death or to detect the presence or absence of disease or injury. When a death has occurred as the result of a suspected crime, an autopsy may be ordered by legal authorities to gather evidence for use in judicial proceedings.

Autosomal dominant traits

Hereditary traits carried by genes that are more likely to be expressed than those of other genes. A dominant trait expresses itself regardless of the function of its corresponding gene. A dominant gene may be inherited, or it may occur due to a spontaneous mutation that causes dominance of a particular gene.

Autosomal recessive traits

Hereditary traits carried by genes that are expressed only when an individual has two copies of the gene. A child needs to inherit the affected gene from both parents for the genetic trait to be expressed. When a disease is inherited as an autosomal recessive trait, the parents do not usually have the disease themselves but are symptomless carriers. Examples of autosomal recessive disorders include Tay-Sachs disease, sickle cell anemia, and albinism. See also AUTO-SOMAL DOMINANT TRAITS.

Avascular necrosis of femoral head

A hip disorder in children. Avascular necrosis causes pain, stiffness and limited range of motion in the affected hip joint. A child with this condition may limp. The condition is caused by the death of bone cells at the top of the thighbone due to a poor blood supply.

Avascular necrosis is diagnosed by creating images of the thighbone, using radionuclide scanning, MRI (magnetic resonance imaging), or X rays, that will show abnormalities in the bone. Medication can reduce the pain and swelling, while physical therapy may help maintain the full range of motion in the hip. In some children, surgery is necessary to repair avascular necrosis or replace the entire hip joint.

Aversion therapy

A technique used to stop or alter an unwanted behavior by coupling that behavior with an unpleasant or painful experience.

Avian flu

A type of influenza first observed in Asia; also called bird flu. Avian flu is known as the strain of influenza caused by the H5N1 virus. Initially, avian flu was transmitted from bird to bird, especially chickens, then to other animals. Then cases were recorded of animal to human transmission, with deaths from avian flu reported in Asia and Europe. Doctors and public health experts have been concerned that if the transmission mechanism changes so that humans can transmit the virus to other humans, a worldwide pandemic (large epidemic) could ensue.

The virus is transmitted only in live or recently killed birds, not in cooked chicken or eggs. Symptoms include fever, aches and pains, coughing, and respiratory distress. Scientists are working on a vaccine for avian flu. Although there is no cure for avian flu, antiviral medications may help relieve symptoms and shorten the course of the flu. Symptoms may also be helped by using nonprescription acetaminophen, nonsteroidal anti-inflammatory drugs such as aspirin, cough syrup, and decongestants.

AVM

See ARTERIOVENOUS MALFORMATION.

Avoidant personality disorder

See PERSONALITY DISORDERS.

Axillary lymph node dissection

Removal of some or all of the LYMPH NODES in the underarm area, typically as part of breast cancer surgery (see MASTECTOMY; LUMPECTOMY). Since cancer cells spread from their point of origin through the LYMPHATIC SYSTEM, testing of the removed nodes can determine whether the cancer has traveled beyond the breast.

B

B cell

A type of white blood cell; B lymphocyte. B cells are formed in the bone marrow and circulate in the blood and lymphatic system. They have an es-

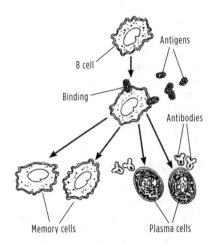

Smart cells

During invasion by a disease organism, certain B cells identify the specific invader (antigen) and bind to it. Then they multiply quickly, becoming either memory cells, which develop antibodies to stop future infections by the same antigen, or plasma cells, which develop antibodies that seek out that antigen in the body and destroy it.

sential role in immunology. Many B cells mature into plasma cells, which manufacture antibodies, proteins necessary to fight infections. Other B cells mature into memory B cells that "remember" the antigen that originally stimulated them to mature. This allows the body to recognize the antigen as a foreign body if it reencounters it in the future and to make antibodies to destroy it. Once antibodies are formed, whenever the body is reexposed to the same bacteria the body recognizes the infectious organism and starts making antibodies to combat it.

Babinski reflex

An abnormal reflex response to stimulation of the plantar (bottom) surface of the foot indicating upper MOTOR NEURON DISEASE (damage to the brain or spinal cord). During a neurological examination, people demonstrating a Babinski reflex will extend and point their great toe up in response to irritating stimulation along the bottom of the foot, which indicates an abnormality in the brain or spinal cord (central nervous system).

Baby bottle tooth decay

TOOTH DECAY in children younger than 3 years caused by sugar-containing liquids. The main cause of bottle dental decay is the practice of allowing a child to suck on a bottle of milk, formula, fruit juice, or other sweet drinks throughout the day or while in bed. These liquids cling to the teeth for hours, especially while the child is sleeping, since saliva flow and swallowing are reduced then. The bacteria in the mouth interact with the natural or refined sugars in the liquid, forming acids that can dissolve the tooth enamel and decay the teeth. Regular dental visits should be started by a child's first birthday.

Back pain

For symptom chart see BACKACHE, page x.

Discomfort, ranging from mild and intermittent aches to constant and severe pain, at any point along the spine. Eight of ten people experience back pain at some point in their lives. Back pain occurs most commonly in the lower region of the spine, which bears the majority of the body's weight. The medical terms describing the different types of back pain are acute, subacute, and chronic. Acute back pain is a mild to severe, short-lived discomfort, possibly caused by an accident or injury, and usually lasting from 1 to 7 days. Subacute refers to pain that is not related to other illnesses or conditions; it is usually mild, though sometimes severe, and lasts from a week to several months. Chronic back pain may be mild to severe; it either lasts a long time or occurs frequently, generally over a period of 3 months or more.

Back pain is most often the result of injuries caused by sudden or unexpected movements of the back, which produce muscle strain. These injuries may result in severely painful muscle spasms that usually last from 2 to 3 days, after which the pain subsides and lingers for a few more days or weeks. Mild back injuries may take up to 4 weeks to heal completely.

Back pain can also be caused by several conditions, among them OSTEOARTHRITIS, a degeneration of cartilage in the vertebrae, as well as degeneration or rupture of the intervertebral disks, which are common components of aging; polymyalgia rheumatica, a joint disorder that can cause pain in the lower back lasting several months or years (see MYALGIA); FIBROMYALGIA, which produces pain and stiffness in muscles and tendons, especially in the neck and upper back; and PAGET DISEASE, a disorder of uneven calcium distribution in the bone. Other causes include SPINAL STENOSIS, the narrowing of the spinal canal; ANKYLOSING SPONDYLITIS; a form of arthritis that causes the joints in the spine to become stiff, producing back pain; OSTEOPOROSIS, a thinning of the bones that may result in small fractures of the spine's vertebrae; REITER SYNDROME, which produces arthritis and back pain, generally in adult men; SPONDYLOLISTHESIS, the forward shifting of one vertebra onto another; infection of the spinal fluid; or spinal tumors.

Back pain is rarely a symptom of a serious illness or disorder, with some exceptions—for example, cancerous tumors of the spine that originated there or in another organ of the body. Also, if a child has back pain that awakens him or her while sleeping, an immediate evaluation should be sought by a doctor because the pain may be due to an infection or a tumor. If a person of any age develops serious back pain after a fall or other physical trauma to the spine, a doctor should be contacted immediately. Timely medical attention should also be sought if the person's symptoms suggest neurological problems such as weakness, numbness, or difficulty urinating.

Mild to moderate back pain may be treated initially by limiting painful activities and using medications to ease discomfort, including ASPIRIN or acetaminophen, prescription NONSTEROIDAL ANTI-INFLAMMATORY DRUGS (NSAIDs), or MUSCLE RELAXANTS. Physical therapy treatments may be prescribed, or in rare cases, TRACTION treatment in a hospital setting may be used to relieve pressure on spinal nerves. Some people with persistent pain that does not respond to treatment may benefit from injections of CORTICOSTEROIDS.

Surgery is usually a last resort in the treatment of back pain, usually only becoming an option when there is constant pain with increasing muscle weakness indicating compression of a spinal nerve. Surgical procedures for back pain include: removal of a herniated disk; LAMINECTOMY, a surgical procedure to remove bone spurs or disk fragments for the purpose of relieving leg pain from nerve cramps; and spinal fusion, a surgical technique that may involve the use of metal implants, which eliminates pain caused by the movement of vertebrae by joining two vertebrae together.

Bacteremia

A bacterial infection in the blood; often called blood poisoning (sepsis). The infection begins in one area, such as a tooth abscess or in the urinary tract, and then spreads. Once infectious bacteria reach the bloodstream, they can travel throughout the body. Symptoms include sudden fever, chills, rapid heartbeat with a drop in blood pressure (septic shock), flushed skin, red streaks leading from a wound, confusion, and mental impairment. Left untreated, bacteremia causes shock and can result in death. A blood culture test is used to diagnose bacteremia. When diagnosed promptly, bacteremia can usually be treated successfully with intravenous antibiotics and other supportive therapy.

Bacteria

A large group of single-celled microorganisms, some of which cause disease in humans. Bacteria, commonly known as "germs," are one of the six principal types of infectious organisms, with the others being viruses, protozoa, rickettsia, fungi, and parasites. Infectious bacteria can enter the body in food, drink, or air; through a wound or opening in the skin; or through a natural opening in the body. Under favorable conditions, bacteria multiply rapidly by cell division. Bacteria are simple organisms that lack a true cell nucleus. Some bacteria have long, whiplike filaments called flagella that allow them to move, while others have short filaments (pili) that do not move but help the bacteria attach to tissue surfaces, such as the lining of the intestine. Many bacteria are surrounded by a protective capsule that help prevent them from being destroyed by the special white blood cells that attack invading microorganisms.

Bacteria normally have no color, so they need to be stained to be seen under a microscope. Bacteria that absorb the dye known as GRAM STAIN appear blue under a microscope and are called gram-positive. Those that do not absorb it are gram-negative. The distinction is important because gram-positive bacteria usually respond to different antibiotics better than gram-negative bacteria do, so whether a bacteria is gram-positive or negative helps guide a choice of med-

ications until more definitive test results are available.

When infectious bacteria invade the body and multiply into large numbers, they release poisons (toxins) that cause disease. Symptoms of bacterial infection depend on the type of bacterium, the site of the infection, and the toxins released by the bacteria. Bacterial toxins from organisms that cause cholera and food poisoning can cause diarrhea, paralysis (from TETANUS and BOTULISM), rash, fever, tissue destruction, and organ failure. The extent of the infection also determines the severity of the disease. Most types of infectious bacteria can be treated effectively with antibiotics, supportive care, and—less commonly—surgery to remove infected tissue or to drain pus from an infected area.

Bacterial vaginosis

See VAGINOSIS, BACTERIAL.

Bacteriology

The branch of biological and medical science that studies BACTERIA, one of the principal causes of infectious disease.

Bagassosis

A lung disease characterized by inflammation of the alveoli in the lungs. Bagassosis is caused by exposure to a certain mold found on sugar cane and sugar beets and their products. The disease is a form of allergic ALVEOLITIS.

Baker cyst

An inflamed and swollen membrane-lined sac, called a bursa, which is located behind the knee. A Baker cyst can be very painful and may involve

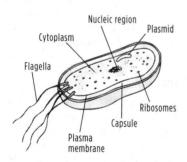

Structure of bacteria

Some bacteria are encased in an outer protective structure called a capsule. Within the capsule, the cell has a rigid cell wall for protection and an inner flexible membrane called the plasma membrane surrounding the fluid interior. Bodies called ribosomes form proteins that are essential to the cell's reproduction. Tails, or flagella, on the bacterium give it mobility.

extensive swelling that spreads down the back of the leg into the calf and ankle. In its normal state, a bursa is flat and contains very little fluid; it functions as a cushion between bones and soft tissues, such as muscles, tendons, ligaments, and skin. A Baker cyst, which is caused by inflammation of the main muscle in the calf and the knee joint, may be due to overuse, injury, infection, or arthritis.

It is important to seek early medical attention if a Baker cyst is suspected because the cyst can rupture and cause symptoms that could be confused with blood clots in the deep veins of the leg. The condition is readily diagnosed by a physical examination of the swollen area and confirmed with ultrasound scanning. Treatment generally includes applying local heat, immobilizing and elevating the affected leg, the use of NONSTEROIDAL ANTI-INFLAMMATORY DRUGS (NSAIDs), possibly drawing fluid out through aspiration, or the injection of a local corticosteroid. Physical therapy may be prescribed.

Balanitis

Inflammation of the foreskin and head (glans) of the penis in an uncircumcised male. The usual cause is bacterial infection from inadequately cleaning under the foreskin. Symptoms can include pain, redness, and swelling of the glans and the foreskin; foul-smelling discharge; a burning sensation on urination; chills and fever; and enlarged lymph nodes in the groin. Ulceration and spread of the infection to deeper tissues of the penis are possible complications. Balanitis is treated with corticosteroid creams to control swelling, antibiotics to fight the infection, and medications to stop pain and fever. If balanitis recurs, circumcision (removal of the foreskin of the penis; see CIRCUMCISION, MALE) may be the best treatment.

Balloon angioplasty

A minimally invasive procedure to open arteries narrowed or blocked by fatty deposits, a disease known as ATHEROSCLEROSIS. The technical name for balloon angioplasty when done on the coronary arteries is percutaneous transluminal coronary angioplasty (PTCA), which means that the procedure is performed through the skin (percutaneous) and inside an artery (transluminal) that feeds the heart (coronary), for the purpose of reshaping that artery (angioplasty).

Balloon angioplasty can be very effective, involves a small incision, is performed under conscious sedation and with a local anesthetic, and allows recovery in days or weeks. Balloon angioplasty is performed for those who have angina (chest pain) during exercise or have had a heart attack. It is usually most effective when only one or two coronary arteries are narrowed or blocked.

During balloon angioplasty, a local anesthetic is injected before a small incision is made to expose an artery. A short tube called a sheath is inserted into the artery, and a hollow, flexible tube called a catheter is threaded through the sheath and down the artery. The guide catheter is passed through until it reaches the heart; the surgical team watches its progress through a televised X ray. Small amounts of dye are injected through the catheter to allow visualization of the diseased artery. Once the catheter is in place, a smaller catheter with a deflated balloon at its tip is passed through the catheter and positioned at the point of narrowing or blockage. The balloon is then inflated, usually for 30 seconds to 2 minutes, to compress the fatty deposit, stretch the artery wall, and increase the artery's diameter.

Balloon catheter

A thin, hollow tube with an inflatable balloon at its tip. A balloon catheter is used to compress the deposits, widen the artery, and restore normal blood flow when an artery is narrowed or blocked by fatty deposits (see BALLOON ANGIOPLASTY). It is also used to open narrowed heart valves in the procedure known as VALVULOPLASTY.

Balloon valvuloplasty

See VALVULOPLASTY.

Barbiturates

Central nervous system (CNS) depressant drugs. Barbiturates, such as phenobarbital or secobarbital act on the brain and CNS to induce drowsiness. Barbiturates can be used to control seizures in diseases such as epilepsy, and they are sometimes used to treat insomnia for short periods. Some short-acting barbiturates are used as general anesthetics.

For many years, barbiturates were used as sedatives, but they have been replaced by safer, less addictive alternatives such as BENZODIAZEPINES. Barbiturates can be addicting, and they are associated with severe side effects when taken in overdose or when abruptly stopped. They should not be used to relieve the anxiety or tension of everyday life.

Bariatric surgery

An operation to aid an obese person in losing weight by controlling appetite and the ability to absorb food. The word *bariatric* means "management of weight" in Greek. Bariatric surgery is not considered cosmetic surgery; it involves a procedure that should only be used to eliminate the serious and life-threatening medical problems caused by morbid obesity. A common procedure involves stapling across the upper part of the stomach to reduce the amount of food that the stomach can hold.

A person is classified as morbidly obese if he or she is 200 percent over his or her ideal weight (or three times as much as it should be). Obese people are at greater risk for medical problems such as diabetes mellitus, hypertension, heart disease, sleep apnea syndrome, degenerative arthritis, an elevated blood cholesterol level,

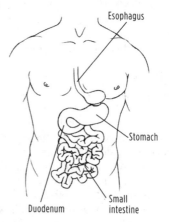

Gastroplasty

Gastroplasty is a procedure in which the surgeon partitions off the upper part of the stomach with a band of silicone mesh to create a small pouch, leaving only a narrow outlet into the rest of the stomach.

and an increased incidence of certain cancers, such as colon and rectum, prostate, uterus, and possibly breast. As a result, the death rate for obese people is much higher than for individuals of normal weight.

The two most commonly used types of bariatric surgery both reduce the amount of food that can be held in the stomach before it passes into the small intestine. Both procedures have the effect of reducing the amount of food that a person can eat at a given meal.

A gastroplasty (also called a gastric partitioning) involves the creation of a small pouch in the top of the stomach—large enough to hold only 1 ounce of food—and restricts the passage of the food through the stomach by stapling a band of synthetic mesh across the bottom of the pouch. Patients feel full after eating only a small amount of food and retain the full feeling longer than they did before surgery. Overeating causes nausea and possibly vomiting.

Less commonly used is the gastric bypass, in which the surgeon constructs a small stomach pouch and then connects this pouch directly to the intestine. With this procedure, food bypasses the remainder of the stomach after it has traveled through the surgically constructed pouch. A gastric bypass can also limit the kinds of food that can be eaten. Possible side effects include low absorption of iron because the gastric bypass eliminates most acid content, which iron needs for absorption.

On average, most people who undergo bariatric surgery lose 50 to 60 percent of their excess weight, with a maximum weight loss reached at 18 to 24 months after the procedure. Some weight-related complications may also be resolved following the weight loss. Patients must continue on a carefully controlled diet, often with vitamin and mineral supplements to ensure proper nutrition, and stay in regular contact with their physician.

Barium enema

Also known as a lower gastrointestinal tract series; an X-ray procedure that uses barium sulfate and sometimes air to outline the lining of the colon and rectum. Barium sulfate, a CONTRAST MEDIUM, is administered rectally and held briefly inside the intestine while a series of X rays is taken.

A barium enema is ordered to check for abnormalities such as tumors, ulcers, obstructions, or polyps of the colon and rectum and to diagnose diverticulosis (the presence of small sacs in the gastrointestinal wall). It is also sometimes recommended as a screening test for colorectal cancer instead of a COLONOSCOPY. In such cases, it may be performed once every 5 to 10 years, starting at age 50 years.

Barium swallow

Also known as an esophagogram or barium meal; an X-ray procedure that uses barium sulfate to outline the pharynx and esophagus. A flavored solution containing barium sulfate, a CONTRAST MEDIUM, is swallowed, and a series of X rays is taken. The barium coats the pharynx and esophagus and appears white on X-ray film, allowing structural and functional abnormalities to show up as dark shapes.

A barium swallow is usually ordered to evaluate the function of the pharynx and the esophagus and to detect abnormalities such as a tumor or a stricture (narrowing) in the esophagus that may be causing difficulty swallowing. It is also used to check for ulcers or other inflammatory conditions in the lining of the esophagus. The procedure is performed by a radiologist in a doctor's office, X-ray facility, or radiology department of a hospital.

The person is given a barium preparation to drink. The barium solution is the consistency of a milkshake and has a chalky taste. During the test, the person will drink about 12 to 14 ounces of the barium solution. The person must remain totally still while the X rays are being taken. The flow of the barium solution is monitored on a fluoroscope, a device that is equipped with a fluorescent screen.

Bartholin glands, diseases of

Disorders affecting the two Bartholin glands, located on either side of the vaginal entrance, that secrete lubricating fluid during sexual arousal. The gland openings can become blocked from infection or injury. As a result, a Bartholin cyst may form, usually causing no symptoms. However, if the cyst (a fluid-filled sac) becomes infected and an abscess appears (Bartholin abscess), the woman may feel pain and tenderness just inside the vagina, where there will be a warm, swollen lump. Treatment includes an antibiotic for the infection. If the abscess does not respond to antibiotics, the doctor may lance and drain it. About 1 percent of all cancers of the vulva are carcinomas of the Bartholin glands. A tumor of the Bartholin glands or duct may resemble a benign Bartholin cyst.

Bartonellosis

See CAT-SCRATCH DISEASE.

Basal body temperature (BBT)

Body temperature taken immediately after awakening in the morning and before getting out of bed. Typically, the BBT is used by women to identify the days during the menstrual cycle when OVULATION (the release of an egg from the ovary) takes place. A woman's temperature often falls by a few tenths of a degree during the 12 to 24 hours before ovulation; then, it rises for several days after ovulation. By measuring the BBT with a special thermometer that is able to detect slight changes and by recording the temperature on a chart every day for several months, an ovulation pattern can be detected. A woman is most likely to become pregnant if she has sex on the days just before, after, or on the day of ovulation.

Basal cell carcinoma

The most common form of SKIN CANCER. Skin cancer is the most common type of cancer in the United States, and basal cell carcinoma accounts for three of four cases. Its principal risk factor is sun exposure. The two other common types of skin cancer are SQUAMOUS CELL CARCINOMA and malignant melanoma (see MELANOMA, MALIGNANT). Of the three, basal cell carcinoma has the best prognosis, with a cure rate of more than 95 percent. Basal cell carcinoma rarely spreads to other parts of the body. However, early diagnosis and treatment are important because, without treatment, basal cell carcinoma will continue to enlarge and can eventually extend below the skin and invade nearby structures.

Basal cell carcinoma most often develops on areas of the body that are frequently exposed to the sun's ultraviolet rays such as the head, neck, hands, and chest, and sun exposure is the main risk factor. Basal cell carcinoma tumors can appear as small, shiny, fleshy nodules (solid masses of tissue) or bumps or as flat, scaly, red areas. They vary from white to light pink to brown. Sometimes blood vessels are visible in the lesions themselves or in the surrounding skin.

For the early detection of skin cancer, doctors recommend regular skin self-examination. It is important to know the regular pattern of freckles, moles, and other marks on skin. It is necessary to get medical attention for a new skin growth; changes in the surface or color of a mole; a spot or bump that is getting larger, scaling, oozing, or bleeding; a sore that does not heal within 3 months; or itchiness or pain in a lesion. In cases of suspected skin cancer, complete personal and family medical histories are taken. The lesion is examined for size, shape, color, and texture, and the rest of the body is checked for other lesions. Diagnosis of skin cancer is made by a skin biopsy (taking a small sample from the lesion and examining it under a microscope).

Most basal cell carcinoma tumors can be cured through minor surgery. The type of treatment depends on factors such as the size, type, depth, and location of the cancer. Surgical options include EXCISION (cutting out the tumor), curettage (scraping), electrodesiccation (burning with an electric current delivered through a probe), and MOHS SURGERY (micro-

scopically controlled surgery removing one layer of skin at a time). Radiation may be helpful for tumors that are difficult to treat surgically and for people unable to tolerate surgery. In the removal of large cancers, skin grafting and reconstructive surgery may be necessary.

It is not uncommon for people who have had a basal cell carcinoma tumor to get another (in the same site or in a new location) within 5 years. Consequently, doctors recommend both monthly self-examinations and regular examinations by a doctor every 6 to 12 months.

The most effective way to prevent basal cell carcinoma is to avoid harmful radiation from the sun. Doctors recommend applying a sunscreen with a sun protection factor (SPF) of at least 15 before going outdoors.

Basal ganglia

A motor control area of the brain. The basal ganglia are clusters of nerve cells (neurons) deep within the brain that help control voluntary movement. In movement disorders such as HUNTINGTON CHOREA (a progressive disorder involving degeneration of nerve cells in the cerebrum), there is an untimely deterioration of nerve cells in the basal ganglia. Parkinson disease is caused by degeneration of dopamine-producing cells in the basal ganglia. Dopamine is an important neurotransmitter that stimulates the nerves in the basal ganglia.

Baseball elbow

An overuse injury common among adolescent pitchers. Similar to tennis elbow, baseball elbow is caused by repeated stress to the elbow as it flexes and extends during overhead throwing. The medial, or inside, portion of the elbow may be injured by the throwing motion made in baseball, while the lateral, or outside, structures of the elbow are compressed by this movement. Baseball elbow is seldom severe, but in the worst cases, the cartilage of the elbow joint may be permanently damaged. A child who plays baseball, especially as a pitcher, and complains of persistent elbow pain should be examined by a doctor. The elbow joint should be rested, and physical therapy may be considered to teach the child appropriate stretching and strengthening exercises.

Baseball finger

An injury resulting from the fingertip being jammed or struck by a thrown ball. Baseball finger, which is sometimes called "mallet finger," causes pain and sometimes discoloration in the joint of the finger closest to the tip. The injury may make it difficult or impossible to fully straighten the finger. X rays are necessary for a diagnosis. Baseball finger is generally treated with a finger splint that must be worn continuously for 1 to 6 weeks, after which a follow-up of orthopedic care is recommended. If proper healing has not occurred, an additional 4 weeks of splinting may be needed. The doctor may suggest appropriate pain medication to relieve discomfort. If healing is not complete within that amount of time, surgical repair may become necessary.

Battery

By law, the illegal application of physical force to another person. Battery need not include force; a mere touch

is sufficient. See ASSAULT, SEXUAL; INCEST; VIOLENCE, FAMILY.

BCG vaccination

Bacille Calmette-Guérin vaccination; a live vaccine derived from a strain of Mycobacterium bovis, a form of bacteria that causes TUBERCULOSIS (TB). BCG vaccination is used to immunize against strains of tuberculosis. Once BCG vaccine is administered, it interferes with the possibility of using tuberculin skin tests to detect TB infection. Therefore, BCG vaccine is not recommended for adults who are at high risk and should be receiving skin tests.

Bed-wetting

Involuntary urination during sleep; also known as nocturnal enuresis. Bed-wetting is common and normal among preschool children, with more than a third of 3-year-olds wetting the bed at night. By age 5, most children are able to control their bladders while sleeping. Bed-wetting is more common in boys than girls. Primary enuresis means the child has never been dry at night. Secondary enuresis refers to the child who has been consistently dry for a number of months before wetting the bed again.

A child usually wets the bed for one of two reasons. His or her bladder may not be sufficiently developed to hold urine through the night, or during sleep the child fails to recognize the need to urinate and sleeps through the impulse. Bed-wetting tends to run in families. A school-aged child who has not achieved nighttime bladder control usually has a parent who experienced the same problem. Bed-wetting may also be related to drinking caffeinated or carbonated beverages, citrus juice, or a great deal of water. A child who has been dry at night and suddenly starts wetting the bed again may be responding to stress. Factors such as a new sibling, a death, or a divorce in the family may be responsible. Enuresis also may be the result of abuse or an underlying disease such as a urinary tract infection. Bed-wetting in a formerly dry child should be evaluated by a pediatrician or family physician. (See also ABUSE, CHILD.)

In the vast majority of children, bed-wetting is not due to a serious underlying medical problem. However, about 1 percent of cases are related to diseases or disorders such as diabetes mellitus, a urinary tract infection, or a structural abnormality. (See also DIABETES MELLITUS, TYPE 1; DIABETES MELLITUS, TYPE 2; and URINARY TRACT INFECTIONS.)

Children need reassurances that bed-wetting is not their fault. They should be praised for staying dry.

For a child of 7 or 8 who is still wetting the bed, the physician may recommend a special pad with an alarm system. Urine on the pad triggers an alarm to wake the child to go to the bathroom. Bladder stretching exercises are sometimes recommended to increase bladder capacity.

Bee stings

Painful injuries caused when stinging insects inject venom into the skin. Stinging insects include female bees, wasps, and ants. A bee sting begins as a sharp pain lasting a few minutes, after which it becomes a dull ache and is likely to itch. The sting site will become red and swollen as the body flushes venom from the area. Most bee stings in the United States involve honeybees, whose stingers usually remain in the skin after the bee stings. It is important to remove the stinger immediately, because venom continues to enter the skin from the stinger for 45 to 60 seconds after the sting. If removed within 15 seconds of the sting, the severity of the reaction is reduced.

In addition to removing the stinger, first aid for bee stings involves washing the wound and applying hydrocortisone cream or calamine lotion to reduce the itching and swelling. An oral antihistamine may help relieve symptoms. A small number of people—one or two out of every thousand—are allergic to bee stings. Allergic reactions to bee stings can include hives, nausea, vomiting, and headaches. Life-threatening allergic reactions such as anaphylactic shock (see SHOCK, ANAPHYLACTIC), dizziness, unconsciousness, and difficulty breathing may also occur immediately after the sting or up to 30 minutes later and may last for hours.

People who know they are allergic to stings should carry sting kits and wear medical identification bracelets or necklaces to inform others about their allergy. Bee stings can be avoided by wearing light-colored clothing that covers as much of the body as possible, choosing unscented soaps and cosmetics, and avoiding flowering plants.

Behavior therapy

A method of treating psychological and psychiatric conditions that focuses on changing outward behavior rather than uncovering emotional conflicts that may help explain that behavior.

Behavior therapy holds that many psychiatric and psychological conditions thought to be illnesses are actually a collection of abnormal behaviors that cause problems in daily life. Since these behaviors are learned just as normal behaviors are, behavior therapy focuses on helping the individual learn new ways of behaving that eliminate or reduce difficulties. Behavior therapy is often combined with techniques aimed at changing thought patterns. Behavior therapy has been shown to be effective for treating specific problems such as abnormal fears (phobias), depression, sexual dysfunction, panic and anxiety attacks, and childhood behavior problems.

Bell palsy

An abnormal neurological condition characterized by weakness or paralysis of muscles on one side of the face. People with Bell palsy cannot move one side of the mouth, close the eye, or furrow the brow on the affected side. Other possible symptoms of Bell palsy include changes in the production of tears and saliva and altered senses of taste and hearing. This condition is caused by damage to or dysfunction of the facial nerve. Nerve inflammation is sometimes the result of a virus, such as the herpes virus that causes cold sores and fever blisters. Possible causes of facial nerve damage that mimic Bell palsy include strokes, tumors, and infections (such as shingles or Lyme disease). Any case of facial weakness or paralysis requires prompt and careful evaluation by a physician. Most cases of Bell palsy resolve without treatment. However, treatment options include CORTICOSTEROIDS, antiviral medica-

tions, and facial massage. Artificial tears or a patch may be necessary to protect the eye from damage. In rare cases, surgery may be recommended.

Bends

See DECOMPRESSION SICKNESS.

Benign

A term that describes a condition that is not malignant (cancerous), invasive, or recurrent and does not metastasize (or spread). A benign tumor is one that is not cancerous.

Benign familial tremor

A neurological disorder characterized by shaking. (See also TREMOR.) Benign familial tremors tend to run in families and are usually harmless. Although they can develop at any age, these tremors become more common as people age. They may manifest themselves as head nodding, difficulty holding small objects, trembling hands, or a quivering voice.

Diagnosis is made on the basis of physical examination. Treatment is often not necessary. Although they affect movement or speech, benign familial tremors seldom cause any other problems. However, if tremors are severe and interfere with daily activities, medications such as anticonvulsants, beta blockers, or tranquilizers may lessen the tremor. It is also helpful to avoid caffeine and other stimulants.

Benign prostatic hyperplasia

See PROSTATE, ENLARGED.

Benzodiazepines

Synthetically produced sedative-hypnotic drugs. Benzodiazepines have replaced barbiturates as the treatment of choice for anxiety and convulsive disorders and for sedation, because they cause less drowsiness and are less likely to be fatal if taken alone in an accidental overdose.

Most benzodiazepines, often referred to as minor tranquilizers, are used to treat anxiety and tension. Three benzodiazepines—diazepam, midazolam, and lorazepam—are used as surgical drugs to sedate patients and prevent them from remembering details of the surgery. Diazepam is also used to treat neurologic conditions involving muscle spasm.

Benzodiazepines should not be taken for long periods, because they can cause physical dependency and severe withdrawal symptoms when stopped. Benzodiazepines can cause an impaired ability to drive. Drinking alcohol increases the sedative effect, so alcohol intake should be avoided when taking benzodiazepines.

Berylliosis

An environmental, chronic, inflammatory disorder of the lungs caused by the inhalation of beryllium dust. Materials that contain beryllium may be found in the aerospace, electronic, and nuclear weapon industries. The symptoms of berylliosis may not develop until several years after exposure. They include chest pain, shortness of breath on exertion, a dry cough, and, occasionally, fever and chills. Berylliosis is often treated with CORTICOSTEROIDS.

Beta blockers

Antihypertensive drugs. Beta blockers are very effective drugs that lower blood pressure by blocking the effects of norepinephrine, thereby easing the heart's pumping action and indirectly widening blood vessels. Current research demonstrates that beta blockers reduce the risk for heart attacks and other cardiovascular events. Beta blockers are inexpensive, safe, and effective for most people with hypertension and no complicating health problems. Beta blockers should be used with caution by people with asthma because they can narrow bronchial airways. Beta blockers can also be useful for people with angina to slow heart rates; they can also be used as eyedrops for glaucoma. Examples of beta blockers include acebutolol, atenolol, betaxolol, carteolol, carvedilol, metoprolol, nadolol, penbutolol, pindolol, and propranolol. Beta blockers may differ in their effects as well as in their side effects; some can cause an impaired ability to drive.

Beta-carotene

A form of CAROTENE, a substance found in plants that is converted to VITAMIN A by the intestines, lungs, and liver.

Bezoar

A ball of indigestible material in the stomach. Bezoars can be composed of hair, fiber, or other indigestible material. Although they are most common in children, bezoars can also occur in adults following partial GASTRECTOMY (surgical removal of part of the stomach). People with diabetes are also more likely to develop bezoars. Trichobezoars are bezoars made of hair only; they develop in children who chew on their hair or pull it out and swallow it. This type of bezoar may also occur in emotionally disturbed adults who eat their hair. A bezoar may produce loss of appetite, nausea, vomiting, and abdominal pain. Treatment usually requires breaking up the bezoar, using a gastroscope. If this is not successful, surgical removal is required.

Bifocal

In optics, eyeglasses made up of two portions, one for seeing near and the other for far distance vision. The upper part is usually used for distant vision, while the lower part is for reading or other close work. Bifocals are generally prescribed for older adults, whose eyes gradually lose the ability to see clearly at close range (called PRESBYOPIA).

Biguanides

Oral hypoglycemic agents; medications for the treatment of type 2 (non–insulin-independent or adult-onset) diabetes. Biguanides make up one of five classes of oral medications used to treat diabetes. Oral hypoglycemic agents are not oral insulin but are medications designed to help reduce blood sugar levels when diet and exercise alone are not enough. Biguanides are effective only if the pancreas is still producing some insulin, as is generally the case with middle-aged and older people with diabetes. People with type 1 diabetes do not secrete enough insulin for the oral medications to be effective.

Bilateral

Having two sides. Bilateral kidney disease, for example, affects both the right and left kidneys.

Bile

A yellow-green liquid that aids digestion. Bile is secreted by the liver and concentrated and stored in the gall-

bladder. The liver produces about 3 cups of bile each day. When a hormone is released by the small intestine, it causes the gallbladder to contract, and bile is released through the bile ducts into the small intestine. The substances in the bile, including bile salts and lecithin, make fats soluble so they can be absorbed by the intestine and pass into the bloodstream.

Another important function of bile is to carry BILIRUBIN (a normal by-product of the breakdown of hemoglobin from aging red blood cells) from the liver to the gallbladder and into the small intestine. The bilirubin is broken down by intestinal bacteria and eventually excreted in the stools. If this process of bilirubin metabolism is interrupted, excess bilirubin accumulates in the bloodstream and causes JAUNDICE (a yellowing of the skin and the whites of the eyes). Jaundice is a symptom of many different liver disorders.

Another component of bile is CHOLESTEROL, a fatlike substance that is excreted by the liver. Cholesterol is an important constituent of cells; however, high levels of serum cholesterol in the bloodstream increase the risk of ARTERIOSCLEROSIS, a disease in which the walls of arteries become inflamed and thickened with plaque. Excess cholesterol can also lead to the formation of GALLSTONES.

Bile duct

One of several tubes that carry bile from the LIVER to the gallbladder and then to the first section of the small intestine (duodenum). A system of bile ducts (the biliary system) starts in liver tissue, in units called lobules, and channels bile into successively larger ducts. Two large tubes, the hepatic ducts, leave the liver and join to form the common hepatic duct. From the common hepatic duct, bile flows either into the gallbladder for storage or into the common bile duct to be carried toward the small intestine.

Bile duct cancer

Cancer in the ducts that carry BILE from the liver to the gallbladder and small intestine. Bile duct cancer occurs most frequently between ages 50 and 70. People who have a history of colitis or gallstones are more likely to develop the disease. JAUNDICE, a yellowing of the skin and the whites of the eyes, is the primary symptom of bile duct cancer. Symptoms may also include itching, weight loss, abdominal pain, nausea, vomiting, and an enlarged liver. Diagnosis is made by physical examination, blood tests, and imaging studies.

Treatment consists of surgery to remove the cancer. Often, the tumor spreads to the liver, from which the tumor may be difficult or impossible to remove. If bile ducts become blocked, they can be treated by inserting tubes through the blockage by using ERCP (endoscopic retrograde cholangiopancreatography), a procedure that utilizes X rays for guidance and a special viewing tube that can perform some surgical procedures. When surgery is successful, periodic CT (computed tomography) SCANNING is necessary to detect cancer should it recur. Doctors may also recommend CHEMOTHERAPY or RADIATION THERAPY. See also BILE DUCT OBSTRUCTION.

Bile duct obstruction

A condition in which BILE is blocked from entering the intestines, creating pressure in the bile ducts. Bile duct obstruction may be due to scar tissue from inflammation, GALLSTONES (hard masses that can form in the gallbladder), BILE DUCT CANCER, or pancreatic tumors (see PANCREAS, CANCER OF THE).

The primary symptoms of bile duct obstruction are JAUNDICE (a yellowing of the skin and the whites of the eyes), itching, and BILIARY COLIC (severe pain in the upper abdomen). The pain may also radiate to the back and is often accompanied by nausea and vomiting.

Bile duct obstruction is diagnosed by ultrasound examination, CT (computed tomography) SCANNING, or ERCP (endoscopic retrograde cholangiopancreatography), the most invasive procedure. ERCP can usually identify the cause and site of the blockage and can be used to treat some types of obstruction. Further treatment varies according to the underlying cause of obstruction.

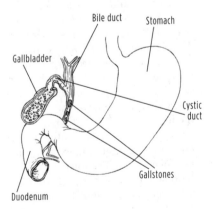

Blocked bile ducts

As bile passes from the liver and gallbladder into the intestine, it travels through a series of ducts. Its passage can be blocked by gallstones, scar tissue, or cancer. Gallstones are hardened masses of cholesterol or salts.

Bilharziasis

See SCHISTOSOMIASIS.

Biliary atresia

A potentially fatal disorder in newborns, in which the bile ducts inside or outside the liver fail to develop or develop abnormally. Biliary atresia causes JAUNDICE (a yellowing of the skin and the whites of the eyes) and CIRRHOSIS (a severe liver disease). The symptoms of biliary atresia appear from 2 to 6 weeks after birth. Jaundice is the primary symptom. An infant may also experience pale stools, dark urine, an enlarged and hardened liver, and a swollen abdomen. Some babies develop an intense, uncomfortable itching that can make them very irritable. The cause of biliary atresia is not known.

Several tests are performed to diagnose biliary atresia definitively, including blood and urine tests, LIVER FUNCTION TESTS, a test for blood-clotting function, ultrasound scanning, X rays, and a liver BIOPSY.

When ducts are completely obstructed, surgery is necessary to drain bile from the liver. In babies who respond to the surgery, bile starts to flow several days following surgery. This surgery is not effective when obstructed bile ducts are inside the liver.

Complications frequently occur after surgery. If the surgery is not successful and complications of cirrhosis become life-threatening, a liver transplant may be considered.

Biliary cirrhosis

An uncommon type of cirrhosis that causes gradual, progressive destruction of bile ducts in the liver. Because its normal excretion is interrupted, bile accumulates in the liver and can damage liver cells. This chronic liver disease is classified as either primary biliary cirrhosis (PBC) or secondary biliary cirrhosis.

Primary biliary cirrhosis

The major problem in the initial stages of PBC is liver inflammation. As time goes on, continuing inflammation around damaged bile ducts leads to severe scarring and eventually life-threatening CIRRHOSIS; PBC may exhibit no symptoms for many years. Often, the first symptom is intense itching. Eventually, such signs as JAUNDICE (a yellowing of the skin and the whites of the eyes), fatigue, cholesterol deposits in the skin, fluid accumulation, and darkening of the skin arise. Related disorders include impaired function of the salivary glands (that causes dry mouth) and of the eyes, arthritis, thyroid problems, and thinning of the bones that can lead to fractures.

Doctors believe that the cause of PBC has a genetic component. The disease may also be caused by a disturbance in the immune system. PBC more commonly affects women than men and usually occurs between the ages of 40 and 60. Because initially there are few symptoms, abnormal laboratory test results (such as liver function tests) are often the first indication of PBC. Treatment begins with the elimination of potentially harmful foods or drugs. Specific symptoms also are addressed. For example, salt restriction or diuretics can reduce fluid buildup. Other medications relieve severe itching. Doctors are also investigating the use of medications, such as colchicine and methotrexate, to slow the course of PBC. In severe cases, a liver transplant may be considered.

Secondary biliary cirrhosis

This form of the disease is also characterized by accumulation of bile in the liver (cholestasis). Secondary biliary cirrhosis results from long-term BILE DUCT OBSTRUCTION or from BILIARY ATRESIA, a congenital condition in which the bile ducts are abnormal or fail to develop. Symptoms include intense abdominal pain, enlarged liver, fever and chills, and some blood abnormalities. Treatment is as for bile duct obstruction or biliary atresia.

Biliary colic

Severe, constant pain in the upper abdomen. Pain may radiate to the right shoulder and the back and can mimic the pain of a heart attack. Biliary colic is often accompanied by nausea and vomiting. Attacks occur intermittently and generally last for hours. GALLSTONES (solid masses that form in the gallbladder) are the most common cause of biliary colic. At times, a stone leaves the gallbladder and becomes lodged in the bile duct. Colic occurs as the gallbladder and bile duct muscle clamp down in an attempt to expel the stone into the intestines. CHOLECYSTITIS (inflammation of the gallbladder) may also develop.

Ultrasound scanning, X rays, or CHOLECYSTOGRAPHY (a type of imaging procedure for the gallbladder and common bile duct) may be used to find out the cause of the pain. In people with recurrent biliary colic or severe symptoms, removal of the gallbladder is usually recommended. See CHOLECYSTECTOMY.

Biliary system

The organs in which bile is formed, concentrated, stored, and transported to the small intestine. The biliary system removes waste products from the liver and carries bile to the intestine. The biliary system is composed of the bile ducts, gallbladder, bile, and various other structures. The gallbladder, a small pouch that lies under the liver, stores and concentrates BILE, which flows through the bile ducts from the liver into and out of the gallbladder. A hormone released by the small intestine causes the gallbladder to contract and release bile into the small intestine, where it helps neutralize stomach acid and make fats soluble to permit their digestion. See also BILE DUCT.

Bilirubin

A breakdown product of hemoglobin, the blood pigment that transports oxygen. When red blood cells are destroyed, the bilirubin that results from the breakdown of hemoglobin is transported to the liver and excreted as part of the bile into the gallbladder and small intestine. A small amount of the bilirubin reenters the bloodstream after it is taken up by the small intestine; later it is excreted in the urine. Measuring the amount of bilirubin in the blood and urine, tests provide information about whether the liver and gallbladder are functioning normally. If an obstruction is blocking the bile ducts or gallbladder, the level of bilirubin in the blood increases. Abnormally high levels of bilirubin can cause jaundice, a yellowish discoloration of the skin and the sclera (whites of the eyes), that can be a sign of liver or gallbladder disease. In addition to liver and gallbladder disease, hemolytic anemia can cause bilirubin levels to rise.

Billroth operation

A type of partial GASTRECTOMY (surgical removal of all or part of the stomach). The Billroth operation was developed by the Austrian surgeon Christian Billroth in the 19th century and became the first successful operation on the stomach. It is still used today in the treatment of some types of peptic ulcers and for gastric cancer.

Bioavailability

The degree to which a drug or other substance is absorbed; the fraction of the oral drug that reaches central blood circulation. Bioavailability measures the extent to which a drug or dietary supplement becomes available to work on the body tissue after it is taken.

Biofeedback

A technique in which sight or sound signals allow a person to become aware of and control specific bodily functions that are not normally controlled voluntarily, such as heart rate, blood pressure, muscle tension, and brain wave activity. Biofeedback has been used successfully to treat a wide variety of conditions, including migraine and tension headaches; chronic pain; and high blood pressure (hypertension).

Biopsy

A diagnostic test in which a specimen of tissue is removed for microscopic examination or testing. Methods of tissue removal vary from biopsy to biopsy. For example, in a NEEDLE BIOPSY, a needle is inserted through the skin to remove tissue that may be diseased; in a punch biopsy, a small cylinder of skin is removed. During a bone marrow biopsy, a needle is placed in a pelvic bone to remove and analyze the bone marrow. Biopsy is used to diagnose cancer or certain infections.

Bioterrorism

The intentional use of chemical or germ (infectious biological) agents on a population as a weapon. Health care workers are usually the first to recognize when such an outbreak has occurred. The infectious agents are usually invisible, odorless, colorless, and tasteless, but are highly potent and capable of doing great harm.

Most bacterial and viral agents, such as ANTHRAX and SMALLPOX, need to be inhaled or ingested to cause disease, while chemical agents usually can cause disease through inhalation or by entering through the skin.

Response to such outbreaks is usually coordinated through the military, the Centers for Disease Control and Prevention (CDC), and local departments of public health.

Biotherapeutic agents

Medically useful drugs whose manufacture involves microorganisms or enzymes produced by microorganisms. Most biotherapeutic agents are produced by genetic engineering, or bioengineering. Because biotherapeutic agents are either identical or similar to proteins produced naturally in the body, they are expected to have less potential to cause side effects than traditional drugs. This is particularly important in cancer therapy. Some dietary supplements are biotherapeutic agents, among them acidophilus and Saccharomyces cerevisiae (brewer's yeast).

Biotin

Vitamin H. A vitamin found in a variety of foods, including liver, salmon, bananas, carrots, cereals, and peanuts. Biotin aids the action of various enzymes in cells. Its functions include helping to form proteins from amino acids, breaking down fats, and forming new fatty acids and glucose.

Bipolar disorder

A mental illness characterized by swings in mood from extreme elation and energy (mania) to abnormal sadness and lethargy (DEPRESSION). The swings may be brief (minutes) or long (years). Bipolar disorder is also known as manic-depressive illness. If a person with manic-depressive illness loses contact with reality, the disease is considered a PSYCHOSIS.

Mania is characterized by a persistently euphoric mood, decreased need for sleep, high physical energy, increased sexual activity, rapid speech, agitation, loss of self-control and judgment, unrealistic beliefs in one's powers and abilities, racing thoughts, and disturbed appetite. Drug abuse, particularly of alcohol, cocaine, or sleeping medications, is common.

Depression is characterized by sadness, melancholy, crying, slowed mental processes, and changes in such physical patterns as eating and sleeping. People with depression sometimes have thoughts about suicide and may attempt to kill themselves. Medically, depression is defined as the daily presence for 2 weeks of at least five of the following nine symptoms: melancholy mood or sadness (sometimes experienced as apathy or irritability) for most of the day; loss of pleasure in practically all activities, particularly ones the person previously enjoyed; disturbed appetite or either weight gain or loss; disturbed sleep, particularly the inability to sleep through the night (insomnia); slowed or agitated physical activity; fatigue or very low energy, often leading to a diminished or nonexistent sex drive; feelings of worthlessness, low self-esteem, or inappropriate guilt; difficulty concentrating and thinking; and morbid or suicidal thoughts or actions.

Bipolar disorder is equally common in men and women. In men, the disease usually begins with a hypomanic or manic episode. In women, depression is usually the first symptom. Ongoing episodes of mania, hypomania, or depression tend to worsen in the few days before a woman with the disease begins her menstrual period. In both men and women, changes in the sleep-wake schedule, such as air travel across time zones or sleep deprivation, may precipitate an episode or exacerbate an ongoing period of depression or mania.

The precise cause of bipolar disorder remains undetermined. Evidence suggests that genetic inheritance has a role.

Some people with bipolar disorder experience a less severe mood disturbance known as hypomania, an abnormally expansive, elevated, highly energized, or irritable mood that comes on quickly. People with hypomania can function well in family, school, and job settings, but those with mania have more problems.

Untreated bipolar disorder usually leads to repeated bouts of illness, with hospitalization likely. Most people with bipolar disorder respond well to medication for the disease.

Birth

The process in which a baby is delivered from the mother. In an uncomplicated vaginal delivery, the baby is pushed out of the uterus and through the vaginal passage known as the BIRTH CANAL by involuntary contractions (see DELIVERY, VAGINAL). Usually, the baby is delivered head first, but sometimes babies are born buttocks first (BREECH DELIVERY) or feet first (footling breech delivery).

Under certain conditions, the doctor may perform a surgical operation called a CESAREAN SECTION (or C-section), in which the baby is delivered through an incision in the mother's abdomen. A cesarean section may be needed when the baby is in a BREECH PRESENTATION or in serious distress; the labor is not progressing or is abnormally long; there is a dangerous infection; the birth canal is not large enough for the baby's passage; or in another situation in which a cesarean is thought to be safer for the mother or baby. See also CHILD-BIRTH; LABOR; and NATURAL CHILD-BIRTH.

Birth canal

The passage from the cervix to the vaginal opening through which a baby moves during CHILDBIRTH. When the cervix is fully dilated (open), the baby's head enters the birth canal, at the top of the vagina, and continues down and out of the body through the vaginal opening. See also REPRODUC-TIVE SYSTEM, FEMALE.

Birth control

See CONTRACEPTION.

Birth control pill

See CONTRACEPTION, HORMONAL METHODS.

Birth defects

Physical problems or abnormalities present in a baby at birth. Birth defects, also known as congenital anomalies, can affect the baby's appearance or how his or her brain or other organs function. The cause of most birth defects is unknown. However, some birth defects, called genetic disorders, are inherited from the baby's parents; others may be acquired prenatally, for example, when a woman contracts a specific infection (such as RUBELLA, TOXOPLASMOSIS, CYTOMEGALOVIRUS, or SYPHILIS), or if the fetus is exposed to a chemical substance (such as drugs or alcohol) during pregnancy. Birth defects may also be acquired during labor and delivery.

When planning a family, a couple concerned about possible birth defects can get GENETIC COUNSELING to learn their risks. During pregnancy, to assess the risk of a baby having certain genetic problems, such as DOWN SYNDROME, or structural defects, such as SPINA BIFIDA, maternal serum screening tests, such as an alpha-fetoprotein (AFP) test, are performed. If the AFP level is abnormal, the doctor may conduct more tests. Further investigations may include ultrasound imaging; AMNIOCENTESIS, in which the amniotic fluid surrounding the fetus is analyzed; or CHORIONIC VIL-LUS SAMPLING (CVS), in which a sample of tissue from the placenta is analyzed.

Birth rate

The number of live births within a population in 1 year divided by the average or midyear number of people in that population. If total population (that is, males and females of all ages) is used, the result is called the crude birth rate.

Birth weight

The weight of a baby immediately after birth. Newborns usually weigh between 5½ and 9 pounds. The average full-term infant birth weight in the United States is 7½ pounds. Newborns weighing from 3⅓ to 5½ pounds are considered to be low-birth-weight babies, and those weighing less than 3⅓ pounds at birth are very low-birth-weight babies. See also PREMATURE BIRTH.

Birthmark

An area of discolored skin that is present from birth or appears during the first few weeks of life. Vascular (relating to blood vessels) birthmarks are common and usually benign (not cancerous). They are composed of blood vessels bunched together in the skin. They can be brown, pink, tan, blue, or red, and they can be flat or raised. The most common types are capillary and cavernous HEMANGIOMA and PORT-WINE STAIN, both of which are reddish purple birthmarks caused by an abnormal distribution or malformation of blood vessels.

Births, multiple

See TWINS; MULTIPLE BIRTHS.

Bisexuality

The condition of being erotically attracted to individuals of both sexes.

Bismuth

An element of bismuth subsalicylate, which is commonly used to treat mild diarrhea. Bismuth subsalicylate is the active ingredient in such commonly used products as Pepto-Bismol and Bismatrol. It is available without prescription in tablets, chewable tablets, and liquid. It can cause dark stools and discoloration of the tongue.

Bisphosphonates

A class of nonhormonal drugs used to treat bone and calcium metabolism diseases. Bisphosphonates are used to prevent and treat OSTEOPOROSIS and to treat PAGET DISEASE of bone as well as certain bone cancers. The drugs work by inhibiting bone resorption, preventing a loss of bone density. Bisphosphonates can lead to an increase in bone mass.

Bites and stings

Wounds delivered to people through contact with humans, animals, and insects. Bites and stings can be minor or serious. Medical treatment should be sought if the person bitten develops swelling, redness, or pus or has not had a tetanus shot in 10 years, or if the wound requires stitches.

Bites, animal

Animal bites are usually puncture wounds and are most often from pets, particularly dogs. Cat bites are more serious than dog bites, because they tend to be deeper and thus much more likely to become infected.

Bites from wild animals are potentially more serious than those caused by pets because of the risk of rabies infection transmitted by the animal's saliva. Rabies is a rare but potentially fatal disease carried primarily by raccoons, bats, skunks, and foxes. Although there is no cure for rabies once symptoms set in, people can be vaccinated after having been exposed to the disease, thereby becoming immune (see RABIES). Any person bitten by an unknown or wild animal should seek immediate emergency medical assistance.

Bites, human

Human bites pose a high risk of infection because of the many types of bacteria and viruses found in the human mouth. Human bites may also cause injury to tendons and joints, especially if the wound extends below the skin. Human bites may be deliberate, or they may happen accidentally, as when someone injures his or her knuckles on another person's teeth during a fight.

First aid for a human bite includes thoroughly stopping the bleeding with pressure on the site, washing the affected area with soap and water, and applying a bandage. The doctor's office will advise whether a tetanus shot is needed.

Bites, insect

Insect bites involve the injection of venom or other agent into the skin, which triggers an allergic reaction. Most reactions are mild, involving only an annoying itching or stinging sensation and mild swelling. Delayed reactions can occur, including fever, painful joints, hives, and swollen glands. A small percentage of people develop severe allergic reactions to insect venom, and many have difficulty breathing, faintness, rapid heartbeat, confusion, or swelling of the lips or throat. A severe reaction must be considered a medical emergency.

The most troublesome insect bites are those caused by bees, hornets, wasps, yellow jackets, and fire ants.

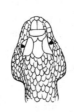 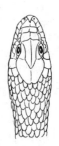

Poisonous   **Nonpoisonous**

Snakes with fangs
Generally, snakes with fangs are poisonous and leave fairly obvious fang marks on the skin when they bite. A pit viper has a short jaw with long, prominent fangs in the front.

Mosquitoes and biting flies generally cause only mild bites. Mild bites are usually treated by removing the stinger, applying ice or a cold pack to the bite area to reduce pain and swelling, applying hydrocortisone cream to the area, and taking an oral dose of a mild antihistamine. See also BITES, TICK.

Bites, reptile

Most reptiles, such as turtles and snakes, are not poisonous, and their bites can be treated with first aid, including thorough washing of the area, applying antibiotic cream or ointment, and bandaging. The best way to reduce the risk of being bitten by a reptile is not to handle them. Only people with proper training in the handling of reptiles should pick them up.

In the event of a reptile bite it is vital to determine if the reptile is poisonous. If the skin in the area of the bite changes color, swells, or is painful, the reptile is probably poisonous. Poisonous snakes in the United States include the cottonmouth (water moccasin), copperhead, coral snake, and rattlesnake. In this case, the person should lie down quietly, taking care to keep the bite area lower than the heart, to limit circulation of the venom. If the bite is on an arm or leg, that limb should be bandaged tightly above the bite, between it and the heart, to slow the spread of the venom. Emergency medical care should be sought, either at a hospital or on the scene of the injury if the person cannot be moved. See also SNAKEBITE.

Bites, spider

Only a few spiders in North America are poisonous to humans; these include the black widow spider and the brown recluse spider. Both prefer warm climates and dark, dry places where flies are plentiful; they often live in outdoor toilets, wood, rock, and brush piles or in dark garages and attics. Bites usually occur on the arms or hands of people looking for something in these places. Often, the person does not realize he or she has been bitten until a swelling or bite mark is noticed.

The symptoms of a black widow spider bite include intense pain and stiffness within a few hours, with or without nausea, fever, severe abdominal pain, and chills. The bite of a brown recluse spider causes intense pain within 8 hours and a fluid-filled blister that forms at the site of the bite and then falls off, leaving a deep, growing ulcer. Mild fever and nausea may occur. First aid measures to be taken in the case of a bite from either spider include placing a snug bandage above the bite to slow the spread of the venom, applying a cold compress or ice bag to the bite, and obtaining emergency medical aid.

Bites, tick

Ticks are often very tiny and hard to see. Some ticks transmit organisms that cause serious illnesses, including LYME DISEASE and ROCKY MOUNTAIN SPOTTED FEVER. If a person is bitten by a tick, the first thing to do is to remove it promptly and carefully, using tweezers while wearing protective rubber gloves, if possible, to grasp it by its head and gently pull it out. Once the tick has been removed, the area should be washed with soap and water, and antibiotic ointment or an antiseptic should be applied. The person handling the tick should wash his or her hands. If part of the tick stays in the skin, or if the person develops a rash or flulike symptoms, medical help should be sought. The symptoms of infection caused by a tick bite may not appear until days or weeks after the bite.

Blackhead

A pimple that has darkened at the top due to exposure to the air. Blackheads typically develop as the plug of greasy material (keratin) blocking a sebaceous gland (see SEBACEOUS GLANDS) is exposed over time to oxygen in the air. Blackheads are often a characteristic of acne and usually appear on the face, chest, shoulders, and back.

Bladder

The sac that holds urine produced in the kidneys until it is expelled from the body. The bladder, one of the organs in the urinary tract, is located inside the pelvis. Two tubes called ureters lead from the kidneys into the back of the bladder. At the base of the bladder, a circular muscle forms a sphincter that can be opened to allow urine to flow into a tube called the urethra, which exits the body in the genital area. The walls of the bladder are muscular and can stretch or expand to hold as much as a pint of urine and then contract to expel it. In an infant, bladder function is entirely reflexive.

Bladder cancer

Abnormal growth and cell division of the tissues of the bladder, the hollow organ that holds urine. Most bladder cancers are transitional cell carcinomas, which are cancers that begin within the layers of the cells lining the inner wall of the bladder. When bladder cancer is confined to the surface layer, it is called superficial bladder cancer. If superficial bladder cancer spreads through the lining of the bladder and invades the muscular wall of the bladder, it is called invasive bladder cancer. Invasive bladder cancer may spread to nearby organs.

If bladder cancer reaches the lymph nodes surrounding the bladder, it may eventually metastasize, or spread, to other organs such as the lungs or bones. The affected organs will have the same kind of abnormal

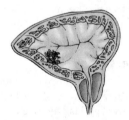

Stage A of bladder cancer
To plan treatment for bladder cancer, a doctor needs to know the extent of the growth of the cancer cells. At an early stage (A), cancer cells are present only in the inner lining (mucosa) of the bladder.

cells that constitute the tumor that originated in the bladder.

Symptoms of bladder cancer may include blood in the urine, pain during urination, difficulty urinating, or the urge to urinate frequently. A medical evaluation should be sought if these symptoms persist longer than 2 weeks. However, bloody urine and urination problems are also symptoms of less serious conditions such as bacterial infections and kidney stones.

Initially, a doctor may suspect a person has bladder cancer based on the person's symptoms. Very rarely, a doctor may be able to feel a bladder tumor through the vagina or rectum. A physician may observe the bladder directly through a specialized instrument called a cystoscope. During a CYSTOSCOPY, a biopsy sample may be taken to definitively diagnose bladder cancer. In some cases, the entire tumor may be removed at the time of biopsy.

Bladder tumors may be benign (noncancerous) or malignant (cancerous). Examples of a benign bladder tumor include transitional cell papilloma, which is very rare and occurs in the lining of the bladder, and nephrogenic ADENOMA, which is a rare, tumorlike lesion of the bladder.

After the stage of bladder cancer has been determined, treatment may include surgery, radiation therapy, chemotherapy, and biological therapy.

Blastomycosis

A chronic infection caused by a fungus inhaled into the lungs and transported by the bloodstream to other organs, principally the skin and bones. The fungus that causes blastomycosis is found in the soil, primarily in the southeastern United States and the Mississippi Valley. The infection is common in dogs, but it is not known to be transmitted from animals to humans. It occurs mostly in middle-aged men.

Blastomycosis often has no symptoms and usually improves on its own. When the infection first occurs in the lungs, the symptoms may be similar to those of a mild cold. It may eventually affect the lungs and the skin, causing symptoms that may include cough, weight loss, chest pain, skin lesions, localized swelling, and coughing up blood. The skin lesions are most common on the exposed skin of the face, hands, wrists, and lower legs. If the infection spreads throughout the body's system, it may affect the urinary tract, skin, liver, spleen, bone, lymph nodes, heart, adrenal glands, gastrointestinal tract, and pancreas.

Because the symptoms tend to vary, blastomycosis is difficult to diagnose. Blastomycosis is usually treated with antifungal medications.

Bleaching, dental

A cosmetic process to whiten teeth that have become discolored. Dental bleaching is considered safe for the teeth and gums when supervised by a dentist. The most immediate results involve applying a bleach solution to the teeth, followed by exposure to a high-intensity heat lamp for 5 minutes, and then applying a fluoride gel to reduce sensitivity. Laser bleaching can also be performed by a dentist in his or her office.

Bleeding

Loss of blood from blood vessels. Bleeding can occur internally or externally through a natural opening, such as the nose or vagina, or through a break in the skin. The amount of bleeding is not necessarily a good indicator of how serious an injury is, because some relatively minor injuries, such as scalp wounds, bleed profusely. Some very serious injuries do not bleed much at all, such as puncture wounds, which are dangerous because of the risk of infection, including TETANUS. Internal bleeding may not be noticeable externally, but it can cause physiological shock, in which the skin becomes clammy and the blood pressure drops severely.

First aid measures to be taken depend on whether the bleeding is mild or severe. Most bleeding usually stops by itself within a few minutes, and direct pressure applied to a wound will stop most external bleeding. For severe bleeding, it may be necessary to apply pressure to the vein or artery above the bleeding point in such a way that the vessel is pressed against the bone behind it. Emergency medical assistance should always be sought for severe bleeding and whenever internal bleeding is suspected.

Bleeding disorders

Diseases involving malfunction of the blood's clotting system or other problems that result in prolonged bleeding. Bleeding may result from problems with clotting, the platelets, or fragile blood vessels. Some bleeding disorders are congenital (present at birth), and others develop during illness or are acquired as a result of medical treatment.

In normal blood, clotting, or coagulation, is a complex process that involves the blood cells known as platelets and as many as 20 proteins (coagulation factors) found in the plasma (the liquid portion of the blood). In a bleeding disorder, something goes wrong with the platelets or with one or more of the coagulation factors. The resulting bleeding can range from mild to severe. Symptoms may include easy and extensive bruising, excessive bleeding after injury, uncontrolled bleeding inside the body, heavy and repeated nosebleeds, and abnormally copious menstrual bleeding. Examples of bleeding disorders include HEMOPHILIA; THROMBOCYTOPENIA; and VON WILLEBRAND DISEASE.

Certain diseases cause defects in the blood vessel wall, making the blood vessels more fragile and more prone to bleed than normal blood vessels. Causes include aging, vitamin C (ascorbic acid) deficiency, hereditary abnormalities, and some drugs.

Bleeding gums

See PERIODONTAL DISEASE.

Blepharitis

Inflammation of the edges of the eyelids. The eyelids look sticky, crusty, and reddened, with scales that cling to the bases of the lashes. The eye may feel gritty when blinking and itch or burn. Eyelashes can fall out. Blepharitis has a number of possible causes, including bacterial infection, lice in the eyelashes, or a skin condition known as SEBORRHEIC DERMATITIS, which causes scaling and yellow crusty patches and appears on other parts of the body besides the eyelids, particularly the scalp. The lining of the eye may also become infected, resulting in CONJUNCTIVITIS (pinkeye).

In rare instances of severe infection, the clear outer covering of the eye (cornea) can ulcerate. In most cases, blepharitis does not threaten sight. Crusts are removed by cleaning the eyelids with a clean cloth soaked in warm water; mild baby shampoo can also be used. Antibiotic or corticosteroid ointments may also be prescribed to fight infection.

Blepharoplasty

See EYELID SURGERY.

Blepharoptosis

Drooping of one or both upper eyelids; also called ptosis. The cause is usually weakness in the muscle that raises the lid. In mild cases, the upper range of vision is blocked; in severe cases, the person can see little or nothing out of the eye without raising the eyelid by hand or tilting the head back. In children who are born with blepharoptosis, usually only one eye is affected. The condition also appears as people age, usually as a result of overall loss in muscle tone.

Children born with blepharoptosis are treated surgically since the drooping eyelid limits normal use of the covered eye and can hamper development of normal vision (see AMBLYOPIA, or "lazy eye"). The age at which surgery is performed depends on the severity of the blepharoptosis.

In adults, treatment of blepharoptosis depends on cause. If an underlying disease is causing the eyelids to droop, treatment of that disease may remedy the condition. Blepharoptosis from aging can be treated surgically, either for cosmetic reasons or to improve vision (see EYELID SURGERY).

Blepharospasm

Repeated, involuntary twitching or quivering of the eyelid. Usually the upper eyelid is affected. Although annoying, temporary blepharospasms cease on their own without treatment. The usual causes are stress and fatigue. Rest and gentle massage often help relieve the condition.

Severe, persistent blepharospasm may also be caused by certain eye diseases, such as GLAUCOMA, inflammation of the eyelids (blepharitis), dry eyes, infection, or inflammation within the eye. Treatment of the underlying disease often alleviates the spasm.

Less common is a condition known as essential blepharospasm, which causes progressively more severe spasms of the eyelids and may also involve other muscles of the face and neck. Essential blepharospasm usually begins after age 50 and is more common in women than men. Essential blepharospasm typically begins with increased blinking or squinting and progresses to repeated strong closing of the eyelids followed by difficulty in opening them. Treatment by injecting medication into the eyelid is successful in some cases. Surgery to remove the involved muscles is also used.

Blind loop syndrome

A condition resulting from alterations in the structure of the intestine. In blind loop syndrome, one or more nonfunctioning segments of intestine are created either inadvertently or purposely by a surgical procedure. For example, a blind loop occurs following a partial removal of the stomach. Blind loop syndrome can also be present at birth.

Blind loop syndrome can lead to bacterial overgrowth and to complications, such as an intestinal obstruction, MALABSORPTION SYNDROME (impaired absorption of nutrients through the small intestine), or necrosis (death of tissue cells). Symptoms may include foul-smelling diarrhea, fatigue, and weight loss. Treatment with antibiotics may succeed.

Blind spot

The area on the retina (the light-sensitive layer at the back of the eye) from which the optic nerve emerges; also known as the optic disc. Since this part of the retina lacks light receptors, the optic disc is insensitive to light. In normal vision with both eyes, the blind spot is not perceived since the blind spot of one eye is covered by a seeing area of the other eye. The term "blind spot" is also sometimes used to refer to apparent holes (scotomas) in the visual field in which nothing can be seen. Scotomas can be a result of retinal disease or glaucoma.

Blindness

Total or partial loss of sight caused by a disease or disorder of the eye, optic nerve, or brain. In most cases, blindness refers to a loss of vision that cannot be corrected with glasses or contact lenses. Blindness does not always refer to a total loss of sight. Some people who are legally blind can perceive slow-moving objects or colors. The term "low vision" is used for people who have moderately impaired vision but are not classified as blind. Color blindness is not actually a form of blindness, since it refers only to a lack of perception of certain colors and not to a loss of vision.

Physicians assess vision with two measurements. Visual acuity measures the ability to see details. Normal vision is defined as 20/20. Any loss of visual acuity raises the second number. For example, a person with 20/200 vision must stand 20 feet away from an object that a person with normal vision can see from 200 feet. The second measurement is visual field, which refers to the size of the area around the center of vision.

Blindness can be caused by GLAUCOMA, CATARACT (see also CATARACT SURGERY), diabetic retinopathy (see RETINOPATHY, DIABETIC), MACULAR DEGENERATION, and SICKLE CELL ANEMIA. Injury to the eye or the optic nerve may also lead to partial or total loss of sight.

Blindness caused by cataracts can often be reversed by surgery to remove and replace the cloudy lens. In loss of sight from most other causes, blindness can be prevented only by early detection and treatment of the underlying condition. If blindness does result, it is generally permanent.

Treatment for blindness consists of teaching the affected person how to adapt to a lack of sight. People who have some remaining vision can use vision aids, such as eyeglasses equipped with a telescopic lens, handheld lighted magnifiers, and specially tinted glasses.

Blister

A small swelling of the skin filled with fluid; also known as a vesicle or bulla. Blisters can develop anywhere that the skin experiences friction and frequently occur on the feet. Groups of blisters or blisters involving more than one body location should be evaluated by a doctor for proper treatment. Although they are common and, in most cases, minor injuries, blisters require attention to prevent infection. They must be covered with an adhesive bandage or gauze pad and should not be punctured unless they are painful or prevent a person from performing essential activities such as walking. Large blisters should only be punctured by a dermatologist.

Blood

The fluid that circulates in veins and arteries throughout the body. The blood transports oxygen, nutrients, and other chemicals throughout the body to every tissue and carries away waste materials. It also defends the body against infections. Because blood loss could be so damaging, blood has the capability to help seal damaged blood vessels, create clots at the sites of injuries to stop bleeding, and help repair damaged tissue. The heart pumps the body's blood supply in a continuous cycle through the arteries to the lungs and all other organs and tissues and then back to the heart through the veins. (See CARDIOVASCULAR SYSTEM.)

A typical adult's body contains about 10 pints of blood. At rest, the heart pumps about 10 pints of blood per minute. About 55 percent of the blood's volume is made up of a fluid called plasma, which transports blood cells, proteins, minerals, and nutrients to the body's tissues. The blood cells—including red blood cells, white blood cells, and platelets—account for the remaining blood volume. The three major types of blood cells each have specialized functions (see BLOOD CELLS).

Blood cell count, complete

See BLOOD COUNT; CBC (COMPLETE BLOOD CELL COUNT).

Blood cells

The three major types of cells carried in plasma, the liquid portion of the BLOOD. They have specialized functions. Generally, red blood cells (erythrocytes) carry oxygen to the body; white blood cells (leukocytes) defend against invasions by bacteria, viruses, fungi, and other foreign material; and platelets (thrombocytes) help the blood to clot and repair damaged blood vessels. Most blood cells are manufactured in the bone marrow, and all three types are generated by a series of cell divisions beginning with a single cell called a stem cell. Red blood cells make up about 99 percent of blood cells, while white blood cells and platelets make up about 1 percent.

Blood clotting

The process by which blood turns from a liquid into a semisolid mass to stop bleeding. It begins when an injury to a blood vessel exposes the blood to cells in the blood vessel's lining. The blood cells known as platelets aggregate (adhere to one another) at the site of the injury. As the platelets aggregate, they trigger a cascade of reactions among various proteins known as coagulation factors, which results in the formation of a clot. The clot that seals the point of bleeding is made up of both the aggregated platelets and fibrin. When the wound heals, other proteins help dissolve the clot.

Blood count

A common blood test that provides information on the number and types of cells in the blood; also known as complete blood cell count or CBC. The term "count" refers to the numerical counting of each blood cell type. To do the test, a small quantity of blood is drawn from a vein into a syringe through a needle. Then the number of red blood cells, the number and kind of white blood cells, and the number of platelets in a given volume of the blood are determined. The test also provides data on the total amount of hemoglobin (the oxygen-carrying pigment) in the blood and hematocrit (the fraction of the blood composed of red blood cells).

A blood count is useful for diagnosing and managing many diseases. It can show problems resulting from loss of blood volume (for example, as the result of internal bleeding), abnormalities in blood cells, chronic or acute infection, allergies, and abnormal clotting.

Blood donation

The collection of whole blood or its components from a person. Whole blood donation takes about 10 minutes, while apheresis (in which components of a donor's blood are collected) requires approximately 1 1/2 hours. Blood collection is strictly regulated by the Food and Drug Administration (FDA). Donated blood is used for persons undergoing bone marrow transplant, organ transplant, heart surgery, burn treatment, and treatment after motor vehicle accidents or other trauma. In autologous transfusion, a person donates blood in advance for his or her own use. See also BLOOD TRANSFUSION.

Blood gases

A laboratory test that measures the amounts of oxygen and carbon dioxide in the blood and determines the acidity; also known as arterial blood gas analysis. A sample for blood gases is taken from an artery, usually in the wrist, the groin, or the arm. Blood gas analysis is useful for evaluating diseases that affect breathing, such as pneumonia, chronic obstructive pulmonary disease, and tuberculosis. It also provides information about the effectiveness of oxygen therapy. Information about the acidity of the blood provides a measure of kidney function and can also provide information that can be used to assess the body's metabolism.

Blood groups

A system that classifies blood by the proteins contained in its red blood cells; also known as blood types. Blood group is important in determining the safety of blood transfusions. If blood from one blood group is transfused into a person with a different blood group, antibodies in the recipient's blood will attack the donated blood as a foreign substance. Transfusions between people of the same blood group are almost always successful.

There are four principal blood groups: A, B, AB, and O. The blood groups are further divided by the presence or absence of the Rh factor (see RH INCOMPATIBILITY). Blood with the Rh factor is Rh-positive (+); blood without it is Rh-negative (–). The most common blood group among Americans is O+, followed in order by A+, B+, O–, A–, AB+, B–, and AB–.

Blood groups are inherited in a predictable manner. This makes blood group data useful for identifying the father of a child whose paternity is in dispute.

Blood loss

BLEEDING, or loss of blood from blood vessels, that can occur inter-nally or externally. Direct pressure halts most external bleeding. If bleeding is severe, or if internal bleeding or shock is suspected, emergency assistance should be sought.

Blood poisoning

The popular name for bacterial infection spreading through the blood. See SEPTICEMIA.

Blood pressure

A measurement of the force exerted by the blood against the walls of the arteries. Blood pressure results from two forces. One is the force of the heart as it contracts; the other is the resistance of the arteries to blood flow, which is a function of their flexibility and size. In general, the more blood the heart pumps with each beat and the narrower and less flexible the blood vessels, the higher the blood pressure.

Blood pressure is measured in millimeters of mercury (mm Hg) and given as two numbers written like a fraction, such as 125/75. The first, larger number represents the blood pressure when the heart is contracting, or the systolic pressure. The second, smaller number represents the pressure between beats when the heart is relaxed, or the diastolic pressure.

Blood pressure lower than 120/80 mm Hg is considered optimal for cardiovascular health. Blood pressure of 120 to 139 over 80 to 89 mm Hg indicates that the person has PREHYPERTENSION. Readings that are consistently over 140/90 mm Hg indicate the presence of HYPERTENSION (high blood pressure). Untreated hypertension can lead to damage to the heart, kidneys, and eyes and is a contributing factor to heart attack and stroke. HYPOTENSION (low blood pressure) may cause fainting or dizzy spells. Hypotension is one symptom of shock following serious injury and blood loss, and it may also result from chronic disease or pregnancy.

Blood pressure cuff

The inflatable band placed around the upper arm to measure blood pressure. The blood pressure cuff is part of an instrument called a SPHYG-MOMANOMETER, the most accurate method of measuring blood pressure.

Blood products

The forms in which blood donations are stored before a transfusion. Blood products include whole blood and various blood components, each of which is used for different purposes:

- *WHOLE BLOOD*, which is used to replace blood lost during surgery or following a severe injury, can only be stored for 3 to 4 weeks

- *RED BLOOD CELLS*, which are useful for treating some kinds of chronic anemia that do not respond to medication and for replacing cells lost from bleeding

- *WHITE BLOOD CELLS (GRANU-LOCYTES)*, which can be given to people who have life-threatening infections or abnormally low levels of granulocytes

- *PLATELETS*, which are used to treat people with blood disorders involving clotting

- *PLASMA*, which is used shortly after collection to correct bleeding and clotting disorders, and

- *CLOTTING FACTORS VIII AND IX*, which are used to treat HEMOPHILIA

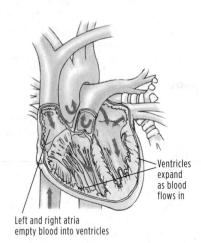

Left and right atria
empty blood into ventricles

Ventricles expand as blood flows in

Diastolic pressure

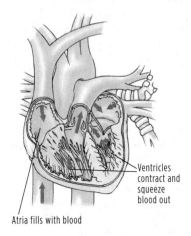

Atria fills with blood

Ventricles contract and squeeze blood out

Systolic pressure

Filling and pumping

Diastolic (dilating) pressure occurs as the heart relaxes and blood flows from the holding chambers (atria) into the pumping chambers (ventricles). Systolic (squeezing) pressure occurs as the ventricles contract and pump blood out of the heart. Blood flows from the right ventricle to the lungs; from the left ventricle to the rest of the body.

Also, immunoglobulins (antibodies) can be concentrated from the plasma of people recovering from viral diseases such as RUBELLA and HEPATITIS B and from the plasma of people who have recently been immunized against diseases such as TETANUS; they can be used to protect people who are unable to produce their own antibodies or who have just been exposed to a viral disease.

Blood smear

A laboratory test that provides information about the number, type, and shape of blood cells; also known as a peripheral smear or differential stain. Once a blood sample has been drawn, the number of white and red blood cells relative to other types of blood cells is counted, any abnormalities in cell shape are noted, and the total number of white blood cells and platelets is roughly estimated. A blood smear also allows doctors to classify the blood by its color and by the shape and size of the cells.

Blood tests

A series of laboratory studies of blood samples used to screen for or to diagnose diseases.

There are hundreds of available blood tests. See BLOOD COUNT; BLOOD GASES; BLOOD SMEAR; CROSSMATCHING. Others include:

- *BLOOD CHEMISTRY* is a group of tests that provides information as to how well major organs are functioning.
- *LIPIDS TESTS*, which measure the blood levels of total cholesterol, high-density lipoproteins, low-density lipoproteins, and triglycerides, all of which have a role in the development of heart disease.

- A *SEDIMENTATION TEST*, which is an indirect evaluation of the body's inflammatory process and may be elevated in cases of infection, inflammation, rheumatoid arthritis, or some cancers (see ESR).

Blood transfusion

The infusion of whole blood or its components directly into the bloodstream to replace blood loss from surgery, injury, or disease. A blood transfusion may also be needed to improve clotting or to enhance the body's ability to transport oxygen to tissues. In a transfusion, a nurse administers the blood intravenously. Before it is transfused, donor blood is carefully screened to make certain it is free from infectious disease organisms and is compatible with the recipient's blood. Incompatibility can provoke serious transfusion reactions such as chills, fever, hives, wheezing, shock, and kidney failure. In autologous transfusion, a person donates blood in advance for his or her own use. In directed donation, family and friends donate the blood for a person's transfusion. See BLOOD DONATION; TRANSFUSION.

Blood urea nitrogen

See KIDNEY FUNCTION TESTS.

Blood vessels

The tubes that carry blood from the heart to the body and back again; a general term for arteries, veins, and capillaries that are structures of the CARDIOVASCULAR SYSTEM.

Blood-brain barrier

A double layer of cells that inhibits substances from crossing from the bloodstream into the fluid that bathes the brain tissues. It protects the brain by slowing or stopping the passage of certain chemical compounds (including some drugs) and disease-causing organisms (such as viruses) from the bloodstream into the brain.

Blow-out fracture

A break in the floor of the bony socket (orbit) surrounding the eye. The usual cause is a hard blow from a nonpenetrating blunt object. The fracture may entrap some of the muscles that move the eye, causing double vision, especially when the person looks up. Other symptoms include bruising around the eye, protrusion of the eyeball, and numbness in the cheek or upper teeth. Tests, including CT (computed tomography) SCANNING, are performed to determine whether eye muscles are involved in the fracture. A blow-out fracture involving muscles requires surgical repair, which is usually performed within 14 days of the injury. If no muscles are involved, if there is no persistent diplopia (double vision), or if no serious cosmetic defect is present, the fracture is allowed to heal on its own.

BMI

See BODY MASS INDEX.

Body mass index

Also called BMI; a measurement of body weight relative to height. The BMI is closely associated with body fat percentage, an important factor that can be difficult to measure. Body weight is more sensitive to fluctuations in muscle mass and water retention than is BMI and, therefore, does not reflect body fat changes as accurately.

When a BMI is above the normal range, a person is considered OVERWEIGHT or obese. A diagnosis of obesity means that an individual weighs 20 percent or more than the average for his or her height. To determine BMI, an individual's weight in pounds is multiplied by 700, divided by the person's height in inches, and divided by the height again. Rather than calculating BMI, health professionals usually consult a table to determine BMI, based on the person's height and weight.

Body piercing

The practice of creating holes in body parts for cosmetic purposes. Body piercing enables people to wear jewelry in such body parts as the earlobes, lips, nose, navel, eyebrows, nipples, and genitals. Body piercing has been practiced in almost every society, chiefly involving ears, nose, and mouth. Nontraditional body piercing has become increasingly popular in Western societies, such as the United States.

Piercing is associated with high infection rates; severe bacterial infections, including TOXIC SHOCK SYNDROME and TETANUS; torn ear lobes and torn nipples; airway obstruction; chipped or cracked teeth; and chewing problems. Body piercing is a potential route of transmission for HIV (human immunodeficiency virus) and other blood-borne diseases if instruments contaminated with blood are used between clients or improperly sterilized.

Boil

A tender, red, inflamed, pus-filled area of skin; also known as a furuncle. Most boils are caused by infection of a hair follicle with staphylococcal (staph) bacteria. Boils most commonly occur on the face, neck, armpits, buttocks, and thighs as painful, red lumps that gradually swell and fill with pus. A head forms with a yellow center, and pain increases as the pressure within the boil increases, until it finally bursts.

Boils should never be squeezed as this can cause the infection to spread. While most boils resolve without treatment within 2 weeks, it is helpful to apply warm compresses to the boil for 30 minutes several times a day. In the meantime, the boil and the surrounding area must be kept clean with antibacterial soap. Applying a sterile dressing prevents spread of draining material, and an antibiotic ointment prevents further infection. A cluster of boils affecting adjacent follicles is called a CARBUNCLE. Carbuncles and severe boils may require

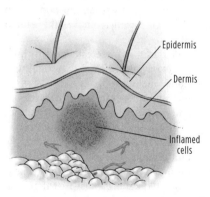

Skin abscess
A boil is an infection deep in the skin, in the underlying layer called the dermis. The dense accumulation of inflamed cells is most often caused by bacteria, but can also result from a clogged pore, inflammation of sweat glands, or in some cases, from prolonged pressure.

surgical draining. In some cases, oral antibiotics are prescribed. People with diabetes, atopic dermatitis, and weakened immune systems are more prone than others to boils, although poor hygiene can be a contributing factor.

Bolus

A relatively large quantity of a substance, such as a dose of a drug; a chewed portion of food; or other substance that is ready to be swallowed. An intravenous bolus is a relatively large volume of fluid or dose of a drug given rapidly and intravenously to speed up or magnify a response.

Bone

The living tissue that makes up the skeleton. Bone is a form of connective tissue (tissue that supports or holds structures of the body together) that is uniquely hard and strong because of a high concentration of the mineral calcium.

A mature bone has several distinct layers: covering the surface except at the ends is a membrane called the PERIOSTEUM; under the periosteum is a layer of hard (cortical) bone tissue. Within the hard bone lies a layer of spongy (cancellous) bone. BONE MARROW lies in the cavities of spongy bone and also in the hollow core of long bones. There are two types of marrow—red marrow, in which blood cells are formed, and yellow marrow that is largely fatty tissue.

Bone tissue contains deposits of calcium and phosphorus that give bone its density and strength. The structure of spongy bone enables it to absorb stress, giving bone considerable resiliency. The bones of the skeleton form a framework that supports parts of the body and protects fragile internal organs and soft tissues. Bone also is the site of the manufacture of blood cells, both red and white. Bone also warehouses calcium and phosphorus and releases these minerals into the bloodstream as necessary.

Bone is continually replacing itself throughout life, a process called remodeling. Bone cells called osteoblasts build up bone by depositing calcium on the structural framework of the tissue, and other cells called osteoclasts break it down and reabsorb it. Until young adulthood, the rate of bone formation exceeds the rate of breakdown, and the density and strength of the bone tissue increases. Between the ages of about 20 and 35, the rate of bone formation starts to fall; after about age 35, the rate of breakdown exceeds the rate of formation, and bone density begins to decrease. See SKELETAL SYSTEM.

Bone abscess

A pus-filled pocket or cavity located on or in the bone and surrounded by inflamed tissue. The bacterial infection that most commonly gives rise to a bone abscess is caused by a staphylococcal infection. (See INFECTION.) Bone abscesses are rare and potentially fatal. They are treated with a surgical procedure to drain the abscess, as well as with appropriate antibiotics. See also OSTEOMYELITIS.

Bone cancer

Cancer that originates in bone tissue. Some cancers can spread to the bones and erroneously are called bone cancer. Also called primary bone cancer, cancer that first develops in bone tissue is uncommon and occurs chiefly in children and adolescents, ages 10 to 25. Cancer can affect any bone, but in adolescence, it typically appears in the long bones of the arms and legs. Bone cancer most often develops in the area around the knee joint. The most common symptom of bone cancer is pain, frequently accompanied by fatigue, fever, weight loss, and anemia. Swelling over a bone can be a sign of bone cancer, particularly if the swelling becomes progressively larger and more tender. Bone cancer can cause bones to fracture.

The condition is assessed by blood tests and by using imaging tools, such as an X ray, a BONE SCAN, CT (computed tomography) SCANNING, or fluoroscopy. Diagnosis is confirmed by a bone biopsy.

Treatment of bone cancer depends on the type, size, location, and stage of the cancer and the age and health of the individual. Surgery is often the primary treatment. Amputation of an affected arm or leg may be necessary, although sometimes surgeons can preserve part of the limb and remove only the cancerous section of a bone, replacing it with an artificial device or a bone graft.

Bone cyst

An abnormal closed cavity or sac lined with tissue and filled with fluid that originates in the bone tissue and is usually noncancerous (benign). Bone cysts are rare, tend to occur in children between the ages of 5 and 15 years, and generally develop in long bones, such as the upper arm bone (humerus) or thighbone (femur), making the affected bones more susceptible to fracture. Bone cysts may be diagnosed by means of X rays, including CT (computed tomography) SCANNING or MRI (magnetic resonance imaging).

Surgery to remove bone cysts may be recommended. Some bone cysts respond to being drained (which is called aspiration) and being injected with a corticosteroid.

Bone density testing

Tests done to evaluate the density of bones. Bone density testing is used to measure bone strength, predict fracture risk, and assess the degree of OSTEOPOROSIS, a condition that results in the bones slowly losing mass and becoming more susceptible to fractures. A certain amount of bone loss is a normal consequence of aging in both men and women. Done periodically, bone density tests can help determine whether and how quickly the bones are losing calcium.

The most accurate imaging technique to measure bone density is DUAL-ENERGY X-RAY ABSORPTIOMETRY (DEXA), an imaging procedure that can detect extremely small degrees of bone loss. DEXA, using a low dose of radiation to detect bone loss, takes only a few minutes.

Bone graft

A surgical procedure to repair lost or damaged bone by replacing it with bone tissue taken from another part of the body or with a compatible synthetic material. Medical procedures that may involve bone grafts include fusion of the spine and of the arm and leg joints, closure of gaps in bones due to trauma or infection, oral or maxillofacial surgery, and the repair of certain bone fractures.

Bone grafts are typically used to fill fracture defects in the growth plate at the end of the long bones in the arms and legs. Generally, the bone tissue or synthetic material is formed to fit into the area needing the graft, and rigid internal fixation is supplied by means of plates, pins, and screws, which hold the grafted, or implanted, material to the healthy bone tissue. Cells of the host bone regenerate on the porous framework of the bone graft, which provides support for the new bone tissue and related structures, stimulating their growth and enabling them to establish new connections between the separated segments of bone.

Bone imaging

Techniques that may use magnetic fields or radiation, often in combination with computers, to record and display images of bone structure. Bone imaging can reveal elements that are important to a complete diagnosis and are not provided by physical examination or laboratory tests. Bone imaging includes conventional X RAYS; CT SCANNING (computed tomography scanning), which sends many X-ray beams from different directions through the area to be observed; and MRI (magnetic resonance imaging), which uses a magnetic field in combination with radio waves to create signals analyzed by a computer to construct an image.

A radionuclide scan, sometimes called a BONE SCAN, is a nuclear medicine procedure that uses a small amount of a radioactive substance as a tracer, and that can indicate if malignant cells have spread from a cancerous tumor to bone tissue. See also ARTHROSCOPIC SURGERY; DUAL-ENERGY X-RAY ABSORPTIOMETRY.

Bone loss

The decline in living bone tissue due to a combination of influences and aging. With age, fat mass increases, while muscle mass and skeletal mass decline. Certain medications can also contribute to bone loss over time by decreasing the body's ability to absorb ingested calcium or vitamin D from the intestines.

Weight-bearing exercise and activities that put stress on bones, including weight-lifting, are known to maintain bone density and may even increase it. Weight training also strengthens muscles, which protect the bones and joints, and may help slow bone loss.

Physicians may advise people who are taking medications that induce bone loss or who are at risk for bone loss to increase their calcium intake or to take a prescription medication that inhibits the breakdown of bone tissue. Women may be prescribed hormone replacement therapy to stimulate greater calcium absorption.

Bone marrow

A soft, organic material rich in blood vessels, found in the cavities and the spongy bone layer of most bones; also known as myeloid tissue. There are two types of bone marrow. Red marrow is the primary production site for blood cells, particularly red blood cells (erythrocytes) and certain kinds of white blood cells (granular leukocytes). Red marrow contains little fat. Yellow marrow gets its color from the large amount of fat it contains; it is usually found in the body's long bones. It produces some types of white blood cells.

Bone marrow biopsy

Microscopic examination of a piece of bone and bone marrow. The procedure can be performed in a doctor's office or outpatient surgery center, using a local anesthetic. Bone marrow biopsy is used to diagnose blood or bone marrow cancers, such as leukemia or multiple myeloma, or to determine if a malignant tumor from another organ of the body has spread to the bone marrow. It is also used to check for infections, to follow up on the effectiveness of treatment, or to find out how well the bone marrow would produce new blood cells if aggressive chemotherapy were to be used.

Bone marrow transplant, allogeneic

The replacement of an individual's defective bone marrow with the bone marrow or stem cells of a healthy donor. Stem cells (cells from which the different types of blood cells develop) are present in normal bone marrow and blood. In an allogeneic transplant, the donor is usually a sibling, other relative, or a nonrelative whose marrow is closely matched to that of the recipient's.

The purpose of a bone marrow transplant is to allow the administration of very large doses of chemotherapy or radiation, doses so large that they may completely destroy the bone marrow. Replacing the damaged bone marrow with new bone marrow helps destroy the cancer and helps the recipient fight off infections. Bone marrow transplant is considered an effective treatment of leukemia and lymphoma.

Bone marrow transplant, autologous

A treatment in which an individual with cancer receives his or her own previously harvested healthy bone marrow or stem cells to replace bone marrow that has been damaged by chemotherapy or radiation. Autologous bone marrow transplant avoids the problems associated with using bone marrow from a donor whose cells may not be a good genetic match for the recipient.

The purpose of a bone marrow transplant is to make it possible to treat someone who has cancer with very high doses of radiation or chemotherapy that may otherwise be fatal.

In the three-step procedure, bone marrow is removed, usually when the disease is in REMISSION or when cancer cells are not detectable, or blood is drawn from the individual. Then the harvested bone marrow or stem cells are frozen in liquid nitrogen and stored; finally, after the individual undergoes high-dose chemotherapy or radiation treatment, which kills all bone marrow cells, the stored healthy bone marrow or stem cells are reintroduced to the patient's body, where they reproduce and replace the destroyed bone marrow. The body will not reject the bone marrow in this instance. However, some cells in the replacement bone marrow may turn out to be cancerous.

Bone scan

A NUCLEAR MEDICINE procedure that uses a radioactive isotope to make an image that identifies areas of bone in which cells are unusually active. The unusual activity could be caused by a tumor, infection, degenerative disorder, or a mending fracture.

Bone scans help doctors identify abnormalities in the bone, but other techniques such as CT SCANNING (computed tomography scanning) and MRI (magnetic resonance imaging) are usually needed to make a definite diagnosis.

Booster

An additional dose of a vaccine administered at determined intervals to promote IMMUNIZATION against a specific disease or diseases and to advance the immune system's ability to defend the body against the disease or diseases. Booster shots for tetanus and diphtheria are commonly recommended for adults at 10-year intervals after the initial vaccination.

Borderline personality disorder

See PERSONALITY DISORDERS.

Bottle-feeding

Feeding of milk or formula to babies usually through sterilized bottles. Most formula is derived from cow's milk that has been fortified with vitamin D and other vitamins, in an effort to make it as much like human milk as possible. Specially prepared formulas are available for infants with milk allergy or specific digestive disorders. See FEEDING, INFANT.

Botulinum toxin, type A

A neurotoxin produced by certain strains of the bacterium Clostridium botulinum, also known as botulism toxin. When consumed in food, botulinum toxin, type A can cause paralysis and death. The neurotoxins produced by *Clostridium* botulinum are among the most potent poisons known. In a purified form, botulinum toxin, type A (known as Botox) has been used to treat blepharospasm (involuntary contraction of the eyelid), strabismus (crossed eyes), and esophageal achalasia (dilated esophagus). When injected under the skin, Botox reduces the appearance of wrinkles for up to 6 months, but then additional injections are needed.

Botulism

A rare, potentially fatal, paralyzing illness caused by a nerve toxin that is formed by certain spores of a bacterium called *Clostridium* botulinum. The bacteria can multiply in low oxygen conditions and form spores that are found in food, most often in home-canned food, raw food, or improperly cooked food; the spores are also present in dust and soil.

There are three basic categories of botulism: food-borne botulism; wound botulism, when an open wound is infected with the bacteria; and infant botulism, which occurs when children younger than 1 year of age consume food containing the spores of the bacteria, which then grow in the intestines and release toxins into the nervous system. It is believed that infants younger than 1 year of age have not yet developed sufficient beneficial digestive bacteria to control botulism spores. Infant botulism may be linked to some cases of SUDDEN INFANT DEATH SYNDROME (SIDS), because breathing is affected in severe cases.

The symptoms of food-borne and wound botulism may include DOUBLE VISION, blurred vision, drooping eyelids, slurred speech, difficulty swallowing, dry mouth, constipation, and muscle weakness. These symptoms generally occur within 18 to 36 hours of eating contaminated food, but may be experienced as soon as 6 hours or as long as 10 days after exposure. Infant botulism causes symptoms including lethargy, poor feeding, constipation, poor muscle tone, and weak crying or sucking. In adults and infants, the symptoms are considered a medical emergency because the illness can be fatal.

A clinical history and physical examination may suggest botulism, but medical tests are essential for ruling out other possible conditions with similar symptoms. The tests may include brain scans, spinal fluid examinations, and ELECTROMYOGRAPHY (EMG). Diagnosis is usually confirmed by testing for the particular bacteria in the stool.

When food-borne and wound botulism are diagnosed early, the treatment of choice is giving the person oral activated charcoal if it can be administered within 1 to 2 hours of the start of symptoms. Adults may also be treated with an antitoxin medication that blocks the action of the toxins circulating in the bloodstream. This treatment can take many weeks. If respiratory failure and paralysis have occurred, treatment may include the use of a ventilator with full-time nursing care for an extended time. Paralysis slowly subsides after several weeks of treatment. Wound botulism may require surgery.

Bougie

A slender, cylindrical instrument inserted into tubular body passages. A bougie may be rigid or flexible, hollow or solid. Bougies are commonly

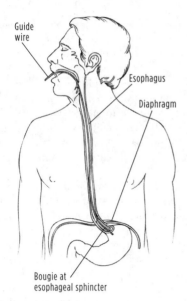

Guide wire

Esophagus

Diaphragm

Bougie at esophageal sphincter

Expanding a passage

To expand an esophagus narrowed by disease, a doctor may insert bougies (cylindrical rods with rounded tips) of increasing size down a guide wire into the passageway.

used to dilate the urethra, to open constricted areas for examination, or to give a person medication.

Bow legs

An outward curving of the bones in the legs. A normal part of development, bow legs are common in children younger than age 2. As a child grows, the curve normally straightens. Bow legs that persist beyond age 2 and into adolescence usually are an inherited trait. In rare cases, they are the result of a more serious underlying condition, such as RICKETS (a vitamin D deficiency that causes bones to soften), a fracture, infection, tumor, or JUVENILE RHEUMATOID ARTHRITIS.

If bow legs persist after age 6, children are usually referred to a pediatric orthopedist for treatment. At this age,

a corrective cast or brace (see BRACE, ORTHOPEDIC) may be required to correct the problem. In severe cases, corrective surgery may be necessary. In younger children, these measures are not recommended and may cause physical or emotional damage.

Bowel

Another name for the INTESTINE, that portion of the canal that extends from the stomach to the anus.

Bowel movements, abnormal

A sign of a disorder in the digestive system. Normal frequency of bowel movements can range from as many as three a day to as few as three a week. Although changes in bowel habits may be due to a harmless condition, a sudden and sustained change may be a symptom of an underlying disease.

Changes in bowel movements that last longer than a week require medical attention. Three or more loose movements a day are considered DIARRHEA. Persistent diarrhea can be a sign of an underlying disorder, such as COLITIS or CROHN DISEASE. In constipation, bowel movements become infrequent and feces are hard and dry. The appearance of blood in stools requires immediate medical attention. Tests that a doctor may order to determine the cause of abnormal bowel movements include a GASTROINTESTINAL (GI) SERIES, GASTROSCOPY, PROCTOSCOPY, SIGMOIDOSCOPY, and COLONOSCOPY.

Bowel sounds

Sounds produced by liquid and air moving through the digestive tract. Doctors use a stethoscope to assess bowel sounds. Normal bowel sounds include irregular, gurgling noises. Loud, rumbling, gurgling noises occur during hyperactive intestinal peristalsis (the wavelike muscle movement that moves food through the digestive tract). Hyperactivity may be the result of GASTROENTERITIS, DIARRHEA, or hunger. Rushed, high-pitched bowel sounds can be an early indication of an intestinal obstruction. The absence of bowel sounds can be a serious symptom of an obstruction.

Bowen disease

The earliest form of SQUAMOUS CELL CARCINOMA, a type of skin cancer; also known as squamous cell carcinoma in situ. In Bowen disease, cancer cells are entirely within the epidermis (the outer layer of skin) and have not yet entered the dermis (the middle layer of skin). Skin cancer is the most common type of cancer in the United States. Its principal cause is long-term sun exposure. Light skin and a family or personal history of skin cancer are additional risk factors. When Bowen disease occurs on the anal or genital skin, it is often related to a sexually transmitted infection with the HUMAN PAPILLOMAVIRUS that causes genital warts.

Bowen disease is characterized by red, scaly, crusted patches on the skin. Patches are often larger than half an inch in diameter. Like other forms of skin cancer, Bowen disease is diagnosed through a biopsy. Early detection is critical. The cancer is removed by fairly minor surgery.

Brace, orthopedic

An appliance that supports a bone or joint structure and its associated muscles, tendons, and ligaments to aid in repair following injury or surgery or that is worn to promote proper positioning of the spine or the extremities. Orthopedic braces may be prescribed for the treatment of instability in the shoulder or knee and to treat conditions including kyphosis (excessive backward curvature of the spine).

Braces, dental

Metal or plastic appliances worn on the teeth that apply steady, gentle pressure over an extended period to move teeth into the proper position. See ORTHODONTICS.

Brachial plexus block

A method of anesthetizing the lower arm and hand for surgery by injecting medication into the bundle of nerves (brachial plexus) in which the branches control feeling in the arm. A brachial plexus block is a form of regional anesthesia (see ANESTHESIA, REGIONAL). In most cases, the injection into the area of the nerve is made with the person under CONSCIOUS SEDATION, a method of controlling pain that leaves the person awake but pain-free.

The complications of brachial plexus block include damage to the nerve, which can cause temporary paralysis, and possibly muscle weakness, which can last up to several months. Injection of an anesthetic agent into a vein may lead to seizures and cardiac arrest.

Brachytherapy

A type of internal radiation therapy used to treat cancer. In brachytherapy, also known as interstitial radiation therapy, a radioactive source is sealed in a container and placed on the surface of the body, near the affected area, or implanted directly into the tumor in the form of small radioactive "seeds" of gold or iodine. This procedure permits a very high but localized dose of radiation to be administered to a tumor without endangering surrounding tissue. Brachytherapy is most often used to treat tumors of the head, neck, prostate, cervix, and breast. It is generally used in combination with external radiation. The usual side effects include inflammation, redness, scarring, and discomfort.

Bradycardia

A slower than normal heartbeat, typically less than 60 beats per minute. When the heart beats too slowly, it fails to provide the body with enough blood to function properly. The usual symptoms of bradycardia are fatigue, shortness of breath, light-headedness or dizziness, or sudden fainting. Since these symptoms can result from conditions other than bradycardia, testing is required to isolate their cause.

There are three principal types of abnormal bradycardia: SICK SINUS SYNDROME, HEART BLOCK (also known as atrioventricular, or AV, block), and BUNDLE BRANCH BLOCK.

When bradycardia requires treatment, the person usually is instructed to stop taking any medication that may slow the heartbeat. In some cases, a PACEMAKER is implanted in the chest to maintain a normal heartbeat.

Brain

The principal and most complex organ in the NERVOUS SYSTEM; the major control center for both basic body system maintenance and the highest levels of thought, emotion, and learning.

The brain and the spinal cord extending down from it together make up the CENTRAL NERVOUS SYSTEM. From the brain and spinal cord, a network of nerves branches out to connect the central nervous system to every part of the body. These nerve pathways are called the peripheral nervous system. A large part of brain activity is largely directed toward regulating such basic, continuous, and vital body functions as breathing and heartbeat.

Because the brain operates continuously to ensure the body's survival, and to direct higher functions such as voluntary movements and conscious thought, it requires an enormous supply of blood. The brain weighs about 3 pounds, but 20 percent of the body's blood supply is channeled to the brain at any time. Blood flows to the brain through four arteries, two on either side of the neck called the carotid arteries, and two running along the spinal

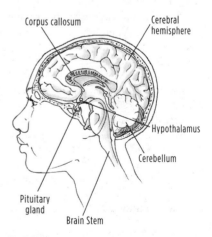

Corpus callosum
Cerebral hemisphere
Hypothalamus
Cerebellum
Pituitary gland
Brain Stem

The Brain

The brain and the brain stem, compared with the other structures in the head and neck, are by far the largest and most complex. The brain is protected by the bony skull.

cord called the vertebral arteries. To protect the soft, gelatinous brain and its blood vessels, three layers of membranes called the MENINGES lie under the skull. (The meninges also cover the spinal cord.)

The brain itself is composed of three main structures: the CEREBEL-LUM, the brain stem, and the forebrain, mostly occupied by the large CEREBRUM, but also including the thalamus, the HYPOTHALAMUS, and the tiny PITUITARY GLAND.

Brain abscess

Also known as a cerebral abscess, a pus-filled cavity surrounded by inflamed tissue in the brain. A brain abscess is a life-threatening medical emergency. Symptoms of a brain abscess include headache, muscle weakness, loss of sensation, vomiting, fever, and seizures. These may come on gradually or suddenly. Diagnosis is made through physical and neurological examination and tests such as a blood culture, chest X ray, ELECTROENCEPHALOGRAM (EEG), CT (computed tomography) SCANNING, or MRI (magnetic resonance imaging). Treatment includes medications such as antimicrobials and antibiotics as well as diuretics and corticosteroids to reduce brain swelling. In some cases, surgery is necessary.

Brain damage

Injury, degeneration, or death of nerve cells within the brain. Damage can be wide and diffuse or localized and specific.

Diffuse brain damage can lead to severe mental or physical handicap. The most significant cause of diffuse damage is hypoxia, or an inadequate level of oxygen reaching the brain. Other causes of diffuse brain damage include encephalitis and some degenerative disorders.

Localized brain damage can result in specific deficits of brain functions such as speech, balance, or coordination and depends on the part of the brain that is affected and the nature and extent of the damage. Head trauma is a common cause of localized brain damage. Other causes include BRAIN TUMOR, BRAIN ABSCESS, STROKE, and ISCHEMIA.

Treatment of brain damage depends on the diagnosis of its underlying cause. Unfortunately, nerve cells do not recover their function after they have been destroyed. However, other parts of the brain can sometimes be trained to compensate for damaged areas. Rehabilitation is a very important part of any treatment plan for people with brain damage.

Brain death

Irreversible cessation of all functions of the entire brain, including the brain stem. This definition of death was developed by Harvard Medical School in 1968. While brain death is diagnosed by a careful clinical examination, the diagnosis is confirmed by a variety of tests that determine an absence of reflexes, unresponsiveness to stimuli, a lack of spontaneous respiration or movement, and the absence of electrical activity of the brain as indicated by a flat ELECTROENCEPHALOGRAM (EEG).

If after 24 hours there is no change in a person's status, he or she is declared dead. This definition of brain death allows for the certification of death even if the lungs and heart continue to function with assistance.

Brain hemorrhage

See HEMORRHAGE, CEREBRAL and HEM-ORRHAGE, SUBARACHNOID.

Brain imaging

The process of making pictures of the brain and its structures. The most commonly used brain scans are CT SCANNING (computed tomography scanning), MRI (magnetic resonance imaging), and PET SCANNING (positron emission tomography scanning). Angiography is useful for imaging the blood vessels of the brain. A relatively new brain scan is called SPECT (single-photon emission computed tomography). New techniques on the horizon include magnetic resonance spectroscopy (to detect abnormalities in the brain's biochemical processes) and near-infrared spectroscopy (to detect oxygen levels in brain tissue).

Brain tumor

An abnormal growth of tissue found inside the skull.

Tumors are classified as benign or malignant (cancerous). In most parts of the body, benign tumors are not especially dangerous. However, any abnormal growth in the skull can put undue pressure on sensitive tissues and impair the function of the nerve tissue.

Tumors are further classified as primary (originating in the brain) or secondary (having traveled to the brain, or metastasized, from another location). The central nervous system (CNS) consists of the brain and spinal cord; brain tumors are more common than spinal cord tumors. Primary CNS tumors such as gliomas and meningiomas are named by their location, the type of cells they are made

of, or both. (See also GLIOMA; MENINGIOMA.)

The symptoms of brain tumors vary according to their size, type, and location. They commonly include headache, seizures, nausea, vomiting, vision or hearing problems, behavioral and cognitive symptoms, motor problems, and balance difficulties. Symptoms generally reflect the particular area of the brain that is damaged by the abnormal growth.

When the medical history, symptoms, and the neurological examination suggest the possibility of a brain tumor, a number of tests can confirm the diagnosis. These include neurological examination, imaging studies, ELECTROENCEPHALOGRAM (EEG), LUMBAR PUNCTURE, and biopsy. Imaging tests may include CT SCANNING, MRI scanning, and PET scanning. A definitive diagnosis requires a biopsy.

Surgery, radiation, and chemotherapy are the three most commonly used treatments.

Bran

The skin or husk of cereal grains such as wheat, rye, and oats. Bran provides one of the most concentrated sources of dietary fiber (see FIBER, DIETARY). A diet high in bran and other fiber-rich foods helps maintain proper bowel function and prevent intestinal disorders ranging from constipation to irritable bowel syndrome.

Braxton Hicks contractions

Mild contractions of the uterus during the final weeks of pregnancy. Braxton Hicks contractions, named for the doctor who first described them, are not true LABOR contractions, although they are often mistaken for them. Mild, irregular, and usually painless, Braxton Hicks contractions last from 30 seconds to 2 minutes. Also known as false labor, they do not indicate the start of true labor but are a sign that the body is preparing for it.

BRCA

Breast cancer genes. When present in a mutated form, these genes indicate that a woman has inherited a tendency to develop breast cancer. Their presence also increases a woman's risk for ovarian cancer.

Antioncogenes normally protect against tumor development. BRCA-1 and BRCA-2 are antioncogenes, and women who have mutations of the BRCA-1 and BRCA-2 genes are less able to keep abnormal cells from dividing. Thus, a woman's risk of developing breast cancer increases significantly if she is born without enough normal antioncogenes or if her antioncogenes mutate later in life. Genetic testing can be done to detect BRCA mutations. Experts recommend that women who have these altered genes should be monitored closely with frequent mammograms and breast examinations.

Breakthrough bleeding

Bleeding (spotting or staining) between menstrual periods. In some women, a small amount of breakthrough bleeding occurs as a normal part of their ovulation. It is important for a woman to report breakthrough bleeding to her doctor, because it can occasionally be a sign of a reproductive system disorder, such as CERVICAL POLYPS, CERVICITIS, ENDOMETRIOSIS, or cancer. Breakthrough bleeding may also occur dur-

ing the first few months after a woman begins taking birth control pills, as her body adjusts to the new levels of hormones. See MENSTRUATION.

Breast

One of the pair of organs attached to the chest consisting of milk-producing glands, blood vessels, fat, and connective tissue. In women, the foremost function of the breasts is to secrete milk to feed an infant. The breast is also sensitive to sexual stimulation.

Breast abscess

An infected area of the breast that fills with pus and forms a lump. Symptoms of a breast abscess include swelling, tenderness, and redness and may include fever. An abscess most commonly occurs in women who are breast-feeding. It may be preceded by MASTITIS, an inflammation of the breast tissue caused when bacteria from the baby's mouth enter the breast tissue through cracks in the nipples. A woman who suspects she has a breast abscess or has a breast lump should see her doctor. For a breast abscess, the doctor may prescribe antibiotics to fight the infection and an anti-inflammatory medication, such as aspirin or ibuprofen, to reduce pain and fever. If antibiotic treatments do not eliminate the abscess, the pus may need to be drained by the doctor.

Breast cancer

For symptom chart see BREAST PAIN OR LUMPS, page xii.

A malignant disease in which cancer cells develop in the breast tissue and can spread to other organs. Breast cancer is the second most common cancer (after skin cancer) among women and the second most common cause of cancer death (after lung cancer) in women. Breast cancer can also occur in men, though infrequently. Women's breast tissue contains fat cells and glandular tissue that form milk-producing lobules. The lobules are separated by fibrous tissue and transport milk through thin tubes called ducts. Breast cancer most commonly develops as a lump in the fibrous tissue or in the ducts.

Breast lumps can be discovered during a monthly BREAST SELF-EXAMINATION or a doctor's annual breast examination. A MAMMOGRAM, a special X ray of a breast, can often detect breast cancers that are too small to feel, although some tumors cannot be detected by a mammogram. Also, although mammography may suggest that a lump is cancerous, it cannot differentiate a cancerous tumor from a benign one with certainty. Besides a lump, other signs of breast cancer include swelling, dimpled skin, breast tenderness, or indentation or nipple discharge.

When a breast lump has been discovered, or the results of a mammogram are abnormal, the doctor usually will conduct other tests, such as aspiration, ULTRASOUND SCANNING, or a BIOPSY to help diagnose or rule out cancer. If the biopsy indicates that a lump is malignant, further evaluation may involve tests to assess the extent or stage of the tumor. Breast cancer stages range from carcinoma in situ at stage 0 to the most serious, stage IV, in which the cancer has spread to other organs in the body.

Treatment options for breast cancer include:

SURGERY Most women with breast cancer have surgery to remove the cancer from the breast. Usually some of the lymph nodes under the arm are also taken out and examined microscopically to see if they contain cancer cells. A newer technique called sentinel node biopsy helps limit the number of lymph nodes that need to be removed for staging. In this technique, a dye is injected into the area where the lump is in order to determine which lymph node drains the area. The dye enables the surgeon to remove those lymph nodes most likely to have cancer but still limit the extent of the surgery.

Two types of operations are performed to treat breast cancer: LUMP-ECTOMY, in which only the lump and surrounding breast tissue are removed, and MASTECTOMY, in which the entire breast is removed.

RADIATION THERAPY High doses of X rays are sometimes used to kill cancer cells and shrink tumors. Radiation may come from a machine outside the body (external radiation therapy) or from introducing radioactive substances (radioisotopes) into the area where the cancer cells are found (internal radiation therapy). Radiation treatments last only a few minutes each time, but typically must be given 5 days a week for about 6 weeks. Radiation therapy is given following a lumpectomy to destroy any cancer cells that may remain in the woman's breast. Side effects of radiation therapy may include nausea or loss of appetite, swelling and redness of the breast, tiredness, muscle pain, and sensitivity to exposure to the sun.

CHEMOTHERAPY If tests show that cancer cells are present in the lymph nodes or have spread to other parts of the woman's body, drugs that kill cancer cells are prescribed. Chemotherapy is most effective in younger (premenopausal) women whose lymph nodes show signs of cancer. Side effects of chemotherapy vary with the types of drugs used, but can include nausea, hair loss, and fatigue.

HORMONAL THERAPY The presence of hormone receptors in breast cancer cells makes it more likely that the cancer cells will respond to hormonal therapy. Hormonal therapy can block hormones from stimulating cancer cells to grow. This is done by using drugs that block the action of hormones (particularly estrogen) or by surgical removal of organs that create hormones, such as the ovaries.

The chance of recovery and choice of treatment depend on the stage of the cancer (whether it is only in the breast or has spread to other organs), the type of breast cancer, specific characteristics of the cancer cells, and whether the cancer has been found in both breasts. A woman's age, weight, general health, desire for future pregnancy, and whether she is still having menstrual periods can all influence the prognosis and choice of treatment.

Breast cancer genes

See BRCA.

Breast enlargement

A surgical procedure to increase the size of the breasts by inserting a fluid or gel-filled implant between the breast tissue and the chest wall. Also called breast augmentation, breast enlargement is typically done on a woman who has lost most or all of a breast to cancer. Breast enlargement surgery is also performed on women who have one breast that is markedly smaller than the other and on women who choose, for cosmetic reasons, to enlarge their breasts.

The implant most commonly used today consists of a silicone shell, filled with saline solution or salt water, that has the consistency of natural breast tissue. For a woman who is having her breast reconstructed after cancer surgery (MASTECTOMY), the surgeon may use tissues from elsewhere in the woman's body during the surgery (see BREAST RECONSTRUCTION). Typically, the surgery takes 1 to 2 hours. The breast enlargement procedure may be combined with a BREAST LIFT to provide the best appearance.

After breast enlargement, mammograms should be continued at the regular intervals recommended by the physician. Breasts that have been surgically enlarged require a special mammogram technique; women should use a mammography facility that is familiar with this technique.

Breast lift

A surgical procedure to restore a more youthful shape to breasts that have sagged due to aging, weight loss, pregnancy, or breast-feeding. A breast lift is also known as a mastopexy. In some cases, the procedure is combined with BREAST ENLARGEMENT to add fullness and volume to the reshaped breast. Breast lifts are most successful in women who have relatively small breasts and do not plan to have any more children.

A breast lift does leave permanent scars. At first, the scars are red and lumpy, but they become less obvious with time and often fade to no more than thin, white lines. Usually the scars are placed so that they cannot be seen while the person is normally dressed. Excessive bleeding and infection of the surgical incision are possible but rare complications of a breast lift. Either condition can widen the scars that remain after the procedure.

Breast lump

A mass in the breast frequently detected by a woman during BREAST SELF-EXAMINATION or by a doctor during an annual examination. Breast lumps are common and usually are not cancerous. In addition to cancer, a breast lump may be a sign of FIBROCYSTIC BREASTS or FIBROADENOMA, or a BREAST ABSCESS. See also BREAST CANCER.

Breast milk

Mother's milk. Beginning with the COLOSTRUM produced the first few days after childbirth, breast milk provides babies with the ideal balance of nutrients in forms readily available to the infant's immature digestive tract, plus valuable protection against disease. See also BREAST-FEEDING.

Breast pump

A device used to extract breast milk without nursing. Breast pumps can be rented or purchased and can be operated manually or electrically by battery or on house current.

Breast reconstruction

A surgical procedure to create a new breast to replace one that has been removed, usually because of cancer (see BREAST CANCER). Breast reconstruction can be performed when the breast is removed in a MASTECTOMY or at a later date. The surgery serves cosmetic and psychological purposes, allowing a woman who has lost a breast to disease to recover a sense of physical wholeness. It does not increase or decrease chances for further breast cancer.

Breast reconstruction requires more than one surgical procedure. Some women and their surgeons decide to begin the series of procedures at the same time that the mastectomy is performed. Others prefer to wait until after healing from the mastectomy is complete and then begin reconstruction.

Two types of reconstruction are available. The choice between them depends on a number of factors, both medical and personal, and should be made by the woman and her surgeon.

The most common technique, called skin expansion, involves stretching the skin to accommodate a synthetic breast implant after mastectomy (removal of the breast). Following traditional mastectomy, the surgeon inserts a balloon expander under the skin of the chest where the breast and skin have been removed. In the other techniques, flap reconstruction, a new breast mound is fashioned from skin and underlying tissue taken from another part of the body, such as the back, abdomen, or buttocks. See BREAST ENLARGEMENT; BREAST LIFT; and BREAST REDUCTION.

Breast reduction

The surgical removal of skin, fat, and underlying tissue to make the breast smaller. Breast reduction is performed most often to solve the problems faced by women with very large, heavy breasts. The excessive weight can cause neck and back pain, skeletal deformities, bra strap indentations in the skin, skin irritation, and even breathing problems. Overly large breasts may create a high degree of self-consciousness.

The procedure is also performed in women who have had a BREAST RECONSTRUCTION following the surgical removal of a breast because of cancer. In this case, the reduction serves to make the remaining natural breast more similar in appearance to the reconstructed breast.

In almost all cases, breast reduction is performed in a hospital with the patient asleep under general anesthesia. The entire procedure takes from 3 to 5 hours, occasionally longer. In the most common procedure, an incision is made that encircles the areola and follows the curve of the crease below the breast. The surgeon then removes excess skin, glandular tissue, and fat and moves the nipple and areola into a new, higher position.

Possible complications include bleeding, infection, the collection of blood under the skin (hematoma), and permanent loss of sensation in the breast or nipple. The nipple and areola may not graft properly because of a disrupted blood supply.

Breast self-examination

For symptom chart see Breast pain or lumps, page xii.

A visual and physical examination of one's own breasts in order to detect breast lumps. Monthly self-examination is recommended. During a self-examination, a woman checks for visual changes in the breasts, including alterations in texture, color, shape, and size. Fingertips are used gently to feel for lumps in the breast tissue. The detection of a new lump requires a visit to the doctor for further evaluation. See BREAST LUMP; BREAST CANCER; and MAMMOGRAM.

Breast-feeding

Nourishing an infant with milk from a woman's breast. Breast-feeding, also called nursing, is the medically preferred way to feed a baby; it is inexpensive, nurturing, and convenient and benefits both the mother and child. Breast-feeding traditionally has been thought to provide protection against pregnancy, but it is not a reliable means of birth control.

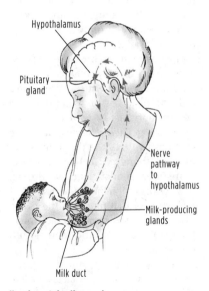

Hypothalamus

Pituitary gland

Nerve pathway to hypothalamus

Milk-producing glands

Milk duct

How breast-feeding works

When a baby sucks on the mother's breast, he or she triggers the let-down reflex. The baby's sucking action stimulates nerve endings in the areola (the pigmented area surrounding the nipple) of the breast. Nerve impulses carry a message to the hypothalamus (a structure at the base of the brain) via the pituitary gland (a gland in the brain that produces and stimulates many hormones) to cause the production of oxytocin. Oxytocin contracts muscles in the alveoli to release milk through the milk ducts in the breast.

Breast milk provides all the nutrients and proteins that an infant needs in the first few months of life. It also contains antibodies that protect babies from illness. Breast-fed babies have fewer infections of the ears and digestive and respiratory tracts than bottle-fed infants; they have a significantly reduced risk for many acute and chronic diseases, develop fewer food allergies, and are less likely to become constipated.

Most pediatricians recommend that breast-feeding be continued at least throughout the first year of an infant's life. If weaning becomes necessary, doctors recommend formula over cow's milk.

Most women can breast-feed. However, prior surgery, medications, or an illness may reduce a woman's milk supply. Breast-feeding may not be appropriate for women who are undergoing chemotherapy, who are HIV-positive (HIV is the human immunodeficiency virus that causes acquired immunodeficiency syndrome, or AIDS), or who have HEPATITIS B (a viral disease that damages the liver). Medications and some types of infection can pass from the mother into breast milk.

For any persistent nursing problems, a doctor, nurse, or lactation specialist should be contacted. La Leche League, an international volunteer group, provides reliable information and support for women who are breast-feeding.

Breath, shortness of

The sensation of having difficulty breathing comfortably. Shortness of breath is also referred to as DYSPNEA and is commonly associated with exercise or physical exertion. See also ASTHMA; BREATHING PROBLEMS; HEART; HEART ATTACK; LUNG.

Breathing

The process of taking air into the lungs and letting it out again. In breathing, air is inhaled into the lungs through the nose or mouth as a result of muscle contractions, and it is exhaled as a result of muscle relaxation.

Breathing exercises

Exercises intended to promote deep, slow, calm breathing to maximize the amount of oxygen in the blood. Breathing exercises enable the breather to use the lungs to their full capacity by emphasizing 'abdominal' or 'diaphragmatic' breathing, in which the diaphragm (the muscle separating the chest from the abdominal cavity) is used to its full potential. Also, many people use breathing exercises to manage stress.

Breathing problems

Difficulties with normal respiration that may be caused by structural irregularities in the respiratory system, acid-base irregularities, or infections that affect the organs involved in breathing. During normal breathing, air is taken in through the nose and propelled to the back of the throat and the larynx, or voice box. The air passes through the windpipe and enters the bronchi, or airways, which distribute the inhaled air to the air sacs of the lungs, where oxygen and carbon dioxide are exchanged. Any inflammation, abnormality, or obstruction in these structures can inhibit the flow of air and produce breathing problems.

Movements of the diaphragm, the ribs, and the muscles between the ribs allow the chest to expand during this process. Abnormalities that inhibit these movements can decrease the flow of air and result in breathing problems.

Breathing problems can be a symptom of an underlying medical condition. WHEEZING, the high-pitched whistling or purring sound that occurs on exhalation, may be caused by a respiratory infection (such as the common cold [see COLD, COMMON]), allergies, ASTHMA, exposure to toxic fumes, an obstruction in the airways, PNEUMONIA, or a genetic abnormality of the lungs. Wheezing should be evaluated medically.

Breech delivery

A birth in which the baby proceeds through the cervix in a BREECH PRESENTATION, buttocks-first or feetfirst. At birth, most babies are in a head-down position, facing the mother's spine; about 3 or 4 percent of babies are born in a breech position. A breech baby can be delivered vaginally, but a CESAREAN SECTION is often performed if labor does not progress, the woman's pelvis is too narrow for the baby to pass through it, or the baby shows signs of distress. The decision may also depend on the physician's level of experience in breech delivery.

Breech presentation

A condition in pregnancy or labor in which, instead of the head, the baby's buttocks, foot, or feet, are positioned against the mother's cervix. In most deliveries, the baby moves into a head-down, facing-back position. But about 3 to 4 percent of babies are in a breech presentation at delivery. A breech presentation is more likely in

pregnancies with a small fetus, more than one fetus, or too much or too little amniotic fluid. Women who have had several children are also at greater risk for a breech presentation because the muscles of the abdomen and uterus are more relaxed and permit the fetus to move more easily into a breech position.

Three types of breech presentation occur. In a frank breech position, the baby's buttocks present with the hips bent and legs extended. In a complete breech, the buttocks present with the hips and knees flexed. In a single- or double-footling breech, one or both of the baby's feet present before the buttocks. See also BREECH DELIVERY.

Bridge, dental

A dental appliance of false teeth that is attached to natural teeth on either side. A fixed bridge is attached to the teeth that have been filed down in order to be fitted with crowns (see CROWN, DENTAL). Fixed dental bridges are more commonly used than removable, partial denture bridges, except in cases in which there are several adjacent teeth missing or the span of empty space is relatively wide. Unlike partial dentures, fixed dental bridges cannot be taken out by the person wearing them.

Bronchiectasis

A condition that refers to the dilation (widening) of portions of the airways, called the bronchi, that branch off the lower part of the windpipe. Bronchiectasis occurs as a result of damage to tissue of the bronchial wall. The bronchial tissue becomes chronically inflamed, thickened, and flaccid. Parts of the tissue are damaged or destroyed, weakening the bronchial wall. Excess mucus is produced and collects in the bronchi, which promotes the growth of bacteria in the area. Infected secretions from the bacterial infection continue to pool and further damage the tissue of the airway wall. The infection and inflammation can spread to the lung tissue, resulting in bronchial pneumonia (see BRONCOPNEUMONIA).

A chronic cough with mucus may be the first and only symptom. Coughing up blood may also occur, and the amount of blood can be massive if the damage has also eroded the blood vessels in the bronchial wall. Coughing spells commonly occur early in the morning and late in the day. Wheezing and shortness of breath (see BREATH, SHORTNESS OF) are symptoms of widespread bronchiectasis. Severe disease may cause low levels of oxygen that cause heart strain. The heart strain may in turn cause swelling in the feet and legs and labored breathing.

Causes of bronchiectasis include respiratory infections, airway obstructions, inhalation of toxic substances, aspiration of stomach acid or food particles, certain genetic conditions such as CYSTIC FIBROSIS, and abnormalities in immune function.

Bronchiectasis is diagnosed on the basis of characteristic symptoms, X-ray findings, and indications of associated conditions such as chronic bronchitis, emphysema, and asthma.

Underlying infections are generally treated with antibiotics, often prescribed for long-term use to prevent recurrent infections. Anti-inflammatory medications, including corticosteroids, may be prescribed, as may medications that thin the pus and mucus to help drain the accumu-lated fluid. Oxygen therapy is useful if the blood oxygen concentration is low, and diuretics may be used to control swelling associated with heart failure. Bronchodilator medications often prove helpful in alleviating shortness of breath and wheezing. In rare cases, surgery is suggested.

Bronchioles

Small airways in the lungs that branch off the bronchi (large tubes) within the lung. The bronchioles terminate in clusters of air sacs called alveoli, deep within LUNG tissue.

Bronchiolitis

Inflammation of the bronchioles, usually due to a viral lung infection. Bronchiolitis is most commonly caused by respiratory synctial virus (RSV). It generally occurs in children younger than 2 years who usually contract the infection during the winter and early spring. Older people, people with heart or lung disease, and people who have immune deficiency disorders may also be susceptible. The virus is contracted when infectious material comes in contact with mucous membranes of the eyes, mouth, or nose. It is spread by the respiratory secretions of infected persons, either by contact with airborne droplets from their coughs or sneezes or by contact with contaminated surfaces and objects. The virus can be destroyed by washing the hands with soap and water and by using disinfectants on contaminated surfaces.

Initial symptoms of bronchiolitis include excess nasal mucus and a low fever for 2 to 3 days. This is followed by coughing, labored breathing, and wheezing for the next 2 to 3 days. Symptoms last for about 7 to 15 days, and most children completely recover. Some young children may require hospitalization, particularly infants younger than 6 months.

The most common approach to treatment of mild infections in children is alleviating symptoms: acetaminophen is generally given to reduce fever, increased liquids are given to relieve dehydration, a mild cough syrup is given to decrease cough, a steam-filled bathroom from hot running water in a shower or tub may also quiet coughing, and a cool-mist vaporizer may be used in the bedroom during sleep to keep airways moist.

Bronchitis

An illness caused by inflammation of the mucous lining of the airways, called bronchi. Bronchitis occurs when the bronchial tubes become irritated. The irritation may be caused by cigarette smoking or by bacterial or viral respiratory infections. The viral infections responsible for the common cold (see COLD, COMMON) are the most frequent cause of bronchitis, which occurs when the virus spreads to the airways. The walls of the airways respond to the irritation by secreting copious, thick mucus, which clogs the inflamed, swollen airways and obstructs the flow of air through them.

Symptoms of acute (sudden) bronchitis include a productive cough and possibly a feeling of tightness in the chest, chills, or a low fever. Symptoms of chronic (long-term) bronchitis include a persistent cough that produces mucus for three months a year for at least two years.

When medical consultation is sought, the diagnosis is generally based on the discolored sputum that is produced by coughing. In some cases, one of the BRONCHODILATORS may be prescribed to open the narrowed airways. Otherwise, treatment is generally based on self-help strategies, including aspirin for fever (do not use aspirin for children), bed rest, and increased fluids. Over-the-counter cough medicine may be helpful if coughing interferes with sleep. Avoiding inhaled irritants, especially cigarette smoking and secondhand smoke, is essential. The use of a vaporizer may be beneficial because warm, humid air helps ease the irritated airways.

Chronic bronchitis is diagnosed by the characteristic cough and its ongoing occurrence over several years. The diagnosis may be confirmed by a medical history, a physical examination, and an evaluation of lung function test results and chest X rays. If detected early and if the person does not smoke, he or she may expect a good survival rate. However, survival rates are low for people with severe forms of this illness that go untreated and for those who continue smoking.

The first line of treatment is to stop smoking. Care must be taken to avoid respiratory infections that will exacerbate chronic bronchitis.

If the sputum of a person with chronic bronchitis abruptly changes in amount, color, quantity, or density, a broad-spectrum antibiotic may be prescribed for 7 to 10 days. If wheezing is present or reversible bronchial constriction is detected on lung function tests, a bronchodilator may be prescribed.

Bronchodilators

Drugs that dilate (widen) the bronchial airways to improve air flow. Bronchodilators are prescribed for people with asthma who have wheezing or breathing difficulties. All bronchodilators relieve coughing, wheezing, shortness of breath, and troubled breathing. They are available in liquid, tablet, and extended-release form for long-term treatment. The medications are also available in injectable and inhaled forms, and generally, the inhaled form is preferable, particularly for acute attacks.

Bronchopneumonia

An infection of the tissues of the lungs that occurs principally in the smaller branches, called bronchioles, of the airways, or bronchial tubes. Bronchopneumonia, which is also called bronchial pneumonia, may be caused by bacteria such as pneumococci, staphylococci, and streptococci or by viruses such as the influenza virus. The disease may develop as a complication of a common cold (see COLD, COMMON) or influenza. Some forms of bronchopneumonia are contagious.

The disease occurs when infection produces pus and mucus, which clog and inflame the air sacs and bronchioles. Symptoms can include a cough that produces blood-streaked sputum, chest pain, fever, chills, and difficulty breathing. In severe cases when insufficient oxygen is delivered to the body, the skin may acquire a bluish tinge and mental confusion can occur. Death may occur within 24 hours to those who are particularly susceptible and have severe infection.

People who contract bronchopneumonia require medical attention and monitoring. Hospitalization is sometimes necessary. If bacteria are the cause of disease, antibiotic medications are prescribed. Fluoroquino-lones are the first-line agents used to treat older people and those with severe symptoms. Macrolides and doxycycline can be used to treat younger persons and those who are less severely ill. Penicillin is also used. If oxygen levels in the bloodstream are low, oxygen therapy may be required.

Pneumococcal vaccination is considered protective against some of the organisms that cause pneumonia and is recommended for healthy people older than 65 and for people with chronic heart or lung disease, compromised immune systems, or alcoholism. The vaccine is also recommended for those who have had their spleens removed.

Bronchopulmonary dysplasia

A chronic lung disease in newborns marked by inflammation of the airways. Infants with respiratory distress syndrome usually require mechanical ventilation to provide enough oxygen for survival and to prevent tissue damage. A VENTILATOR controls their rate of breathing and amount of oxygen intake. Bronchopulmonary dysplasia occurs when the infant's lungs and airways are damaged by protracted exposure to oxygen and the pressure of the ventilator. An affected infant may experience shrill wheezing and noisy, rapid, labored breathing. The skin may turn blue from lack of oxygen. The baby may experience lung infections, impeded growth, and problems with feeding.

Bronchopulmonary dysplasia is diagnosed when chest X rays reveal damage to the lungs. An infant with this condition continues to need oxygen therapy, often with a ventilator, in order to breathe (see OXYGEN, SUP-

PLEMENTAL). With good nutritional support, such as feeding the baby intravenously or with a tube that passes through the nose or mouth into the stomach, the baby's lungs will begin to heal. The oxygen levels and pressure can be slowly decreased as the baby recovers, usually over many months.

When the infant no longer needs the ventilator, oxygen may be administered through a mask or a tube in the nose. Treatment may also include medications to open airways or prevent fluid buildup in the lungs.

Bronchoscopy

A technique that uses a rigid or flexible fiberoptic instrument for the visual examination of the airways, or bronchial tubes. The procedure can be used to obtain samples of tissue from the bronchial tubes and air sacs of the lungs.

Bronchospasm

A narrowing and constriction of the muscles surrounding the airways, or bronchi, reducing the flow of air. Bronchospasm may be associated with ASTHMA, inflammation caused by infection, chronic BRONCHITIS, or exercise. Bronchospasm is generally treated with one of the BRONCHODILATORS, which relaxes smooth muscle and opens the airways to permit normal breathing.

Bronchus

A tube that is an airway from the trachea (windpipe) into each LUNG. The main bronchus in the lung branches into smaller passages called segmental bronchi, which in turn branch further into smaller tubes called bronchioles.

Bruise

A collection of blood in unbroken tissue; also known as a contusion. Most bruises fade slowly within 10 to 14 days. As a bruise fades, the changing colors represent chemical changes in the hemoglobin of red blood cells as they are broken down and reabsorbed into the bloodstream. If bruises do not fade, if they appear for no reason, or if they are accompanied by persistent pain or headache, medical attention is needed.

Bruit

An abnormal sound heard when a stethoscope is placed over an artery. A bruit (pronounced "broowe" or "broot") is a sign of partial obstruction of the artery by fatty deposits and can be a sign of increased risk for heart disease and stroke (see ATHEROSCLEROSIS).

Bubonic plague

An acute, infectious disease caused by a bacterial organism found in wild rodents and transmitted to humans by fleabites or the ingestion of flea feces. Bubonic plague, also called plague, can be transmitted from one infected person to another by the spread of infected droplets from coughing, which is produced when the infected person contracts PNEUMONIA. When this occurs, it is referred to as pneumonic plague.

Initial symptoms of bubonic plague are headache, nausea, vomiting, aching joints, and general malaise. Lymph nodes of the groin, armpit, or neck become painful and swollen. Body temperature, pulse rate, and respiration rate are increased. Death can occur within 4 days. In nonfatal cases, the infection can improve within 2 weeks.

In pneumonic plague, death may occur within 3 days of the first appearance of symptoms.

Tests that may indicate a plague infection include culturing the lymph nodes, sputum, and blood. Immediate treatment with antibiotics is essential to prevent death. Oxygen, intravenous fluids, and respiratory support may be necessary. Infected persons must be isolated.

Plague is rare in developed countries, but pneumonic plague bacteria is considered a possible weapon of bioterrorism.

Bulimia

A behavioral illness characterized by recurrent episodes of binge eating and extreme countermeasures to reduce the effect of the food, often by self-induced vomiting.

To be classified as bulimia, binges and countermeasures have to occur an average of twice weekly over a period of 3 months. Most people with bulimia have body weights within or near the normal weight range, but they perceive themselves as fat and put extreme emphasis on body image. The disorder usually begins in late adolescence or early adulthood, and about nine in every ten people with bulimia are female. The exact cause of bulimia is unknown.

Most people with bulimia are aware that their eating is abnormal and are secretive about their behavior. The illness is often associated with symptoms of depression (such as low self-esteem and bouts of crying), heightened anxiety, and substance abuse. Purging behavior can produce a variety of physical symptoms, such as imbalances in metabolism, abnormal heart rhythm, and significant and permanent loss of tooth enamel from acid in the vomit. In a small number of cases, hospitalization is required. Death from bulimia is rare, but it does occur.

Treatment may include behavior therapy (in which the person monitors eating and is rewarded for normal behavior), family therapy, individual counseling, and group therapy. If the person has depression, antidepressant medications may be used. Naltrexone hydrochloride and lithium are also used.

BUN

Blood urea nitrogen. See KIDNEY FUNCTION TESTS.

Bundle branch block

A delay or obstruction in the passage of electrical impulses through the ventricles (lower chambers) of the heart. The delayed signal makes a detour around the damaged area, so that the affected ventricle still beats but slightly slower than its counterpart. Bundle branch block may have the effect of slowing the heartbeat (see BRADYCARDIA).

Bundle branch block is a common abnormality. It is often present at birth or develops later in life for no known reason. In some people, bundle branch block is caused by aging, hypertension (high blood pressure), past heart attack, viral infection, disease of the heart valves, heart failure, or chronic obstructive pulmonary disease.

In many cases, bundle branch block produces no symptoms and does not require treatment. The condition is usually detected with an electrocardiogram (ECG), which measures the electrical activity of the heart. If the blockage is severe and the heartbeat very slow, the individual may experience periods of fainting or near-fainting. Surgical implantation of a PACEMAKER usually remedies the problem.

Bunion

A painful, inflamed, bony protrusion at the base of the big toe. A bunion is caused by an abnormal enlargement of the joint of the big toe, which is forced inward against the other toes and may overlap the toe next to it. Symptoms may include swelling, soreness, and redness near the toe joint; an inflamed bursa and calluses at the affected area; and persistent or intermittent pain. Mild cases may be treated with protective devices, orthotics in their shoes, or nonsteroidal anti-inflammatory medications. In severe cases, an orthopedic surgeon or podiatrist can correct the condition with a surgical procedure.

Burkitt lymphoma

A malignancy of the lymph glands, often in the jaw or the abdomen. Burkitt lymphoma is a fast-growing cancer that can eventually invade the CENTRAL NERVOUS SYSTEM and the BONE MARROW. The disorder was first discovered in Africa, where it is very common. It chiefly affects children in areas of tropical Africa and New Guinea and is currently thought to be associated with the EPSTEIN-BARR VIRUS, which also causes infectious mononucleosis (see MONONUCLEOSIS, INFECTIOUS). Burkitt lymphoma is rare in the United States, except as an AIDS-related cancer.

Burns, chemical

Injury to the skin caused by corrosive chemicals. Chemical burns are reactions that occur when a person's skin comes in contact with acids, alkalis, or other corrosive agents, in which chemical energy is converted into heat. Chemicals will usually continue to burn the skin as long as they are in contact.

Chemical burns should always prompt a person to seek emergency medical care, because the depth of injury may be difficult to assess. First aid measures that may be started include brushing off any powdered chemicals and flushing the area with large amounts of cool, running water. For burns affecting a person's eye, it is important when flushing that eye with cool water to make sure that the water does not run into the unaffected eye. If possible, the person should cover the burn with a cool, wet cloth. Ointments are not recommended.

Burns, electrical

Injury caused by contact with electricity. Sources of electricity that can cause burns when an unprotected portion of a person's body comes in contact with them include power lines, lightning, defective household electrical equipment, and unprotected electrical outlets. As electrical current goes into the body, it is converted to heat that can cause extensive damage to blood vessels, nerves, bone, and muscle.

There are three types of burns associated with electricity: contact burn injuries, when the current passes through the body and leaves two burns (one where the electrical current entered the body and the other where it exited); electrical flash burn, an electrothermal (heat generated by electricity) injury caused by the arcing of the current; and flame burn, which occurs when electricity ignites clothing or surrounding material.

Any person with an electrical burn should receive emergency medical care. It is never wise to approach a person injured by electricity unless the power source has been turned off.

Burns, heat

Injury caused by exposure to dry heat sufficient to damage the skin. Heat burns, also called thermal burns, can have many causes, including contact with an open flame, hot objects, explosions, and the sun. Heat burns are classified according to degree of severity. About 2 million people in the United States receive burns each year; 300,000 of them are serious injuries. Burns are the third-largest cause of accidental death in the United States.

The goals of first aid for burns are to remove the person from smoke or fumes, to reduce the effect of heat on the skin, to relieve pain, to prevent fluid loss, to prevent infection, and to summon emergency medical help when necessary. Correct first aid can be important in hastening recovery. In the case of small burns, cool water will lessen pain and stop tissue damage. The person should remove any constricting jewelry and cover the burn area with a dry, sterile bandage or clean cloth. For burns covering a large surface area, the person may be in shock and should lie flat, if injuries permit, with feet elevated, until medical help arrives. Second-degree burns cause damage to the layer of skin below the surface of the body

and should be cooled as quickly as possible with cold water; these burns may take 2 or 3 weeks to heal. Third-degree burns destroy all layers of skin and are a medical emergency; aid for the person should be summoned by dialing 911 or the emergency number for the area.

Burns, scald

See SCALDS.

Bursa

A fluid-filled, enclosed sac of connective tissue designed to reduce friction between moving body parts. Bursae are located between the skin and bone and between tendons and bones, muscles and bones, and ligaments and bones to cushion the movements of one body part over the other.

Bursitis

An inflammation of a BURSA, the fluid-filled sac that serves to reduce friction against moving bones. Bursitis most commonly affects bursae of the shoulder, the elbow, the hip, and areas directly above and below the knee. Repeated movement can cause persistent friction between a bursa and the muscles and bones surrounding it. The ongoing friction causes irritation, swelling, and inflammation of the bursa, which becomes enlarged and puts pressure on nearby tissues. Movement increases the pressure, causing more pain.

Joint movement near the inflammation is limited by the pain. The entire area affected by bursitis eventually becomes painful. The pain may radiate to nearby muscles and tendons. The site may also feel hot to the touch and become red and swollen. When bursitis persists, the bursa can become calcified, and deposits may form, limiting movement of the tendons.

Bursitis is diagnosed by physical examination and the use of imaging, which can reveal the enlarged bursa and possible calcified deposits. The condition can be managed by avoiding activities that put pressure on or irritate the bursa.

Self-help techniques include applications of ice to treat pain and swelling, wrapping to control swelling and provide support, and range-of-motion exercises to aid in maintaining joint mobility. Medical treatments may include acetaminophen for pain and anti-inflammatory drugs to ease discomfort from inflammation. Corticosteroids may be injected into the bursal area, and if infection is present, antibiotics may be prescribed.

Bypass surgery

A procedure to detour around obstructions in the arteries providing blood to the heart. Bypass surgery, known technically as coronary artery bypass grafting (CABG), is used to treat ATHEROSCLEROSIS, a disease in which deposits of fat and other materials clog the arteries, causing ANGINA (chest pain) and often leading to HEART ATTACK. Bypass surgery is the treatment of choice when a simpler approach to treating blocked arteries, such as medication or BALLOON ANGIOPLASTY, is insufficient. A major procedure performed under general anesthesia, bypass takes about 3 to 6 hours to complete, depending on the complexity of the case. Most commonly, bypass surgery is recommended for people with debilitating angina, blockage of the left main coronary artery, impaired function of the left ventricle (the heart's main pump), or multiple blockages in the coronary arteries.

The chest is opened by cutting through the skin and splitting the breastbone to expose the heart. The person is then connected to a heart-lung machine, a device that circulates and oxygenates the blood and performs the work of the heart and lungs. The heart itself is stopped to make it easier for the surgeon to work.

Two methods of creating the bypass are commonly used. In one, a section is taken from the saphenous vein in the leg. One end of the vein graft is stitched into the aorta (the artery that carries oxygenated blood from the heart to the body), and the other end is stitched into the blocked coronary artery downstream from the blockage. The second method uses one or both of two arteries known as the internal mammary arteries, which arise from the subclavian arteries and lead to the inside of the chest well.

In recent years a procedure known as minimally invasive direct coronary artery bypass surgery has been developed as an alternative to the standard bypass operation. Minimally invasive direct coronary artery bypass surgery causes less trauma and postoperative pain and requires less medication than standard bypass surgery; however, it seems to carry a greater risk of heart attack or stroke. In addition, it cannot be used for people with multiple blockages or, in most cases, with blockages on the right side of the heart.

Coronary artery bypass surgery is one of the most commonly performed operations in the United States. Fewer than 1 percent of those undergoing bypass surgery die of heart attack or stroke during or shortly after the procedure. The risk is highest for older people, people with diabetes mellitus, those with other major health problems, and people undergoing a second bypass procedure. Complications, such as high blood pressure or irregular heart rhythm, can result but are often temporary or can be controlled with medication. Most people experience rapid relief of their symptoms. See also ANGIOGRAM; CARDIAC STRESS TESTING; CHEST PAIN; CORONARY ARTERY DISEASE; and ELECTROCARDIOGRAM (ECG).

C

C-reactive protein

A protein produced in the liver and released into the bloodstream when INFLAMMATION is present in the body. An increased level of CRP may indicate an increased risk of heart disease and stroke in some people. See also HEART DISEASE, ISCHEMIC.

CA-125 test

A blood test used in the diagnosis of cancer of the ovary (see OVARY, CANCER OF THE). Elevated levels of the protein CA-125 are suggestive of ovarian cancer, but also can be elevated with several noncancerous conditions such as fibroid tumors, liver disease, endometriosis, and pelvic infections, in addition to the presence of other cancers, including those of the liver, lung, cervix, breast, stomach, and colon. As a result, doctors must use other tests and procedures to diagnose the cause of an elevated CA-125 level.

Cachexia

General ill health marked by extreme weight loss and a wasted appearance. Cachexia is associated with chronic infections and malignant conditions, such as cancer and AIDS.

Café au lait spots

Benign (not cancerous), cream-colored to brown spots found on the skin; the color is produced by melanin. Spots are present at birth or develop in childhood. In some cases, café au lait spots are a sign of the inherited disorder NEUROFIBROMATOSIS.

Calciferol

Vitamin D2. A fat-soluble, crystalline unsaturated alcohol that occurs naturally in fish liver oils, spinach, broccoli, soybeans, and other dried beans. Calciferol helps the body use calcium and is used in the treatment of osteomalacia, osteoporosis, rickets, and hypocalcemic disorders. See also VITAMIN D.

Calcification

The buildup of calcium salts that occurs normally in bone development. Calcification may also refer to the accumulation of calcium salts and calcium deposits in tissues that normally do not have a buildup of calcium. For example, in a person with persistent BURSITIS, a calcium deposit may affect the shoulder, elbow, hip, or knee area, causing pain and inflammation. Calcification or accumulation of calcium in blood vessels can occur with ATHEROSCLEROSIS.

Calcinosis

Calcification of the skin and other soft tissues, which particularly affects the skin of the hands. Calcinosis is characterized by swollen hands, pinpricks of red coloration on the skin of the hands, thickened nails, and sores on the fingers. Calcinosis is one of five elements in a form of scleroderma called CREST SYNDROME. The "C" in the acronym CREST stands for calcinosis.

Calcium

An element found in food that is essential for neurotransmission, muscle contraction, bone formation, tooth formation, and proper heart function. Imbalances of calcium can lead to many health problems, and an excess of calcium in nerve cells can cause their death.

Calcium channel blockers

A class of drugs used to treat hypertension (high blood pressure), chronic angina pectoris (chest pain), and cardiac arrhythmias and to prevent migraine headaches. Calcium channel blockers lower blood pressure by decreasing contractions of the heart and relaxing the smooth muscle found on the blood vessel walls, which reduces resistance to blood flow.

Calculus, dental

A mineralized, porous deposit that hardens and adheres to the crowns and roots of the teeth. Dental calculus, also called TARTAR, is caused by the accumulation of plaque (see PLAQUE, DENTAL).

Calculus, urinary tract

A stone that forms in the organs that produce and transport urine, including the kidneys, ureters (tubes connecting the kidneys and bladder), and the bladder. These stones form from crystalline materials normally present in the urine. (See URINARY TRACT.)

Urinary tract calculi usually cause no symptoms until the stones obstruct and irritate the urinary tract. The first symptoms are often severe pain, nausea, and blood in the urine. Location of the pain depends on the position of the calculus. There may also be an urgent need to urinate, with a burning sensation upon urination. Infection with fever and chills may also be present; the combination of urinary tract calculi with fever is a medical emergency.

The presence of calculi must be established by the person's medical history, a direct physical examination, analysis and testing of the urine, and X rays.

Most small stones pass out of the urinary tract without medical intervention, usually within 6 weeks after symptoms begin. Patients are advised to drink large amounts of water to help flush the calculi out. When stones do not pass on their own, LITHOTRIPSY is a procedure to help break up stones.

If these approaches do not succeed, or if the calculus completely blocks the flow of urine, the obstruction must be removed and any accumulated urine must be corrected. In addition to lithotripsy, stones may be removed by cystoscopy. During this procedure, a urologist may use snares to retrieve the stone or crush the stone into smaller pieces so they can pass out of the body in the urine.

Occasionally, surgery is required to remove stones.

Callus, bony

The newly formed soft bone that develops after a bone fracture and during the bone's healing process. Bony callus may also refer to a thickening of the surface layer of the skin over a bony prominence, usually on the feet, but also on the hands. Such a callus usually forms in response to pressure. Symptoms include pain with pressure. In most cases, these do not require medical attention, unless they become very painful.

Callus, skin

An area of tough, thickened skin caused by pressure or friction. Calluses commonly develop on the palms, fingertips, and soles of the feet. Calluses are most often associated with specific types of work and sport. Calluses can cause tenderness or pain under the skin. Self-treatment of calluses includes using a file, pumice stone, or towel to rub away excess skin when the skin is damp. Medical treatment includes paring the thickened skin with a scalpel. In some cases surgery may be needed.

Caloric test

A procedure used to determine whether abnormalities or disease are present in the inner ear of a person experiencing dizziness, balance problems, or hearing loss. The test is usually part of a group of diagnostic methods called electronystagmography (ENG) that evaluates the function of the vestibular system (inner ear nerve system essential to balance) and associated areas of the brain.

Calorie

A measurement of energy provided by food for use by the body. A difference exists in how the term is used popularly and in the scientific community. Scientifically, a calorie is $1/1,000$ of a kilocalorie. Popularly, however, the term calorie is used sometimes interchangeably with the scientific term kilocalorie. Scientifically, a kilocalorie is a measure of the amount of heat required to raise the temperature of 1 kilogram of water 1 degree Celsius (centigrade). This measurement is used because it can be determined readily.

Mildly active adults need about 25 calories (kilocalories) per kilogram of body weight per day to meet their basic energy needs.

Calorie requirements

The amount of energy required by the body for normal function, growth, repair, and physical activity. Daily calorie requirements vary from person to person and depend largely on how active an individual is. To maintain health, sedentary women and older people must take in about 1,600 calories a day. Active women, children, teenage girls, and sedentary men require approximately 2,200 calories. Very active women, teenage boys, and active men need about 2,800 calories daily.

A calorie is a measurement of energy. The three basic components of the diet—proteins, carbohydrates, and fats—provide different amounts of energy or calories, as do alcohol and soluble fiber. Carbohydrates and fats are the body's main sources of energy. Every gram of fat contains more than double the number of calories in a gram of protein or carbohydrate. In the average, healthful daily diet, 50 to 60 percent of calories should derive from carbohydrates, no more than 30 percent (and preferably less) from fat, and 10 to 20 percent from protein. However, the typical diet consumed by the average American has a much higher percentage of calories derived from fats.

Calvé-Perthes disease

See OSTEOCHONDROSIS.

Campylobacter

A type of bacteria that is the most frequent cause of bacterial DIARRHEA in the United States. Stomach cramps and fever are additional symptoms of *Campylobacter* infection. Infection is usually caused by eating foods, such as undercooked chicken, that have been contaminated by *Campylobacter*.

Cancer

Any of a group of diseases characterized by an uncontrolled, abnormal growth of cells that can spread throughout the body. The terms malignancy and neoplasia are often used interchangeably with cancer. Cancer is thought to develop from a single cell or a small set of cells after changes have occurred in their DNA, the genetic material that instructs cells how to behave. Some cancers result from inherited genetic abnormalities, and others are triggered by carcinogens, environmental agents capable of causing genetic mutations (see CARCINOGEN). Sometimes, viruses interact with genes in cells and make them more likely to become cancerous. Often, the reason that a cell becomes cancerous is unknown.

Cancer cells cause harm in several different ways. They can deprive normal cells of nourishment or space; they can form a mass, or TUMOR, that may eventually invade and destroy normal tissue; and they can metastasize (spread) by traveling through the bloodstream or the lymphatic system to other parts of the body. Most cancers take years to develop; cancer that is detected and treated before it has invaded adjacent organs or spread throughout the body has the best chance of being cured.

Cancer is classified into five major groups. About 80 to 90 percent of cancer cases are carcinomas. A CARCINOMA is a tumor that originates in the surface tissue of an organ. A SARCOMA is a tumor that originates in the bone, cartilage, muscle, connective tissues, or fatty tissues. Myeloma originates in the plasma cells of the bone marrow. LYMPHOMA originates in the lymph system, and LEUKEMIA originates in the blood-forming cells of the bone marrow.

A number of investigations or workups can be done to help identify cancer. However, a tissue biopsy, which involves taking a sample of affected cells for analysis under a microscope, is the only absolutely accurate method of diagnosing cancer.

There are four general types of treatment for cancer: surgery, RADIATION THERAPY, CHEMOTHERAPY with anticancer drugs, and biological therapy, which helps the body's own immune system to fight the cancer. Many people with cancer will receive treatments that combine some or all of the available therapies. Quitting smoking significantly reduces the risk of developing cancer. For information about specific types of cancer, see the entry for the site of cancer— for example, BREAST CANCER or COLON, CANCER OF THE.

Cancer screening

Tests performed on people without symptoms to identify possible cancer at an early stage. Screening tests have been used effectively for cancers of the breast (see MAMMOGRAM), cervix (see PAP SMEAR), colon (see FECAL-OCCULT BLOOD TEST, COLONOSCOPY, and SIGMOIDOSCOPY), and prostate gland.

Candidiasis

See YEAST INFECTIONS.

Canker sore

A small, painful sore or ulcer that occurs inside the mouth. It is usually surrounded by an area of redness less than a few millimeters (around an inch) in diameter. Canker sores commonly first appear when a person is in his or her 20s or 30s. The sores tend to disappear in 1 to 2 weeks. Recurrences are common and may be induced by trauma, eating spicy or citrus foods, and menstruation.

Canker sores appear to run in families and are believed to be associated with immune system disorders or conditions, nutritional deficiencies, or gastrointestinal problems. There is no cure for canker sores.

Capillary

A microscopic blood vessel that connects the smallest arteries (arterioles) and the smallest veins (venules) to complete the circulation of blood at a cellular level. The capillary walls are membranes through which nutrients and oxygen pass from the blood into body cells, while waste such as carbon dioxide passes out. See also HEART.

Capsulitis, adhesive

See FROZEN SHOULDER.

Car restraints

Safety devices used in motor vehicles to minimize the risk of injury or death during accidents. Car restraints include lap and shoulder safety belts, child safety seats, and air bags. The use of lap and shoulder seat belts provides the greatest possible protection against being thrown out of a vehicle during an accident. The use of lap and shoulder seat belts reduces the risk of fatal injury to front-seat occupants of cars by 45 percent and the risk of moderate to critical injury by 50 percent.

Carbohydrates

Essential nutrients that are the body's main source of energy. There are two primary types of carbohydrates: simple (SUGAR) and complex (starch). Starches and sugars in fruits, vegetables, and grains are all examples of carbohydrates.

Simple carbohydrates (sugars) are found in many forms beyond sucrose, the simple white table form that is spooned into coffee. Natural sugars, such as fructose, glucose, and lactose, occur in fruit and milk.

Complex carbohydrates (starches) provide more lasting sources of energy than simple carbohydrates because they are absorbed more slowly. The foods that are rich in complex carbohydrates—starches such as potatoes, pasta, rice, and beans—are often rich in vitamins, minerals, and fiber. For highest nutritional value, it is best to eat complex carbohydrates in unrefined forms, such as brown rice rather than white rice.

Carbon dioxide

A colorless, odorless, tasteless gas formed from carbon and oxygen. Carbon dioxide is found in nature, both as part of the atmosphere and in combination with other elements as carbonates. Carbon dioxide is what produces the bubbles in natural mineral waters and carbonated soft drinks. Carbon dioxide also causes bread dough to rise and is used in fire extinguishers. Carbon dioxide is a product of the burning of fuels that contain carbon, such as coal, oil, gasoline, and natural gas. The presence of carbon dioxide in the atmosphere has been growing steadily, thus upsetting the natural balance of the ecosystem and leading to the greenhouse effect and GLOBAL WARMING. It can accumulate in indoor areas that have poor ventilation. Too much carbon dioxide in these areas can cause headaches, difficulty concentrating, and shortness of breath. Carbon dioxide may also be a cause of SICK BUILDING SYNDROME.

Carbuncle

A cluster of painful, pus-filled boils (see BOIL) on the skin. A boil results when a hair follicle becomes infected with staphylococcal (staph) bacteria. In a carbuncle, boils in adjacent follicles expand and join to form a mass with multiple drainage points.

Both the carbuncle and the area surrounding it must be kept clean with antibacterial soap. Many carbuncles resolve by applying warm compresses for 30 minutes several times a day for about 2 weeks and keeping the area scrupulously clean. This helps decrease inflammation. Some carbuncles are deep in the skin and cannot drain on their own; they require surgical drainage.

Carcinogen

An agent capable of causing or promoting cancer. Carcinogens, such as cigarette smoke, can be created by humans, or they may exist naturally in the environment (for example, ultraviolet radiation from the sun). Smoke, sunlight, X rays, and viruses are all known carcinogens, as are asbestos, air pollution, fatty foods, and certain chemicals used to preserve food. Carcinogens cause cancer in different ways. Some change normal cells into cancer cells, while others create conditions that enable other factors to cause cancer.

Carcinogenesis

The origin or development of cancer in previously healthy cells.

Carcinoma

A cancerous tumor arising from cells in surface tissues or the linings of organs. Carcinoma is one of the five basic kinds of CANCER and the most common form, accounting for about 80 to 90 percent of all cancers. Carcinomas tend to invade nearby tissues and metastasize (spread). Cancers of the lungs, skin, breast, cervix, and prostate gland are usually carcinomas.

Cardiac arrest

A sudden and immediate cessation of the heartbeat. Breathing stops, and, since blood flow to the brain is cut off, the person loses consciousness. Unless a normal heart rhythm is reestablished within 4 to 6 minutes, the person will die of irreversible brain damage.

Cardiac arrest almost always occurs in a heart affected by underlying heart disease (see HEART DISEASE, CONGENITAL; HEART DISEASE, IS-CHEMIC), such as coronary artery disease, or by damage to the heart muscle, which is often the result of a previous HEART ATTACK. Cardiac arrest is commonly preceded by VEN-TRICULAR FIBRILLATION.

Warning: Cardiac arrest is a medical emergency requiring immediate response, so someone should call 911 or the local emergency number. Until paramedics arrive, CARDIOPULMO-NARY RESUSCITATION (CPR) can help maintain blood flow to the brain until adequate medical help arrives. A device called a DEFIBRILLATOR is often used to restart the heart with an electrical shock. A person who has survived cardiac arrest is at increased risk of another cardiac event.

Cardiac output

The amount of blood the heart pumps per minute. Cardiac output is reduced in people with heart failure or those who have had a heart attack that injured the heart muscle. Cardiac output gives doctors a sensitive indicator of changes in the heart's functioning efficiency and provides an early warning of developing problems.

Cardiac rehabilitation

A medically supervised program designed to speed recovery and improve mental and physical functioning in people with heart conditions. Cardiac rehabilitation is commonly recommended after a heart attack, heart surgery (such as balloon angioplasty or bypass surgery), or diagnosis of

heart disease (for example, congestive heart failure (see HEART FAILURE, CONGESTIVE), hypertension, or congenital heart disease). Most programs include exercise in physical therapy, counseling in diet and nutrition, and stress management.

Cardiac stress testing

Procedures that measure and compare heart function at rest and during exercise. Faster heart rates make it easier to detect impaired blood flow to the heart or abnormal heart rhythms. Cardiac stress testing is performed to diagnose a heart condition, monitor progress in those who have had a HEART ATTACK or have undergone heart surgery, and determine safe exercise levels for people who have heart disease or are at risk for developing it.

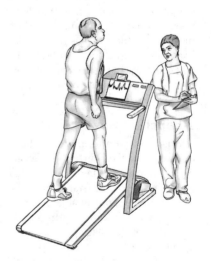

Exercise stress test in action
For those able to exercise, the heart rate is monitored with electrode leads attached to the chest while the person walks or runs on an elevated treadmill. Alternatively, a stationary bicycle may be used.

Cardiac stress testing includes several testing options. The stress ECG, a variation of the standard ELECTROCARDIOGRAM (ECG), measures the electrical patterns of the heart while at rest. The stress test compares the patterns of the heart during exercise to see if the increased stress causes changes.

A pharmacological stress test, which is also known as the chemical stress test, is used for those who cannot perform a physical activity like walking on a treadmill or riding a bicycle. The person to be tested is injected with a drug such as dobutamine or adenosine, which causes the heart rate to speed up.

A stress ECHOCARDIOGRAM allows doctors to visualize the heart as it is moving and to observe its main pumping chambers, the shape and thickness of the chamber walls, the valves, and the outer covering and major vessels of the heart. It is also possible to determine the volume and direction of blood flow through the heart. Echocardiogram images of the heart are taken while it is at rest and under stress and then compared. This testing is usually combined with ECG stress testing for more sensitive results than are obtained with ECG stress testing alone.

A nuclear stress test determines which parts of the heart muscle have good blood flow and which do not. An extremely small amount of a radionuclide (radioactive substance), usually thallium, is injected into the person. The thallium, which travels through the bloodstream, can be detected by a gamma camera. Areas of the heart with good blood supply appear dark on the gamma camera because of the presence of the thallium, while areas with reduced or absent blood flow appear gray or white.

Cardiology

The branch of medicine that specializes in studying the structure and function of the heart and the diseases that affect it. A cardiologist is a physician who specializes in cardiology.

Cardiomegaly

Enlargement of the heart. The heart can increase in size as a result of disease that places extra workload on it, such as hypertension (high blood pressure), congestive heart failure (see HEART FAILURE, CONGESTIVE), or excessive alcohol use. This condition is known as pathological cardiomegaly. Cardiomegaly can cause a number of symptoms, such as EDEMA (swelling) in the lower extremities, shortness of breath, weakness, dizziness, cardiac arrhythmias (irregular heart rhythms), and palpitations (fast, irregular heartbeat). Treatment consists of treating the causative condition and making necessary lifestyle changes, such as abstaining from alcohol.

Cardiomyopathy

A type of heart disease in which the heart muscle is abnormally enlarged, thickened, or stiffened, reducing its ability to pump effectively.

There are two basic types of cardiomyopathy: ischemic (resulting from a lack of oxygen to the heart muscle) and nonischemic (not resulting from a lack of oxygen). Ischemic cardiomyopathy is caused by CORONARY ARTERY DISEASE. Nonischemic cardiomyopathy is less common than ischemic cardiomyopathy. It is a progressive disease and often occurs in young adults and even children. People with nonischemic cardiomyopathy often require heart transplantation.

TYPES AND SYMPTOMS

Nonischemic cardiomyopathy can have numerous causes, including infections, endocrine disorders, metabolic disorders, alcoholism, or exposure to substances that damage the heart. Many cases are idiopathic, which means the cause cannot be identified. There are three principal varieties of nonischemic cardiomyopathy:

DILATED CARDIOMYOPATHY This type refers to overall dilation (enlargement) of the heart, particularly the ventricles (lower chambers), which do most of the work of pumping blood into the lungs and the body. As the heart weakens, it pumps out a smaller portion of the blood in its chambers. Heart failure sets in, and fluid accumulates in the legs, abdomen, and lungs. Shortness of breath caused by fluid accumulation in the lungs is a common symptom. Swelling in the liver often causes pain in the abdomen. Blood clots can form in the enlarged heart chambers, break loose, travel through the bloodstream, and block arteries, particularly in the legs, lungs, kidneys, or brain.

HYPERTROPHIC CARDIOMYOPATHY This type results from abnormal thickening of the heart wall, most often the septum (wall) between the ventricles. It can also affect just the tips of the ventricles or the entirety of one or both ventricles. The thickening decreases the amount of blood the heart can pump with each beat, leading to an inadequate supply of oxygen-rich blood to the body. In advanced disease, the thickening may actually block the aorta (the main artery leaving the heart), so that little or no blood actually reaches the body.

The major symptoms of hypertrophic cardiomyopathy are shortness of breath; ANGINA (chest pain), which is often long-lasting and occurs after rather than during exercise; and loss of consciousness or lightheadedness with exertion. Heart rhythm may also be affected, producing palpitations (uncomfortably fast, irregular heartbeat). Sudden death due to cardiac arrest can occur as a result but is rare.

RESTRICTIVE CARDIOMYOPATHY This is the least common type of cardiomyopathy. The heart muscle becomes so stiff that during the relaxation phase between heartbeats little blood enters the ventricles. Since the heart can only pump the blood it actually receives, the flow of blood into the lungs and the body decreases. A person with restrictive cardiomyopathy is likely to complain of fatigue, have swollen hands and feet, and experience difficulty breathing during exertion. Pain in the upper right abdomen, nausea, bloating, and loss of appetite are also common. Angina may occur as well. Congestive heart failure (see HEART FAILURE, CONGESTIVE) and cardiac arrhythmias (heart rhythm problems) can result.

Diagnosis and treatment

Depending on symptoms, a number of tests may be needed to determine whether cardiomyopathy is present and, if so, in which form. A chest X ray can show the size of the heart and reveal any pulmonary congestion. An ELECTROCARDIOGRAM (ECG) and an echocardiogram may be needed.

Treatment of cardiomyopathy depends on the type and severity of disease and its symptoms. A number of medications may be useful, including diuretics, beta blockers, and vasodilators, digitalis, anticoagulants, or antibiotics.

For some cardiomyopathies, surgery is a treatment option. The most common surgical procedure is removal of part of the thickened septum in hypertrophic cardiomyopathy, a procedure called a myectomy. A PACEMAKER is often implanted in people whose cardiomyopathy causes irregularities in heart rhythm. In some cases when the heart muscle is severely damaged, transplant surgery may be recommended.

Cardiopulmonary resuscitation (CPR)

Lifesaving techniques used to maintain oxygen and blood flow to people who are unconscious and whose heart or breathing have stopped.

CPR is performed in emergencies involving cardiac arrest, choking, or drowning. Death can occur in 8 to 10 minutes when a person has stopped breathing, and brain death can occur in as few as 4 to 6 minutes. CPR should be given only by people who have been trained in CPR.

Recently CPR procedures were revised to put more emphasis on chest compressions than on rescue breathing.

If an unresponsive person is not moving or breathing, chest compressions can keep the blood flowing until help arrives. By placing the hands over the chest, with elbows straight and weight centered above the person's chest, the person performing CPR can push on the person's chest at a rate of about 100 times per minute. After 30 chest compressions, two rescue breaths should be given; and the person's pulse and breathing should be checked after every four cycles of 30 compressions and two breaths.

The airway is opened to ensure that there is nothing blocking the windpipe; mouth-to-mouth rescue breathing is necessary to get oxygen to the person's lungs; and chest compressions replace the missing heartbeat to maintain blood flow to the brain and other organs.

Cardiorespiratory fitness

The capacity of the heart and lungs to function during physical activity. Cardiorespiratory fitness is measured using equipment that records a person's heart rate, blood pressure, and respiration.

The test's measurements reveal the heart rate, respiratory rate, oxygen uptake by the lungs, and concentration of oxygen and carbon dioxide in the exhaled air. The analysis of these measurements can establish the level of a person's cardiorespiratory fitness, or ability to exercise.

Cardiothoracic surgery

Any procedure used to treat a disease, abnormality, or injury in the chest (thorax), particularly in or around the heart. This includes coronary artery bypass and valve surgery of the heart; removal of lung tumors and abscesses; and repair of injuries to the heart, lungs, and chest walls.

Cardiovascular

Pertaining to the heart and blood vessels.

Cardiovascular fitness

The ability of the heart to sustain exertion without undue stress. Cardiovascular fitness is promoted by regular exercise—at a minimum, 20 to 30 minutes a session, at least 3 times a week—that strengthens the heart and lungs.

Cardiovascular system

The HEART and the BLOOD VESSELS, also called the circulatory system, which transports the BLOOD that carries oxygen, carbon dioxide, nutrients, antibodies, enzymes, and waste materials throughout the body. This vast system is vital to maintaining life.

Cardioversion

A procedure in which an electrical shock is administered to the heart in an attempt to restore an abnormal heart rhythm to normal. Cardioversion is similar to the emergency procedure known as DEFIBRILLATION, except that it uses a smaller amount of electricity, is rarely used in an emergency, and is applied most often to cardiac arrhythmias (heartbeat abnormalities) that are not immediately life-threatening. Cardioversion is a standard treatment for ATRIAL FIBRILLATION (the upper chambers of the heart quiver rather than contract, causing an abnormally fast and rapid heartbeat) and ventricular tachycardia (a fast heartbeat that begins in the lower heart chambers rather than the upper; see TACHYCARDIA, VENTRICULAR). In chemical cardioversion, medications are used in place of electric shock to produce the same effect on an abnormal heartbeat.

Carotene

An orange pigment found in plants that is converted to VITAMIN A by the liver, lungs, and intestines. Orange fruits and vegetables such as cantaloupe, papaya, carrots, sweet potatoes, and pumpkin are rich in carotene. This substance is also found in dark green, leafy vegetables such as spinach and kale. Vitamin A is essential for growth and development and helps maintain healthy eyes, skin, and mucous membranes and normal bone structure. Carotene is an antioxidant chemical that may prevent damaging changes in cells.

Carotid artery

One of four major blood vessels of the neck and head. In the lower neck, there are two common carotid arteries (left and right), with two branches (internal and external). The left common carotid artery leads from the aorta and runs up the neck on the left side of the trachea (windpipe). Just above the larynx (voice box) it divides in two, forming the left internal carotid and the left external carotid arteries. The right common carotid artery leads out from the subclavian artery, itself a branch of the aorta, and then divides in a similar fashion on the right side of the neck.

Carotid endarterectomy

A surgical procedure used to remove the buildup of fat and cholesterol in the principal artery supplying blood to the brain, to restore the normal blood flow and lower the risk of STROKE. Fat and cholesterol deposits (plaques) form as a result of ATHEROSCLEROSIS.

Carotid endarterectomy is usually

performed in those who have already had a stroke or a temporary stroke-like event (see TRANSIENT ISCHEMIC ATTACK) and who have at least a 50 percent blockage in the carotid artery. The procedure is sometimes used to treat persons who have not experienced a stroke or transient ischemic attack but who have 80 percent or greater blockage in the carotid artery.

Carpal tunnel syndrome

Compression of the median nerve that causes numbness, tingling, weakness, or pain in the wrist or hand, particularly the thumb and index, middle, and part of the fourth fingers. These sensations are often more pronounced at night and may cause wakening. As the disease progresses, there may be burning, cramping, and weakness of the hand. Decreased hand grip can cause dropping of objects. Sometimes shooting pains are experienced in the forearm. Chronic carpal tunnel syndrome can eventually lead to wasting or atrophy of hand muscles.

Carpal tunnel syndrome is an example of a nerve entrapment syndrome and is by far the most common compression syndrome. See also COMPRESSION SYNDROME; NERVE ENTRAPMENT; and PINCHED NERVE. In some individuals, carpal tunnel syndrome is the result of a REPETITIVE STRAIN INJURY, which is caused by activities such as uninterrupted computer keyboard use.

Physical examination usually reveals signs or carpal tunnel syndrome. The doctor may order a nerve conduction study or ELECTROMYOGRAM or wrist X rays may provide additional useful information.

Most cases of carpal tunnel syndrome can be treated with braces or splints to relieve or minimize pressure on nerves. In some cases, NON-STEROIDAL ANTI-INFLAMMATORY DRUGS (NSAIDs) are prescribed to reduce inflammation and swelling. If splints and NSAIDs fail to control an individual's symptoms, a corticosteroid injection may reduce inflammation and swelling, which in turn lessens the nerve compression. A small number of people require surgery to relieve the pressure.

Carrier

A person in whom the specific organisms of a disease reside, but who does not show any apparent symptoms of the disease. A carrier is capable of transmitting the infection to another person. In genetics, a carrier is a person who has a recessive gene and therefore though they may not have symptoms of a disease, they can still transmit the trait to offspring.

Cartilage

A smooth, fibrous, and dense connective tissue that is an important component of the skeleton. It is not as hard as bone, but is composed of the same material, a structural protein called collagen. Cells in cartilage also secrete a gelatinous substance that gives cartilage some of its flexibility. Cartilage lacks its own blood supply, which is why it heals slowly when torn or damaged in a sports injury or trauma. Slower, wear-and-tear damage to cartilage in joints will also gradually repair itself.

Castration

Surgical removal of the testicles in a man or the ovaries in a woman; most often performed as part of cancer surgery. Castration may be used in the treatment of some breast and prostate cancers since estrogen stimulates the growth of some breast cancers and testosterone stimulates the growth of prostate cancer. See ORCHIECTOMY for the male surgery and OOPHORECTOMY for the female.

Cat-scratch disease

An uncommon disease caused primarily by the *Bartonella* bacteria, which are transmitted among cats by fleas. Cat-scratch disease (CSD) is usually but not always associated with a history of a cat's scratch or bite. The disease is generally mild and improves without treatment. It most frequently affects people younger than 17 years.

The symptoms of CSD typically include a small reddish lesion at the site of a cat scratch or bite on the skin, swollen lymph nodes, and sometimes a fever. Swelling in the lymph nodes (armpit, neck bone, and above the collarbone) may persist for months. Headaches, joint pain, and eye redness may occur.

Treatment of CSD is not always required, but may include antibiotics or surgery. Although associated problems rarely occur, they may include TONSILLITIS, ENCEPHALITIS, HEPATITIS, PNEUMONIA, and other serious diseases.

Cataplexy

A sudden loss of voluntary muscle control. Cataplexy is a classic symptom of NARCOLEPSY (a sleep disorder characterized by sudden and irresistible collapses into sleep). Signs of cataplexy include slight weakness, a nodding head, garbled speech, sagging facial muscles, buckling knees, and limp arm muscles. In some cases, there is a total collapse, during which a person appears unconscious but remains awake and alert. Attacks last from several seconds to 30 minutes.

Cataract

A cloudiness or opacity in the normally clear lens of the eye. The lens is made of water and protein, which are arranged in a specific way to preserve the clarity of the lens. A cataract forms when alterations in the proteins occur and form a cloudy or opaque area in a portion of the lens.

In the early stages, a cataract has little effect on vision. As the cataract grows, vision may become blurred or cloudy. Lights can look too bright, appear to be surrounded by halos, and may cause increased glare, an effect that often hampers the ability to drive at night. Colors may seem muted, and overall night vision often worsens. Vision can become double or multiple. In advanced cases, the pupil of the eye is visibly milky or white rather than black.

In most cases, cataracts are identified during a professional eye examination, often before the individual has noticed any change in vision. The only lasting treatment is surgery, which involves removing the cloudy lens (see CATARACT SURGERY).

Cataract surgery

A procedure to restore vision lost because of cloudiness in the normally clear lens of the eye (see CATARACT for more information about this disease). The cloudy lens is removed and usually replaced with an artificial lens implant placed inside the eye.

Rarely, when an implant cannot be placed, contact lenses or glasses with thick lenses are used.

Surgery is indicated only when cataracts cause difficulty with reading, driving, and other basic visual tasks. Cataract surgery has become more common over the past decade because of its safety, ease, and excellent outcome.

Following cataract surgery, itching and mild discomfort in the eye are normal. The eye may leak fluid and be sensitive to light and touch. For a few days after surgery, drops to control pressure inside the eye may be prescribed. Most activity is permitted during recovery, except bending and lifting, which raise pressure inside the eye.

People who have received a lens implant and who wear contact lenses or glasses typically need a new prescription a few weeks after surgery. If no intraocular lens has been placed in the eye, special contacts or glasses will be prescribed.

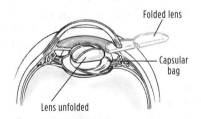

Replacement of damaged lens

Phacoemulsification is a type of cataract surgery that requires only a tiny, self-healing incision and an ultrasonic probe. The first step is to make the incision in the cornea and insert the probe to break up and suction out the old lens. The second step (shown above) is to insert a new lens, folded to fit through the incision, and smooth it out into its proper position in the eye.

Complications from cataract surgery are not common. These include infection, bleeding, inflammation, loss of vision, light flashes, or retinal detachment. Prompt medical attention resolves most problems.

Catatonia

An extreme expression of physical activity in which the individual is either completely immobile or frantically overactive. A person immobilized by catatonia may hold a bizarre posture for hours or resist being moved; those who are hyperactive engage in frantic behavior that has no apparent purpose. Symptoms may also include resistance to all instructions, inability to talk (mutism), stupor, strange gestures or grimaces, unusual mannerisms, purposeless repetition of a word just spoken by someone else (echolalia), and repeated imitation of someone else's movements. People with catatonia may pose a risk to themselves or others and require supervision.

Catatonia may be a symptom of major DEPRESSION, BIPOLAR DISORDER, or SCHIZOPHRENIA. Patients are usually treated in an inpatient psychiatric facility. Tranquilizers or electroconvulsive therapy may be used.

Cathartics

Agents that cause bowel movements by stimulating the movement of food through the digestive system.

Cathartics are sometimes given to people who have been poisoned because they accelerate the expulsion of the poison from the digestive tract. Cathartics should never be given to a person who has been poisoned without the advice of a doctor or a specialist at a poison center.

Catheter

A flexible, hollow tube inserted into various body cavities. Catheters are commonly used to empty the bladder through the urethra (see CATHETERI-ZATION, URINARY) or to enter the heart through a vein in the arm or leg for examination (see CATHETERIZA-TION, CARDIAC). Catheters are also used in PERITONEAL DIALYSIS for treatment of kidney failure.

Catheterization, cardiac

A minimally invasive procedure that involves threading a catheter (thin tube) through a blood vessel into the heart to obtain diagnostic information about the heart, coronary arteries (the arteries on the surface of the heart), and the aorta (the main artery leaving the heart). The doctor tracks the passage of the catheter through the circulatory system to the heart on a fluoroscope, an X-ray device that displays its image on a monitor. By injecting a special dye through the catheter, the doctor can take accurate X-ray pictures of the heart and its arteries.

Cardiac catheterization is performed primarily for three reasons. The first is to help make a diagnosis in cases in which symptoms, such as breathlessness or chest pain during exercise, suggest heart disease and preliminary test results are inconclusive. The second reason is to assess the need for surgery. The third reason cardiac catheterization is performed is for treatment (for example, BALLOON ANGIOPLASTY and STENT placement).

Catheterization, urinary

Insertion of a thin, flexible tube (catheter) into the bladder to drain urine. Catheters may be used temporarily, such as during surgery and recovery, or continuously in people who cannot retain urine normally or empty their bladder (see INCONTINENCE, URINARY). Typically, the catheter has a balloon tip that is inflated with air or sterile liquid to hold it in place after it is inserted. The balloon is then deflated to remove the catheter. The urine drains into a bag that is emptied periodically.

Caudal

A term that usually refers to a position toward the end of the spine; literally means "of the tail."

Cauterization

The use of a hot instrument, an electrical current, a corrosive chemical, or some other agent to destroy tissue or to stop bleeding. Cauterization can be used, for example, to seal blood vessels cut during surgery or to remove tonsils or other diseased tissue.

Cavernous sinus thrombosis

A potentially fatal condition caused when a blood clot in the cavernous sinus becomes infected with bacteria, which accumulate in the blood and produce toxins. Cavernous sinus thrombosis is usually a consequence of bacterial sinusitis. The infection may spread into other sinus areas through associated veins. Symptoms may include headache, a high fever, seizures, and loss of consciousness.

A person with cavernous sinus thrombosis may have a red, swollen, bulging eye with loss of movement. CT (computed tomography) SCANNING of the sinuses and brain may be performed to confirm the diagnosis.

Treatment includes intravenous antibiotics at high doses and surgical drainage of the infected sinuses. The prognosis is considered grave, even with prompt treatment.

Cavity, dental

A hole in a tooth caused by decay. A cavity is caused by the formation of dental plaque (see PLAQUE, DENTAL), which is made up of bacteria, food particles, and saliva. The bacteria interact with sugars in food particles that remain in the mouth and on the teeth to form acid, which dissolves the calcium and phosphate in the enamel of the tooth. This damage to the structure of the tooth is the first stage in the development of a dental cavity. If the cavity is not treated, it can reach the inner structures of the teeth, inflame the pulp of the tooth, and cause persistent pain, especially after consuming foods that are sweet, hot, or cold.

Dental cavities are treated by a dentist who removes the decayed tissue by using a dental drill. He or she then fills the prepared tooth with an amalgam or composite filling. See also TOOTH ABSCESS; TOOTHACHE.

CBC (complete blood cell count)

The number of red blood cells, white blood cells, and platelets in one cubic millimeter of blood. This laboratory test is commonly used to diagnose disease, especially infections and anemia. It is also used to guide decisions about the TRANSFUSION of red blood cells and platelets. See also DIAGNOSIS; MYELOPROLIFERATIVE DISORDERS.

CCU

See CORONARY CARE UNIT.

CD4 cell

A designation that refers to specific molecules present on the surface of immune cells called helper T lymphocytes, which are critical for the body's defenses in a variety of infections. During HIV (human immunodeficiency virus) infection, the virus binds to the CD4 molecules on the helper T cells. This allows the virus to attack the helper T cell, making it incapable of activating other immune cells, which decreases the immune system's function and makes a person more susceptible to infection by other pathogens.

Infection with HIV is characterized by a significant decline in the number of CD4 cells and in their ability to function. When T-cell function is sufficiently impaired, the infection progresses to AIDS (acquired immunodeficiency syndrome).

Cecum

The saclike first section of the large INTESTINE, located in the lower right abdomen. The small intestine ends at the cecum, and the appendix branches from it.

Celiac disease

A disorder in which the lining of the small intestine is damaged by an immune reaction to gluten, a protein found in grains, such as wheat, rye, and barley. Celiac disease leads to MALABSORPTION SYNDROME (the impaired absorption of nutrients in the small intestine).

Common symptoms include abdominal bloating and pain, weight loss, chronic diarrhea, and flatulence. Stools often are greasy, pale, bulky, and foul-smelling. In children, malnutrition may result, causing anemia, delayed growth, and FAILURE TO THRIVE. In some cases, the symptoms are not limited to the digestive system. They may also include fatigue, bone pain, behavioral changes, muscle cramps, joint pain, seizures, rash, numbness or tingling in the legs, sores in the mouth, tooth discoloration, and menstrual irregularity. In other cases, symptoms are virtually absent. There is an increased rate of intestinal cancer among individuals who have celiac disease.

Celiac disease is an autoimmune disorder (see AUTOIMMUNE DISORDERS), which means it is caused by a malfunction in the body's own immune system. It can be an inherited disorder, can occur at any age, and can be triggered by a stressful event. Because the symptoms mimic those of many other digestive disorders, establishing an accurate diagnosis can be difficult.

The only effective treatment is a change in diet. Avoidance of all foods that contain gluten is prescribed. Left untreated, celiac disease can lead to complications, such as CANCER, OSTEOPOROSIS, miscarriage, congenital defects, short stature in children, or seizures.

Cell

The fundamental structural unit of all body tissue and all living things. The human body is composed of billions of cells, specialized to carry out specific roles in the vast system of processes that keep the body functioning.

The cell centers on its nucleus, contained within the cytoplasm by a nuclear membrane. The nucleus directs the manufacture of cell proteins, and the type and quantity of proteins determine the structure and function of the cell. Amino acids are the chemical compounds that are the structural building blocks of proteins. The cell nucleus contains DNA, which provides the master pattern for these amino acids, as well as the mechanism for reproducing the same pattern for a new cell.

The genetic material of the cell, a chemical compound called DNA, is in the nucleus. The DNA is the chemical blueprint, or master plan, for the cell. The DNA is organized on stringlike structures called chromosomes, and each chromosome contains smaller units known as genes. The DNA (close to a particular gene on the chromosome) directs the formation of a related chemical called RNA, which carries an encoded message for the making of a specific protein. In this manner, the cell is able to accurately and efficiently pass along its unique characteristics to a new cell. See also CHROMOSOMES; GENE; and HEREDITY.

Cellulitis

An acute, spreading infection of the skin. Cellulitis often follows trauma to the skin; it is usually caused by a staphylococcal or streptococcal infection in otherwise healthy individuals. Common symptoms include redness, warmth, and tenderness of the affected area, as well as fever, chills, and malaise. Cellulitis is a serious disease because infection can spread via the lymph system or the bloodstream. Cellulitis is diagnosed by appearance, and the organism responsible for causing the condition may be identified in some cases by cultures of the blood. Cellulitis is treated with antibiotics.

Celsius scale

A temperature scale based on the difference between the freezing and boiling points of water. In the Celsius scale, the freezing point of water is 0° (32° Fahrenheit), and the boiling point is 100° (212° Fahrenheit).

Central nervous system

The BRAIN and the SPINAL CORD, which together monitor and control all the body's functions, responses, and behaviors, both conscious and unconscious. The central nervous system (CNS) works together with the peripheral nervous system, composed of the nerves emanating out from the CNS to all parts of the body. See NERVOUS SYSTEM.

The sensitive structures of the CNS are armored in bone: the brain lies within the SKULL, and the spinal cord is encased inside the bones of the spine.

The brain and spinal cord receive, process, and send information in the form of electrochemical impulses transmitted between individual nerve cells called neurons. The complex nerve pathways that make up the CNS are entirely composed of these specialized cells. See NERVE; NEURON.

Cephalosporins

A class of antibiotic drugs used to treat infections caused by bacteria. Cephalosporins work by damaging the cell walls of some bacteria and killing them. Cephalosporins are used to treat urinary tract infections, tonsillitis, celulitis, and respiratory tract infections such as pneumonia. Cephalosporins will not work for colds, flu, or other viral infections.

Cephalosporins should be used with caution for people who are allergic to penicillin-type antibiotics. The risk of cross allergy is about 15 percent. Allergic reactions may include rash, itching, fever, and very rarely, a severe ANAPHYLACTIC REACTION.

Cerclage, cervical

A surgical procedure that places a stitch called a cerclage in the cervix to hold it closed during pregnancy. The cerclage is used to try to stop PRETERM LABOR as a result of an INCOMPETENT CERVIX or a cervix that is unable to resist the pressure of the growing pregnancy. In the most common approach, the cerclage is a stitch placed by the physician that draws the cervix closed like a drawstring. The procedure is usually performed between the 13th and 16th weeks of pregnancy; the stitch is removed at about the 37th week, allowing labor

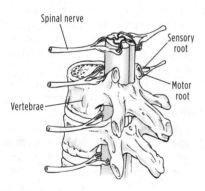

Spinal nerve

Sensory root

Motor root

Vertebrae

The spinal cord

The spinal cord, which links the brain to the rest of the body, is enclosed within the bony vertebral column for protection. Extending out from the spinal cord are the spinal nerves, including the sensory roots that convey information to the brain about body sensations and the motor roots that send information from the brain or spinal cord to muscles and organs.

and delivery to proceed normally thereafter. It is not clear how effective the cerclage is in stopping preterm labor.

Cerebellum

A portion of the BRAIN, located in the lower back of the skull and connected to the brain stem. This two-hemisphere structure coordinates balance and muscular movement.

Cerebral contusion

Damage to the surface of the brain and its underlying tissues from an acute head injury, such as that sustained in a fall. This results in a bruise on the brain as opposed to a concussion, which results in an alteration in consciousness but no structural damage.

Cerebral hemorrhage

See HEMORRHAGE, CEREBRAL.

Cerebral palsy

The term for a group of chronic disorders that impair control of movement, appear in the first few years of life, and generally do not worsen over time.

Acquired cerebral palsy is usually the result of brain damage from head injury or infection such as bacterial meningitis. Congenital cerebral palsy is present at birth, although it may not be diagnosed until some months later. Causes of congenital cerebral palsy include infections during pregnancy, jaundice in a newborn infant, RH INCOMPATIBILITY, and severe oxygen shortage in the brain or trauma to the head during labor and delivery.

Symptoms of cerebral palsy include seizures, muscle contractions, delayed development, mental retardation, gait abnormalities, spasticity, speech difficulties, vision problems, and hearing abnormalities. The initial signs of cerebral palsy usually occur before age 3 years. Parents are often the first to notice that an infant is not developing on schedule. This is usually known as DEVELOPMENTAL DELAY.

As time goes on, poor control of the muscles of the throat, mouth, and tongue can cause drooling. Difficulty with eating and swallowing may lead to a FAILURE TO THRIVE. Another common complication is incontinence in older children. About 50 to 70 percent of children with cerebral palsy have some intellectual impairment.

Diagnosis of cerebral palsy is based on medical history and the examination of a baby's motor skills. Doctors check for slow development, abnormal muscle tone, and unusual posture. The doctor may order tests such as CT (computed tomography) scanning, MRI (magnetic resonance imaging), ultrasound, or ELECTROENCEPHALOGRAM (EEG). Intelligence and vision tests are sometimes also recommended.

There is no cure for cerebral palsy. However, proper management of neurological problems can enable people with cerebral palsy to lead productive lives. Treatments include medication to control seizures and spasms; special braces to compensate for muscle imbalance; mechanical aids such as computers to overcome impairments; counseling for emotional and psychological needs; and physical, occupational, speech, and behavioral therapy. Surgery is sometimes recommended for contractures, conditions in which muscles become fixed in a rigid, abnormal position causing distortion or deformity.

Cerebral thrombosis

A clot or thrombus that forms in and blocks an artery in the brain. When the clot completely blocks the artery, cutting off blood and oxygen to the brain, brain cells die and a STROKE occurs. This can cause permanent damage to that area of the brain or death. Stroke is the third leading cause of death in the United States.

A stroke is a life-threatening condition for which immediate emergency treatment is required. Hospitalization is necessary and may include lifesaving interventions and supportive measures. There is no cure for a stroke. The goal of treatment is to limit the damage to the brain, control symptoms, and maximize an affected person's ability to function. Even with prompt treatment, death may occur. A person may also recover completely or suffer permanent BRAIN DAMAGE.

Cerebrospinal fluid

Also known as CSF, the clear, watery fluid that circulates inside and around the brain and spinal cord. In a diagnostic test called a LUMBAR PUNCTURE, a sample of CSF is removed for analysis in order to diagnose problems such as bacterial or viral meningitis, inflammation, tumors, hemorrhages, brain abscesses, and neurosyphilis.

Cerebrovascular accident

The sudden rupture or blockage of a blood vessel within the brain, leading to acute neurological damage; commonly referred to as STROKE. Cerebral infarctions, or thrombotic strokes, result from blockage caused by thrombosis (clot formation) or embolism (interruption of blood flow as a result of obstruction by a clot or plug of insoluble material carried in the bloodstream). An embolism usually results in a sudden onset of symptoms, while a thrombotic stroke usually begins more gradually.

Cerebrovascular disease

Any disease affecting an artery within and supplying blood to the brain. Risk factors for cerebrovascular disease include HYPERTENSION (high blood pressure), cigarette smoking, heart disease (see HEART DISEASE, ISCHEMIC; HEART DISEASE, CONGENITAL), warning signs or history of stroke, and diabetes (see DIABETES MELLITUS, TYPE 1; DIABETES MELLITUS, TYPE 2).

Cerebrum

The most developed, complex, and largest portion of the brain; the site of most conscious and intelligent activity. The cerebrum has two hemispheres (cerebral hemispheres) composed of white matter, covered by a thin, deeply wrinkled layer of gray matter (the cerebral cortex). The cerebral cortex is the site of language, sensation, voluntary movement, memory, emotion, and imagination.

Certification, board

The process through which a physician's qualifications in a medical specialty are recognized by one of the specialties that make up the American Board of Medical Specialties (ABMS). To become certified in a specialty (for example, pediatrics or surgery), a physician must generally complete an approved residency training program and pass a comprehensive examination.

Cerumen

See EARWAX.

Cervical cap

A barrier method of birth control that keeps sperm from entering the cervix. A cervical cap is a firm rubber dome that fits over a woman's cervix and is held in place by suction and a flexible ring. See CONTRACEPTION, BARRIER METHODS.

Cervical dysplasia

The presence of abnormal cells on the surface of the cervix. They are not cancerous, but have characteristics similar to early cancer cells when viewed under a microscope. Symptoms can include bleeding from the vagina between menstrual periods (see BREAK-THROUGH BLEEDING), after having sex, or after menopause, or a heavy vaginal discharge. Cervical dysplasia is often linked to HUMAN PAPILLOMAVIRUS (HPV), a sexually transmitted disease that causes venereal warts.

Cervical dysplasia is usually detected during a routine PAP SMEAR, a screening test for abnormal cell growth on the cervix. When abnormal cells are present, the doctor usually performs a COLPOSCOPY (a greatly magnified visual inspection of the cervix), and often a biopsy (removal of cells for examination under a microscope). Many mild cases of cervical dysplasia resolve on their own, while more severe cases usually require removal of the abnormal cells.

Cervical incompetence

See INCOMPETENT CERVIX.

Cervical intraepithelial neoplasia

See CIN.

Cervical polyps

Grapelike growths of tissue that may protrude from the opening of the cervix. The usual symptoms of polyps are bleeding during and after intercourse or a bloody discharge from the vagina.

While cervical polyps are usually harmless, a woman who has the symptoms of polyps should report them to her doctor because similar symptoms can be caused by cancer of the cervix (see CERVIX, CANCER OF). The doctor will likely perform a PAP SMEAR and BIOPSY to rule out cancer.

Cervicitis

An inflammation of the CERVIX, the lower part of the uterus. Symptoms may include an abnormal vaginal discharge, pain during sexual intercourse, bleeding after sexual intercourse, aching in the lower abdomen, frequent or painful urination, burning, itching, or fever. To diagnose cervicitis, a doctor performs a pelvic examination, a PAP SMEAR (to rule out the possibility of cervical cancer), and tests to culture for infectious organisms. The doctor may also perform a COLPOSCOPY (a magnified examination of the surface of the cervix).

Cervicitis is usually caused by a bacterial or viral infection, such as a sexually transmitted disease. If tests show that an infection is causing the cervicitis, antibiotics or other medications may be given. In cases in which a foreign object has caused the irritation, simply removing the object may be all that is needed. A woman who suspects that she may have cervicitis should contact a doctor; untreated cervicitis can lead to PELVIC INFLAMMATORY DISEASE or fertility problems.

Cervix

A small, cylindrical organ made up of fibrous tissue and muscle located between the uterus and the vagina. An opening in the middle of the cervix connects the cavity of the uterus with the vagina. This passage is large enough to allow menstrual fluid to pass out of the vagina, but is too small to allow foreign objects to enter. Glands inside the cervix produce mucus that helps prevent microorganisms from infecting the vagina. The cervix has a circular muscle that expands in size and shape during pregnancy and childbirth. During childbirth, the cervix can expand to about 4 inches wide. See also REPRODUCTIVE SYSTEM, FEMALE.

Cervix, cancer of

A curable, slow-growing cancer that initially develops in the cervix and, if untreated, can spread to the other reproductive organs. Cancer of the cervix chiefly occurs in women between the ages of 30 and 55 and is nearly 100 percent curable when caught in the precancerous stage. It is one of the few cancers that has well-defined, recognizable precancerous stages. Before the cancer appears, abnormal changes occur in the cells on the surface of the cervix. The precancerous condition, CERVICAL DYSPLASIA, is categorized in various stages. The mildly abnormal cells may return to normal or may eventually develop into cancer. Severe dysplasia and early cancer can be treated and entirely cured.

The warning signs of cancer of the cervix may include vaginal bleeding after sexual intercourse or between periods, genital warts, an abnormal vaginal discharge, and pain during intercourse. However, the precancerous stage (dysplasia) usually exhibits no symptoms. Diagnosis of cancer of the cervix starts with a PAP SMEAR. If dysplasia is detected, another pap smear may be done, or a colposcopy (examination of the cervix under illuminated magnification) or biopsy (taking a tissue sample) may be performed.

If an area of abnormal cell growth persists, or if early cancer is diagnosed through colposcopy or biopsy, treatment is necessary. A local anesthetic will be given, and the doctor can use one of several methods—laser surgery (using extreme heat) or cryosurgery (using extreme cold)—to destroy the abnormal cells. If cancer has been diagnosed, the affected tissue may be removed in a cone biopsy. In more advanced cases, radiation may be used to kill or shrink the cancer cells. Chemotherapy may be given either orally or intravenously, or surgery may be performed.

A localized tumor may be treated by a hysterectomy, possibly combined with radiation, while more extensive surgery is needed if the tumor has spread beyond the cervix. Once cervical cancer has spread to the lungs, liver, and other organs, only palliative therapy (treatment that relieves the symptoms but does not cure the disease) is available.

Cesarean section

A surgical procedure in which a baby is delivered through incisions in the mother's abdominal and uterine walls. It is performed in situations where it has been judged the safest method of CHILDBIRTH. A cesarean section may be performed if labor fails to progress (the contractions are not adequately dilating the cervix); in a multiple pregnancy; or if a baby is in distress, in a BREECH PRESENTATION, or is too big to pass safely through the mother's birth canal. A cesarean section may also be needed if the mother has a serious medical condition, such as diabetes, blood pressure problems, ECLAMPSIA, or active genital herpes. A woman who has had a cesarean section may deliver vaginally in a future pregnancy.

Chalazion

An inflamed, tender lump on the eyelid caused by the blockage of a small gland that produces the oil layer of tears. A chalazion appears some distance from the edge of the eyelid, unlike a stye, which occurs close to the eyelashes. A chalazion may cause discomfort in the eye, sensitivity to light, and increased tearing. Over

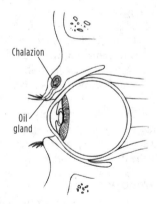

Inflamed oil gland
A chalazion differs from a stye in that it does not contain an active bacterial infection. It forms when debris blocks the natural drainage of oils from glands in the eyelid. A chalazion tends to be less painful than a stye but often is more long-lasting, taking a month or more to diminish.

time a chalazion forms a cystlike swelling, which may put pressure on the eyeball and distort vision (ASTIGMATISM) or become infected. In many cases, chalazions resolve on their own within a few months. Applying warm compresses (a clean cloth soaked in hot water and wrung out) for 10 minutes four times a day may speed healing. If swelling continues, a chalazion can be drained surgically under local anesthesia in the doctor's office.

Chancre

A painless, ulcerated lesion that may be produced by an inflammatory reaction that occurs 10 to 60 days after exposure to SYPHILIS. Chancres are usually located on the genitals and tend to heal spontaneously, although the syphilis infection persists.

Chancroid

A sexually transmitted disease (STD) caused by the bacterium *Haemophilus ducreyi* when it enters the body through a scrape, sore, or crack on the surface skin of the genitals. Chancroid is spread via direct contact with a chancroid sore during sexual contact, including vaginal, anal, or oral sex.

Generally, within 2 to 5 days of sexual contact, the initial symptom of chancroid appears in the genital area as one or more small, painful, open, red sores, which may bleed when touched. The sores may produce pus and a bad odor and can spread to the thighs and abdomen. If they become infected, they may cause the lymph nodes in the groin to become painful and swollen.

Untreated, the infection can produce chronic sores on the genitals that may persist for months. Chancroid is successfully treated with antibiotics. Chancroid is contagious for as long as a person has open sores.

Charcot joint

The chronic degeneration of a joint that may not cause any discomfort because of a neuropathy (loss of sensation) affecting the joint. Charcot joint is usually caused by neurological disorders, such as diabetic neuropathy (see DIABETES MELLITUS, TYPE 2), leprosy, and syphilis. It is characterized by swelling, hemorrhage, heat, instability, and atrophy of joints, such as the knee. Early diagnosis and treatment can sometimes prevent further damage. However, in severe cases, joint replacement may become necessary.

Charcot-Marie-Tooth disease

A group of inherited neuromuscular disorders characterized by weakness and loss of muscle tissue in the lower legs, feet, and hands. Charcot-Marie-Tooth disease (CMT) occurs when the insulating tissue surrounding peripheral nerve fibers or the nerve fibers themselves degenerate. The disease is named for the three French doctors who first identified it. CMT chiefly affects muscular and sensory function in the limbs and is one of the most common hereditary neurologic disorders.

Individuals with CMT slowly lose normal use of their hands, feet, arms, and legs as the nerves to the extremities degenerate. CMT is also associated with foot deformities, such as high arches or flexed toes. Often, a high-arched foot is the first sign of the disorder. Mild loss of sensation can often occur. The leg and foot problems usually allow people to live active lives and only rarely are so disabling that the person needs to use a wheelchair.

A doctor experienced with the disease will suspect CMT based on a characteristic pattern of foot, leg, and hand weakness. A family history and tests will be used to confirm the diagnosis. Tests may include an ELECTROMYOGRAM (EMG), which records the electrical activity of muscle cells and shows characteristic changes of CMT; a nerve conduction velocity test, which measures the speed at which nerve impulses travel along the nerves; and DNA studies.

Treatment may involve physical therapy, lightweight lower leg braces, shoe inserts, and sometimes surgery to correct foot deformities. There is no cure for CMT.

Chelation therapy

Traditional treatment for people poisoned with heavy metals. Chelation is the process of removing undesirable metals from the body by administering substances called chelating agents, which bind chemically to the metals in the blood. The metal and the chelating substance form a compound that can be excreted in the urine.

Chelation therapy is a standard medical treatment for people poisoned with lead, iron, arsenic, mercury, copper, zinc, aluminum, manganese, and other metals. Chelation therapy is recommended by some alternative medicine practitioners as a treatment for heart and arterial disease, but there is no scientific evidence for any benefits with heart disease.

Chemical peel

The use of a caustic agent, usually an acid, to remove the damaged, outer layers of the skin and to improve and smooth its texture. Chemical peels are used for people with wrinkles caused by sun exposure, aging, blemishes, acne scars, and uneven pigmentation. A chemical peel can be applied to the entire face or to specific areas.

Chemotherapy

Treatment with drugs, especially for cancer. Cancer chemotherapy includes any and all medications used to treat cancer, whether the drugs are antineoplastic (anticancer) or cytotoxic (cell-killing). Chemotherapy is often used in comprehensive cancer therapy because it reaches throughout the entire body. Localized treatment, such as surgery and radiation, target a specific area. Chemotherapy can treat cancer cells that have spread beyond the original site of the disease to other parts of the body.

Chemotherapy drugs are divided into several categories based on how they affect chemicals in cancer cells, the specific cellular processes the drug interferes with, and the phase of the cell cycle the drug affects.

• *ALKYLATING AGENTS* These drugs work directly on DNA to prevent the cancer cell from reproducing. They are used to treat chronic leukemia, non-Hodgkin lymphoma, multiple myeloma, and some cancers of the breast, ovary, and lung.

• *NITROSOUREAS* Nitrosoureas inhibit enzymes needed for DNA repair. Because these drugs can travel to the brain, they are used to treat brain tumors. They also are used to treat non-Hodgkin lymphomas, multiple myeloma, and malignant melanoma.

• *ANTIMETABOLITES* These drugs interfere with the growth of RNA and DNA. They are used to treat chronic leukemias and tumors of the breast, ovary, and gastrointestinal tract.

• *ANTITUMOR ANTIBIOTICS* These drugs have both antimicrobial and cytotoxic activity. They also interfere with DNA by inhibiting certain cellular activities, and they work in all phases of the cell cycle.

• *MITOTIC INHIBITORS* These drugs can inhibit cell division (mitosis) or interfere with other parts of cell reproduction.

Chest pain

For symptom chart see CHEST PAIN, page xiv.

Any pressure, squeezing, or general discomfort in the chest. Chest pain is not a condition in itself but a symptom of an underlying cause that can be serious, such as heart attack, or trivial, such as indigestion or a strained muscle.

The most common type of chest pain related to the heart is ANGINA, which is caused by insufficient blood flow to the heart. Examples of other heart-related causes of chest pain include malfunction of the heart's mitral valve (MITRAL VALVE PROLAPSE (MVP)) or aortic valve (AORTIC STENOSIS), inflammation of the tissue surrounding the heart (PERICARDITIS), and inflammation of the heart muscle itself (MYOCARDITIS).

About one in five people who see a doctor for chest pain are experiencing difficulty with the esophagus, the tube that leads from the throat to the stomach. The most common disease of the esophagus that causes chest pain is HEARTBURN, which can be a symptom of ESOPHAGEAL REFLUX (acidic stomach contents entering the esophagus) or HIATAL HERNIA (a portion of the stomach protrudes through the diaphragm muscle).

Since chest pain is not a condition but a symptom, treatment depends on the source of the problem. The principal diagnostic objective is to determine whether the pain originates in the heart or in another organ.

Chest tube

A medical instrument used to drain accumulations of fluid in the pleural space, a condition called PLEURAL EFFUSION.

Chest X ray

The most common diagnostic tool for producing images of the structures, organs, and tissues inside the chest. When X-ray beams are passed through the chest, dense structures such as bone do not allow many X rays to pass through them. Tubular structures such as the blood vessels in the chest are outlined more clearly on X-ray film if they are filled with a CONTRAST MEDIUM. Chest X rays may be used to diagnose lung diseases such as cancer or pneumonia or to help identify conditions such as an enlarged heart, congestive heart failure, and other consequences of heart disease.

Cheyne-Stokes

An abnormal respiratory pattern characterized by alternating episodes of APNEA (in this case, a temporary cessation of breathing) and deep, rapid breathing. Causes of Cheyne-Stokes respiration include cerebrovascular disease, brain tumors, metabolic disturbances affecting the brain, and head trauma. See also SLEEP DISORDERS.

Chickenpox

An acute, highly contagious illness caused by the varicella-zoster virus, which also causes SHINGLES, a later reactivation of the virus. Chickenpox is transmitted by direct contact with a person who has the illness or by respiratory exposure to infected droplets. The incubation period is 14 to 16 days, and it can be transmitted within 10 to 21 days following exposure. To prevent transmission to another person, the individual who has chickenpox should be isolated until all the skin lesions have crusted over.

An itchy rash of red-outlined, fluid-filled bumps, often described as dew drops on a rose petal, is the first symptom of chickenpox. Moderate fever, mild headache, and general malaise may also be present.

Diagnosis is made on the basis of a physical examination and medical history and confirmed by detection of viral antigens in the lesions or blood. In mild cases, only the symptoms of chickenpox are usually treated. Wet compresses may be applied to control itching and scratching. To prevent infection of the lesions, frequent bathing with soap and water and frequent changes of underclothing are recommended. In more severe cases, antiviral medications, oral antihistamines, or pain relievers are sometimes given. The risk of severe, even fatal, disease is higher in adults and in persons with depressed T-cell immunity (for example, those with AIDS [acquired immunodeficiency syndrome]) or people taking CORTICOSTEROIDS or receiving CHEMOTHERAPY. A vaccine is recommended for all healthy children who have not had chickenpox, beginning at the age of 12 to 18 months, or between 19 months and 13 years of age.

Child abuse

See ABUSE, CHILD.

Childbirth

The process of giving birth to a child, involving the three stages of LABOR. Usually, babies are delivered with the help of a medical caregiver. Some women cannot deliver their babies by vaginal delivery (see DELIVERY, VAGINAL) and must have them by CESAREAN SECTION (C-section), a surgical procedure in a hospital in which the baby is born through an incision in the abdomen.

Chiropractic

The practice of physical manipulation to diagnose, treat, and rehabilitate disorders of the neuromusculoskeletal system. Chiropractic is based on the ideas that the human body has an innate self-healing ability and that it seeks balance. Chiropractors believe that small internal misalignments, called vertebral subluxations, interfere with proper functioning of the nervous system and the body's ability to maintain a healthy balance. Chiropractic seeks to bring a misaligned body back into balance through the manual manipulation of the spine, joints, and muscles.

The manual manipulation of the spine practiced by chiropractors is widely considered to be effective for the relief of acute lower back pain.

Chlamydia

The most common bacterial sexually transmitted disease (STD; see SEXUALLY TRANSMITTED DISEASES) in the United States. Chlamydia is caused by the bacterium *Chlamydia trachomatis* and is usually transmitted by sexual activity. The bacteria that cause the infection are carried in the blood, semen, or vaginal fluid of an infected person, entering the body via contact with these fluids.

In men, chlamydia can cause nonspecific urethritis (NSU), with symptoms including a discharge from the penis and pain when urinating. Chlamydia may also cause a swelling of the testes.

Women often have no symptoms of chlamydia. If symptoms occur, they may include a yellow-green vaginal discharge, pain during urination, persistent lower abdominal pain, pain during sexual intercourse, spotting between menstrual periods, and possibly nausea and fever.

Without treatment, chlamydia may persist for as long as 15 months, during which time it is communicable to sexual partners. The infection can eventually spread to the upper reproductive tract in women and result in serious complications, including inflammation of the fallopian tubes (SALPINGITIS) or the cervix (CERVICITIS) and PELVIC INFLAMMATORY DISEASE (PID). These conditions can cause INFERTILITY. In pregnant women, the bacteria can be passed to the fetus.

Chlamydia may be diagnosed by culturing cells, but more commonly, newer tests are used that detect chlamydial DNA or that use immuno-fluorescent antibodies to detect chlamydia. A 7-day course of oral antibiotics is generally prescribed to treat chlamydia.

Choking

A breathing emergency caused by an airway that has been blocked by food or another object. Choking is a common emergency, usually the result of inadequately chewed food that has become lodged in the throat or windpipe.

Choking is usually accompanied by panic, with a visible expression of terror on the person's face. He or she may turn purple, the eyes may bulge, and the person may wheeze or gasp. If the person is turning blue and is able to communicate only through hand gestures, he or she is most likely choking. The HEIMLICH MANEUVER may be used by trained persons to dislodge the obstruction. Even if the blockage is removed and the person's breathing restored, emergency medical assistance should always be sought, because complications can arise from both the emergency and the first aid measures taken.

Cholangiocarcinoma

A cancer of the bile ducts, the tubes that carry bile from the liver and gallbladder to the small intestine. Symptoms of this uncommon cancer include jaundice (yellowing of the skin), pale stools, and dark urine, often accompanied by weight loss and fatigue. No effective treatments have been developed, and the prognosis is usually poor. Complete surgical removal of the affected duct is some-times attempted if the cancer is small and localized.

Cholangiopancreatography

A diagnostic procedure performed to evaluate diseases of the bile ducts of the liver such as stones or narrowing. In conventional ERCP (endoscopic retrograde cholangiopancreatography), a CONTRAST MEDIUM is injected directly into the bile ducts. In magnetic resonance cholangiopancreatography (see MRI), the bile ducts are visualized without the use of a contrast medium during an abdominal magnetic resonance examination.

Cholangitis

Inflammation of the bile ducts, the channels that carry bile from the liver to the gallbladder and to the intestines. (See BILARY SYSTEM.) Cholangitis is most commonly the result of obstruction of bile flow and consequent bacterial infection. The most common symptoms of cholangitis are abdominal pain, fever, and jaundice (a yellowing of the skin and the whites of the eyes). In some cases, abdominal symptoms are minimal, but chills and fever are present.

When the symptoms suggest cholangitis, it is important to discover the underlying cause and location of obstruction to avoid recurrence. Cholangitis is diagnosed by ultrasound and CT (computed tomography) SCANNING or ERCP (endoscopic retrograde cholangiopancreatography). Balloons can be inserted to open up blockages.

Cholecystectomy

Surgical removal of the gallbladder. A cholecystectomy is performed in severe cases of CHOLECYSTITIS, or inflammation of the gallbladder. Cholecystitis is usually the result of GALLSTONES (solid masses, primarily of cholesterol, formed in the gallbladder). Cholecystectomy is also indicated for patients with recurrent symptoms due to gallstones.

Today, laparoscopic cholecystectomy is the preferred surgical treatment of symptomatic gallstones. It has largely replaced open cholecystectomy, which requires a long abdominal incision.

Cholecystitis

Inflammation of the GALLBLADDER. Cholecystitis is usually the result of GALLSTONES (solid masses, primarily of cholesterol, which form in the gallbladder). When a gallstone in the cystic duct blocks the flow of bile from the gallbladder to the intestine, acute cholecystitis occurs and requires immediate treatment. Very often, surgical removal of the gallbladder (CHOLECYSTECTOMY) is necessary.

A stone that lodges in the cystic duct can cause extreme cramping pain in the upper abdomen. The pain may radiate to the right shoulder and the back and can be mistaken for a heart attack. As the gallbladder becomes increasingly inflamed, nausea and vomiting occur. Left untreated, jaundice (a yellowing of the skin and the whites of the eyes) and CHOLANGITIS (inflammation of the bile ducts) may develop. A rare but extremely serious complication of cholecystitis can be rupture of the gallbladder. This causes a severe form of peritonitis (inflammation of the peritoneum, the membrane that lines the abdominal cavity). A life-threatening emergency, peritonitis requires immediate medical treatment.

In some cases, a stone that obstructs the bile duct may pass on its own into the duodenum or fall back into the gallbladder. However, in most cases, gallstones must be removed by using an endoscope or by surgery.

Cholecystography

An X-ray procedure for examining the gallbladder and common bile duct, which cannot be seen in a normal X ray. In cholecystography, a contrast dye that can make the organs visible in an X ray is administered either orally or intravenously. The dye can reveal the presence of gallstones or blockages; failure of the dye to become concentrated in the gallbladder may indicate a diseased gallbladder. Cholecystography can help to diagnose problems such as CHOLECYSTITIS (inflammation of the gallbladder that is most often caused by GALLSTONES) and BILIARY COLIC. Cholecystography has been replaced by ultrasound scanning as the first choice for imaging the gallbladder. It is now used when ultrasound scanning fails to provide a definite diagnosis.

Cholera

An acute intestinal infection that is caused by the bacterium *Vibrio cholerae*. In epidemics, the organism is spread by water contaminated directly or indirectly with feces or vomit from people who are infected. The organism that causes cholera is able to grow well in some foods, including rice, but it cannot grow or survive in acidic foods, including carbonated beverages, and is killed by heat.

People infected with cholera may have only mild diarrhea or no symptoms at all. In severe cases, death may occur within hours of becoming infected. Profuse watery diarrhea and vomiting cause a rapid, life-threatening loss of vital fluids and salts, with the possibility of circulatory collapse and shock. Cholera can be fatal if it is not diagnosed and treated promptly.

For milder cases, treatment is generally based on having the person drink an oral rehydration solution or, in more severe cases, administration of intravenous solutions until the person is able to ingest fluids.

Cholesteatoma

A benign mass or tumorlike growth formed by an accumulation of dead cells in the middle ear and/or mastoid (the prominent bone behind the ear). The condition is caused by repeated or chronic middle ear infections and inflammation and is usually associated with poor eustachian tube function. Cholesteatomas are formed when the skin of the eardrum grows into the middle ear. This skin forms a ball-shaped pocket that fills up with dead cells shed by the eardrum. The pocket erodes the bone that lines the middle ear cavity, often damages the delicate bones of hearing in the middle ear, and may become infected.

Mild to moderately severe hearing loss and a recurring discharge from the ear are usually the symptoms of cholesteatoma. Headache, earache, weakness of the facial muscles, and dizziness are less common symptoms that may precede serious complications.

The first phase of medical treatment for cholesteatoma with drainage concentrates on drying the fluid that is causing the infection within the ear. If there are polyps (growths of in-flamed tissue) in the ear canal, they may have to be surgically removed before the infection will clear up. Once the infection has cleared up and the ear is dry, MICROSURGERY and complete removal of the cholesteatoma by an ear surgeon are usually recommended.

Cholesterol

A chemical that is an essential component of cells and is a building block for many hormones. Cholesterol, a sterol, is a form of lipid (see LIPIDS). A certain amount of cholesterol is required by the body. Elevated levels of this waxy, fatlike substance are associated with an increased risk of ATHEROSCLEROSIS, a condition in which blood vessels are narrowed by fat deposits, which can compromise the blood flow to vital organs. Eventually, there may be sufficient blockage of an artery to cause a HEART ATTACK or STROKE. Eating too much fat, especially saturated fat, can raise blood cholesterol levels. See also FATS AND OILS.

A person's cholesterol levels are determined by a combination of genes and lifestyle. When blood cholesterol is high, lifestyle changes, such as diet and exercise modification, may bring it under control.

When the total blood cholesterol level is elevated, tests can detect the levels of the different types of blood cholesterol. Cholesterol does not float freely in the bloodstream, but is attached to special carriers called lipoproteins. The two most important carriers are low-density lipoprotein (LDL) and high-density lipoprotein (HDL). The levels of LDL and HDL have opposite effects on the heart. High levels of LDL, referred to as "the bad cholesterol," are associated with a buildup of plaque (fat deposits) in the arteries, leading to atherosclerosis and heart disease. High levels of HDL, "the good cholesterol," reduce the risk of disease.

Cholesterol in foods

Dietary cholesterol is present in all animal products (meat, poultry, dairy products, eggs, cheese, butter, and fish). Red meats (beef, pork, and lamb) contain the most cholesterol, while fish and poultry generally contain lesser amounts. There is no cholesterol in any plant product or the oils made from them.

Saturated fat from both animal and plant products is a major factor in raising blood cholesterol levels and may be even more damaging than foods high in cholesterol such as egg yolks. Saturated fats are found in meats, poultry, dairy products, certain tropical vegetable oils (palm, palm kernel, coconut), and solid vegetable fats that are hard at room temperature; they should be avoided.

Like saturated fats, trans-fatty acids (also known as trans fats) raise levels of harmful LDL cholesterol, promote clogged arteries, and increase the risk of heart disease. They may be present in stick margarine, crackers, cookies, and deep-fried foods.

Unsaturated fats

Unsaturated fats such as fish oils and pure vegetable oils are healthier choices than saturated fats and hydrogenated oils. Some unsaturated fats even lower cholesterol levels and may reduce the risk of cardiovascular disease.

Canola oil and avocado oil are good sources of monounsaturated fats, as are a variety of nuts: almonds, hazel-nuts, macadamias, pecans, and pistachios. Monounsaturated fatty acids lower levels of harmful LDL cholesterol and have no negative effect on the helpful HDL variety. Polyunsaturated fats are found in corn, safflower, soybean, and sunflower oils. Omega-3 fatty acids, another type of polyunsaturated fats, are found in fish.

Cholesterol-lowering drugs

Drugs used to lower cholesterol levels and reduce the risk of heart disease. Most people with high cholesterol levels are able to reduce their levels with improved diet and increased exercise, but for some, these measures are not enough, and cholesterol-lowering drugs must be prescribed. There are four types of drugs used to lower cholesterol levels.

Statins

These drugs lower levels of total cholesterol, LDL (low-density lipoprotein) cholesterol ("bad" cholesterol), and to a lesser degree, triglycerides. Statins work by interfering with the manufacture of cholesterol in the body, blocking an enzyme called HMG-CoA reductase that is needed by the body to manufacture cholesterol. Less cholesterol in the body stimulates the liver to remove LDL cholesterol from the bloodstream, thus lowering the risk of clogged blood vessels and heart disease.

Bile acid sequestrants

Bile acid sequestrants are synthetic substances that lower both total cholesterol and LDL cholesterol levels. The body does not absorb these drugs, so they are relatively free of serious side effects. They work by binding to the acids in the intestine and prevent their reabsorption, causing their elimination in the stool. With fewer bile acids in circulation, the liver is forced to convert cholesterol into bile acids, thereby removing LDL from the blood.

Bile acid sequestrants have side effects, including constipation, gas, bloating, nausea, and heartburn. The constipation associated with this therapy tends to diminish over time.

Niacin (nicotinic acid)

Niacin is one of the B vitamins and is needed for carbohydrate metabolism. When taken in very large quantities, niacin becomes an effective, versatile, low-cost drug that lowers LDL cholesterol and triglyceride levels while raising HDL (high-density lipoprotein) cholesterol ("good" cholesterol) levels. When combined with a bile acid sequestrant, niacin can reduce LDL cholesterol levels by as much as 40 to 60 percent.

There are disadvantages to niacin. Some forms of it must be taken three times a day, and the sustained-release form can have toxic effects on the liver. Niacin can also raise the blood sugar level so it should be taken with caution by people with diabetes.

Fibric acid derivatives

Fibric acid derivatives lower the levels of triglycerides and very low-density lipoproteins. Although fibric acid derivatives raise HDL cholesterol levels, they do not lower LDL cholesterol levels as effectively as other drugs. These drugs are chiefly used to treat people with exceptionally high levels of triglycerides. They work by reducing the production of triglycerides in the liver or by preventing their synthesis.

Side effects of fibric acid derivatives include dizziness, drowsiness, blurred vision, chest pain, flulike symptoms, and liver disorders.

Cholesterol absorption inhibitor

This is a newer class of drug that inhibits the uptake of cholesterol by the large intestine, or colon. Ezetimibe is the first drug developed in this category, and it is often given with the statin drug simvastatin in a combination drug. Side effects may include stomach pain, feeling tired, or allergic reactions such as throat swelling. The doctor should be notified promptly if these side effects occur.

Chondromalacia

The progressive softening and erosion of cartilage, most commonly appearing in the undersurface of the kneecap (patella). The principal symptom of the condition is tenderness or pain behind and around the kneecap(s). Activities that involve repeated or prolonged bending of the knee, such as walking on an incline, climbing and descending stairs, squatting, or sitting for a long time, intensify the pain.

Treatment provided by a physician specializing in sports medicine generally includes applying heat and taking anti-inflammatory medication, such as aspirin, ibuprofen, or other NONSTEROIDAL ANTI-INFLAMMATORY DRUGS (NSAIDs).

Chondromatosis

A condition in which benign cartilage masses or tumors covering a movable joint become detached and remain in the joint space. These free bodies are sometimes called "joint mice." Chondromatosis most commonly affects the knee joint. The symptoms include limited range of motion in the affected joint, and, if the condition persists over time, there is an increased risk of degenerative joint disease. The cause is unknown.

Chorioamnionitis

In pregnancy, inflammation of the amniotic membranes typically after their rupture. The cause is an infection by bacteria that reach the uterus through the vagina. Symptoms in the mother include fever, abdominal pain and cramping, a drop in blood pressure, and tenderness of the uterus. Symptoms in the fetus include a higher than normal heart rate.

Chorioamnionitis generally occurs at the end of a pregnancy, when more than 24 hours have elapsed between rupture of the membranes and delivery, permitting bacteria to multiply. To avoid the risk of infection, doctors will choose to induce labor if it has not begun spontaneously within 12 to 36 hours of membrane rupture. In rare instances, an infection occurs when there has been no obvious rupture of the membranes and sometimes may cause PRETERM LABOR. AMNIOCENTESIS may be used to confirm the presence of an infection.

Chorioamnionitis is treated in a hospital with antibiotics given intravenously. Because the antibiotics cannot penetrate the placenta to treat the fetus, immediate delivery is recommended. If the baby is born with an infection, antibiotics may be given intravenously.

Chorionic villi

During pregnancy, tiny fingerlike projections attached to a membrane that eventually becomes the part of the PLACENTA closest to the baby. The fetal blood vessels project into the villi, which are surrounded by the mother's blood.

Chorionic villus sampling

A prenatal test that detects genetic abnormalities in a fetus. In chorionic villus sampling (CVS), a small sample of chorionic villi (projections in the placenta that absorb nutrients from the mother's blood) is taken from the placenta.

Chorionic villus sampling can detect most of the same defects as AMNIOCENTESIS, but it can be performed earlier. The test is usually performed in a hospital, between the 9th and 12th weeks of the pregnancy, with results available in about 10 days.

Chorionic villus sampling is not

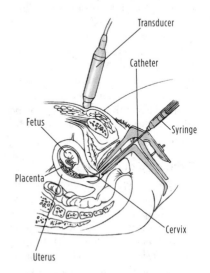

Prenatal testing

For chorionic villus sampling (CVS), the doctor inserts a catheter into the uterus via the vagina and, guided by ultrasound transducer, extracts cells from a part of the placenta called the chorionic villi.

without risk, including the risk of injury or infection of the cervix. The risk of miscarriage is greater with CVS (1 in 100) than with amniocentesis (1 in 200). Rarely, the test causes harm, such as limb deformities to the fetus, especially when performed before the 10th week of pregnancy.

Chromium

A gray, metallic element essential for energy in the human diet. In its active form, chromium helps insulin to move glucose, or blood sugar, from the bloodstream into the cells where it can be metabolized. A diet that is low in chromium can affect the ability of insulin to process carbohydrates, proteins, and fats. The best dietary source for chromium is brewer's yeast grown in chromium-rich soil.

Chromium picolinate

A complex mineral important for converting carbohydrates and fat into energy and maintaining normal blood sugar levels. Chromium picolinate is naturally present in whole grains, brewer's yeast, nuts, and dried beans. Only trace amounts are required by the body.

Chromosomal abnormalities

Variations from normal in the number or structure of chromosomes, which may or may not cause genetic defects. Chromosomes carry genes, which determine an individual's characteristics. About one in 500 newborns has a chromosomal abnormality. Abnormalities generally occur while egg and sperm cells are forming.

Chromosomal abnormalities are diagnosed through KARYOTYPING, a process for analyzing chromosomes through a blood, skin, bone marrow, or other tissue sample. The chromosomes are examined under a microscope where they are counted and structural defects are identified. Prenatal testing is available to diagnose a chromosomal abnormality in a fetus when there is a high risk or the suspicion of a problem.

Types of abnormalities

Chromosomal abnormalities can range from very severe and lethal, to disorders that involve mental retardation, to relatively mild disorders, depending on which chromosomes are involved.

Sometimes a fetus can inherit the wrong number of chromosomes, and instead of receiving the normal 46 (23 from each parent), it will receive an extra set, for a total of 69 chromosomes. Sometimes a fetus inherits a single extra chromosome from a parent or may be missing a chromosome. Various conditions, such as DOWN SYNDROME (trisomy 21 syndrome), trisomy 18 syndrome, and trisomy 13 syndrome, involve having an abnormal number of chromosomes. Abnormalities can also occur due to structural changes within chromosomes. These types of changes can result in mental retardation and other birth defects. It is unknown why such breaks occur.

Birth defects

Birth defects associated with chromosomal abnormalities can be divided into two categories: those that occur in sex chromosomes and those that occur in the other chromosomes. Most human chromosomal abnormalities occur in the autosomes, the 22 pairs of chromosomes that are the same in males and females. The most common serious autosomal abnormality is Down syndrome, which occurs occurs in one of every 800 births. Both autosomal and sex chromosomal abnormalities usually can be diagnosed before birth by AMNIOCENTESIS and CHORIONIC VILLUS SAMPLING.

Chromosomes

Genetic material in the nucleus of cells where genes are located. Chromosomes consist of highly compacted threads of DEOXYRIBONUCLEIC ACID (DNA) and associated proteins. Each species normally has a characteristic number of chromosomes in each cell; 46 chromosomes are found in human cells, including two that determine the sex of the individual.

Chronic

Long-lasting; long-term; always present. In medicine, a chronic condition is one lasting 3 months or more.

Chronic fatigue syndrome

A serious, often disabling illness characterized by persistent, unrelenting, and severe exhaustion, as well as muscle pain and cognitive disorders that are sometimes referred to as "brain fog." Chronic fatigue syndrome (CFS) is not associated with significant muscle weakness, psychological disorders, or physical illness. The condition affects women three times more often than men. Adolescents may be affected, but less frequently than adults.

The earliest symptom of CFS may be a strong, noticeable feeling of exhaustion that comes on suddenly and persists or continually comes and goes. A good night's sleep does not alleviate the feeling of tiredness.

Two criteria are used in the medical diagnosis of chronic fatigue syndrome: the person diagnosed must have experienced severe and chronic fatigue for 6 months or longer without other known medical conditions that have been clinically diagnosed. In addition, the person must have four or more of a set of specific symptoms at the same time, including substantial impairment in short-term memory or concentration, sore throat, tender lymph nodes, muscle pain, multijoint pain without redness or swelling, headaches different from those previously experienced, unrefreshing sleep, and malaise lasting more than 24 hours after exercise. Further diagnostic evaluation for chronic fatigue syndrome is usually based on the exclusion of other possible illnesses. True CFS, in which a person meets the diagnostic criteria, is rare. Since the cause of CFS is unknown, treatment is aimed at relieving symptoms.

Chronic obstructive lung disease

See CHRONIC OBSTRUCTIVE PULMONARY DISEASE.

Chronic obstructive pulmonary disease

An obstruction of the airways that progressively affects the ability to breathe. Chronic obstructive pulmonary disease, or COPD, is caused by chronic bronchitis or emphysema or a combination of the two. Emphysema is defined by anatomical changes in the lung and characterized by destruction of the tissue that makes up the walls of the air sacs, or alveoli, which results in overinflation of the air sacs. Chronic bronchitis is defined by clinical symptoms and characterized by a daily cough and sputum production for 3 months or longer. Cigarette smoking is the primary cause of COPD, although not all smokers get COPD. COPD is irreversible; however, if a person stops smoking, the disease progression is slowed.

Symptoms of COPD begin with a cough that produces mucus and usually occurs upon awakening in the morning. When a person who has COPD acquires a common cold (see COLD, COMMON), the infection tends to progress quickly to the chest area. Frequently, the mucus coughed up during chest colds is yellow or green.

If COPD progresses, shortness of breath (see BREATH, SHORTNESS OF), generally becomes more pronounced over time. At first, shortness of breath occurs with physical exertion, but people with advanced COPD may experience labored breathing even at rest. In the early stages of COPD, chest X rays are usually normal; in advanced stages of COPD, they may demonstrate changes that are not specific to COPD but are characteristic of it. Spirometry, a test that measures airflow, can confirm the diagnosis. Analysis of arterial blood gases is needed.

There is no cure for the condition, but several strategies may be helpful. Smoking cessation is the first and most important approach.

Since bouts of INFLUENZA or PNEUMONIA can intensify the symptoms of COPD and because a person who has the condition may be more susceptible to these infections, annual influenza vaccinations and a pneumococcal vaccination every 6 years are recommended. When bacterial infections occur, antibiotics may be prescribed early to help control the intensified COPD symptoms these infections can cause.

Some of the conditions produced by COPD, including bronchospasm, spasm of the muscles lining the airway, inflammation, and excessive secretions, can be improved. BRONCHODILATORS in metered-dose inhalers or oral medications can relax constricted bronchial airways and help relieve the wheezing associated with bronchospasm. In some people with COPD, CORTICOSTEROIDS may decrease inflammation. Increased fluid intake is helpful for thinning secretions so they may be expelled more efficiently, and RESPIRATORY THERAPY is sometimes used to loosen chest secretions in people who have severe COPD.

Very low oxygen levels in the blood associated with extreme disease may be treated with long-term oxygen therapy (see OXYGEN, SUPPLEMENTAL) used continually throughout the day.

Although surgery to reduce lung volume is a complex procedure, it may be an option for people with severe COPD. Lung transplantation is considered for some people younger than 50.

When airway obstruction is mild and treatment strategies, including smoking cessation, are adhered to, the prognosis can be favorable. When the obstruction is moderate to severe, the risk of death becomes greater, but with proper care and appropriate lifestyle changes, good survival rates can be achieved.

Circulatory system

See CARDIOVASCULAR SYSTEM.

Circumcision, male

Surgical removal of the foreskin (prepuce) of the penis. Circumcision is performed routinely on many newborn males for social or cultural reasons. There is no medical reason for routine circumcision of infants. However, in later life, conditions may develop in uncircumcised males that require circumcision. These include inability to pull the foreskin back from the head of the penis, inability to return the retracted foreskin to its normal position, and repeated infections of the foreskin and glans (BALANITIS). These conditions usually develop because of poor hygiene.

Cirrhosis

A chronic disease in which healthy, functioning liver cells degenerate and are gradually replaced by scar tissue. As scar tissue replaces healthy tissue, the liver is less able to remove toxins from the bloodstream and carry out its normal functions. Eventually, if enough liver cells are damaged, liver failure and death result. The scarring can also cause portal hypertension (an increase in the pressure of the blood system of the liver). Portal hypertension can cause ESOPHAGEAL VARICES (the dilation of the veins of the esophagus), a potentially life-threatening condition in which the veins are prone to bleeding. Cirrhosis also increases the risk for liver cancer.

The early stages of cirrhosis cause few symptoms. Eventual symptoms may include loss of appetite, weight loss, indigestion, weakness, and fatigue. Spidery red lines called angiomas (see ANGIOMA) may appear on the face, arms, and upper trunk. In the late stages of cirrhosis, as the tissue damage becomes severe, there are signs such as ASCITES (an abnormal accumulation of fluid in the abdominal cavity), bleeding in the digestive tract, and, sometimes, jaundice (the yellowing of the skin and the whites of the eyes).

Alcoholism, fatty liver, and hepatitis C (a viral infection) are the most common causes of cirrhosis in the United States. Additional causes of cirrhosis include other viral infections, autoimmune disease, malnutrition, parasites, drug reactions, toxic chemicals, metabolic defects, and congestive heart failure (see HEART FAILURE, CONGESTIVE).

Because many liver diseases cause similar symptoms, a number of tests may be needed to make a definitive diagnosis of cirrhosis. In addition to conducting a physical examination and taking a medical history, the doctor may order blood and urine tests, liver function tests, ultrasound scanning, X rays, and a liver biopsy.

In the early stages of cirrhosis caused by alcohol, it is often possible to halt the progression of cirrhosis by completely avoiding alcohol. As cirrhosis progresses, medications can be prescribed to treat symptoms. A liver transplant may be recommended.

Claudication

Pain or cramping in the limbs, usually the feet and legs, caused by ATHEROSCLEROSIS (narrowing or blockage of the arteries by deposits of fat and other materials). People with severe claudication may have to use a cane, walker, or wheelchair and are at increased risk of developing gangrene, for which amputation may be required.

Possible signs of claudication include cold or numb feet, loss of hair on toes or legs, impotence (erectile dysfunction) in men, cyanosis (bluish skin) or paleness, sores on feet or legs that do not heal, and thickened toenails. Since similar symptoms can arise from other conditions (for example, a pinched nerve in the spine), tests that measure blood flow to the limbs are required for accurate diagnosis and to assess how severe the disease is. Risk factors for claudication include ARTERIOSCLEROSIS, HYPERTENSION (high blood pressure), high blood cholesterol levels, high blood homocysteine levels, diabetes mellitus, smoking, obesity, lack of exercise, and being age 60 or older.

Lifestyle changes are important in the treatment of claudication. These include regular exercise, eating a heart-healthy diet low in cholesterol and fat, avoiding tobacco, and increasing the intake of B vitamins and folic acid to reduce homocysteine levels. Medications may also help the symptoms of claudication. However, people with severe symptoms will need more aggressive treatment. One option for certain types of blockage in a major artery is angioplasty (see BALLOON ANGIOPLASTY).

Claustrophobia

A fear of confined areas or enclosed spaces that can lead to extreme anxiety or panic. Often part of PANIC DISORDER, claustrophobia may be treated with therapy and the use of a mild tranquilizer.

Clavicle

See COLLARBONE.

Cleft lip and palate

Birth defects in which the lip or the roof of the mouth fail to close. Cleft lip and palate can occur in combination or separately.

Cleft lip and palate may be caused by genetic factors or by a teratogen (an agent such as a drug or a chemical that causes abnormalities in develop-

ing fetuses) or by a combination of genetic and environmental factors.

Babies born with cleft lip or palate have immediate problems with feeding. A special device, called an obturator, can be fitted over the palate so the baby can be fed. A cleft palate may interfere in normal speech development, even with corrective surgery.

Cleft lip is usually closed surgically at 1 or 2 months of age. A cleft palate is generally closed surgically during the first year of life to allow the baby to develop speech.

Clicking jaw

A symptom of temporomandibular joint or TMJ syndrome, which in-

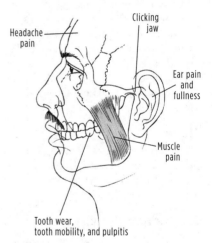

Symptoms of TMJ
The symptoms of temporomandibular joint (TMJ) syndrome go far beyond the clicking jaw. Other symptoms include muscular pain in the sliding joint between the skull and the lower jaw, especially when chewing; tooth wear from grinding of the teeth, movement of teeth, and inflammation of the inner pulp of the teeth (pulpitis); ear pain and ringing in the ears; headache in the temples and the back of the head; and sensitivity to light and blurred vision.

volves an irregular functional relationship between the jaw joints and the supporting muscles and ligaments. Other possible symptoms of TMJ syndrome include limited jaw movement, headache, and facial pain.

Clinical trial

A test or study of a medical treatment to determine whether it is safe and effective.

Clitoridectomy

Removal of the CLITORIS. It is not performed in the West today except in cases of cancer of the vulva.

Clitoris

A small, rounded, highly sensitive structure that is part of a woman's external sexual organs (see REPRODUCTIVE SYSTEM, FEMALE). The clitoris, which is richly supplied with nerves and blood vessels, is above the opening to the vagina, where the labia majora join.

Clone

A group of genetically identical cells or organisms derived from a single original cell or organism by asexual reproductive methods.

Clostridium difficile

An organism that causes an acute inflammation of the colon. *Clostridium difficile* (*C. difficile*) is found in dust, soil, vegetation, and the gastrointestinal tracts of humans and animals. A pathogenic strain of this bacteria produces toxins that cause diarrhea and COLITIS, often after antibiotic treatment.

Antibiotic therapy, which may produce an imbalance in the normal flora of the intestines, is usually the cause of the overgrowth of *C. difficile* in the colon. Antibiotics inhibit the growth of many bacteria but permit certain bacteria, including *C. difficile*, to flourish in the intestines, which may lead to antibiotic-associated colitis. Symptoms include diarrhea, abdominal cramps, and low-grade fever.

The symptom of diarrhea generally begins within 4 to 10 days of starting antibiotic treatment, but sometimes develops after the medication has been discontinued. Symptoms usually stop when antibiotic therapy is discontinued.

Diagnosis is made by performing tests on a stool sample for the presence of a toxin produced by *C. difficile*.

Treatment is based on stopping the antibiotic treatment that may be causing the diarrhea.

Clubbing

A condition often caused by chronic lung disease in which the tips of the fingers or toes become enlarged and the area where the nail emerges from the nail bed becomes rounded.

Clubfoot

See TALIPES.

Coarctation of the aorta

A birth defect in which the aorta, the main artery leading from the heart into the body, is severely narrowed. Usually the narrowing occurs just past the point where the subclavian artery, which supplies the upper body, branches off the aorta. This narrowing causes a discrepancy in blood pressure between the upper body (which will have higher blood pressure) and the lower body (which will have lower blood pressure). Other complications include HYPERTENSION (high blood pressure), congestive heart failure (see HEART FAILURE, CONGESTIVE), enlarged heart, kidney failure, premature development of blockages in the coronary arteries, ANEURYSM (ballooning) and possible rupture of the aorta, stroke, or heart attack. Left untreated, coarctation of the aorta usually results in death before age 40.

Signs of the disease include cyanosis (a bluish tint to the skin) in the lower body, high blood pressure in the arms but not the legs, and a weak pulse in the groin along with a strong pulse in the carotid arteries. Symptoms can include dizziness, headache, cramps in the legs with exercise, fainting, and nosebleeds.

Surgery is the usual treatment. The procedure may be performed as soon as the condition is detected or, if diagnosed in infancy, delayed until childhood.

Coccidioidomycosis

A potentially fatal fungal infection caused by *Coccidioides immitis*, a fungus that lives in the semiarid, sandy soil common to the southwestern United States, Mexico, and Argentina. Coccidioidomycosis is caused by inhaling an airborne form of the fungus at a certain stage in the organism's life cycle. Construction and agricultural workers, as well as archeologists in endemic areas, are particularly vulnerable.

The symptoms of coccidioidomycosis include flulike malaise with fever, fatigue, cough, headaches, rash, muscle aches, and weight loss. Symptoms may also begin as acute pneumonia or, rarely, as chronic pneumonia. One form may affect the skin, bone, and meninges, which are the membranes lining the brain and spinal cord.

Diagnosis is made by discovering the fungus in a person's saliva or from a culture made from the main airways of the lungs.

Long-term treatment with medication may be effective in curing coccidioidomycosis if treatment begins early and there are no complications.

Cochlea

The fluid-filled, snail-shaped structure in the inner EAR that translates sounds into electrical impulses and relays them to the brain.

Cochlear implant

An electronic device designed to restore partial hearing to children and adults who are severely hearing impaired due to damage to the COCHLEA (inner ear) and are unable to benefit from HEARING AIDS. Cochlear implants involve several components, including a surgically implanted transmitter, which is activated by a device worn outside the ear. Cochlear implants differ from hearing aids in that they do not enhance sound to make it louder or clearer. Instead, the cochlear implant bypasses damaged parts of the hearing system, converts speech and environmental sounds into electrical signals, and directly stimulates the hearing nerve.

Most individuals who are profoundly hearing impaired find they are better able to receive some sound with the implants. Normal hearing is not entirely restored, but many implant recipients can successfully talk on the phone.

Codependence

A pattern of behavior found in a person who enables someone addicted to alcohol, drugs, or compulsive gambling to maintain his or her ADDIC-TION. The behavior is usually unwitting. The codependent person honestly wishes to help but does so in ways that prevent the person who is addicted from recognizing the addiction for what it is. Treatment consists of helping the codependent person recognize the pattern of enabling behavior and take steps to change it.

Coitus

The sexual union of two people of the opposite sex, in which the man's penis enters the woman's vagina. See SEXUAL INTERCOURSE.

Coitus interruptus

A birth control method commonly known as withdrawal. Coitus interruptus relies on a man withdrawing his penis before he ejaculates into a woman's vagina. Coitus interruptus is extremely unreliable because semen containing sperm can be released before a man has an orgasm and ejaculates. Pregnancy can occur after a drop or two of semen enter the vagina. See CONTRACEPTION, OTHER METHODS.

Cold injury

An abnormal and potentially serious physical condition that is caused by exposure to cold temperatures. Cold injuries range from FROSTBITE and pernio to HYPOTHERMIA.

The best course of action is preventing cold injuries. The head, face, and neck should be covered because much of a person's body heat is lost there first due to of the large blood supply in those areas.

Cold remedies

Prescription or nonprescription medications that relieve some of the symptoms of the common cold. Cold remedies cannot prevent or cure the viral infections that cause the cold, but they can sometimes make the person who has a cold feel more comfortable. These cold remedies fall into several general categories: ANTIHISTAMINES; DECONGESTANT DRUGS; nose sprays, which are are decongestants directly applied to the inside of the nose; COUGH REMEDIES; pain relievers; and multisymptom or combination "cold and flu" preparations.

Cold sore

A small, highly contagious blister around the mouth caused by the herpes simplex virus (see HERPES, OROLABIAL); also known as a fever blister. Although factors, such as stress, sun exposure, fever, injury, colds, or other illness, can trigger an outbreak, one can occur without an apparent trigger.

There is no known cure for the virus that causes cold sores. They generally resolve without treatment in 7 to 14 days, but doctors can prescribe oral antiviral agents to shorten the duration. To be most effective, treatment should start when the tingling begins.

Cold, common

Infection of the respiratory tract, caused by any one of more than 200 different viruses. Sometimes called a head cold, the infection causes inflammation of the mucous membranes lining the nose and throat. Nasal congestion, sore throat, and sometimes other symptoms, usually confined to the nose and throat, are produced by the inflammation. The larynx (organ in the throat that contains vocal cords) may also become involved, causing laryngitis.

The symptoms of the common cold usually include nasal congestion and nasal discharge. At first the nasal discharge may be thin and watery, later becoming thick and greenish yellow. Sneezing, watering eyes, sore throat, hoarseness, coughing, a congested feeling in the head and chest, and headache are other common symptoms. Sometimes a person with a cold experiences achiness, mild fatigue, and fever.

A common cold generally lasts from 7 to 14 days. A physician should be consulted if the symptoms of a cold persist for more than 10 days. Specific symptoms that require a doctor's attention include earache, pain in the face or forehead, or a fever lasting longer than 4 days or going above 102°F. A combination of symptoms including persistent hoarseness or sore throat, shortness of breath and wheezing, and a dry, painful cough may indicate PNEUMONIA and require immediate medical attention.

There is no effective prescription drug treatment for the common cold. A physician will not usually prescribe antibiotics for a person with a cold because the virus causing the cold does not respond to antibiotic medication. However, people who have recurrent bouts of SINUSITIS or BRONCHITIS or frequent ear infections should see a physician.

While there is no medical treatment for the virus causing the common cold, the symptoms of the infection can be relieved to decrease the discomfort of the person who has a cold. Among the treatments doctors recommend are bed rest, drinking plenty of fluids, gargling with warm salt water for sore throats (1/2 teaspoon in 6 ounces of warm water), and applying petroleum jelly to soothe a raw nose. Nasal sprays may reduce sneezing and nasal congestion.

Because most colds are passed hand to hand, doctors recommend frequent hand washing during cold season as possibly the simplest and most effective way to keep from getting a cold.

Colectomy

The surgical removal of all or part of the colon. A colectomy is performed to treat serious diseases, such as colon cancer (see COLON, CANCER OF THE), DIVERTICULAR DISEASE, and severe COLITIS.

The surgeon begins by making an incision in the abdominal wall. Next, the tumor or diseased part of the colon is removed. When possible, only part of the colon is excised, allowing the healthy remaining sections to be joined together to maintain a passageway for stools. Usually the operation involves a large incision and scar.

Colic

Gastrointestinal pain experienced by infants. Continual, intense crying, along with fussiness and irritability, are the hallmarks of colic. Almost all affected infants will have the onset of symptoms by 3 weeks of age. Colic usually occurs at least three times a week and lasts for 3 hours or more. It rarely lasts beyond the first 3 months of an infant's life. Colic can be a sign of a more severe medical problem. A colicky baby who is vomiting or whose bowel movements contain blood or mucus needs to be seen by a pediatrician or family physician. The doctor will examine the child to exclude a more serious problem.

Colicky symptoms generally improve as the child matures. The pediatrician or family physician can suggest a number of calming techniques. Researchers believe that food sensitivity may have a role in some cases of colic (see FOOD INTOLERANCE).

Colitis

Inflammation of the lining of the colon. Colitis may affect the entire colon or only parts of it. One type of colitis is caused by bacterial infection. A more serious type of colitis, ulcerative colitis, shares many similarities with CROHN DISEASE, and both diseases are considered types of INFLAMMATORY BOWEL DISEASE. Shallow and widespread bleeding ulcers are typical of ulcerative colitis.

The most common symptom of colitis is blood in the feces (see FECES, BLOOD IN THE). Other symptoms may include abdominal pain, persistent diarrhea, fever, and weight loss. Ulcerative colitis may also have symptoms in other parts of the body; for example, iritis (an inflammation of the muscles controlling the pupil) or arthritis pain.

Colitis is diagnosed by a complete physical examination and tests, such as stool analysis, blood tests, a lower gastrointestinal (GI) series (an X-ray procedure also called a BARIUM ENEMA), sigmoidoscopy, and colonoscopy. A BIOPSY (analysis of a tissue sample) can confirm the presence of ulcerative colitis. Anti-inflammatory drugs are the main treatment for ulcerative colitis.

Chronic ulcerative colitis can increase the risk of colon cancer. In some cases, surgical removal of all or part of the colon (a COLECTOMY) becomes necessary.

Colitis, antibiotic associated

See CLOSTRIDIUM DIFFICILE.

Collagen diseases

Disease of the connective tissue, which is an essential part of every structure in the body. Collagen diseases are sometimes referred to as connective tissue diseases, immunologic rheumatic diseases, or AUTOIMMUNE DISORDERS. The characteristic symptom of all the disorders in this group is the inflammation that damages the connective tissues of the body, many of which are composed of collagen. With collagen diseases, the body's antibodies begin to attack the affected person's own body cells and their components, instead of attacking bacteria, viruses, and other invaders as antibodies normally do.

All the body's systems may be affected. The soft tissue or joints are often involved, but there is often little damage to the affected bone and cartilage. For some people, the symptoms appear and disappear at intervals. For others, the disease ends independently and never recurs. Many people lead active lives despite their disorder; others are profoundly affected and do not regain full health. Although there is no cure, certain medications such as CORTICOSTEROIDS are used to treat the symptoms and delay the progression of the condition. See CONNECTIVE TISSUE DISEASE, MIXED. Also see specific collagen diseases: LUPUS ERYTHEMATOSUS, SYSTEMIC; SCLERODERMA; SJÖGREN SYNDROME; POLYCHONDRITIS, RELAPSING; and POLYMYALGIA RHEUMATICA.

Collagen injections

Placing a natural protein substance under the skin to fill in the wrinkles, creases, furrows, and other changes in the skin caused by aging or sun damage.

Collagen injections are not suitable during pregnancy, in people who are allergic to beef or to lidocaine, and in people with AUTOIMMUNE DISORDERS.

Collar, orthopedic

A therapeutic device worn around the neck to provide support for the neck. An orthopedic collar may be made of rigid plastic for firm support during daily activities. During sleep, a softer, more comfortable, cotton collar may be worn. Orthopedic collars may be the first line of treatment for cervical osteoarthritis when there is persistent pain. The collar may also be a component of ongoing treatment for OSTEOARTHRITIS, as well as for a prolapsed disk in the neck portion of the spinal column.

Collarbone

The bone that spans the top of the chest from the upper sternum (breastbone) to an extension of the shoulder blade (scapula). Because the collarbone (also called the clavicle) functions as a strut that forces the shoulder blade out and back to form the shoulder, it is subject to stress and fracture.

Colles fracture

A transverse break in the two bones of the forearm, called the radius and ulna. A Colles fracture is generally caused when a person's outstretched hand bears the brunt of the body's full weight in a forward fall. This kind of fracture may be treated with a cast for 5 to 8 weeks to immobilize the bones and allow repair. Surgery

involving internal fixation appliances is sometimes indicated for severe fractures. If the ligaments are injured, chronic pain may result. Later complications of Colles fracture include CARPAL TUNNEL SYNDROME.

Colon

The largest portion of the large INTESTINE extending from the end of the small intestine to the rectum.

The colon functions as a storage area for solid wastes before they are passed out of the body in a bowel movement. See DIGESTIVE SYSTEM.

Colon cancer, hereditary nonpolyposis

A form of colon cancer that does not develop from polyps and arises in individuals who have an inherited susceptibility to it.

Hereditary nonpolyposis colon cancer occurs in two forms. HNPCC type 1 is characterized by the development of carcinomas in only the colon and the rectum, while HNPCC type 2 develops in other locations in addition to the colon and the rectum, including the stomach, larynx, bladder, ovary, and bile ducts.

Colon cleansing

A controversial procedure intended to flush toxic substances from the bowel. Colon cleansing, which is also called colonic irrigation, is a method of detoxification based on the idea that impacted fecal material can stick to the lining of the colon instead of being excreted in the normal manner. Most doctors object to the procedure on the grounds that irrigation removes essential protective bacteria that naturally occur in the intestines.

Colon, cancer of the

Cancer of the large intestine, which is made up of the colon and rectum. Colon and rectal cancers are often grouped together as colorectal cancer (see also RECTUM, CANCER OF THE). Although colon cancer is the second most common cause of cancer death in the United States, it has a very high cure rate when detected early.

Warning signs include blood in the stool and a sudden change in bowel habits, whether constipation or diarrhea. Other possible symptoms include frequent gas pains, a change in the diameter of bowel movements, and a feeling that the bowel has not emptied completely after a bowel movement. There may also be tenderness or a mass in the abdomen. In some cases, bloating, discomfort, rumbling, and gurgling occur. Sometimes, there are no symptoms until the intestine ruptures or the cancer causes an intestinal obstruction See INTESTINE, OBSTRUCTION OF.

Colon cancer usually arises from polyps, abnormal growths that protrude from the colon walls that over time can become cancerous. As cancer cells multiply, a tumor can develop in the intestinal lining that gradually enlarges and may become bloody and ulcerated and constrict bowel movements. Left untreated, the cancer can spread to nearby organs.

When polyps in the colon are identified at an early stage, they can be removed during a COLONOSCOPY before they become cancerous. Other diagnostic tests include a FECAL-OCCULT BLOOD TEST (a test for traces of blood in the stool), a rectal examination, blood tests, and stool sample analysis. Tests commonly used to identify polyps include a lower GASTROINTESTINAL (GI) SERIES, SIGMOIDOSCOPY, and COLONOSCOPY. A lower GI series or BARIUM ENEMA uses the chemical barium sulfate, which is visible on X rays, to enable doctors to see the inside of the colon and rectum.

Surgery is the best treatment for colon cancer. In a procedure known as a colectomy, tumors are removed and the healthy remaining sections of the colon are joined together.

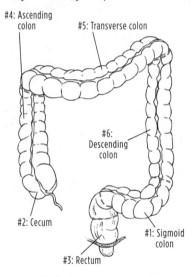

#4: Ascending colon
#5: Transverse colon
#6: Descending colon
#2: Cecum
#1: Sigmoid colon
#3: Rectum

Frequency of colon cancer

Cancer of the colon (large intestine) occurs with greater frequency in some parts of the colon than others (see numbers). Most cancers occur in the front portion that leads from the small intestine up the right side of the abdomen (ascending colon) or, even more frequently, in the latter portion (sigmoid colon) leading down the left side of the abdomen toward the anus.

Colon, irritable

See IRRITABLE BOWEL SYNDROME.

Colon, spastic

See IRRITABLE BOWEL SYNDROME.

Colonoscopy

A diagnostic examination of the inside of the colon by inserting a long, flexible instrument called a colonoscope through the rectum. A colonoscope is a type of endoscope used specifically to examine the colon and has attachments such as lenses, a light, and a small video camera.

Colonoscopy is used to check for inflammation, polyps, and other abnormalities of the colon. For example, it can locate bleeding sites, ulcers, polyps, and colorectal cancer (see COLON, CANCER OF THE; and RECTUM, CANCER OF THE). Most physicians now recommend a baseline colonoscopy at age 50.

The person undergoing the procedure lies on his or her left side on an examining table. The colonoscope is gently inserted into the rectum and slowly threaded all the way up the colon.

While slowly withdrawing the tube, the doctor examines the inside of the colon directly through the scope or on a video monitor. Inflamed tissue, abnormal growths, bleeding, ulcers, and even muscle spasms can be seen.

Colorado tick fever

A viral infection transmitted by the bite of a wood tick. Symptoms generally begin within 4 to 5 days of the tick bite, but may not appear for as

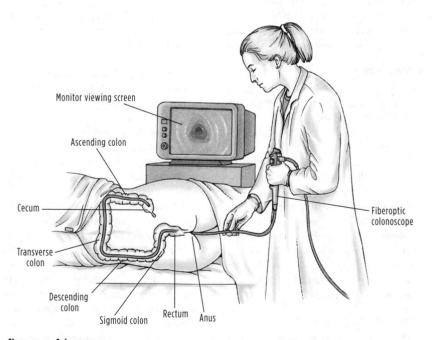

Monitor viewing screen

Ascending colon

Cecum

Transverse colon

Descending colon

Sigmoid colon

Rectum

Anus

Fiberoptic colonoscope

Close-up on Colonoscopy

Colonoscopy is a procedure in which the inside of the colon is examined using a fiber-optic colonoscope, an elongated flexible viewing tube that transmits images to a monitor. Bleeding sites, inflamed tissue, ulcers, polyps, and colorectal cancer can be easily visualized and identified using colonoscopy.

long as 20 days following a bite. General malaise with high fever and a fine, red rash are the usual symptoms. Recovery is usually within a week to 10 days, but the virus can live in the red blood cells for several months.

Cases of Colorado tick fever affecting the liver or central nervous system have been reported. Hallucinations and memory loss may occur with severe infection. Rarely, the infection causes pathological changes in the heart, brain, and lungs and can be fatal.

There is no vaccine for Colorado tick fever. Preventive steps should be taken to avoid getting wood tick bites, including tucking long pants into socks to protect the legs while hiking through tick-infested areas and wearing shoes and long-sleeved shirts.

Colostomy

A surgical procedure in which a STOMA, an artificial opening, is created in the abdominal wall to allow the discharge of feces into a bag attached to the skin.

A colostomy can be temporary or permanent. If it is temporary, the stoma will be closed in a second procedure once the intestine has recovered from initial surgery. A permanent colostomy requires keeping the stoma clean and regularly emptying the bag that collects the waste. People who have colostomies usually return to a normal bowel routine.

Colostrum

The first breast milk produced after childbirth. Low in fat and carbohydrates and high in protein, colostrum is easy to digest and is rich in antibodies that defend the newborn against infection. Colostrum has a laxative action and is the ideal first food for the newborn. After 3 to 5 days, colostrum is replaced by mature milk. See BREAST-FEEDING.

Colposcopic biopsy

Removal of tissue from one or more sites on the CERVIX during COLPOSCOPY in order to examine it for abnormal cells.

Colposcopy

A procedure to examine the surfaces of the vaginal walls and the cervix for abnormal cells, using a colposcope, a lighted magnifying instrument.

Coma

A profound or deep state of unconsciousness. A coma may occur as an outcome of an underlying illness, or it may be caused by trauma. A person in a coma lacks both wakefulness and awareness. In addition to providing treatment to reverse the coma, medical care includes providing nutrition and preventing infection (especially pneumonia) and pressure sores. Physical therapy may be used to prevent permanent muscular contractions and orthopedic deformities.

Comas rarely last longer than 2 to 4 weeks. The prognosis for a person in a coma depends on its cause and the nature of neurological damage. In some cases, a prolonged coma is followed by a persistent VEGETATIVE STATE, in which a person has lost cognitive neurological function and awareness of the environment, yet retains noncognitive function and a sleep-wake cycle.

Common cold

See COLD, COMMON.

Compartment syndrome

An acute or chronic condition caused by exercise or injury and characterized by pain and swollen muscle tissue. The swelling produces an increased pressure of the fluids within the closed muscle compartment and persists after the exercise session is over. The condition most commonly occurs in the leg, especially in the front of the lower leg, but may also affect the forearm, thigh, and buttocks.

The symptoms include severe pain, swelling, numbness, motor loss, or weakness in the affected muscle. Many people experience a gradual onset of aching and a sensation of fullness in the affected muscle or muscles after starting to exercise or after reaching a certain level of intensity. The pain may occur on one side of the body or both, sometimes with more severe pain on one side.

The symptoms of compartment syndrome are generally relieved when a person stops exercising or rests. Compartment syndrome may be acute (coming on suddenly) or chronic (persistent for a long time).

Treatment may include exercising on a different surface, changing footwear, and adjusting a person's training intensity. The use of orthotics, special shoe inserts for extra support, as well as exercises, may be recommended. In severe and persistent cases of compartment syndrome, a surgical procedure called fasciotomy, which relieves the pressure on muscles, may be recommended.

Complication

In medicine, a disease or problem arising in addition to the original condition or following surgery.

Compress

A pad of cloth or other material that is pressed firmly against a body part for a period of time as part of therapy. Compresses may be dry or wet, and they may be cold, lukewarm, or hot. Wet compresses may contain medications and are used chiefly to relieve inflammation. Dry compresses are often used to stop bleeding.

Compression fracture

A break in a vertebra, or bone of the spine, caused by a collapse of the bone tissue in one or more vertebrae. The symptoms of a compression fracture depend on the area of the back affected. If the fracture occurs in the lower back, walking may make the pain worse. Most compression fractures do not affect the nerves. However, if the fracture puts pressure on the nerves or spinal cord, symptoms may include numbness, tingling, or weakness. The causes of compression fractures include OSTEOPOROSIS, SPINAL INJURY, and malignant growths, such as tumors. The treatment depends on the underlying cause.

Compression syndrome

A collection of symptoms caused by pressure on a nerve or nerves that supply the muscles and carry sensations from a particular area of the body. Symptoms of a compression syndrome include weakness, numbness, tingling, and pain. CARPAL TUNNEL SYNDROME (compression of the median nerve at the wrist) is by far the most common compression syndrome. Possible treatments for a compression syndrome include identifying and avoiding the activity that contributes to the problem and wearing a splint. NONSTEROIDAL ANTI-INFLAMMATORY DRUGS (NSAIDs) are often recommended to reduce inflammation. If symptoms are severe or persistent, surgery may be needed to relieve the pressure on the nerve.

Computed tomography scanning

See CT SCANNING.

Conception

The fertilization of an egg by a sperm that initiates pregnancy. During sexual intercourse, 300 million or so sperm are ejaculated into the vagina. About 3 million of them penetrate the cervix to get to the uterus; the rest are killed by vaginal secretions or are excreted from the body. The sperm that reach the egg secrete an enzyme that breaks down the outer covering of the egg. Once a single sperm has penetrated the egg, the outer covering immediately changes, to prevent other sperm from entering. The nucleus in the head of the sperm and the nucleus of the egg fuse to form a fertilized egg, also called a ZYGOTE. The zygote is made up of a unique combination of genes, half of which come from the man's sperm and half from the woman's egg. See also OVULATION.

Concussion

A brief loss of consciousness following a head injury. The length of time the person is unconscious may relate to the severity of the concussion. A concussion may be accompanied by headache, faintness, nausea or vomiting, slightly blurred vision, and difficulty concentrating.

As a general rule, concussion is a minor, temporary injury that does not cause permanent damage to the brain. However, any head injury is potentially serious, so any head injury that results in a person losing consciousness should receive medical attention. About one-third of all people with concussion may experience symptoms after the event, including insomnia, irritability, restlessness, depression, moodiness, or the inability to concentrate. Concussion is usually self-healing, although the doctor may prescribe a pain reliever other than aspirin for any headache.

Condom

A thin sheath usually made of latex and placed over a man's erect penis to prevent sperm from entering a woman's vagina, helping to prevent pregnancy. Latex condoms also help prevent spread of disease through sexual intercourse. Other names for a condom include rubber and prophylactic. A polyurethane female condom that lines the vagina is also sold. See CONTRACEPTION, BARRIER METHODS.

Condyloma

See HUMAN PAPILLOMAVIRUS.

Condyloma acuminatum

A sexually transmitted viral infection that is caused by the HUMAN PAPILLOMAVIRUS (HPV) and produces genital warts (also known as venereal warts). Condyloma acuminatum is currently one of the most common sexually transmitted diseases among men and women living in the United States. The virus is transferred during vaginal sexual intercourse, oral sex, and anal sex.

Once a person is infected, the warts may appear within 2 weeks, within several months, or even within several years. In women, the warts appear in the vagina, around the opening of the vagina, on the cervix, and in or around the anus. The infection may also cause itching and a vaginal discharge. In men, the warts are located on the penis and are usually too small to be observed by visual examination. The warts may cause itching, irritation, or bleeding.

A PAP SMEAR will reveal the presence of the wart virus in women. A COLPOSCOPY to examine the vagina and cervix through a magnifying lens may also be used in the diagnosis of condyloma acuminatum in women. Men may be diagnosed by applying a weak solution of acetic acid to the penis and looking for warts with the aid of magnification.

Some warts improve without treatment. Treatment procedures to remove warts include using liquid nitrogen to destroy the warts by freezing the tissue; applying one of the topical chemicals bichloroacetic acid (BCA), trichloroacetic acid (TCA), or podophyllin, which is later washed off; laser treatments; or burning off the warts with an electrical instrument.

It is important that an infected person advise his or her sexual partners so they can be examined and treated if necessary. Condoms should be used until the virus is completely cured.

Cone biopsy

A procedure in which a cone-shaped or cylindrical section of tissue is removed from a woman's cervix with a scalpel or a laser for diagnosis or treatment of cervical DYSPLASIA or localized cancer of the cervix. It is performed when a woman has had a PAP SMEAR that is more than moderately abnormal.

Confidentiality

The protected privacy of identifiable personal health information. The medical profession generally extends the promise of confidentiality to people who seek medical care.

In terms of access to medical records, the need for privacy among people receiving medical care and the release of personally identifiable information must be weighed against the benefits that the availability of medical data can offer in certain situations. Having access to the medical records of people who are unconscious and have been brought into hospital emergency departments may save lives.

State law requires that certain medical information be reported to state and local governments. This information is maintained in databases and includes the reporting of sexually transmitted diseases to public health agencies, informing child-welfare agencies of child abuse, and advising law-enforcement agencies of injuries caused by firearms.

Confidentiality may also be breached if there is a potential for harm to a third party. For example, a psychiatrist has a duty to warn authorities about a patient's homicidal tendencies.

The Health Insurance Portability and Accountability Act (HIPAA) further protects medical record information. HIPAA regulations require that this information not be released by health care personnel, providers, or payers for medical services (such as insurance companies) without the authorization of the person receiving medical care.

Congenital

Any condition existing at birth. Congenital conditions usually exist before birth and may or may not be inherited. A congenital abnormality is a structural abnormality present at birth.

Congestive heart failure

See HEART FAILURE, CONGESTIVE.

Conjunctiva

The thin mucous membrane that lines the inside of the eyelids and covers the white, exposed surface (sclera) of the EYE. Cells in the conjunctiva produce a fluid that helps lubricate the lids and the cornea to keep the eye moist.

Conjunctivitis

Inflammation of the membrane lining the eyelids and the exposed outer surface of the eye (CONJUNCTIVA). Popularly known as pinkeye, conjunctivitis is the most common eye disease in the Western hemisphere. The disease's severity ranges from mild to severe. Symptoms can include redness, irritation and pain, excessive tearing, itching, blurred vision, a grainy or gritty feeling in the eye, increased sensitivity to light, and crusts that form on the eyelids overnight.

Conjunctivitis can result from a number of different causes: viral infection, various kinds of bacteria, allergies (usually to pollen, house dust, or pet dander), exposure to chemicals (including swimming pool chlorine), and certain systemic diseases. Wearing contact lenses, particularly extended-wear lenses, increases the risk of conjunctivitis. Typically, the overnight formation of crusts on the eyelids that create the sensation that the eye is glued shut is a sign of bacterial infection.

Conjunctivitis can also arise in newborns as a result of exposure to bacteria during passage through the birth canal. If the inflammation comes from the bacterium that causes GONORRHEA (see also SEXUALLY TRANSMITTED DISEASES), it can result in blindness. Prompt treatment is required. In most states, drops are placed in a newborn's eye shortly after birth to prevent this infection.

Treatment of conjunctivitis depends on the cause. Viral conjunctivitis clears up on its own. Bacterial conjunctivitis is treated with antibiotic drops or ointments.

Connective tissue

Any tissue that connects, binds, or supports a structure of the body. Different connective tissues are derived from different combinations of cells, fibers, and substances found in bones, arteries, and veins.

Connective tissue disease, mixed

A chronic inflammatory autoimmune disease. Mixed connective tissue disease (MCTD) is a term used to describe overlapping groups of collagen diseases that cannot be individually categorized as one of the specific disorders. MCTD is characterized by symptoms including muscle weakness and pain in the joints. There may be other symptoms relating to disorders of the heart, lungs, and skin. Kidney disease and a dysfunction of the esophagus, including swallowing problems, may be associated with the abnormalities in the body. See also COLLAGEN DISEASES.

Conscious sedation

A method of controlling discomfort during surgery in which the patient is awake but drowsy and insensitive to pain. Conscious sedation is sometimes used alone for minor procedures. It can also be combined with regional or local anesthesia to provide additional pain control for more extensive surgery.

Constipation

For symptom chart see CONSTIPATION, page xvi.

Infrequent or irregular bowel movements in which feces are hard and dry. Although most people have one bowel movement a day, as many as three movements a day or as few as three a week are considered normal. Regularity and ease of defecation are more important than frequency. Doctors recommend that anyone who experiences constipation after years of regularity seek medical help. This is especially important when constipation is accompanied by other symptoms, such as weight loss, abdominal pain, or rectal bleeding (see FECES, BLOOD IN THE).

Diagnostic tests to determine the cause of constipation include a lower GASTROINTESTINAL (GI) SERIES (an X-ray procedure also called a BARIUM ENEMA) and SIGMOIDOSCOPY or COLONOSCOPY (examinations of the rectum and colon using flexible viewing tubes passed through the anus).

Treatment depends on the cause. Doctors generally recommend adding fiber-rich vegetables, fruits, and bran to the diet, drinking adequate fluids, and responding promptly to the urge to defecate. Because constipation is a side effect of many medications, the doctor will review all medications that a person is taking and adjust them as necessary. Laxatives should be used cautiously and infrequently.

Contact dermatitis

A skin reaction caused by exposure to an external agent. In allergic contact dermatitis (see also SKIN ALLERGY), there may be no apparent inflammation the first time a person is exposed to the substance. But on subsequent occasions, after the skin has become sensitive or allergic to the substance, exposure produces a skin eruption. Allergic contact dermatitis differs from irritant contact dermatitis. Irritant contact dermatitis is a rash caused by contact with any substance, such as strong soaps or detergents, that produces skin inflammation in most people. Many substances can be both irritants and allergens.

Symptoms of contact dermatitis vary from person to person but may include redness, itching, inflammation, blistering, crusting, scabbing, scaling, thickening, and pigment (color) changes. It may be difficult to distinguish contact dermatitis from other forms of dermatitis. A doctor will ask about any exposure to irritants or a history of ALLERGIES. Diagnosis is based on skin examination and PATCH TEST results that indicate sensitivity to commonly encountered substances. Treatments to control symptoms may include corticosteroids and antihistamines. Scratching should be avoided.

Contact lenses

Small, thin, plastic disks shaped to correct visual defects and designed to be worn on the surface of the cornea (the clear outer covering on the front of the eye) over the iris and pupil. Contact lenses float on the thin layer of liquid that lubricates the cornea.

There are two basic types of contact lenses. Hard lenses are made from a relatively rigid plastic. Modern hard lenses are fitted with grooves that make it easier for oxygen to pass to the cornea; such lenses are called gas-permeable. Soft lenses use a plastic with a higher water content, which makes them more flexible and also allows oxygen to reach the cornea. Oxygen is important for preserving the health of the cornea under the lens.

Daily-wear contact lenses are designed to be replaced daily. Extended-wear lenses can be worn for longer periods without removal and cleaning; in the United States, Food and Drug Administration rules limit this period to 7 days (or 30 days for silicone hydrogel lenses).

Contact lenses can be made with a single-vision correction, or they can be designed as bifocals, with one part of the lens for distance vision and another for close. Astigmatism is corrected with toric contact lenses, which are usually hard. Toric lenses compensate for the asymmetry in the cornea and remove or reduce the resulting distortion in vision.

Contact lenses raise the risk of eye infection, particularly if the lenses are not removed and cleaned regularly and properly. In rare cases, infection with a bacterium or a fungus can cause an ulcer on the cornea (see CORNEAL ULCER). This condition is serious, and it may threaten sight.

Giant papillary conjunctivitis is a common reaction among soft-lens wearers who are prone to allergy. It is believed that lipid deposits on the lens cause the membrane (conjunctiva) of the upper eyelid to become bumpy and inflamed.

If too little oxygen penetrates the contact lens, problems can arise in the cornea. In corneal vascularization, tiny blood vessels grow into the normally vessel-free cornea. In extreme cases, the new blood vessels cloud vision. Switching to another type of contact lens or to eyeglasses usually resolves the problem.

Contagious

An infection or disease that is communicable by contact. A contagious disease is one that is transmitted by contact with a person infected with it, with that person's bodily fluids, or with objects and surfaces touched by the infected person.

Continuing care retirement communities

See LONG-TERM CARE FACILITY.

Contraception

Also called birth control. The deliberate prevention of pregnancy or conception by various means. Common methods of contraception include barrier and hormonal methods, intrauterine devices (IUDs), coitus interruptus (withdrawal), natural family planning, spermicides, and sterilization. Each method of birth control has benefits and drawbacks.

Contraception, barrier methods

Methods of contraception that prevent pregnancy by keeping sperm from entering a woman's uterus. There are several types of barrier contraceptives, including condoms (both male and female), diaphragms, and cervical caps.

All barrier methods of contraception should generally be used with a spermicide, which is a chemical that kills sperm on contact. Some barrier methods also offer protection from SEXUALLY TRANSMITTED DISEASES (STDs). Barrier methods are not as effective as some other contraceptives, such as hormonal methods (see CONTRACEPTION, HORMONAL METHODS) and intrauterine devices (IUD; see IUD).

- *CONDOM* A thin sheath placed over a man's erect penis to contain the semen and prevent sperm from entering a woman's vagina. Condoms provide the best possible protection against the spread of STDs but they are not 100 percent perfect. Used condoms should always be discarded.

- *THE FEMALE CONDOM* A polyurethane sleeve that lines the vagina, the female condom shields the vagina and cervix from semen. At the upper end, the sleeve has a round cap, braced by a light ring; a much larger ring opens the sheath for penile penetration of the vagina.

- *DIAPHRAGM* A flexible rubber dome that is propped against the pubic bone to cover the cervix and part of the uterus. To obtain a diaphragm, a woman must see a doctor to determine proper fit and to get a prescription for the device and spermicide to use with it. The diaphragm must hold the spermicide firmly against the cervix. After intercourse, a diaphragm must be left in place for 6 hours before it can be removed and cleaned.

- *CERVICAL CAP* A firm rubber dome that fits snugly over a woman's cervix. Like a diaphragm, a cervical cap can only be obtained by prescription and requires a doctor's examination to determine the correct size. Similarly, a cervical cap must always be used with a spermicide. After intercourse, the cap must stay in place for at least 6 hours; it can remain inserted for up to 36 hours.

- *CONTRACEPTIVE SPONGE* Made of absorbent polyurethane foam that has been impregnated with a spermicide, the round sponge works by bracing spermicide against the cervix while blocking the cervical opening. Sponges can be inserted up to 24 hours before intercourse and must stay in place for 6 hours after intercourse. The sponge is available without a prescription. Its failure rate is relatively high.

Contraception, emergency postcoital

Birth control that a woman may use after having unprotected sex or having been the victim of sexual assault. Two common methods are used, either oral medication or insertion of an intrauterine device (IUD). Both require a visit to a doctor or clinic.

Morning-after pills are a series of birth control pills containing estrogen and progestin, which inhibit the growth of the lining of the uterus (endometrium), making it impossible for a fertilized egg to grow there.

Contraception, hormonal methods

Methods of preventing pregnancy by changing the levels of female hormones in a woman's body. Hormonal birth control methods include birth control pills, hormone implants or injections, an intrauterine device (see IUD) impregnated with hormones, and morning-after pills. Hormonal birth control methods are easy to use, highly effective, and relatively inexpensive. Hormonal methods work by preventing ovulation. They also cause changes in a woman's cervical mucus and uterus that help prevent pregnancy. Hormonal birth control methods are relatively safe, but not every woman may be able to use them. Women with certain health conditions, such as high blood pressure or an inherited tendency to develop blood clots, may not be good candidates for using hormonal contraception. Hormonal methods do not protect against SEXUALLY TRANSMITTED DISEASES; they should be used in combination with condoms in a non-monogamous relationship.

Birth control pills are safe and effective when taken daily, as prescribed. The failure rate for birth control pills rises if a woman misses taking pills. If that happens, a backup form of birth control should be used for the remaining part of the monthly cycle.

Other hormonal methods

Hormonal implants are a safe and very effective form of birth control. Available only by prescription, implants are small, soft-plastic capsules that are placed beneath the skin, usually in a woman's upper arm. They release a steady but low-dosage stream of hormones. Hormonal injections are another safe and effective form of birth control, available only from a doctor. The intramuscular injections work primarily by preventing ovula-

tion. Each injection provides birth control for 3 months, although contraceptive protection appears to extend somewhat past the deadline.

Contraception, other methods

Other methods of birth control include the rhythm method (natural family planning), spermicides, coitus interruptus (the withdrawal method), intrauterine devices (IUDs), and sterilization. Each method works in a different way to prevent pregnancy.

The rhythm method is based on the assumption that pregnancy can be avoided by not having intercourse around the days a woman ovulates, the time of the month when she is most fertile. This method works best when women have regular cycles and ovulate predictably and when it is used with a spermicide or a barrier method. Even in the best circumstances, rhythm is only about 80 percent effective.

Spermicides contain a chemical that kills sperm or makes them unable to fertilize an egg. Inexpensive and easy to use, spermicides are widely available without a prescription. Spermicides are most effective at preventing pregnancy when used with a barrier method, such as a diaphragm. Using a spermicide may offer some protection against some sexually transmitted diseases.

Coitus interruptus, more commonly known as the withdrawal method of birth control, relies on a man withdrawing his penis before he ejaculates into a woman's vagina. This behavior method of contraception is ineffective because sperm can be released before a man ejaculates.

Sterilization involves surgical procedures for both women and men.

Sterilization should be considered a permanent method of birth control. Sterilizing women involves a procedure called a TUBAL LIGATION, in which the fallopian tubes are clipped or banded closed, cut and tied off, or burned (cauterized) with an electric current and cut. For men, sterilization is done with a VASECTOMY.

Intrauterine devices are small devices containing copper or hormones that are placed in the uterus to interfere with ovulation and conception. A hormonal IUD must be replaced every year; the copper version can be kept in place for up to 12 years. See IUD.

Contraceptive

A device or agent used to prevent conception, the fertilization and implantation of an egg in the uterus. See various CONTRACEPTION entries.

Contraceptive foam and jelly

See CONTRACEPTION, OTHER METHODS.

Contraceptive implant

See CONTRACEPTION, HORMONAL METHODS.

Contraction stress test

In pregnancy, a test in which contractions (see CONTRACTIONS, UTERINE) are induced in the mother's uterus, and the heart rate of the fetus is monitored electronically to measure the fetal response to the contractions. Monitoring the baby's heartbeat assesses the baby's health and can help the doctor decide whether to let the pregnancy go on or to induce labor.

Contractions, uterine

The strong, rhythmic tightening of the muscles of the uterus, increasing in intensity, frequency, and duration, that accompanies labor. Uterine contractions cause the cervix to dilate (widen) so the baby can pass into the vagina. See also LABOR.

Contracture

A deformed or distorted joint caused by abnormal shortening of muscles and tendons surrounding the joint or by the shrinking of scars in the connective tissue capsule or skin associated with the joint.

Contraindication

A factor in a person's condition that makes it inadvisable to participate in a particular treatment, such as taking a certain medication or undergoing surgery.

Contrast medium

A substance used in radiography to increase the contrast of an image. The contrast medium can be introduced either in or around the structure. Usually, a contrast medium is a substance through which X rays cannot pass, such as barium. Other commonly used agents are iodine-based mediums for INTRAVENOUS PYELOGRAPHY, CT SCANNING (computed tomography scanning), and ANGIOGRAPHY and gadolinium for MRI (magnetic resonance imaging).

Controlled substance

A substance regulated by U.S. federal law to prevent abuse. Controlled substances are divided into five schedules, based on their medicinal value, harmfulness, and potential for abuse or addiction.

Contusion

See BRUISE.

Conversion disorder

A mental illness that is not due to any physical cause, but in which a distressed person develops physical symptoms that mimic a disease of the nervous system or a general medical condition. The symptoms are due to a psychological conflict and are not faked. The symptoms are severe enough to significantly impair the person's ability to function in family life or work and can include difficulty walking, paralysis or localized weakness, inability to speak, difficulty swallowing ("lump-in-the-throat" feeling), inability to urinate, loss of sense of pain or touch, blindness, double vision, deafness, hallucinations, and seizures.

Treatment consists of a physical examination by a doctor to rule out any underlying disease, followed by psychiatric treatment to help the person understand the emotional basis of the disorder.

Convulsion

Involuntary jerking movements, now called a SEIZURE.

COPD

See CHRONIC OBSTRUCTIVE PULMONARY DISEASE.

Copper

A mineral that is essential for manufacturing collagen (a protein that is a major component of connective tissue) and for enabling oxygen to bind to hemoglobin, an oxygen-carrying protein in red blood cells. Copper deficiency causes an anemia that resembles iron deficiency anemia. Copper is also necessary for healthy functioning of the heart, efficient energy production, and absorption of iron from the digestive tract. Dietary copper is found in whole grains, nuts, liver, and oysters.

Cor pulmonale

Enlargement of the right ventricle (lower right chamber of the heart) because of disease in the lungs. Cor pulmonale is a Latin phrase meaning "lung-affected heart." The right side of the heart pumps blood into the lungs, where it takes on oxygen for transport into the rest of the body. In a healthy person, little pressure is required to pump blood into the lungs. As a result, the muscle of the right ventricle is not as strong as the left, which pumps blood into the body. However, if the lungs are impaired by diseases such as EMPHYSEMA or PULMONARY FIBROSIS, the heart must work much harder to deliver blood. The right ventricle enlarges to accommodate this overload. At first the heart can compensate, but over time it fails.

Cor pulmonale is a serious disease that can shorten a person's life. In some cases, it is acute and reversible; more often than not, it is chronic. In addition to treating the underlying respiratory disease, the doctor may recommend using supplemental oxygen, restricting salt and water intake, and taking diuretic medications to reduce fluid accumulation in the lungs and lessen the heart's workload.

Cordotomy

An operation performed to divide bundles of nerve fibers within the spinal cord. Cordotomy is done to relieve persistent pain that has failed to respond to other measures, such as strong analgesic medication or TENS (transcutaneous electrical nerve stimulation). It is most often performed for severe, unremitting pain associated with cancer in the lower trunk and legs.

Cornea

The transparent, curved structure forming the front of the eyeball. Covered by the CONJUNCTIVA (the lining on the surface of the eye and inside the eyelids), the cornea contains five layers of clear tissue that help to focus light onto the retina. It joins the sclera (white of the eye) at its outer rim, and the black pupil and colored iris lie under it. The cornea itself is difficult to see because of its transparency.

The cornea helps focus light rays onto the retina at the back of the eye and protects the front of the eye. The top layer of the cornea is extremely sensitive to the slightest scratch, in order to protect the structures beneath it.

The front of the cornea is curved outward, much like the lens of a camera. See also CATARACT SURGERY.

Corneal abrasion

An injury to the thin skin (epithelium) overlying the transparent covering (cornea) of the eye. Symptoms may include severe pain in the eye, sensation of a foreign body in the eye, abnormal vision, sensitivity to light, redness, and swollen eyelids. Treatment consists of removing any foreign body that may be present, lubrication with artificial tears or ointment, and antibiotic drops or ointment in the eye if infection poses a risk. Most doctors recommend covering the eye with a patch to allow healing and relief of pain. Corneal injuries heal quickly with treatment, and the eye typically returns to normal within 24 to 48 hours.

Corneal transplant

See KERATOPLASTY, PENETRATING.

Corneal ulcer

An open sore on the transparent outer covering of the eye (cornea). Signs and symptoms include impaired vision, severe pain, redness, a visible white patch on the cornea, sensitivity to light, and increased tearing. Corneal ulcers usually arise from infection by bacteria, often through contamination of an injury to the cornea.

Corneal ulcers are serious and can lead to vision loss if left untreated. A medical examination is conducted, and laboratory tests of tissue from the ulcer are performed to determine the cause of the infection. If a corneal ulcer is present, then the appropriate antibacterial, antiviral, or antifungal agent is prescribed, usually in the form of eye drops. If the ulcer erodes through the cornea, surgery is required.

Coronary artery bypass

See BYPASS SURGERY.

Coronary artery disease

Narrowing or blockage of the arteries that nourish the heart by deposits of cholesterol, calcium, and other materials (see ATHEROSCLEROSIS); also known as coronary heart disease. Even though blood flows through the heart, the heart muscle itself gets the oxygen it needs from the coronary arteries, which branch off from the base of the aorta (the main artery carrying oxygen-rich blood out of the heart). The coronary arteries travel over the surface of the heart, encircle the top, and branch out toward the bottom, forming the pattern of a crown (corona means "crown" in Latin).

The symptoms of coronary artery disease vary from one person to another. The most common is ANGINA, diffuse chest discomfort or pain often described as a feeling of tightness or heaviness that is brought on by exertion but relieved by rest. Critical vessel narrowing may cause pain even when resting. Other symptoms can include shortness of breath, especially after stress or exercise; cardiac arrhythmia (irregular heartbeat); nausea or upset stomach; severe sweating; weakness or fatigue; and (in women) breast pain or a feeling in the upper abdomen that is comparable to indigestion. When coronary artery disease produces no symptoms, it is said to be silent.

Coronary artery disease, with or without angina, can result in a HEART ATTACK when a blood clot forms in a narrowed artery and blocks it.

Coronary artery disease can impair the heart muscle's ability to pump blood, which can cause congestive heart failure (see HEART FAILURE, CONGESTIVE). The weakening heart cannot meet the body's demand for blood, and fluid can accumulate in the lungs or other parts of the body.

If coronary artery disease is suspected, one or more of several tests may be used to check for abnormality, including a resting ELECTROCARDIO-GRAM (ECG) to record the electrical activity of the heart; an ECHOCARDIO-GRAM to visualize the structure and function of the heart and the major arteries; or myocardial perfusion imaging, which allows doctors to observe the pattern of blood flowing through the coronary arteries. A stress test may also be needed.

If the results of any of these tests are abnormal, the person who has been tested is likely to undergo a minimally invasive procedure known as cardiac catheterization (see CATHETERIZA-TION, CARDIAC) to obtain diagnostic information about the heart, the coronary arteries, and the aorta.

Treatment of coronary artery disease depends on the severity of the disease, the location of the narrowed arteries, the symptoms, and a person's overall health. The doctor treating the person with coronary artery disease has a number of options, including recommending lifestyle changes, prescribing medication, and performing surgery or less invasive interventional techniques such as BALLOON ANGIOPLASTY or stenting.

The major surgical treatment is BY-PASS SURGERY.

Coronary care unit

A part of the hospital dedicated to treating people with serious acute heart disease; commonly abbreviated as CCU. The CCU combines specialized equipment for constant electronic monitoring of heart function with highly trained personnel who can detect the signs and symptoms of heart problems and intervene as needed.

Coronary heart disease

See CORONARY ARTERY DISEASE.

Coronary thrombosis

Partial or complete blockage by a blood clot of one of the arteries that nourish the heart. Since the surface arteries (coronary arteries) provide the heart with oxygen-rich blood, the clot cuts off the oxygen supply to the heart muscle downstream. The result is myocardial infarction, or HEART ATTACK.

Medications called thrombolytic agents, which can dissolve the clot when administered a short time after it has formed, can be used to treat coronary thrombosis. Anticoagulant medication is used as a follow-up treatment to prevent the formation of subsequent blood clots.

Corpus luteum cyst

An ovarian cyst in which a fluid-filled sac develops from a persistent corpus luteum, the yellow pouch that remains after an egg has been released from a follicle (egg sac) in the ovary. If the egg is not fertilized, the body normally resorbs the corpus luteum. Corpus luteum cysts usually go away in a few weeks but can grow as large as 4 or more inches in diameter and can cause pain in the woman's lower abdomen, usually on only one side. A corpus luteum cyst may cause delayed menstrual periods or bleeding between menstrual periods. If a woman develops symptoms of a corpus luteum cyst, her doctor will usually perform a PELVIC EXAMINATION and may order tests such as ULTRASOUND SCANNING, to rule out conditions such as cancer, ECTOPIC PREGNANCY, or other noncancerous ovarian growths.

Corpuscle

Most often refers to two types of blood cells. Red blood corpuscles, or erythrocytes, are iron-rich cells that transport oxygen through the bloodstream. White blood corpuscles, or leukocytes, have key roles in defending the body against invasion by viruses, bacteria, and fungi.

Corticosteroid hormones

The group of three types of hormones produced by the adrenal cortex (the outer layer of the ADRENAL GLANDS). The steroid group of hormones includes androgens and estrogens, the two SEX HORMONES that affect sexual development and reproduction; glucocorticoids, which maintain glucose (sugar) regulation, suppress the immune and inflammation responses, and increase in concentration in response to stress; and mineralocorticoids, which include ALDOSTERONE, a hormone that regulates sodium and potassium balance, controls sodium levels in the urine, and maintains blood volume and blood pressure. Corticosteroid hormones are essential to life. Synthetic corticosteroids are used to treat various skin disorders, chronic upper respiratory conditions, arthritis, autoimmune disorders, and inflammatory bowel disease. They are also used after kidney transplantation. See also CORTICOSTEROIDS.

Corticosteroids

Steroids produced by the adrenal glands in response to the release of adrenocorticotropic hormone (ACTH) by the pituitary gland. Corticosteroids are used for hormonal replacement therapy if the body does not produce sufficient amounts naturally; for suppression of ACTH secretion by the pituitary gland; to suppress the immune response; and as anticancer, antiallergy, and anti-inflammatory agents.

Corticosteroids have many uses and forms. In paste form, they are used by dentists to relieve the discomfort of some mouth and gum conditions. Corticosteroids are inhaled to help prevent the symptoms of asthma. As a nasal spray, corticosteroids are used to treat the symptoms of allergy.

As eye drops, corticosteroids are used to treat certain eye diseases and to relieve discomfort, redness, and irritation of the eye. Corticosteroids are used to treat ulcerative colitis, hemorrhoids, and other rectal problems. As a skin cream, corticosteroids are used to relieve redness, swelling, itching, and discomfort of many skin problems. Corticosteroids suppress the immune system, and they are important for treatment or prevention of asthma, rheumatoid arthritis, and organ and tissue transplant rejection.

Side effects from prolonged use include weight gain, susceptibility to infections, easy bruising, osteoporosis, and muscle weakness. Chronic use of corticosteroids needs to be monitored closely by a doctor because steroids may cause side effects.

Cortisol

A glucocorticoid hormone produced in the adrenal cortex (the outer layer of the adrenal glands); also known as hydrocortisone. Cortisol is a potent hormone that regulates the metabolism of glucose (sugar), other carbohydrates, proteins, and fats. Cortisol also helps maintain blood pressure and cardiovascular function, helps balance the effects of insulin in breaking down sugar for energy, and helps slow the inflammatory response produced by the immune system when diseases or injuries occur.

Cortisol has a part in so many vital functions within the body; in healthy people the amount produced and released is precisely balanced.

Increased levels of cortisol may be associated with physical stress, HYPERTHYROIDISM (overactivity of the thyroid gland), obesity, and ACTH-producing tumors. CUSHING SYNDROME is caused by excessive production and release of cortisol by the body or caused artificially by taking large doses of cortisol to help control some other medical condition.

The failure to produce normal levels of cortisol is called adrenal insufficiency or Addison disease. It may be caused by an autoimmune disorder of the adrenal glands or inadequate secretion of ACTH by the pituitary gland. Low thyroid conditions, hypopituitarism, tuberculosis, fungal infections of the adrenal glands, adrenal hemorrhage, or certain medications are other factors that may impair the body's ability to make cortisol.

Cosmetic surgery

Any procedure to enhance the appearance or beauty of a person rather than to resolve a medical problem. Common examples are face-lift, CHEMICAL PEEL, and EYELID SURGERY.

Costochondritis

An inflammation of the cartilage attaching the front of the ribs to the breastbone, causing localized pain and tenderness. The area affected is generally the second or third rib attachment. The pain, which may be severe, tends to become more intense with movement or exercise and may be mistaken for a heart attack. Pressure applied directly to the site can make the pain worse. Redness and swelling are not usually present. Diagnosis may require tests that exclude other possible causes, including chest X rays, electrocardiograms, and certain blood tests. Costochondritis is primarily treated with medication to relieve the associated discomfort.

Cough

A reflex that produces a sudden burst of air through the airways. Coughs clear material from the airways and help expel material from the lungs, including inhaled particles and sputum. Sputum, which is also called phlegm, is composed of a mixture of mucus, debris, and cells that have been shed from the lungs. Dry coughs do not produce sputum, but a productive cough indicates sputum production. Sputum that is yellow, green, or brown may indicate a bacterial infection. When it is white, clear, or watery, a virus, allergy, or irritant is generally the cause.

In evaluating a cough, a doctor may need to know the length of time it has been present, the time of day it occurs, the presence of accompanying symptoms, the amount of sputum if any is produced, and the appearance or color of sputum.

Coughs may be related to several conditions, including infection, allergy, or fluid in the lungs. Treatment is usually directed at the underlying cause rather than at suppression of the cough, especially if large amounts of sputum are produced.

Cough remedies

Products available without prescription to help alleviate a cough. Coughing is a useful process in which secretions (mucus) are cleared from the throat and the lungs (a "productive" cough); productive coughs should generally not be suppressed, since they serve a valuable purpose. However, a dry or unproductive cough that hurts the throat or interferes with sleep may benefit from treatment with a cold remedy.

Cough remedies are divided into three categories. Cough suppressants control a dry cough, usually in the early stage of a cold. Expectorants loosen mucus congesting the lungs so the person can cough it up. Cough-cold combinations relieve the cough associated with colds, flu, or hay fever. These combination drugs may also contain antihistamines, decongestants, and pain relievers.

Cough, chronic

A noisy expulsion of air from the lungs, usually sudden and involuntary, that is recurrent and may either produce a dry, hacking sound or bring up phlegm. When a cough recurs and is persistent for more than 3 weeks, it is termed a chronic cough.

A physician should be consulted when a cough continues to get worse after about a week. This prolonged duration of coughing, together with other possible symptoms, may indicate the presence of a serious medical problem. Laboratory tests or imaging studies may be necessary to diagnose the underlying cause.

Coughing up blood

Expelling sputum that contains blood, also called hemoptysis. While coughing up blood may be alarming, it is not always serious. Flecks of blood in the sputum may indicate acute or chronic bronchitis. However, when large amounts of blood are coughed up, or blood-flecked sputum persists, a prompt medical evaluation is necessary to exclude a serious underlying condition. These conditions include tumors of the respiratory tract, particularly lung tumors; blockage of a blood vessel in the lungs, a condition called pulmonary embolism; heart failure, lung infections, and bronchiectasis.

Diagnosing the underlying cause when a person coughs up blood is crucial. The first step is a chest X ray, which may help identify the underlying cause. Often an examination called BRONCHOSCOPY, which uses a viewing instrument to observe the bronchial tubes to identify the cause of bleeding, may be needed. Antibiotics may be prescribed.

If the bleeding occurs in a major blood vessel and a large amount of blood is coughed up, urgent treatment to stop the bleeding and to remove any clots blocking the airway is usually necessary. Bleeding caused by heart failure or pneumonia generally subsides when the condition is medically treated.

Surgery may be required to remove a diseased area of the lung if this is causing coughed up blood. If a tumor is discovered that is inoperable, treatment with radiation and chemotherapy should be considered.

Couples therapy

Counseling or psychotherapy that focuses on the interactions between two people in a long-term relationship.

Coxsackievirus

Any of a group of viruses that cause a variety of infectious diseases, including a mild form of MENINGITIS and HAND-FOOT-AND-MOUTH DISEASE. The most common symptoms of an infection include flulike malaise, fever, and muscle aches. There may also be coughing, nasal congestion, diarrhea, and vomiting.

Coxsackieviruses can cause a mild form of meningitis, called aseptic meningitis, and, rarely, transient paralysis. The symptoms of aseptic meningitis include pain and stiffness in the neck and back, muscular aches, fever, malaise, loss of appetite, and vomiting. The symptoms may disappear within a week, but fatigue and irritability may persist for a month or longer.

When the virus causes hand-foot-and-mouth disease, most commonly in infants and children, a skin rash develops on the face, neck, and chest. Fever may develop, and the infection may progress to aseptic meningitis.

Inflammation of the heart muscle (MYOCARDITIS) and inflammation of the membranous sac that encloses the heart (PERICARDITIS) may also be caused by a coxsackievirus. Myocarditis in newborns produces symptoms including a sudden fever and feeding difficulties. It can be fatal to infants. In adults, the symptoms of myocarditis are fatigue, shortness of breath, and chest pain, but complete recovery is common.

Coxsackievirus infections are diagnosed by isolating the virus from the throat or stool specimens. Because it is a virus, medical options are limited and treatment is directed toward managing symptoms.

Crab lice

Small, crablike organisms that attach themselves to human hairs. Crab lice usually live in pubic hair, but may also become attached to eyelashes, eyebrows, and hair in the armpits or on the face. The lice may be transmitted by direct physical contact with a person who has crab lice or contact with an infested person's bed linens, towels, or clothes.

There may be no symptoms of infestation, or symptoms may appear immediately or may take several weeks to become noticeable if the eggs have not hatched. In most instances, the lice cause itching, which becomes worse at night. A bluish rash is sometimes observed at the site of the bites. If lice are in the eyelashes or eyebrows, the eyes may become inflamed.

When an infestation of crab lice is suspected, medical attention should be sought. The nits cannot be banished by soap and water washing as they cling tightly to the hair shafts. Destroying them requires an over-the-counter medication, usually lindane or pyrethrin solution.

Cradle cap

A condition in babies in which thick, yellow scales form in patches over the scalp. A form of SEBORRHEIC DERMATITIS, cradle cap is common during the first 3 months of life but infrequent after 1 year of age. Cradle cap usually resolves on its own without any special treatment by age 12 months. Remedies include using over-the-counter medicated shampoos, massaging mineral oil into the scalp, and using a soft toothbrush to remove scales.

Cramp

A sudden, painful spasm in a muscle due to an excessive and prolonged contraction of the muscle fibers. Common causes include overuse, muscle stress, and dehydration. Any unexplained cramp that is not relieved by simple self-care measures should be evaluated by a doctor.

Cranberry

A natural substance used to treat urinary tract infections. Components of cranberry prevent bacteria from adhering to the lining of the bladder. Cranberry is available in pill form as well as in sweetened juice products.

Cranial nerves

Twelve pairs of nerves originating in the brain that control most of the functions in the head and face, including the sense organs. Some of the cranial nerves carry only sensory signals from the sense organs, others carry motor messages to move the muscles of the organs and structures of the head, and some carry autonomic (involuntary) messages for functions such as heartbeat. Some of the cranial nerves have all three capabilities.

Craniofacial dysostosis

A birth defect comprising a characteristic group of deformities that involve an abnormal fusion, or joining, between some of the bones of the skull and face (see BIRTH DEFECTS). The fusion does not allow the craniofacial bones (bones of the skull and face) to grow normally, which affects the shape of the head and the appearance of the face as well as the positioning of the teeth.

Craniofacial dysostosis varies in severity. The major associated problem is an underdevelopment of the upper jaw, causing a facial deformity characterized by bulging eyes and a sunken middle portion of the face.

An abnormal relationship between the upper and lower jaws, called malocclusion, is also a feature of the syndrome. Dental and plastic surgery specialists can monitor facial growth. Mental retardation is not usually a feature of the syndrome. It is recommended that parents of an infant born with craniofacial dysostosis contact a craniofacial center for a complete evaluation of the child, as well as for treatment planning and comprehensive related services.

Craniopharyngioma

A slow-growing, calcified, cystic tumor of the brain that is usually benign (not cancerous), develops near the pituitary gland, and usually affects children or older adults. A craniopharyngioma may be associated with increased pressure within the cranium. The tumor usually develops in the pituitary stalk and projects into the hypothalamus. In rare instances, it may develop in or migrate to the opening between the nose and throat or extend into the cervical spine.

There may be no symptoms of these tumors. If there are symptoms, they are the result of the pressure the tumor applies to tissues surrounding the pituitary gland. A common symptom is a slowly progressive, dull, and localized headache.

A craniopharyngioma is diagnosed by general physical examination, a neurologic evaluation, and MRI (magnetic resonance imaging). Other tests may include those for pituitary function.

If a craniopharyngioma causes excessive pressure on the brain or other conditions that are considered serious and possibly life-threatening, surgical removal of the tumor may become necessary, followed by radiation therapy. If the tumor adheres to surrounding blood vessels, it may be impossible to remove it entirely.

Craniosacral technique

See VISUALIZATION.

Craniosynostosis

Premature or early closure of one or more of the openings in the skull of a newborn. Babies are normally born with the seven bones of the skull separated by fibrous borders (sutures). The soft spot where sutures intersect is called a FONTANELLE. The fact that the bones of the skull are not solidly fused at birth enables the shape of the infant's head to mold as it passes through the birth canal and later permits the skull to expand as the brain grows in early infancy. In craniosynostosis, the sutures close too early. A deformed skull, pressure on the brain, and vision problems can result.

Craniosynostosis is usually first suspected by a pediatrician, family physician, or geneticist, who may refer the child to a pediatric neurosurgeon or a craniofacial surgeon. The suture ridges and fontanelles are examined.

The fusion of a single suture may not need treatment. However, the treatment of more extensive craniosynostosis requires procedures performed by teams that specialize in craniofacial surgery. Most surgery for craniosynostosis is done between 3 and 6 months of age.

Craniotomy

A procedure to remove a section, or flap, of the skull to expose and operate on the tissues underneath, usually the brain. A craniotomy is used to repair aneurysms and ruptured blood vessels, remove tumors of the brain, fix malformed arteries and veins, and treat blockages in the flow of cerebrospinal fluid (a condition called HYDROCEPHALUS).

Cranium

The part of the SKULL that encloses the brain; sometimes used to refer to all the bones of the skull.

Creatinine clearance

See KIDNEY FUNCTION TESTS.

CREST syndrome

A form of the disease SCLERODERMA, an autoimmune disorder in which the body's immune system attacks its own tissues.

CREST is an acronym that includes the following syndromes: calcinosis, which is a calcification in the skin; Raynaud phenomenon, which causes a sequence of color changes in the fingers and toes caused by blood vessel spasms in response to cold; esophageal dysfunction, which may be gastroesophageal reflux or difficulty swallowing; sclerodactyly, which is a narrowing and hardening of the skin of the fingers or toes; and telangiectasia, which is a dilation of the tiny blood vessels, especially those in the skin.

Creutzfeldt-Jakob disease

A rare fatal condition characterized by a rapidly progressive mental deterioration and muscle wasting. See also MAD COW DISEASE.

CRH

Corticotropin-releasing hormone. A hormone produced by the hypothalamus that stimulates the pituitary gland to release ACTH (adrenocorticotropic hormone).

Cricothyroidotomy

An emergency intervention to provide a breathing passage for an individual with great difficulty breathing because of a blockage in the upper respiratory system around the voice box. A needle is inserted into the TRACHEA (windpipe) through the skin and a membrane called the cricothyroid, which lies just below the prominent bulge of the LARYNX (voice box). A breathing device attached to the hollow needle then sends air in and out of the lungs.

Crisis intervention

Providing immediate care or advice to people with acute physical or psychological problems.

Critical

Pertaining to a period of crisis in a person with a life-threatening medical condition.

Critical care

Assessing and treating the health of a person at immediate risk of dying. Critical care, also known as intensive care, covers the whole process of treating seriously ill patients.

The INTENSIVE CARE UNIT of the hospital provides state-of-the-art, 24-hour care by doctors and nurses who are trained to take aggressive and immediate action to intervene, whenever necessary, to save the life of a patient.

Crohn disease

Chronic inflammatory disease of the digestive tract. Crohn disease is also known as enteritis, ileitis, and regional enteritis. Although it can occur anywhere in the digestive tract, from the mouth to the anus, this disease most frequently affects the junction of the colon (large intestine) and the ileum (small intestine).

Abdominal pain and diarrhea are the most common symptoms of Crohn disease. Frequently, these problems follow a meal. Other signs include fever, joint pains, loss of appetite, and weight loss. Inflammation of the lining of the intestine, anal fissure (a tear or ulcer in the lining of the anal canal), anal fistula (an abnormal channel formed between the anal canal and a tiny hole in the skin surrounding the anus), or an abscess may also develop. The disease usually develops between ages 20 and 30.

Diagnosis is based on a complete physical examination and tests, such as stool analysis, blood tests, a lower gastrointestinal (GI) series (an x-ray procedure also known as a barium enema), and SIGMOIDOSCOPY or COLONOSCOPY.

Treatment is with anti-inflammatory drugs to suppress the inflammatory response so the body can heal itself. Powerful corticosteroids, immunosuppressants, and antibiotics may also be prescribed. Severe attacks generally require hospitalization and intravenous administration of medication.

When medication cannot control the symptoms or a complication develops, a COLECTOMY (surgical removal of all or part of the colon) becomes necessary.

Crossed eyes

See STRABISMUS.

Crossmatching

A laboratory test to determine a person's blood group by identifying the proteins on the red blood cells; also known as blood typing and ABO typing. Crossmatching is important for determining the safety of blood transfusions (see TRANSFUSION). Crossmatching is also important for women during pregnancy (see RH INCOMPATIBILITY).

Cross-tolerance

Resistance to the effects of a drug that develops through the repeated use of another, similar drug.

Croup

An inflammation of the voice box and windpipe that narrows the airway just below the vocal cords, resulting in difficult and noisy breathing. Croup is a common illness in young children, especially those aged 6 months to 3 years. After the age of 3, the windpipe is more developed and swelling is less likely to interfere with breathing. Croup occurs most frequently between October and March.

There are two types of croup; both often begin with a common cold (see COLD, COMMON). Spasmodic croup is caused by mild upper respiratory infection or allergy and begins suddenly, often at night. The symptoms include gasping for breath, hoarseness, and a distinctive barking cough. Usually there is not a fever with spasmodic croup, and it can reoccur.

Viral croup usually develops from a cold and progresses to a barking cough. It is caused by a viral infection in the voice box and windpipe. The child's airway swells and more fluid is secreted, causing labored, noisy breathing, a condition called STRIDOR. If stridor occurs when a child is resting and not crying or moving, it may indicate severe croup. Low fever often accompanies symptoms of viral croup, but the child's temperature may get as high as 104°F. For milder cases of croup, using a humidifier at home may be effective.

The danger of croup in young children is that the inflammation may cause progressive swelling and obstruct breathing. A doctor should be called if there is a suspicion of croup, and emergency medical services should be sought if any of the following symptoms develop: extremely labored breathing, a whistling sound with breathing that increases in volume with each breath, pallor with blue coloration at the mouth and fingertips, wheezing when inhaling during rest, and drooling, with great difficulty swallowing saliva.

Crown, dental

The visible part of the tooth that normally protrudes above the gum line. A dental crown is also the name for the artificial replacement placed over a dental implant or the remaining structure of a natural tooth, most often because of a fracture or tooth decay. The purpose of a crown is to replace the structure of a tooth, to im-

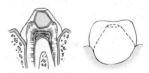

Tooth filed to a stub   Crown fitted over stub

Crowning a tooth

If a tooth is severely decayed, broken, or fragile, the dentist may construct an artificial crown. First, the dentist removes any decay and files the natural tooth down to make room for the crown. The new crown (shown above) is cemented in place and filed to duplicate the bite of the original tooth.

prove the appearance of a tooth or teeth, or to replace missing teeth with a dental bridge, including a pontic (a false tooth attached to one or more crowns).

Crush syndrome

The consequence of prolonged continuous pressure on the limbs, which decreases the blood supply to skeletal muscles and may damage muscle tissue. The damaged muscle can release breakdown products such as myoglobin into the bloodstream, which can be toxic to the kidneys.

Cryopreservation

The use of extremely low temperatures to preserve sperm or embryos for use at a later time. Frozen sperm can be thawed and used for ARTIFICIAL INSEMINATION or ASSISTED REPRODUCTIVE TECHNOLOGY.

Cryosurgery

Using a temperature below freezing to remove abnormal or diseased tissue. Cryosurgery is used to remove lesions, such as warts, from the skin and to treat cancer or precancerous conditions of the CERVIX. The freezing agent used is typically liquid nitrogen, which has a temperature of approximately –256°F. Depending on the location of the abnormal tissue, the nitrogen can be applied with a cotton-tipped applicator or a metal probe.

Cryotherapy

Also known as CRYOSURGERY; the use of very low temperatures to destroy tissue by freezing. Cryotherapy is used to control pain or bleeding, reduce the size of brain lesions, remove lesions of the uterine cervix, and treat malignant and benign tumors and common skin conditions (such as skin tags and warts). In this procedure, cold is given through a probe that has liquid nitrogen flowing through it.

Cryptococcosis

An infection that is contracted when soil contaminated with a specific yeast, often from pigeon droppings, is inhaled. Cryptococcosis infections may be limited to the lungs, or they may spread to the meninges (the membrane surrounding the brain), the skin, the bones, or other areas of the body.

Diagnosis of cryptococcosis is made by identifying the yeast in sputum, urine, blood, cerebrospinal fluid, or other body secretions. If treatment becomes necessary, antifungal therapy is usually prescribed.

Cryptorchidism

See TESTICLE, UNDESCENDED.

Cryptosporidiosis

An infection caused by a microscopic parasite that lives in the intestines of humans and animals. It is transmitted by eating or drinking food or water that is fecally contaminated. The symptoms generally begin within 2 to 14 days of exposure and last between 2 and 14 days. They often include profuse watery diarrhea, abdominal cramps, nausea, and a moderate fever. The gallbladder may also be infected. Sometimes, the infection may not cause symptoms and improve on its own, but in people with weakened immune systems, cryptosporidiosis can be severe and even fatal.

There is no vaccine currently available, and no antiparasitic drug has been discovered to treat cryptosporidiosis.

C-section

See CESAREAN SECTION.

CT scanning

Computed tomography scanning; formerly known as CAT (computerized axial tomography) scanning. A diagnostic imaging technique in which multiple projections of X rays (passed through the body from several angles) are analyzed by a computer to produce cross-sectional images of structures, including bone, organs, muscles, and tumors. The digital images obtained through CT scanning are more detailed than the images obtained through standard X rays. The procedure is a painless, noninvasive method of visualizing detailed views of internal organs and structures; in many cases, it can eliminate the need for more invasive procedures.

CT scanning can aid in surgery and in the diagnosis of many different conditions. It may be used in association with treatments such as radiation therapy, in which knowing the precise density, size, and location of a tumor is essential to providing the correct dosage of radiation. CT scans of the blood vessels can be performed to locate and detail precisely the nature of conditions such as an aneurysm (abnormal ballooning of a weakened area in the wall of an artery).

For some CT scans, an intravenous contrast medium containing iodine may be administered to make the blood vessels show up more clearly, or a flavored barium drink may be given to provide contrast to internal structures. The person being scanned lies on a narrow table that slides into the scanner.

Culture

The process of taking a sample of material from the body and then placing it in a medium conducive to the growth of microorganisms. The type of specimen depends on the suspected site of infection in the patient. For example, urine is cultured to detect a kidney or bladder infection.

Cunnilingus

Oral stimulation of a woman's clitoris and vagina with a partner's mouth and tongue. See ORAL SEX.

Cushing syndrome

A rare hormonal disorder produced by chronically increased levels of the hormone cortisol in the bloodstream; also known as hypercortisolism.

Cushing syndrome has varying symptoms. The disorder is generally characterized by the wasting of muscles, thinning of skin, severe fatigue, high blood pressure, hyperglycemia (high blood sugar), and weakened bones. In most cases, there tends to be obesity (especially around the waist), rounding of the face, and an increase in fat tissue in the neck area. This is offset by thin arms and legs. The skin bruises easily and heals poorly. There may be dark pink or purple stretch marks on the abdomen, thighs, buttocks, arms, and breasts. Weakened bones may interfere with routine movements; lifting objects, bending down, or simply getting up from a chair can cause backaches or fractures of the ribs or spine. An affected person may experience anxiety, depression, and irritability.

Cushing syndrome is diagnosed on the basis of medical history, physical examination, and laboratory tests. Common screening tests for Cushing syndrome include the overnight dexamethasone suppression test, in which a dose of dexamethasone is given at midnight and a fasting cortisol level is checked the next morning, and also the 24-hour urinary free cortisol level, for which the person's urine must be collected for a day to check the output of cortisol.

Treatment of Cushing syndrome is related to the cause of excess cortisol production and may include surgery, radiation, chemotherapy (if the disorder is due to cancer), and the use of cortisol-inhibiting drugs.

Cutaneous

Pertaining to the skin.

Cutdown

An incision through the skin to identify a vein and insert a catheter for intravenous infusion. A cutdown is performed when an infusion cannot be begun by VENIPUNCTURE (piercing of a vein with a needle).

CVS

See CHORIONIC VILLUS SAMPLING.

Cyanide

A poisonous, colorless liquid with the odor of bitter almonds. Only a few milligrams of cyanide can be rapidly fatal to humans. Cyanide prevents the use of oxygen by body tissues, and if a large dose is consumed, death will occur almost immediately.

As with any suspected poisoning, the first thing a person should do is call a POISON CENTER and follow the instructions or go to the nearest hospital emergency department.

Cyst

A small, closed sac filled with liquid, semisolid, or solid material. A cyst can become inflamed, infected, and painful. If cysts become infected or are otherwise troublesome, they can be removed through draining or EXCISION (cutting). See also DERMOID CYST and EPIDERMAL CYST.

Cystectomy

Surgical removal of the bladder. BLADDER CANCER, which invades the muscular bladder wall, is the most common reason for cystectomy. In men, the prostate gland and seminal vesicles are also removed; in women, the urethra, uterus, cervix, and the front wall of the vagina are removed. Lymph nodes in the area are also removed and checked for cancer. To replace the role of the bladder in storing urine, a new reservoir is created surgically from a portion of the small or large intestine.

Depending on the surgery, a person who has undergone radical cystectomy either must wear a urine collection bag at all times or can drain the internal reservoir periodically. In some cases, a section of intestine may be brought down to the urethra, allowing the patient to urinate normally. Radical cystectomy is an effective treatment for bladder cancer.

Cystic fibrosis

An inherited disease characterized by thick, sticky mucus in the lungs and other organs and increased salt content in sweat.

The first sign of CF in an infant may be intestinal blockage. Some babies with CF may have bulky stools, poor weight gain, or slow growth, all the result of low levels of digestive enzymes in the intestines. Children with CF may also have chronic coughs, wheezing, or respiratory tract infections. People with CF tend to become dehydrated because they lose too much salt in their sweat. Often parents of children with CF report that their infants taste salty when they kiss them. Chronic lung infections associated with the disease gradually destroy lung tissue, eventually leading to death. The average life expectancy for people with CF is 20 to 30 years.

Even though CF remains incurable, various treatments can relieve discomfort and slow the deterioration of tissue. Intestinal blockage in newborns can be removed surgically. Malabsorption can be improved by giving pancreatic enzymes with meals. To compensate for their inadequate digestive system, most people with CF must eat a high-calorie diet. Respiratory infections are treated with antibiotics and bronchodilators.

Cystitis

Inflammation of the interior lining of the bladder; the most common urinary tract infection in women. Cystitis occurs when bacteria from the colon that live on the skin near the rectum or in the vagina enter the urinary tract through the urethra. The bacteria travel up the urethra, infecting the bladder. Sexual intercourse can precipitate cystitis in women. In men the urethra is farther away from the bladder than in women, so cystitis is less frequent in men. Symptoms can include more frequent urination, a burning sensation while urinating, and blood in the urine. Even though the urge to urinate may be strong, only small amounts of urine are released, and they may have a strong smell. Fever and soreness in the lower abdomen or back may also occur.

Cystitis is very common; the risk of cystitis may be reduced by drinking plenty of fluids, wiping from front to back after urination or a bowel movement (in women), and by emptying the bladder immediately before and after sexual intercourse. Drinking about 2 quarts of water or other fluids for a day may relieve symptoms. Cranberry juice is sometimes thought to help prevent cystitis. A physician should be consulted when symptoms persist or are severe. Antibiotics or other drugs may be prescribed.

Cystocele

A protrusion of the bladder into the vagina. A cystocele, which is sometimes called a fallen or dropped bladder, is caused by the stretching and weakening of the pelvic muscles and most often occurs after childbirth. Symptoms can include pressure or aching in the vagina, difficulty in urinating, and problems with penetration during sexual intercourse. Stress

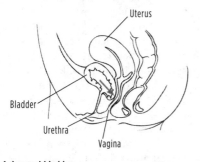

A dropped bladder

In a woman whose pelvic muscles have been weakened, most often by childbirth, the base of the bladder may drop against the vagina—a condition called a cystocele (arrow indicates area of pressure).

incontinence, in which urine leaks out when a woman laughs or coughs, is also common. Some women with cystoceles are predisposed to developing urinary tract infections. Problems may not arise until after menopause, when the loss of estrogen weakens pelvic muscles even further.

A doctor can easily detect a cystocele during a routine pelvic examination. In mild cases, symptoms may be relieved with regular practice of KEGEL EXERCISES. Postmenopausal women may find that HORMONE REPLACEMENT THERAPY will reverse some of the weakening of the pelvic muscles. Insertion of a vaginal PESSARY may provide temporary support of the bladder and urethra and improve urinary control. If symptoms are severe or interfere with daily activities, a surgical procedure can correct a cystocele by pushing the bladder upward and sewing it into position.

Cystography, voiding

A detailed X-ray study of the bladder. The test may be performed when an infection, tumor, bladder stones, or reflux of urine into the kidneys is suspected. The patient first empties his or her bladder by normal urination. Then, a thin, flexible tube (catheter) coated with anesthetic jelly is inserted through the urinary tract. The bladder is filled with dye through the catheter, and X rays are taken with the patient in different positions. The patient voids the dye by urinating, and another X ray is taken.

Cystoscopy

Visual examination of the inside of the lower urinary tract and bladder through a special viewing instrument tipped with a light (cystoscope). Cystoscopy is performed for a number of reasons, including blood in the urine, inability to control urination (incontinence), infection, congenital abnormalities, calculi, and tumors.

Cystotomy

A surgical incision made into the bladder, usually to inspect or repair the bladder or for placement of a tube to aid in urination.

Cystourethrocele

A condition in which the tissues supporting the bladder and urethra are weakened in women. The weakness can cause stress incontinence, in which urine can leak out when the woman sneezes, coughs, jumps, or lifts heavy objects.

A doctor can detect a cystourethrocele during a routine pelvic examination. Treatment can include KEGEL EXERCISES in mild cases, medications that increase the tone of the muscles around the urethra, hormone replacement therapy in women who are past menopause, or surgery.

Cytomegalic viral retinitis

Infection of the light-sensitive layer (retina) at the back of the eye with CYTOMEGALOVIRUS (CMV). CMV infection usually produces no symptoms, except in people with compromised immune systems. Cytomegalic viral retinitis (also called cytomegalovirus retinitis) occurs in approximately one of every four people with AIDS and may lead to blindness. Symptoms include floaters (small, moving shapes in the visual field), impaired vision, blind spots, and loss of vision to the sides. Treatment is difficult, since antiviral medications stop the virus

from reproducing but do not destroy it. Recently, intraocular injections and implants with antiviral drugs have shown great benefit without the side effects of systemic drugs.

Cytomegalovirus

A member of the herpesvirus group, which also includes herpes simplex virus types 1 and 2, varicella-zoster virus (the virus that causes CHICKENPOX), and EPSTEIN-BARR VIRUS (the virus that causes infectious mononucleosis; see MONONUCLEOSIS, INFECTIOUS). Cytomegalovirus (CMV) can survive in the body in a dormant state for months to years after a person has been infected. Once infected, a person retains the living virus within his or her body for life.

After an initial infection, the majority of adults and children who contract cytomegalovirus have few or no symptoms and no long-term health consequences. A prolonged infection follows, during which time a person does not experience clinical illness and is generally unaware of the presence of the virus.

When reactivated, the virus may or may not produce symptoms. If there are symptoms, they may include a mononucleosislike syndrome with prolonged fever, sore throat, fatigue, and swollen glands. Mild HEPATITIS may be experienced. People with weakened immune systems can develop eye infections, PNEUMONIA, COLITIS, and ENCEPHALITIS.

Cytomegalovirus is spread via bodily secretions, including saliva, urine, feces, blood, tears, breast milk, semen, and cervical secretions.

There is no treatment for CMV infection in an otherwise healthy person at this time. Several antiviral medications are available for infants and persons with weakened immune systems who develop serious infections.

The very small percentage of women who contract CMV for the first time during pregnancy are at risk of having a baby who has symptoms at birth or who may develop disabilities at a later time. CMV remains the most significant cause of congenital viral infection in the United States. Infants who are infected by their mothers before birth may have a generalized infection with symptoms that are apparent at birth. These may range from jaundice caused by moderate enlargement of the liver and spleen to fatal disease.

D

D and C

Dilation and curettage. A procedure in which the ENDOMETRIUM (the lining of a woman's uterus) is scraped away with a spoon-shaped instrument called a curet. A D and C may be done as a diagnostic or therapeutic procedure to treat a variety of disorders, such as excessive bleeding during menstrual periods. A D and C is also commonly performed after a woman has a miscarriage or for an abortion. In this outpatient procedure, a local anesthetic is given to numb the cervix; a sedative may be given for relaxation. A SPECULUM is

used to expand the vagina, and then the cervix is gradually opened with a series of plastic or metal wedges called dilators. The doctor inserts a curet through the cervix into the uterus to remove the surface of the endometrium. The scrapings are then examined under a microscope for abnormalities, such as cancer or polyps.

Complications, although rare, may include perforated tissue, excessive bleeding, or infection. Until the cervix contracts to its normal size, a woman is at increased risk for bacterial infection.

D and E

Dilation and evacuation. A procedure in which a woman's cervix is dilated and the contents of the uterus are removed by suctioning. Almost always an outpatient procedure, D and E is typically performed as part of an abortion procedure or after a miscarriage. When performed during the first trimester of pregnancy, the procedure may be referred to as vacuum aspiration, vacuum curettage, suction curettage, or suction D and C.

Dacryocystitis

Inflammation of the tear sac and the tear duct leading from the eye to the nose. The cause is usually bacterial, but viruses or fungi may be the cause. Symptoms include warm, painful swelling of the lower eyelid close to the nose, oozing of pus from the eye when pressure is applied to the swollen area, and fever. Since tears normally drain from the eye through the tear duct into the nose, blockage of the duct from dacryocystitis may cause tears to stream from the eye.

Applying a warm compress (a clean cloth soaked in very warm water and then wrung out) can help relieve pain and promote drainage. In infants, gentle massage of the tear duct four times a day for up to 9 months can help drain the blockage and create normal flow. Antibiotic ointments or oral medications can be used against infection. In some cases, a tiny tube is inserted into the tear duct and the duct is flushed with a sterile saltwater solution.

Date rape

Sexual contact that is forced on a person who is acquainted with the rapist. Date rape, also known as acquaintance RAPE, is most common among women between the ages of 16 and 24 years. The use of alcohol and drugs also can be a factor, especially when the man puts drugs in a woman's drink or food without her knowledge.

de Quervain disease

A painful inflammation of the sheath surrounding the tendon that is attached to the bone at the outside of the wrist. It is seen in individuals who use their thumbs and hands in a repetitive manner. The sheath is enclosed in a narrow tunnel, and the tendon becomes compressed when the sheath is swollen. This puts excessive pressure on the tendon, which causes the severe wrist pain commonly produced by de Quervain disease. Pressure on the nerve can cause numbness and tingling over the thumb and index finger.

Treatment may include limitation of activities involving movements of the wrist and the use of a thumb brace to rest and support the area. Ice and NONSTEROIDAL ANTI-INFLAMMATORY DRUGS (NSAIDs) may be recom-

mended for pain management. A thumb splint may also be used for 3 weeks. A cortisone or anesthetic injection in the area is sometimes helpful. If the pain persists, outpatient surgery is needed.

Deafness

An inability to hear, which may affect any age group, with consequences ranging from minor to severe. A small proportion of hearing-impaired persons in the United States are considered profoundly deaf, meaning their hearing loss is so severe they cannot benefit from hearing aids or other forms of mechanical sound amplification. A much larger proportion of people who are hearing impaired can benefit, in varying degrees, from the use of amplification devices.

Deafness is usually caused by illness or accidents. It may also run in families and be inherited. Certain conditions such as rubella (German measles) during a woman's pregnancy create a risk that her baby will be born deaf.

There are four general categories of hearing loss: conductive hearing loss, sensorineural hearing loss, mixed hearing loss, and central hearing loss. Conductive hearing loss is caused by diseases or obstruction in the outer or middle ear; this condition is not generally severe and can be helped by a hearing aid, by performing surgery on the eardrum or middle ear, or simply by cleaning earwax or other obstructions from the ear canal. Sensorineural hearing loss results from damage to the sensory nerves or hair cells in the inner ear and ranges in severity from mild to profound. Because this type of hearing loss affects certain sound frequencies more severely than others, a person with sensorineural hearing loss perceives distortions in sound, even when the sound is amplified. In such cases, hearing aids may not help a person with sensorineural hearing loss. Mixed hearing loss is caused by problems in the outer or middle ear, as well as in the inner ear. Central hearing loss is caused by damage to or impairment of centers or connections in the brain.

An evaluation of the degree and type of hearing loss is made with the help of hearing tests (see AUDIOMETRY). A person with hearing loss will be evaluated and fitted with various kinds of hearing aids and other mechanical sound amplifiers, including assistive listening devices.

Communication systems are frequently used to benefit people who are deaf. American Sign Language (ASL) is a language system formed by making distinctive shapes and movements with one or both hands. Individual hand signs are related in both concrete and abstract meaning of spoken words. Finger spelling is a system based on forming shapes with the hands that correspond to the letters of the alphabet. Oral communication is a system taught to deaf children using speech as an expressive skill for articulating thoughts to another person. Lip-reading is used along with oral communication.

Death

The end of life. By medical definition, death generally occurs when a person has sustained irreversible cessation of circulatory and respiratory functions. When a person's heartbeat and respiration are being maintained mechanically, death occurs when there is an irreversible cessation of all functions of the entire brain, including the brain stem.

Death rate

The number of deaths within a group of people in 1 year divided by the average or midyear population of that group. If total population is used, the result is called the crude death rate. Death rate can also be calculated for the population within certain age groups; the result is the age-specific death rate. Death rate may be measured in people with a specific disease or condition, such as a gunshot wound (homicide rate) or heart disease.

Debridement

Surgical removal of foreign material or damaged, dead, or contaminated tissue from a severe wound or injury. Surgical debridement usually requires an anesthetic because it involves cutting away the damaged tissue with sharp instruments or a laser. Debridement helps promote healthy healing of badly damaged skin, tissue, muscle, and bone.

Decerebrate

The state of being without a functioning cerebrum (the main controlling part of the brain). This condition occurs when the brain stem is damaged. When in response to stimulation the arms of a comatose person are extended and internally rotated, he or she is said to be in decerebrate posture. See also COMA.

Decompression sickness

The health problems caused by nitrogen bubbles in a scuba diver's bloodstream, which can block the flow of blood. Decompression sickness, also called "the bends," usually results from an ascent to the surface of the water that is too rapid to allow the release of excess nitrogen absorbed with oxygen during the descent into the water. Nitrogen, which is an inert gas, is not metabolized by the body and may be especially retained in fatty tissue. All of it must be released from the body through exhalation as a diver ascends. When the ascent is too rapid, the nitrogen cannot escape, and this can result in nitrogen bubbles forming in the diver's blood, preventing normal blood flow. The side effects of this blockage may range from discomforts such as headaches, to more severe impairment including confusion and paralysis, to dire outcomes, such as coma and death. The treatment for decompression sickness is hyperbaric oxygen therapy. See DIVING MEDICINE.

Decompression, spinal cord

A surgical procedure to relieve pressure on the spinal cord or on a nerve root emerging from the cord. Spinal cord decompression is performed to treat conditions such as disk prolapse (a ruptured disk; see SLIPPED DISK), SPINAL STENOSIS (narrowing of the spinal canal), a tumor, or a vertebral fracture. Surgery is usually indicated when the problem becomes disabling or interferes with walking or bladder or bowel control.

Decongestant drugs

Drugs used to relieve nasal congestion. Decongestants are widely available in many forms to treat a congested (stuffy) nose typical of colds and allergies. Decongestants relieve only a stuffy nose and are not ef-

fective against other symptoms of colds or allergies. Decongestants cannot cure colds.

Even though decongestants are widely available without prescription, they are drugs that can cause problems. Nasal sprays and nose drops, for example, should never be used for longer than 3 days, because they can cause rebound congestion, in which the nose remains stuffy or gets worse with every dose.

Some decongestants that are combined with antihistamines can cause drowsiness and should not be used by people who are driving or operating machinery. Decongestants alone do not cause sleepiness but can cause a jittery feeling, palpitations, and increased blood pressure.

Decubitus ulcers

See PRESSURE SORES.

Defecation

The elimination of FECES or stool from the body in a bowel movement. Food is first broken down in the digestive tract. Toward the end of the tract, as waste passes through the colon, most of the remaining fluid is absorbed. The solid waste that remains is composed of a mixture of undigested and indigestible material, including vegetable fibers (roughage), bile pigments, mucus, bacteria, and dead cells.

Repeatedly ignoring the urge to defecate is a common reason for CONSTIPATION. Regularity and ease of defecation are considered more important than frequency.

Defibrillation

An emergency procedure used to stop an uncontrolled, rapid, and ineffective heartbeat by administering an electric shock to the heart. The machine used to provide the shock is known as a DEFIBRILLATOR. An uncontrolled, rapid, and ineffective heartbeat (ventricular fibrillation) often follows a heart attack. If left untreated, it can lead to brain damage or sudden death. The sooner defibrillation is given after ventricular fibrillation sets in, the more likely it is to be effective at preventing death or brain damage.

Defibrillator

A device used to administer an electric shock to the heart to stop an uncontrolled, rapid, and ineffective heartbeat. (See DEFIBRILLATION.)

There are three basic types of defibrillators. The manual defibrillator is used in a hospital setting to administer a high-energy electrical charge to a person experiencing ventricular fibrillation or cardiac arrest (no heartbeat). Handheld paddles are placed against the chest wall on both sides of the heart. Manual defibrillators are also used for the nonemergency procedure known as CARDIOVERSION,

which is used to regulate an abnormal but not immediately life-threatening heart rhythm.

An automatic external defibrillator (AED) can be used by people who are not doctors, such as firefighters and emergency medical technicians. The AED device not only administers the electric shock but also reads and interprets the heart rhythm and determines the proper amount of electricity to provide.

The third type of defibrillator is the implantable cardioverter defibrillator (ICD), which is placed surgically in the chest to monitor the heartbeat and administer electric shock as needed to correct an abnormal heartbeat. The ICD contains an electronic memory of adverse events that can be retrieved and analyzed. An ICD is similar in size and mechanics to a PACEMAKER, but while pacemakers are generally used for people with bradycardia (abnormally slow heartbeat), ICDs are typically used for those with tachycardia (a tendency toward overly fast heart rhythms). Some people benefit from the insertion of a combined pacemaker-ICD device.

Defoliant poisoning

The effects of exposure to herbicide defoliant chemicals on animals and humans. Exposure to defoliants, especially AGENT ORANGE, has been linked to chemical acne, non-Hodgkin lymphoma, HODGKIN DISEASE, and soft-tissue SARCOMA.

To prevent defoliant poisoning among agricultural workers, US law requires that any persons handling defoliants wear protective clothing, face masks, and gloves. In addition, agricultural workers and others using

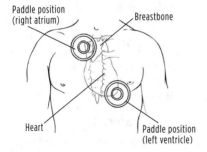

Paddle position (right atrium)

Breastbone

Heart

Paddle position (left ventricle)

Placement of external paddles
An external defibrillator has paddles that are positioned on the chest to deliver one or more shocks to a person with sudden cardiac arrest.

defoliants must pass a course on the safe handling of such chemicals.

Degenerative joint disease

See OSTEOARTHRITIS.

Dehydration

A decrease in the body's water level below that required for adequate circulation. Dehydration has many symptoms, including increased thirst, anxiety, weakness, confusion, and fainting. A decrease in urine output, dry and pale skin without the normal elasticity, sunken eyes, and decreased tears are also signs of dehydration.

Severe dehydration must be treated quickly to avoid cardiovascular collapse and death. A fluid loss of up to 5 percent of normal body weight is considered mild; a loss of between 5 and 10 percent is considered moderate; and a loss of 10 to 15 percent is considered severe. The best treatment for dehydration is prevention. Adequate fluids must be consumed at all times, particularly during illness.

Delirium

A state of mental confusion that develops over a few hours or days and tends to fluctuate, often rapidly. Delirium involves changes in consciousness, such as reduced awareness of the person's surroundings, a loss of attention or concentration, impaired memory, disorientation to time or place, and impaired use of language (such as difficulty naming objects).

Delirium is caused by a disturbance in brain function and may be due to many medical conditions including general medical illness, certain chemical substances, infections, medica-tion side effects, and alcoholism. Treatment of delirium depends on the underlying cause and often involves hospitalization and medication (usually tranquilizers) to control mood or stabilize brain function. In most cases, delirium lasts approximately 1 week, although it may take several weeks or even months for cognitive function to return to normal. Full recovery depends on the cause and pre-existing medical and neurological conditions. If delirium occurs in older people, it may be a sign of a serious medical illness.

Delirium tremens

A disorder involving severe physical and psychological symptoms that can occur when alcohol is withdrawn from a person dependent on it (see ALCOHOL DEPENDENCE); commonly abbreviated to DTs. Individuals who drink the equivalent of 7 or 8 pints of beer, or 1 pint of distilled alcohol (for example, whisky or vodka), every day for several months or who have been alcohol-dependent for more than 10 years are most at risk for DTs.

The disorder usually begins within 72 hours of the last drink, but may not occur for 7 to 10 days. There are physical and psychosocial symptoms. The disorder is a medical emergency. Once the person survives the acute episode, treatment for alcohol dependency can begin.

Delivery, vaginal

The passage of a baby through the vagina, or birth canal, and out of the mother's body. Vaginal delivery is the most common type of birth. When a vaginal delivery is not considered safe or possible, a CESAREAN SECTION, in which the baby is removed through an abdominal incision, is performed.

Delusion

A persistent, unshakable, and false belief that is held despite obvious evidence to the contrary. Delusions can take many forms: persecution (that others are plotting against the individual); grandeur (that a person is a well-known figure); or jealousy (that one's lover or spouse is unfaithful).

Delusions can be caused by the abuse of substances such as crack cocaine, a general medical condition such as Alzheimer's disease or systemic lupus erythematosus, or underlying mental illness. Treatment depends on the underlying cause.

Dementia

A syndrome marked by a progressive loss of memory and other intellectual functions. Although it can occur at any age, dementia is most common in older people. Its early signs may be as subtle as simple forgetfulness and confusion. However, an affected person gradually cannot function normally and eventually becomes incapacitated. Dementia is not a normal consequence of aging. More than half of all cases are caused by Alzheimer's disease and are irreversible. Among the potentially reversible causes of dementia are deficiencies in thyroid hormone and vitamin B_{12}.

Memory impairment, especially for recent events, is the hallmark of dementia. Other cognitive symptoms may include confusion, decreased judgment and understanding, disorientation, impaired speech, an inability to name objects, and difficulty concentrating. Emotional problems may follow. Eventual symptoms may include agitation, anger, frustration, aggression, paranoia, restlessness, and wandering.

As the condition progresses, the person's ability to reason and comprehend is increasingly impaired. Over time, basic functions such as eating, dressing, washing, and using the toilet become more difficult or even impossible.

Dementia results from diseases that damage normal brain cells. Damage to brain cells can occur from a variety of causes such as multiple strokes, ALZHEIMER'S DISEASE, HUNTINGTON CHOREA, PARKINSON DISEASE, Lewy body dementia, and PICK DISEASE. The diagnosis of dementia is based on a complete physical examination, medical history, and test results.

An important part of the diagnosis in a person suspected of having dementia is ruling out other possible causes of a person's symptoms. For instance, depression can cause pseudodementia, a syndrome that resembles dementia.

Most forms of dementia are irreversible. However, if a potentially treatable underlying cause is identified, appropriate management may lessen the symptoms of dementia or in rare instances it may be cured. Some form of daily supervision is necessary to ensure the comfort and safety of a person with dementia, even in its early stages. There is no known cure for Alzheimer's disease, the leading cause of dementia. However, in its early to middle stages, medications can slow the progression of the disease and may lessen some of the cognitive symptoms.

Demyelination

Breakdown of the fatty sheaths that surround and insulate nerve cells. See MULTIPLE SCLEROSIS.

Dendritic ulcer

See HERPES KERATITIS.

Dengue

An acute viral illness that is characterized by high fever and transmitted by the *Aedes aegypti* mosquito, usually found in tropical or subtropical regions and especially in urban areas. People living in or traveling to these areas are at risk of contracting the illness. Dengue, also called dengue fever, has rare, but severe forms that may be fatal.

In addition to a sudden fever, dengue symptoms include chills, severe frontal headache, pain behind the eyes, and muscle and joint aches.

Densitometry

The measurement of bone density using special X-ray techniques. Dual photon absorptiometry (DPA) and DUAL-ENERGY X-RAY ABSORPTIOMETRY (DEXA) are often ordered to measure the density of the vertebrae in the lower back and hip.

Dental dam

A barrier device commonly used in dental procedures that may also be used during oral sexual activity to prevent possible transmission of SEXUALLY TRANSMITTED DISEASES (STDs). The use of a dental dam is recommended by health professionals for use during oral-vaginal sex, oral-penile sex, or oral-anal sex. The use of dental dams has not been clinically tested to prove their effectiveness, but their use is recommended as one component of safer sex.

Dental dams are generally 6-inch squares of latex, although hygienic nonlatex dental dams are also available. Before use, the device must be rinsed to remove the powdery talc coating, then patted dry with a lint-free towel or air dried. Before oral-vaginal sex, the dam is spread over the entire vaginal opening and clitoris. The edges of the dam are held with the hands. Before oral-anal contact, the dam is used to cover the anus. A new dental dam should be used for each oral sexual activity, and only one side of the device should be used before discarding it. A dental dam used in the anal region should not be used for oral-vaginal activity, as organisms from the anus can be harmful to the vagina.

Dental examination

An exploration and analysis of the mouth, teeth, and gums by a dentist. A dental examination may be performed as a routine yearly checkup or to assess a complaint.

During the examination, the dentist looks at the overall condition of the entire mouth, the teeth, the gums, and the supporting structures.

At the first dental examination and at periodic intervals thereafter, dental X rays may be taken to look for conditions that cannot be observed visually, such as the status of wisdom teeth (see WISDOM TEETH), the effects of possible PERIODONTAL DISEASE, and for cavities between teeth and under existing fillings.

Dental hygienist

A dental professional trained to examine, clean, and scale the teeth; take and develop X rays; and offer instruction on proper dental care. The primary responsibility of the dental hygienist is professional cleaning of the teeth.

Dentin

The main tissues located beneath the enamel of the surface of the tooth. Dentin, which is primarily composed of calcium, is less brittle than enamel and softer, which makes it more vulnerable to infection and TOOTH DECAY. When exposed, dentin is very sensitive to touch or pressure, heat, cold, foods that are either sweet or sour, and even airflow.

Dentist

A person who has received specialized training in dentistry and has met the necessary legal qualifications to practice in the field. Dentists are educated at university-affiliated dental colleges and graduate with a DDS degree (doctor of dental surgery) or a DMD degree (doctor of dental medicine). After passing an examination, they are licensed by the state where they practice dentistry.

Dentistry

The medical profession concerned with the health of the teeth, gums, and tissues of the mouth. Dentistry involves preventing, diagnosing, and treating disorders in these structures; dentists are practitioners of this profession.

Dentures

An artificial replacement for missing natural teeth and adjacent tissues in the upper jaw, the lower jaw, or both. Dentures are made of a strong acrylic resin, sometimes in combination with various metals. Partial dentures replace one or several missing permanent teeth (see BRIDGE, DENTAL), and a full denture (false teeth) replaces all the teeth. Saving the permanent teeth may be impossible if a person has serious PERIODONTAL DISEASE or severe TOOTH DECAY, although some teeth can be saved by a ROOT CANAL TREATMENT and dental crown (see CROWN, DENTAL).

Deoxyribonucleic acid

Commonly known as DNA, the fundamental genetic component of all cellular organisms and some viruses. DNA is the material that forms the structure of genes. With the exception of identical twins, each person's DNA is unique. In any one individual, DNA is a component of each cell and is identical in every cell, whether a skin cell, bone cell, or other cell. DNA gives cells their specialized functions.

The DNA molecule is continuous, double-stranded, and shaped like a twisted ladder with the footholds representing nucleotide bases, the substances that form genes. Specific genetic instructions depend on the sequence (code) in which the nucleotide bases appear within a gene. DNA instructions are carried out by RIBONUCLEIC ACID (RNA), a chemical messenger that transports the DNA's orders into the part of the cell where proteins are made.

Depression

An abnormal and persistent mood state characterized by sadness, melancholy, slowed mental processes, and changes in such physical patterns as eating and sleeping. While feelings of being blue or down usually improve on their own after a few days, depression continues.

In very severe cases, depressed people may develop psychotic symptoms, such as hearing voices that tell them to kill themselves. Depression impairs a person's ability to function in family relationships, school, and job roles. In about 5 percent of cases, depression may alternate with periods of high excitement and energy (mania); in this case, the disease is BIPOLAR DISORDER. The most serious complication of depression is suicide.

Depression is a common disorder and usually recurs. In some people, depression becomes chronic. Depression often accompanies other disorders, such as anorexia nervosa, bulimia, obsessive-compulsive disorder, and substance abuse.

The precise cause of depression is unknown. Imbalances in certain brain chemicals (neurotransmitters) appear to be involved. Depression tends to run in families, indicating a genetic component. Stressful life events can also be causes. Older people are at increased risk of depression.

Because depression may lead to suicide, the disorder can be life-threatening. About one in seven people with untreated depression kill themselves.

Depression can be treated effectively in almost all cases. The most common approaches are psychotherapy and antidepressant medication, sometimes used alone or in combination with psychotherapy.

A variety of effective ANTIDEPRESSANTS are available, all of them effective. The choice of medication and the dosage depend upon the person's symptoms and any side effects caused by the particular drug.

Dermabrasion

The removal of the surface layer of the skin by high-speed planing or sanding. Originally, dermabrasion was performed to improve the appearance of scars that resulted from injury or disease. It is now also used to treat acne scars, remove tattoos, and correct sun-related skin damage such as fine wrinkles and age spots.

Dermatitis

Inflammation of the skin; dermatitis is the general term for noninfectious skin rashes. Dermatitis can be due to an allergen or irritant or a genetic predisposition. Symptoms vary from person to person but may include redness, itching, inflammation, blistering, crusting, scabbing, scaling, thickening, and pigment (color) changes.

Diagnosis of dermatitis is based on the appearance of the skin, patch test results, tissue biopsy, and personal and family medical history. Treatment depends on the underlying cause. Doctors may prescribe medications such as corticosteroids and antihistamines. Some cases of dermatitis respond well to PHOTOTHERAPY (treatment with light). It is important to identify and avoid irritants.

Dermatitis, atopic

Inflammation of the skin. This form of DERMATITIS is closely linked with atopy, an inherited predisposition to become hypersensitive or allergic to substances such as pollen, ragweed, dust mites, molds, and animal scales or droppings. It is often associated with other atopic disorders such as hay fever and asthma. Atopic dermatitis affects approximately one in ten infants and young children. Some outgrow it, although their skin usually remains dry and easily irritated throughout life. Environmental influences can bring on the symptoms of dermatitis.

Itching is the primary symptom of dermatitis. Very often there are also cracks behind the ears and rashes on the cheeks, arms, and legs.

There is no single test to diagnose atopic dermatitis. Diagnosis is based on the typical appearance of the rash and a thorough medical history.

Treatment varies according to severity. The regular use of moisturizers on dry, atopic skin is helpful, along with medications such as topical corticosteroid creams, antihistamines for itching, drugs to control any secondary infections, or—in more severe cases—immunosuppressant medications. Many people respond well to PHOTOTHERAPY (treatment with light).

Dermatitis herpetiformis

An intensely itchy skin eruption that is associated with gluten-sensitive enteropathy (a disorder in which the lining of the small intestine is damaged by an allergic reaction to gluten, a protein found in grains such as wheat, rye, and barley). Dermatitis herpetiformis is a chronic skin disease characterized by clusters of papules (small, superficial bumps on the skin) or blisters that occur in a symmetrical pattern on the elbows, knees, buttocks, scalp, and shoulders. Although there are usually no gastrointestinal symptoms, treatment is with a gluten-free diet and medications.

Dermatology

The study of the skin, including its anatomical, physiological, and pathological characteristics. Dermatology encompasses the diagnosis and treatment of skin, hair, and nail disorders. Special concerns include treating and preventing damage to the skin and performing cosmetic procedures to improve the appearance of the skin. A physician who specializes in the skin is called a dermatologist.

Dermatophyte infections

Infections such as JOCK ITCH and ATHLETE'S FOOT caused by moldlike fungi (dermatophytes). See also TINEA.

Dermoid cyst

A cyst that is lined by skin. Dermoid cysts can contain a variety of tissues such as hair, sebaceous (oily) material, sweat glands, and, depending on where they occur in or on the body, even cartilage or bone. Dermoid cysts that occur in the ovary develop from embryo cells that can even grow teeth within the cyst. Dermoid cysts are usually benign (not cancerous). The most common locations for dermoid cysts are the eyebrows, nose, and scalp.

Desensitization, allergy

A therapy that involves repeatedly, and in a controlled manner, exposing a person's body to small amounts of extract from a substance (called an ALLERGEN) that causes allergies in the person, with the goal of eventually building up a tolerance to the allergy and reducing the allergic reaction in that person. More commonly known as allergy shots.

People who receive allergy desensitization usually benefit within 1 to 2 years of treatment, and most continue the therapy at longer intervals for the following 3 to 5 years.

Side effects are uncommon but can be severe. A rare, but extremely severe allergic response to this form of exposure to an allergen is anaphylactic shock, which is characterized by a swelling of body tissues including those in the throat, difficulty breathing, and a sudden fall in blood pressure. Because of this risk, allergy shots should be given only by a physician and a medical staff trained in immunology and the management of potential complications.

Detoxification programs

A medical process, usually in a hospital setting, in which a person addicted to alcohol or drugs is withdrawn from the addictive substance under the care of a physician. Detoxification is not a treatment for the addiction; rather, it is designed to manage the serious, even fatal physiological effects of stopping drug use, such as DELIRIUM TREMENS in alcohol-dependent people.

Developmental delay

The condition in which a child in his or her early years of life has not attained the physical, intellectual, or social development considered normal for his or her age. In the first 5 years of life, children continually change, achieving skills in four areas: movement, language, intellect, and sociabil-

ity. While individual children vary, defined developmental milestones exist within which normal children develop certain skills such as sitting up or walking.

The causes of developmental delay generally are categorized chronologically. Prenatal causes include chromosomal abnormalities or infections, such as rubella, that occur during pregnancy. Perinatal causes refer to problems at birth such as oxygen deprivation. Postnatal causes are infections or injuries that occur after birth.

Often, a developmental delay will be detected at an infant's or a child's regular examination. When a delay is found, the next step is finding its cause. Investigation may involve a neurologist, psychologist, speech pathologist, occupational therapist, or physical therapist. Specific treatments may involve eyeglasses, hearing aids, regular therapy, or enrolling the child in a special school.

Developmental disorder, pervasive

Severe and extensive impairment in social interaction, language skills, and motor skills beginning in childhood. Often some degree of mental retardation accompanies these problems. The exact cause of the disorders is unknown. Often the term pervasive developmental disorder is mistakenly used interchangeably with AUTISM. However, it is a general term referring to autism and several other more rare disorders including RETT SYNDROME and ASPERGER DISORDER. See also DEVELOPMENTAL DELAY.

DEXA

See DUAL-ENERGY X-RAY ABSORPTIOMETRY.

DHEA

Dehydroepiandrosterone. A chemical naturally produced by the adrenal glands. DHEA is related structurally to the hormones ESTROGEN and TESTOSTERONE. After age 30, the body begins to make less DHEA. This has led manufacturers to produce and market DHEA supplements as antiaging remedies. Claims have been made that DHEA supplements increase muscle, decrease fat, and boost immunity, energy, and strength. However, reliable evidence is lacking to support these claims, and liver damage may result from using them even briefly.

Diabetes, insipidus

A disease of the pituitary gland or kidneys characterized by the passage of large amounts of urine. It can be distinguished from diabetes mellitus (see DIABETES MELLITUS, TYPE 1 and DIABETES MELLITUS, TYPE 2) in two ways: it does not involve insulin production, and there is no excessive glucose (sugar) in the urine.

Diabetes insipidus is caused by an insufficient amount of ADH (antidiuretic hormone) or by the resistance of the kidneys to the effects of ADH. Without ADH, a person's urinary output may be ten times greater than the normal urine output.

When diabetes insipidus is due to insufficient ADH, the causes may include pituitary gland surgery, serious head injury that involves the hypothalamus or pituitary gland, or tumors of the pituitary gland or brain. Often the cause of inadequate ADH is not identifiable. When the disease is caused by a failure of the kidneys to respond to ADH in the blood, the underlying cause may be a genetic disorder, inadequate potassium in the blood, excess calcium in the blood, or certain medications.

Diabetes mellitus, type 1

The less common of the two main groups of conditions characterized by an abnormally high glucose (sugar) level in the blood; formerly known as insulin-dependent diabetes or juvenile-onset diabetes. Type 1 diabetes mellitus is due to little or no insulin production by the pancreas. People with type 1 diabetes require insulin injections to live. Type 1 diabetes most often occurs in children and young adults, but it can also develop in people older than 40 years.

Causes and symptoms

The cause of the inability of the pancreas to produce insulin is thought to be an autoimmune disorder. This disorder results when the infection-fighting mechanism in the body, the immune system, begins to destroy the insulin-producing beta cells in the pancreas.

Frequent urination (especially noticeable at night), excessive thirst, and weight loss are the classic symptoms of type 1 diabetes and relate to the elevation in blood sugar and the excess amount of sugar in the urine. The inability of the body to metabolize glucose can result in other symptoms, including fatigue, blurred vision, and slow healing.

Because the person's ability to metabolize glucose is compromised, glucose is unavailable to be used as fuel, so the body breaks down stored fats and proteins. The body converts the broken-down fats into waste products called ketones, which may build up in the blood and be released into the urine. Ketone levels in the blood can increase to produce a life-threatening condition called ketoacidosis. The symptoms of ketoacidosis are abdominal pain, vomiting, rapid breathing, and extreme tiredness or drowsiness. Severe cases of ketoacidosis may cause mental confusion or even coma.

Diagnosis and treatment

Diagnosis is made on the basis of the fasting plasma glucose test, along with the symptoms of frequent urination and frequent thirst. The normal range for a fasting blood glucose level is between 70 and 100 milligrams per deciliter (mg/dL) of blood.

Daily insulin medication is essential for treating type 1 diabetes. Since insulin is destroyed by digestive enzymes and cannot be taken orally, it must be delivered directly into the tissues by insulin injection or by an insulin pump.

In the future, it may be possible to inhale insulin to treat diabetes.

Several different insulin preparations are available with different onset and duration of action. The amount of insulin required is determined by a doctor and is based on a number of factors, including the person's age, height, weight, food intake, and exercise level.

Monitoring the blood glucose level

Once a person has been diagnosed with type 1 diabetes, frequent self-monitoring of the blood glucose level is needed to adjust the insulin dose and maintain a near-normal blood sugar level.

Self-monitoring is best accomplished using a blood glucose meter to provide accurate measurement of blood sugar levels.

A person with type 1 diabetes should also have a test for the percent of glycosylated hemoglobin in the bloodstream (hemoglobin A1c test) every 3 to 6 months. This test measures the amount of glucose attached to hemoglobin A, a protein found in red blood cells. The percentage of glucose attached to hemoglobin depends on the average glucose concentration and is a good measure of diabetic control for the preceding 3 to 4 months.

Risks and complications

The two main acute risks for people with type 1 diabetes are hypoglycemia and hyperglycemia, both of which are caused by an imbalance between insulin and the blood sugar level in the blood. If too much insulin is taken, the sugar in the blood may become depleted, causing hypoglycemia. When there is too little insulin in the blood, the glucose level may become too high, producing hyperglycemia. Each of these conditions carries the potential for serious medical emergencies.

Recent studies show that maintaining tight control of the blood sugar level reduces the risk of diabetic complications, which can include damage to the large blood vessels, leading to an increased risk of heart attack, stroke, and blockage of the blood supply to the legs and feet.

It is important for women with type 1 diabetes who wish to become pregnant to make sure the blood sugar level is kept under tight control before and during pregnancy to reduce the risks of major birth defects. See also HYPEROSMOLAR HYPER-

GLYCEMIC NONKETOTIC SYNDROME, sometimes mistakenly called diabetic coma.

Diabetes mellitus, type 2

The more common of the two main groups of conditions characterized by an abnormally high glucose (sugar) level in the blood; formerly known as non–insulin-dependent diabetes or adult-onset diabetes. Type 2 diabetes, which accounts for 90 to 95 percent of all people with diabetes, is characterized by INSULIN RESISTANCE that causes interference with the ability of the body to metabolize glucose (sugar) for energy, leading to above normal levels of glucose in the blood. Many people with type 2 diabetes do not require daily insulin therapy. Although type 2 diabetes usually begins in adults older than 40 years and is most common in people older than 55 years, it is becoming increasingly common in younger people.

Causes

Most people with type 2 diabetes have insulin resistance, along with an inability of the pancreas to secrete sufficient amounts of insulin to compensate for the insulin resistance. Two possible causes of insulin resistance have been identified. The first involves the receptors with which insulin must bind in order to function. People with type 2 diabetes may not have enough of these receptors or may have defects on the receptors. The second possible cause involves the inability of the cells to properly process insulin's signal to metabolize glucose.

Risk factors for type 2 diabetes include heredity, ethnic background, and increased age. Certain medications—including diuretics used to treat high blood pressure and corticosteroids—can also contribute to an elevated blood sugar level.

Symptoms

Many people with type 2 diabetes do not have any symptoms at first. In time, they may develop symptoms such as recurrent infections, vision difficulties, or neuropathy (nerve damage). Other common complications include fatigue, a general ill feeling, sudden inexplicable weight loss, frequent urination (especially noticeable at night), and excessive thirst. These symptoms are the result of the excess sugar in the blood and the inability of the body to process and use glucose. Inability to concentrate and loss of coordination may also be a problem. Rarely, loss of consciousness or coma from an extremely abnormal blood sugar level occurs.

Diagnosis

Diabetes is diagnosed by measuring the blood glucose level. If the glucose level is 126 milligrams per deciliter (mg/dL) or higher on the results of two fasting plasma glucose tests, a diagnosis of diabetes is confirmed. The diagnosis also can be established if the glucose level is over 200 and the person has classic symptoms such as blurred vision, thirst, or fatigue.

Treatment

The goals are to normalize the blood sugar level, eliminate symptoms, and prevent long-term complications caused by diabetes. In treating type 2 diabetes, diet and weight loss are generally the first approaches to controlling the blood glucose level. Often modest weight loss can significantly improve blood sugar levels.

In addition, people with type 2 diabetes derive many benefits from physical activity. Not only does regular exercise in combination with the proper diet help weight reduction efforts by burning extra calories, but it can also improve the way the body responds to insulin.

Medications for people with type 2 diabetes are used in combination with diet and exercise when those elements of treatment alone are not sufficient to control the diabetes. People with type 2 diabetes who still produce some insulin may be treated with sulfonylureas. These agents are oral hypoglycemics and work by stimulating the pancreas to produce more insulin. The chemical names for the sulfonylureas include glyburide, glipizide, glimepiride, and chlorpropamide.

Nonsulfonylurea agents are another group of medications used to treat diabetes. These are the insulin-sensitizing agents such as metformin.

Another class of agents, the glucosidase inhibitors, such as acarbose, work by inhibiting the breakdown of sugars by intestinal enzymes. As a result, they slow digestion and absorption of sugar, making these medications most useful for people experiencing marked elevations in the blood sugar level after eating.

Oral medications cannot control the blood sugar level in all people with type 2 diabetes, even when people diet and exercise; some may require insulin. In other people, over time, oral medications lose their effectiveness and insulin may be needed. Insulin doses are keyed to the person's blood sugar levels. See the above entry, DIABETES MELLITUS, TYPE 1, for information on monitoring blood sugar levels.

Risks and complications

Hypoglycemia (low blood sugar) may be experienced when the effects of insulin or oral medicine are intensified by insufficient food intake, excessive activity, stress, illness, or drinking alcoholic beverages.

It is important that type 2 diabetes be diagnosed and treated as early as possible because it can cause severe health problems over time, in some cases before a person realizes that he or she has the disorder. Specifically, the heart, blood vessels, eyes, kidneys, and nerves are at risk from conditions produced by type 2 diabetes. See also HYPEROSMOLAR HYPERGLYCEMIC NONKETOTIC SYNDROME, often mistakenly called diabetic coma.

Diabetes, gestational

A condition of INSULIN RESISTANCE in pregnant women in which the effects of the hormone insulin, which is produced by the pancreas, are partially blocked by other hormones produced by the placenta. These hormones—including estrogen, cortisol, and human placental lactogen—are essential for a healthy pregnancy. However, they induce a resistance to insulin, resulting in an increase in the insulin requirement. If the pancreas is incapable of making enough insulin to meet the increased requirement during pregnancy, gestational diabetes develops. Most cases of gestational diabetes develop during the latter half of pregnancy and resolve after childbirth, when the placenta is delivered and the hormone elevations associated with pregnancy drop.

There are several complications of gestational diabetes, but most can be prevented by early diagnosis of the condition and keeping the blood sugar level as near normal as possible for the remainder of the pregnancy through diet, exercise, and possibly insulin injections. A pregnant woman can monitor her own blood sugar level by using a glucose meter at home.

Complications associated with gestational diabetes can affect both the baby and the mother. Complications that impact the baby include: an excessively large fetus, which may preclude a normal vaginal delivery and necessitate a CESAREAN SECTION; and hypoglycemia (low blood sugar) in the baby immediately after delivery if the mother's increased blood sugar level raised the fetus's insulin level.

Gestational diabetes may increase the chances of the pregnant woman's developing PREECLAMPSIA, a complication characterized by high blood pressure, protein in the urine, and swelling of the face and extremities.

Diabetes, insulin-dependent

See DIABETES MELLITUS, TYPE 1.

Diabetes, non–insulin-dependent

See DIABETES MELLITUS, TYPE 2.

Diabetic retinopathy

See RETINOPATHY, DIABETIC.

Diagnosis

The act or process of determining a disease process by history, physical examination, and often laboratory testing (such as blood studies, urinalysis, and imaging studies). For some diseases (such as breast cancer or colon cancer), early diagnosis can make the difference between cure and serious illness or death.

Diagnostic imaging

Techniques that allow internal areas of the body to be visualized through X rays, magnetic fields (MRI scanning), and radio-frequency waves and sound waves (ultrasound) to produce pictures of the structures and tissues of the body.

Dialysis

A medical therapy for eliminating toxic waste products that accumulate in the bloodstream because of inadequately functioning kidneys. Dialysis uses a membrane that permits different substances to diffuse or pass through at different rates, filtering and purifying the blood. Dialysis is necessary in cases of KIDNEY FAILURE. It is also used to remove drugs from the body after a poison is ingested or after a drug overdose.

There are two types of dialysis, HEMODIALYSIS and PERITONEAL DIALYSIS.

Dialysis machine

Also known as an artificial kidney, dialyzer, or hemodialyzer; a machine used for DIALYSIS that takes over the function of the kidneys when they are unable to filter toxic waste products from the blood.

Diaphragm muscle

The large sheet of muscle that divides the chest (thorax) from the abdomen

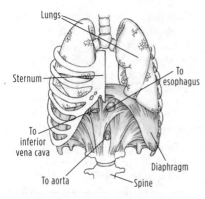

Muscular sheet

The diaphragm arches over the abdominal cavity, forming the powerful, muscular floor of the chest cavity. Three openings in the diaphragm provide passage for the esophagus, the aorta, the inferior vena cava (vein from the abdomen and lower limbs to the heart), and several nerves.

and provides most of the power that moves air in and out of the lungs. The diaphragm is attached to the spine, ribs, and sternum, forming the floor of the chest cavity.

Diaphragm, contraceptive

A birth control device that fits over a woman's cervix and keeps sperm from entering. See CONTRACEPTION, BARRIER METHODS.

Diarrhea

For symptom chart see DIARRHEA, page xviii.

Abnormal increase in the frequency, fluidity, and volume of bowel movements. More than three soft, loose, or watery bowel movements in a day constitute diarrhea. In a healthy adult, most cases of diarrhea last from 24 to 48 hours and are not serious. Diarrhea can be more dangerous to infants and older people because of an increased risk of dehydration, upsetting body chemistry and depleting important body salts. Left untreated, it can lead to shock. Persistent or severe diarrhea requires medical attention.

Most frequently, acute diarrhea is due to a viral infection or a change in diet. Other causes include food poisoning, GASTROENTERITIS, CELIAC DISEASE, LACTOSE INTOLERANCE, MALABSORPTION, DIVERTICULAR DISEASE, INFLAMMATORY BOWEL DISEASE, IRRITABLE BOWEL SYNDROME, anxiety, overconsumption of alcohol, and reaction to medications. See also DIARRHEA, E. COLI; DIARRHEA, TRAVELER'S.

For treatment, doctors advise resting and drinking clear fluids until diarrhea subsides. Because watery diarrhea can rapidly cause a loss of body fluids and crucial body salts, oral rehydration fluid may be needed. Other over-the-counter medications may relieve symptoms. In severe cases, the doctor may prescribe drugs that slow intestinal activity and ease cramping, or the person may need intravenous fluids.

Diarrhea, E. coli

Escherichia coli (E. coli) diarrhea, frequent, liquid bowel movements caused by *E. coli* bacteria, which normally inhabit the digestive tract of humans without harm. However, a strain of *E. coli* (enterohemorrhagic) that is most commonly associated with contaminated hamburger meat causes bloody diarrhea and sometimes death. Another type of *E. coli* bacteria is responsible for many cases of traveler's diarrhea (see DIARRHEA, TRAVELER'S).

Symptoms generally last for a week, followed by spontaneous recovery.

However, a life-threatening complication called HEMOLYTIC-UREMIC SYNDROME (HUS) occurs in about one in ten cases. This syndrome, which affects primarily very young children and older people, can lead to KIDNEY FAILURE.

Dehydration due to *E. coli* diarrhea is treated with oral rehydration fluid that is available over-the-counter at pharmacies. In severe cases, intravenous fluids are required. Medications to slow diarrhea should not be used in cases of bloody diarrhea.

Diarrhea, traveler's

Diarrhea caused by ingesting contaminated water or food while traveling in areas with poor sanitation. Abdominal cramps, fever, dehydration, nausea, and vomiting may also occur. In many cases, over-the-counter medications control diarrhea. DEHYDRATION can be treated by drinking adequate clear liquids.

Persistent diarrhea may require testing to determine its cause. If a bacterial infection or parasite is the cause, the doctor will prescribe medication. (See also DYSENTERY; AMEBIC DYSENTERY.) To prevent diarrhea, doctors recommend that travelers use bottled water, avoid fresh fruits, and eat only thoroughly cooked foods.

Diastolic blood pressure

A measurement of the force exerted by the blood against the walls of the arteries when the heart relaxes between beats. The first measurement is called systolic blood pressure and is the top number or first number in a reading. Diastolic blood pressure is the second measurement (or bottom number) given in a blood pressure reading. See BLOOD PRESSURE.

Diathermy

Producing heat in a part of the body with a high-frequency electrical current, ultrasonic wave, or microwave radiation to relieve pain in joints and muscles, to coagulate bleeding vessels, or to separate tissues without causing bleeding.

Diet, balanced

A diet that consists of adequate amounts of the seven essential substances: proteins, carbohydrates, fats, fiber, vitamins, minerals, and water in appropriate proportions. See FOOD GUIDE PYRAMID.

Dietary assessment

The evaluation of an individual's diet to identify which nutrients are being supplied or neglected in the diet, related behaviors, and habits associated with disease. Dietary assessment is usually conducted by a registered dietician (RD).

Dietary reference intakes

Current standards for the components of a healthy diet in the United States and Canada. The National Academies of Science released new dietary reference intakes (DRIs) in 1997 to update food allowances originally set in 1941.

Dietetics

The study of the kinds and quantities of foods needed to maintain health and manage diseases.

Dietician, registered

A food and nutrition expert who has completed the academic and practice requirements established by the Commission on Dietetic Registration, the credentialing agency of the American Dietetic Association.

Digestive system

The organs that take food into the body, break it down into chemical components, extract nutrients to provide energy for the body's cells, and rid the body of the waste products. Also known as the gastrointestinal system, the digestive system can be considered to be a long tube stretching the full length of the body from the mouth to the anus; related organs such as the LIVER, GALLBLADDER, and PANCREAS, assist in the digestive process along the way.

Digital subtraction angiography

An X-ray procedure used to visualize blood vessels (both arteries and veins) through a series of computer images after they have been injected with a CONTRAST MEDIUM.

Dilation

Enlarging or expanding of something. Dilation takes place when a hollow organ or body cavity stretches or gets bigger.

Dilation and curettage

See D AND C.

Dilation and evacuation

See D AND E.

Dilator

An instrument used to enlarge an opening.

Diphtheria

An acute, contagious, bacterial illness that may affect the respiratory system or the skin. Symptoms of respiratory diphtheria include a characteristic fibrous membrane that forms on the tonsils, in the throat, and in the nose. The condition is spread by direct physical contact or by direct or indirect contact with respiratory secretions of an infected person. Respiratory diphtheria is potentially fatal and carries the risk of complications, including inflammation of the heart muscle.

Symptoms of cutaneous diphtheria include open wounds on the skin that become infected with the diphtheria bacteria; it is spread by contact with an infected person's open sores. Serious complications and death occur much less frequently in the cutaneous form of diphtheria than with respiratory diphtheria.

A vaccine has made respiratory diphtheria rare in the United States, although the illness may be carried without symptoms even in areas where most of the population has been immunized. Active immunization against diphtheria is offered by diphtheria-tetanus-pertussis (DTaP) vaccines, which are routinely given to all children, with boosters available to adults.

People with symptoms of respiratory diphtheria are generally hospitalized in intensive care units. Diphtheria antitoxin medication neutralizes the toxin produced by the bacteria, but only if it is not yet bound to cells. For this reason, this medication must be administered as soon as the illness is clinically diagnosed, without waiting for a laboratory confirmation. The dosage may be given intravenously.

Treatment of cutaneous diphtheria is generally based on regular, thorough cleaning of skin lesions with soap and water and prescribed medication for a 10-day period.

Diplopia

See DOUBLE VISION.

Disability

A physical or emotional condition that impairs the ability to function. Degrees of disability are highly variable.

Disinfectants

Agents that destroy disease-carrying microorganisms. Disinfectants include heat, radiation, and chemicals, which may destroy, neutralize, or inhibit the growth of microorganisms.

Disk prolapse

See SLIPPED DISK.

Disk, intervertebral

The flat, circular structure firmly embedded between the vertebrae (bones of the spine) to serve as a shock absorber for the spine by separating the vertebrae and keeping the bony struc-

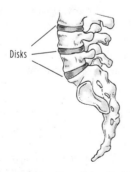

Disks

Shock absorbers

The intervertebral disks act as cushions between the vertebrae. Each disk has a central core of gel, encased in a fibrous capsule. Ligaments running the length of the spine hold the disks in place.

tures from rubbing together when a person moves and bends. The characteristics of intervertebral disks change with advancing age.

Dislocation, joint

An irregularity in the close positioning of the two parts of a joint that prevents the joint from functioning normally. The most common large joint dislocation occurs in the shoulder, but joint dislocations may also occur in the shoulder, hip or spinal vertebrae. Symptoms of a joint dislocation include a misshapen appearance, pain, swelling, discoloration, and an inability to move the joint. A joint that is dislocated because of trauma is a serious injury and should be treated immediately. After giving the person a muscle relaxant, the doctor will gently rotate the dislocated joint back into place. In some cases, traction or surgery may be needed.

Dissociative disorders

A group of related abnormal emotional conditions in which an individual becomes detached from fundamental aspects of waking consciousness, such as personal identity, memory, or awareness of self and body. Dissociative disorders are thought to originate in overwhelming traumatic experiences, such as combat, physical or sexual assault, or severe accidents. Unable to integrate the trauma into his or her normal consciousness, the person detaches from the disturbing experience as a way of coping with it.

Since dissociative disorders usually arise from a traumatic experience, treatment typically consists of psychotherapy focused on that experience.

Distal

In anatomy, the portion of a body part located farther away from the point of origin or attachment. The elbow, for example, is distal to the shoulder, and the distal end of the thigh bone is part of the knee joint. The opposite of distal is proximal.

Diuretics

Drugs that cause the body to excrete water and salt. They are considered useful to treat HYPERTENSION (high blood pressure), especially among older people. Diuretics can significantly reduce the risk of stroke and, to a lesser degree, heart attacks caused by high blood pressure. Diuretics are also used in diseases such as congestive heart failure, in which the person retains excess fluids.

There are three primary types of diuretics: thiazides, which are commonly used to treat high blood pressure (hypertension); loop diuretics, which work on the region of the kidneys called the loop of Henle and increase the excretion of water, sodium, potassium, calcium, and magnesium by decreasing the concentration and dilution of urine; and potassium-sparing agents, which are mild diuretics, too. But the potassium-sparing effects make them useful in offsetting the effects of thiazides and loop-sparing diuretics.

Diverticular disease

The presence of small sacs or pouches (diverticula) in the walls of the lower end of the colon. Diverticular disease includes both diverticulosis and diverticulitis.

Diverticulosis refers to the presence of diverticula in the digestive tract, is very common, and often produces no symptoms. About one in five people with diverticulosis has abdominal pain, bloating, gas, constipation, or diarrhea. Left untreated, diverticulosis can lead to serious complications, such as an abscess.

Diverticulitis is the inflammation or infection of one or more diverticula. Inflammation leads to muscle spasm, severe abdominal pain, nausea, and fever. The cramps and tenderness associated with diverticulosis usually occur on the left side of the abdomen. If diverticula bleed, typically bright red blood appears in the stools. Possible complications of diverticulitis include the development of a stricture, narrowing of the intestine (see INTESTINE, OBSTRUCTION OF); a fistula, an abnormal channel that forms between parts of the intestine; an abscess, a pus-filled sac around the diverticulum; and PERITONITIS.

Diverticular disease is diagnosed by a complete physical examination and tests.

In many cases, diverticulosis responds well to the adoption of a high-fiber diet. In diverticulitis, doctors often prescribe antibiotics, as well as antispasmodic drugs, to control abdominal pain. An attack of diverticulitis may require hospitalization.

Diving medicine

A specialized form of medicine that treats DECOMPRESSION SICKNESS, based on hyperbaric oxygen therapy (HBO). During this therapy, scuba divers who have been affected by unreleased excess nitrogen in the bloodstream enter special hyperbaric chambers and are fitted with oxygen masks. By combining increased air pressure with the inhalation of 100 percent oxygen, HBO allows the body to release the extra nitrogen at a healthful pace.

Dizziness

For symptom chart see DIZZINESS, page xx.

A feeling of faintness or an inability to maintain normal balance while sitting or standing. Dizziness is a common symptom that almost everyone experiences at some time. Most often dizziness is not a serious problem and goes away on its own; however, medical attention is required when dizziness is accompanied by a complete loss of consciousness, when other symptoms are present (such as tingling or chest pain), when the cause appears to be medication-induced, or when light-headedness persists for 3 weeks or longer. If medical examination reveals possible neurological or heart problems, further testing probably will be done.

DNA

See DEOXYRIBONUCLEIC ACID.

Do-not-resuscitate order

A type of advance directive, commonly known as a DNR, made by an individual or the person's physician, stating exactly under which circumstances the person should or should not be resuscitated (see ADVANCE DIRECTIVES).

Donor

A person who leaves instructions for his or her body or organs to be donated for medical use after death. To do this, a person fills out a Uniform Donor Card and has it signed by two witnesses.

Dopamine

A NEUROTRANSMITTER in the brain that is involved in the control of movement. A depletion of dopamine produces symptoms of PARKINSON DISEASE, such as rigidity, tremors, and reduced movement.

Doppler ultrasound

An ULTRASOUND SCANNING technique that produces images of structures inside the body and can provide information about blood flow rate at the same time. Doppler ultrasound creates an image of the area being scanned by processing the echoes produced by harmless, high-frequency sound waves as they strike moving material, such as blood moving through the blood vessels.

Dorsal

In anatomy, on or of the back of the body or an organ. Dorsal describes a position situated on or related to the back surface of the body or a body organ. The opposite of dorsal is VENTRAL.

Dose

The quantity of a therapeutic agent to be taken at one time. Dose may refer to the quantity of a drug or amount of radiation.

Double vision

Seeing two images of a single object. Also known as diplopia, double vision is caused either by a defect in a single eye or by misalignment of both eyes. There are two types of double vision: monocular (single-eye) double vision, in which the person continues to see two images through one eye even if the other eye is covered, and binocular double vision, in which covering one eye stops the diplopia.

Treatment of double vision depends on the cause. Astigmatism or keratoconus is usually remedied with corrective glasses or contact lenses. Abnormal growth of the conjunctiva is repaired surgically, as are dislocated lenses, cataracts, and some problems of the retina. Eyelid swelling may be treated with medicine or surgery, depending on the underlying condition. Strabismus is usually repaired surgically during childhood. Conditions such as myasthenia gravis, Graves disease, and stroke are treated with medication. Microvascular infarctions, which are commonly seen in people with diabetes, often resolve on their own as the nerve regenerates, in which case double vision gradually clears up.

Douche

Cleansing the vagina by flushing it with water or chemicals. Douching is almost never recommended and is not an effective method of birth control.

Down syndrome

A chromosomal abnormality that results in mental retardation and other complications. Down syndrome results from an extra copy of chromosome 21 and is also known as trisomy 21. Pregnant women aged 35 or older have a significantly increased risk of having a baby with Down syndrome.

Children with Down syndrome have a characteristic appearance, often have heart defects, are also more at risk for gastrointestinal abnormalities, and have a much higher than average risk of developing childhood leukemia. They are also at

risk for developing epilepsy, hypothyroidism, and vision or hearing defects. The normal life span of people with Down syndrome is shortened.

The diagnosis is usually suspected after a physical examination and confirmed with blood chromosome analysis. A chest X ray or echocardiogram can detect heart defects, and a gastrointestinal X ray can be used to find intestinal blockages. Down syndrome can be detected in a fetus in early pregnancy through AMNIOCENTESIS or CHORIONIC VILLUS SAMPLING.

There is no specific treatment for Down syndrome. Heart defects or intestinal blockages may require surgery. Special education and training and occupational and physical therapy are available in many communities for mentally retarded children.

DRIs

See DIETARY REFERENCE INTAKES.

Drop attack

A type of SEIZURE that causes a sudden fall. This type of seizure may occur in a severe form of EPILEPSY called Lennox-Gastaut syndrome.

Drowning

Suffocation or near-suffocation from submersion in water or other liquid. The immediate cause of drowning is a lack of oxygen. Symptoms of near-drowning include swollen abdomen; bluish skin on the lips and ears; cold, pale skin; confusion; cough with pink, frothy sputum; fever; failure to breathe; shallow or gasping breathing; and unconsciousness.

In a near-drowning emergency, quick action and first aid can prevent death. Once rescued, ARTIFICIAL RES-PIRATION (or rescue breathing) must be started immediately if the person is not breathing, even if this involves performing this maneuver in the water. It is wise to perform the HEIM-LICH MANEUVER first to clear the airways of water. If the person cannot be aroused or is not breathing or moving, CARDIOPULMONARY RESUS-CITATION (CPR) should be started. As soon as possible, the person must be checked by a doctor.

Drowning, dry

A form of DROWNING in which no fluid enters the lungs. In dry drowning, even though water does not enter the lungs, there is a fatal lack of oxygen. This may be due to a person's strong laryngeal reflex, which diverts water from the lungs to the stomach, but impairs breathing nevertheless.

Drowsiness

A decreased level of consciousness characterized by sleepiness and trouble remaining alert. Abnormal drowsiness may be a sign of a head injury, high fever, HYPOGLYCEMIA (low blood sugar level), HYPERGLYCEMIA (high blood sugar level), MENINGITIS (inflammation of the membranes, or meninges, that surround the brain and spinal cord), or liver failure.

Drug

In medicine, a drug is a compound used to treat disease, injury, or pain. A drug may also be any substance intended for use as a component of a medication. A drug can cause addiction or a change in consciousness. Alcohol and tobacco are legal drugs that are widely abused.

Drug abuse

The use of illegal drugs or the use of a legal drug in excessive quantities or for purposes other than those for which it is normally intended.

Drug abuse may lead to drug dependence (see DRUG ADDICTION), which involves a compulsive craving for the drug, tolerance for its effects, and unpleasant or even dangerous symptoms if the drug is withdrawn. Treatment depends on the drug being used and the level of abuse.

Drug addiction

A disorder involving physical and psychological dependence on a drug or drugs and characterized by tolerance (the need to consume larger and larger amounts of the drug to feel its effects), physical symptoms if the drug is withdrawn, or both. Drug addiction poses serious health risks because of its long-term physical effects, disruption of family and work life, and the symptoms of drug withdrawal, which can range from highly unpleasant to fatal.

Drug addiction can be treated with a variety of medical, behavioral, and supportive therapies. Most programs begin with detoxification, a 4- to 7-day medical process, usually in a hospital setting, in which a person addicted to drugs is withdrawn from the addictive substance under the care of a doctor.

Drug eruption

A skin reaction that is caused by taking a medication. Drug eruptions are caused by a sensitivity or allergy (see ALLERGIES) to some medications. Symptoms range from a mild rash to life-threatening ANAPHY-

LAXIS. Penicillin and related drugs are the most common causes of allergic reactions. Iodine-based drugs used as contrast mediums for X rays also cause reactions in some people.

Treatments to control rashes include corticosteroids and antihistamines. In the case of severe rashes, an underlying infection may need to be controlled.

Drug sensitivity

An individual's response to a drug, or an antibiotic's effectiveness against a microorganism.

Drug treatment programs

A process involving medical, psychological, behavioral, therapeutic, and other interventions designed to help a person abstain from alcohol or drugs and function normally in society. A variety of treatment programs are available.

Types of programs include:

- *OUTPATIENT OR DAY-TREATMENT CENTERS*, which allow the person to live at home and continue with work or school while undergoing a structured program;
- *RESIDENTIAL PROGRAMS*, which offer an intensive, live-in approach based on a modified 12-step approach (see TWELVE-STEP PROGRAM);
- *THERAPEUTIC COMMUNITIES (TCS)*, which are full-time, residential, drug-free programs that use peer support, counseling, and work to help people learn how to live without substances;
- *HALFWAY HOUSES*, which rely on peer-group counseling within a residential setting while residents

make the transition to individual living in the community; and

- *MEDICATION MAINTENANCE PROGRAMS*, which serve people addicted to narcotics, such as heroin.

Drug trial

See CLINICAL TRIAL.

Drunk driving

Using a car or other motor vehicle while impaired by alcohol and not capable of handling the vehicle safely. Most states also apply drunk driving laws to operation of a motor vehicle under the influence of illegal or abused drugs used alone or in combination with alcohol. In the United States, a driver with a blood alcohol concentration (BAC) of 0.08 percent or more is considered to have committed a drunk driving offense. As many as half of all traffic deaths in the United States involve alcohol.

Dry eye

Persistent failure of the tear glands to produce moisture of sufficient quantity or quality to wet and lubricate the eye normally.

Dry eye can result from exposure to extremely dry climates. It may also be caused by certain medications. Dry eye becomes more common with age and to some degree is estimated to affect three of four people older than 65 years. Particularly when accompanied by dry mouth, dry eye may be a symptom of systemic disease, such as RHEUMATOID ARTHRITIS, systemic lupus erythematosus, and SJÖGREN SYNDROME, all of which affect the body's lubricating glands.

Primary treatment consists of artificial tears, which usually contain methylcellulose and are available over-the-counter as eye drops. Sterile ointments may be used at night to prevent drying during sleep.

Dry mouth

A symptom of certain diseases or a side effect of some medications that interfere with the ability of the salivary glands to function properly. The medical term is xerostomia. While dry mouth is a symptom rather than a disease, it can present significant health problems. It may contribute to poor nutrition, tooth decay, and other infections of the mouth. People who experience dry mouth should seek attention from a physician, a dentist, or both.

Dry mouth may be due to any number of medications, diseases, treatments, or other causes. More than 400 different medications may cause dry mouth. Cancer treatments may also play a part.

In addition to recommendations from a doctor or dentist who is treating a person for dry mouth, some self-help treatments may help the symptoms. Most important is drinking fluids frequently and avoiding caffeinated beverages and tobacco.

DSA

See DIGITAL SUBTRACTION ANGIOGRAPHY.

DTaP vaccination

A vaccine typically given at regular intervals during infancy and childhood that offers immunization against diphtheria, tetanus, and pertussis, which is also called whooping cough.

An infant is generally given an initial DTaP vaccination at the age of 2 months. The injections are repeated at the ages of 4 months and 6 months, in the period between 12 and 18 months, and again when the child is 4 years old. A booster vaccination against diphtheria and tetanus is given at age 14 and every 10 years thereafter into adulthood.

Potential adverse reactions have been primarily associated with the pertussis part of the vaccine, and the DTaP vaccination is much less likely to cause any side effects than the older vaccine for pertussis. Although serious side effects are less common, there may be pain, swelling, and redness at the site of the injection, as well as a fever, drowsiness, vomiting, and fussiness in infants.

Dual-energy X-ray absorptiometry

The most complete and accurate imaging technique for measuring bone density. DEXA is a painless procedure that uses very small amounts of radiation and takes only about 15 minutes. It is commonly used to detect a case of OSTEOPOROSIS that is mild or asymptomatic or to assess the bones after a bone fracture has occurred. DEXA also offers physicians a baseline for treatment and is used during ongoing medical care to assess the response to treatment for osteoporosis. See also BONE DENSITY TESTING.

Duct

In anatomy, a tube or other walled passage in an organ of the body. A duct is typically a narrow tubular passage through which fluid passes, such as those found in the gallbladder or glands.

Duodenal ulcer

A sore or wound in the mucous membrane lining the wall of the duodenum, the first part of the small intestine into which the contents of the stomach are emptied.

Upper abdominal pain is the most common symptom of a duodenal ulcer. Other symptoms may include a burning, gnawing pain between the shoulder blades, nausea, vomiting, loss of appetite, and weight loss.

Evidence strongly suggests that infection with the bacterium HELICOBACTER PYLORI is responsible for the majority of ulcers. Other factors that may play a role are the long-term use of nonsteroidal anti-inflammatory drugs (NSAIDs), such as aspirin and ibuprofen, heavy use of alcohol, and smoking.

Diagnosis is usually made after taking a medical history of symptoms and conducting a variety of tests. Pain and nausea are typically eased by food, milk, antacids, or vomiting.

Medications play a vital role in the treatment of duodenal ulcers. Many doctors prescribe drugs that reduce acid secretion, including histamine blockers, anticholinergic agents, and PROTON PUMP INHIBITORS. There are also drugs that coat the lining of the duodenum and stomach with a protective layer that prevents acid from reaching the ulcer. In addition to reducing acid secretion, eradicating an H. pylori infection cures the ulcer; however, no single medication has proven effective against H. pylori. But a medical regimen called triple therapy (the use of three medications at once) can eradicate about 90 percent of cases of the bacteria; in triple therapy, two medications are antibiotics and the third is usually a proton pump inhibitor.

Possible complications of duodenal ulcers include bleeding, scarring, and pyloric stenosis. There is also a small risk that ulcers will penetrate or perforate the duodenal wall. When a duodenal ulcer fails to respond to treatment or if complications develop, surgery may occasionally become necessary.

Duodenitis

Inflammation of the duodenum (the first part of the small intestine into which the stomach empties). In some cases, duodenitis has no symptoms. Sometimes, there may be discomfort in the upper abdomen, indigestion, nausea, or vomiting.

Duodenitis sometimes is accompanied by GASTRITIS (inflammation of the stomach lining). Infection with HELICOBACTER PYLORI, a bacterium, may play a role in duodenitis, or it can be a side effect of treatment with nonsteroidal anti-inflammatory drugs (NSAIDs).

Duodenitis is most commonly diagnosed by endoscopy, in which a lighted tube is inserted down the esophagus and through the stomach to the duodenum, so the tissue may be directly observed by the doctor.

As with duodenal ulcers, antacids, histamine-2 blockers, and proton pump inhibitors may offer relief of duodenitis. If the duodenitis has been caused by H. pylori, a medical regimen called triple therapy (the use of three medications at once) can eradicate most cases. See DUODENAL ULCER.

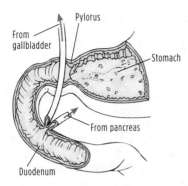

First part of the small intestine

Partially digested food from the stomach empties into the duodenum, the first of the three parts of the small intestine (followed by the jejunum and the ileum).

Duodenum

The first part of the small INTESTINE; the duodenum extends below the stomach, curving around the pancreas before it empties into the jejunum (the second part of the small intestine).

Dupuytren contracture

A disease that produces a rigid deformity of the hand, or hands, most commonly involving the inward bending of the ring finger and little finger, but sometimes progressing to involve all the fingers. Dupuytren contracture is painless and may progress slowly. The cause is unknown but the disease may be associated with alcoholism, liver disease, epilepsy, or diabetes mellitus. Treatment may include surgery.

Durable power of attorney

A legal document signed by a mentally competent adult, delegating decision-making responsibilities for his or her health care or property to another person or agent. It includes a statement specifying that the agent can continue to make decisions when the individual becomes incapacitated (see ADVANCE DIRECTIVES).

Dust diseases

Lung diseases caused by exposure to dust. Dust diseases are caused by industrial and mining dusts that are made up of particles small enough to be inhaled into the lungs and become embedded in lung tissue. These dusts may have varying effects on the body that range from minor to severe injury and in some cases can cause death.

Dust diseases are named for the type of dust that causes them. Examples include SILICOSIS; ASBESTOSIS; Berylliosis, which occurs when beryllium dust is inhaled; BAGASSOSIS; FARMER'S LUNG; siderosis, which may be caused by iron oxide dust; stannosis, which is caused by breathing dust from tin oxide; and byssinosis.

The course of a dust disease may be unpredictable. There may be no symptoms in the early stages of a dust disease, or symptoms may appear soon after onset. The first sign tends to be shortness of breath (see BREATH, SHORTNESS OF). An affected person may then develop a cough.

Dust diseases often weaken resistance to other diseases and make the affected person more susceptible to tuberculosis, lung cancer, pneumonia, chronic bronchitis, and emphysema.

The most effective treatment for dust disease is preventing further dust exposure. In some cases, it may be essential for a person to seek alternative employment; in other cases, wearing a protective face mask while working may be sufficient.

Dust mites

Tiny insects that are related to spiders and ticks and can cause allergic reactions in sensitized people who inhale their microscopic body parts or fecal matter. Dust mites, which live on fabrics such as mattress bedding, upholstered furniture, stuffed animals, and carpeting that collect dust, may produce mild symptoms of allergic rhinitis or bring on bronchial ASTHMA attacks.

The most effective approach to reducing allergic reactions to dust mites is to remove or limit the use of carpeting, especially wall-to-wall carpeting, and upholstered furniture. A home dehumidifier or air conditioner in warm, damp climates may help reduce humid indoor conditions in which dust mites thrive. Dust mites grow poorly when the humidity is below 50 percent. If an air conditioner is used, the filter should be regularly cleaned.

It is important to control dust mites in the bedroom, the area of the house which usually has the highest concentration of dust mites and is also the room where people spend most of their time. Reducing exposure involves regularly washing all bedding in hot water every week to 10 days and cleaning or dusting walls, ceilings, closets, and all furniture surfaces weekly.

DXA

See DUAL-ENERGY X-RAY ABSORPTIOMETRY.

Dying, care of the

See END-OF-LIFE CARE.

Dysarthria

Difficult to understand, poorly articulated speech. A person with dysarthria has trouble speaking because of damage to the muscular systems required for normal speech from stroke, degenerative neurological disorders, alcohol abuse, and poorly fitted dentures. Causes of dysarthria can be diagnosed through a physical examination and tests. Treatment may involve referral to a speech pathologist.

Dysentery

An intestinal infection characterized by bloody diarrhea and abdominal cramps and most common in developing countries with poor sanitation. There may also be fever, dehydration, and excess mucus secretions from the anus. Dysentery is caused by ingesting food or water contaminated with either bacteria or amebae. Diagnosis is made through analysis of a stool sample and blood tests.

Treatment of bacterial dysentery, usually caused by infection with the *Shigella* bacillus or the *Campylobacter* bacterium, is with antibiotics. Treatment of amebic dysentery is with antiamebic drugs. In most individuals, oral fluids can maintain hydration. However, if dehydration is severe, intravenous fluids are needed.

Dysequilibrium

A type of DIZZINESS. In dysequilibrium, a person experiences balance problems when walking or standing (and not when sitting or lying down). This condition most often affects older people and is usually associated with other medical problems, such as a prior STROKE, PARKINSON DISEASE, peripheral neuropathies, severe arthritis of the knee or hip, or visual changes (for example, those following cataract surgery). Diagnosis is usually made through medical history and physical examination. Treatment of dysequilibrium involves correction or care of any underlying medical problems, if possible. Not all causes of disequilibrium are treatable. In such instances, physical therapy is often helpful for maintaining balance and muscle strength. See also OSTEOARTHRITIS.

Dyskinesia

An abnormal, involuntary movement such as twitching, nodding, or jerking. Dyskinesias range from mild to severe and from slow to rapid. These movements may develop as a side effect of a drug, or they may be caused by a brain disorder.

Dyslexia

One of the LEARNING DISABILITIES characterized by difficulty with written symbols. Dyslexia is not necessarily linked with low intelligence.

Although its exact cause remains unknown, dyslexia may have educational, psychological, and biological components. There is some evidence that dyslexia tends to run in families.

Dyslexic children often have trouble with the mastery of early reading skills. In fact, the one trait shared by all dyslexic children is that they read at levels significantly lower than what is typical for their age and intelligence. Other common symptoms of dyslexia include problems with identifying single words, trouble understanding sounds, delayed spoken language, spelling problems, a tendency to transpose letters in words, confusion with directions and distinctions (such as right and left), and problems with mathematics.

Early evaluation and treatment of dyslexia are best; otherwise, a child can quickly fall behind in school. Children suspected of having dyslexia must be tested by trained educational experts.

Dysmenorrhea

A condition in which a woman experiences painful menstruation. See MENSTRUATION, DISORDERS OF.

Dyspareunia

A condition in which a woman experiences painful sexual intercourse. See INTERCOURSE, PAINFUL.

Dysphagia

See SWALLOWING DIFFICULTY.

Dysphasia

Impairment of the ability to speak or sometimes to understand language. Dysphasia is the result of brain injury. Aphasia is the absence of the ability to speak or understand language but is often used interchangeably with dysphasia to describe individuals with any type of language impairment.

Dysphonia

See HOARSENESS.

Dysphoria

A state of feeling unwell or unhappy; the opposite of euphoria.

Dysplasia

Abnormal cells that may precede the development of cancer. Dysplasia most often occurs in cells that reproduce rapidly. Dysplasia is classified as mild, moderate, or severe, depending on how abnormal the affected tissue appears under a microscope.

Dyspnea

The sensation of difficult, labored, or uncomfortable breathing. Dyspnea can vary widely in severity. It may be experienced as the result of many conditions, ranging from overexertion to serious illnesses, such as CHRONIC OBSTRUCTIVE PULMONARY DISEASE (COPD) or asthma. Other conditions that produce dyspnea include anxiety, interstitial pulmonary fibrosis, anemia, neuromuscular disorders, pneumonia, lung cancer, and heart disease.

Treating the underlying disease is the most effective and primary treatment for dyspnea; however, two types of medication, opiates and anxiolytics, may improve symptoms. Opiates can relieve breathlessness and may improve exercise performance, while anxiolytic medications help reduce anxiety, relieve the ventilatory response related to the available amounts of oxygen in the blood, and lower the intensity of the emotional reaction to breathlessness.

Dysthymia

Chronic, persistent depressed mood; essentially a form of mild DEPRESSION. In adults, the depressed mood of dysthymia lasts for at least 2 years and is accompanied by two or more of the following symptoms: poor appetite or overeating, inability to sleep (insomnia) or too much sleep (hypersomnia), low energy or fatigue, low self-esteem, poor concentration, diffi-

culty making decisions, and feelings of hopelessness. Treatment consists of psychotherapy, antidepressant medications, or both.

Dystonia

A neurological movement disorder that results in distorted or impaired voluntary movement. The disorder is often painful and may affect one part of the body, several parts, or the entire body. Focal dystonia, generally appearing during a person's 50s, is the term used to describe the disorder when a single part of the body is affected; an individual may have more than one focal dystonia. When the whole body is involved, the condition is termed generalized dystonia. This form of the disorder usually occurs during childhood. Dystonia may occur as the result of stroke, most commonly affecting an arm and leg on the same side of the body. Otherwise, the cause is unknown. There is no cure at present, although medication may help reduce spasm in selected cases.

Dystrophy

A progressive condition caused by defective nourishment of an organ or system. MUSCULAR DYSTROPHY is a group of disorders characterized by progressive skeletal muscle weakness.

Dysuria

The medical term for painful or difficult urination. Dysuria is often a symptom of disorders such as cystitis, urethritis, or bladder stones or of a sexually transmitted disease, such as gonorrhea. See URINATION, PAINFUL.

E. coli

A bacterium known as *Escherichia coli* that has hundreds of strains, some of which produce a powerful toxin that may cause severe illness. Most strains of *E. coli* are harmless and live in the intestines of healthy people and animals. Strains of *E. coli* are differentiated from one another by specific markers found on their surface. One strain, referred to as diarrheagenic *Escherichia coli* or non–Shiga toxin-producing *E. coli*, causes travelers' diarrhea, which is usually mild and self-limiting. *E. coli* is also a common cause of urinary tract infections. A Shiga toxin-producing *E. coli* can cause severe symptoms and is life-threatening; this *E. coli* was first identified as a cause of food-borne illness in the United States in 1982.

Transmission of *E. coli* may also occur via person-to-person contact in families and child-care facilities, by drinking or swimming in water that is contaminated with fecal material, or by ingesting foods that may have been improperly treated or washed.

Infection with hemorrhagic *E. coli* causes intense bouts of diarrhea, which may be bloody, and abdominal cramps.

To diagnose infection, the stool is cultured and tested for the causative strain of *E. coli* bacterium by SMAC agar, a test that detects the organism. *E. coli* infections in the blood and urine are identified by culturing these body fluids. Most *E. coli* infections are treated by antibiotics, but some strains are resistant to all antibiotics.

E. coli diarrhea

See DIARRHEA, E. COLI.

Ear

The organ for hearing and balance. The structures of the ear are in three parts: the outer ear, the middle ear, and the inner ear. Most of these structures lie inside the skull. See HEARING.

Ear, discharge from

A symptom of infection in or damage to any of several parts of the ear. A discharge of blood or fluid from the ear following increasing pain and HEARING LOSS may indicate a ruptured or perforated eardrum (see EARDRUM, PERFORATED).

Discharge may also be caused by an OTITIS MEDIA (middle ear inflammation that ruptures the eardrum), SWIMMER'S EAR, an injury to the lining of the ear canal, or by a fungus in the ear canal.

A physician should be consulted whenever there is a discharge from the ear. Depending on the type of infection producing the discharge, a doctor may prescribe antibiotics. In cases of swimmer's ear, a physician may remove the ear discharge and clean the ear with a suction device or cotton-tipped probe. Ear drops containing one of the CORTICOSTEROIDS and an antibiotic may be prescribed.

Ear, foreign body in

The presence of any object that is not part of the natural structure of the ear lodged inside the ear canal. Only a physician using the correct instrument should attempt to remove foreign bodies from the ears. Attempts to remove foreign objects from the ear at home are dangerous, especially if a household item is used as a tool. Such attempts can cause serious injury to the ear or push the object farther into the ear and complicate its removal. If a live insect gets stuck in the ear, it is safe to apply a few drops of mineral or baby oil into the ear canal to try to immobilize the insect until a doctor can remove it.

Earache

Pain in one or both ears, medically termed otalgia, which may be sharp and stabbing or dull and throbbing.

When earaches are severe and persistent, an infection may be the cause. A physician should be consulted about a severe earache.

Any number of infections or conditions may cause an earache, including infection of the ear canal, barotrauma, SWIMMER'S EAR, or OTITIS MEDIA. Pain can also be caused by a build-up of EARWAX, a sore throat, or painful neck muscles.

Eardrum, perforated

A hole, rupture, or tear in the tympanic membrane, commonly called the eardrum, which separates the ear canal and the middle ear. A decreased ability to hear and a discharge may accompany a perforated eardrum.

Physical trauma, exposure to very

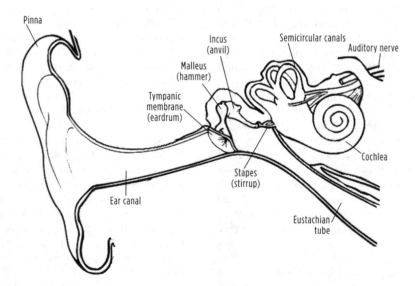

Anatomy of the ear

The structures of the ear gather sound waves and pass them through the hollow outer ear, through the vibrating eardrum and bones in the middle ear, and then into the fluid environment of the inner ear. There they are converted into nerve impulses that travel via the auditory nerve to the brain.

loud noise, infection, or medical procedures are all possible causes of a perforated eardrum. Being exposed to sudden explosions can cause the eardrum to rupture.

The amount of HEARING LOSS is usually related to the size of the perforation and its location in the eardrum.

A physician should be consulted if a perforated eardrum is suspected; he or she can diagnose the condition and recommend the appropriate treatment. A hearing test (see AUDIOMETRY) is generally performed before attempts are made to correct the perforation. Most small perforations of the eardrum will heal on their own, usually within a few weeks but possibly over several months.

In more extreme perforations, surgery (TYMPANOPLASTY) may be necessary to repair a perforated eardrum.

Earwax

Wax in the ear canal that is secreted by special glands in the skin lining the outer part of the canal. This wax, termed cerumen, traps dust and other particles to prevent them from going deeper into the ear where they might injure the eardrum and helps keep the ear canal dry by repelling water. It also has antibacterial properties.

In some people, excessive wax builds up, sometimes as often as every few months. It becomes hardened and blocks the ear canal, causing discomfort. Wax blockage can noticeably impair hearing, create ringing in the ears, make the ears feel plugged, and sometimes even cause EARACHE or dizziness.

A physician may wash out the impacted wax, in a procedure named ear lavage. The accumulated wax is softened, then removed by syringing of the ears with body-temperature water or saline.

Ebola virus

A family of viruses, which has four subtypes, three of which have been identified as a cause of disease in humans and one of which has caused disease in primates. The Ebola virus, which originated in Africa, causes Ebola hemorrhagic fever (Ebola HF), a severe, often fatal illness.

Ebola HF can be diagnosed with blood tests within a few days of symptoms appearing. The most frequent symptoms include high fever, headache, muscle aches, stomach pain, nausea, fatigue, and diarrhea, with upper respiratory symptoms including cough and chest pain.

There is no known cure or vaccine for Ebola HF, and no effective antiviral therapy exists. Treatment is generally based on supportive therapy, including the replacement of blood products and the maintenance of fluid and electrolyte balance, oxygen status, and blood pressure.

ECG

Electrocardiogram; a recording of the electrical activity of the heart as a graph or series of waves on a strip of paper. The machine used to record the electrocardiogram is an electrocardiograph. The ECG is useful in determining whether heart rate and rhythm are normal and in detecting signs of a large number of conditions that affect the heart. For example, changes in the ECG tracing may indicate that a heart attack is occurring or that a heart attack has occurred and is now healed.

Echocardiogram

An image of the heart created by bouncing ultrasound waves off the heart and into a machine that translates the echoes into a computer-generated picture. Echocardiography is a method of visualizing the heart using ultrasound technology.

An echocardiogram is useful for determining the size of the heart, its pumping strength, valve problems, damage to the heart muscle, abnormal blood flow patterns, structural abnormalities (such as enlargement of the heart, or cardiomegaly), and blood pressure in the pulmonary arteries (arteries leading to the lungs) (see HYPERTENSION, PULMONARY). A special technique, called Doppler echocardiography, can be used to measure the speed of blood flow through the heart. Another technique, called the TRANSESOPHAGEAL ECHOCARDIOGRAM, involves inserting a small transducer into the esophagus (the tube leading to the stomach). The transducer emits ultrasound waves that allow better images of the back of the heart.

Eclampsia

A serious and rare condition of late pregnancy in which the mother develops seizures or lapses into a coma. Eclampsia is almost always preceded by a condition called preeclampsia, in which the woman has swelling, high blood pressure, and protein in her urine. In about one pregnancy in 1,000, PREECLAMPSIA leads to eclampsia in late pregnancy, during labor or delivery, or after delivery. Eclampsia can be life-threatening and must be treated aggressively in the hospital to protect the lives of both the mother and the baby.

ECT

Electroconvulsive therapy. Also known as shock or electric shock therapy, ECT consists of an electrical shock administered to the brain to induce a controlled seizure. ECT is used primarily as a psychiatric treatment for major depression that does not respond to antidepressant medication, particularly when there is a risk of suicide.

A great deal of controversy has surrounded ECT, in part because the therapy was used indiscriminately after its introduction in the 1930s.

Although antidepressant medications have made ECT less necessary than in the past, it still remains an effective treatment for severe depression that does not respond to medication. One benefit is that ECT begins to work in a few days, while medications usually take from 4 to 6 weeks to alleviate depression.

Ectopic pregnancy

A condition in which a fertilized egg implants outside the uterus. Most ectopic pregnancies occur in the fallopian tubes, but can occur (less often) on the ovaries, cervix, and in the abdominal cavity. Some factors increase a woman's risk of having an ectopic pregnancy, including inflammation of the fallopian tubes (known as SALPINGITIS), damage to tissues inside a tube, previous tubal surgery, or use of an intrauterine device.

Symptoms of an ectopic pregnancy may include lower abdominal pain (usually concentrated on one side), vaginal bleeding, nausea, and vomiting. However, an ectopic pregnancy may cause no symptoms. Women with ectopic pregnancies often do not even know they are pregnant. Symptoms typically are experienced 6 weeks or more after a woman's last menstrual period. The greatest risk to the woman is when an ectopic pregnancy ruptures, and severe internal bleeding occurs. Abdominal pain will increase as blood builds inside a woman's abdominal cavity; she may experience shoulder pain, weakness, dizziness, or fainting.

When an ectopic pregnancy is suspected, a doctor performs a pelvic examination and usually orders blood tests and ULTRASOUND SCANNING. A woman with a ruptured ectopic pregnancy needs immediate surgery to remove the embryo and repair or remove the damaged tissues of the fallopian tube. If an ectopic pregnancy has not ruptured or caused severe bleeding, and the fallopian tube has not ruptured, the embryo can usually be removed surgically by performing a LAPAROSCOPY. If, as a result of an ectopic pregnancy, a woman's fallopian tube has ruptured, it can sometimes be repaired. If damage to the tube is considerable and cannot be repaired, the tube will be removed in a procedure called SALPINGECTOMY.

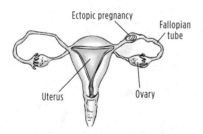

Location of ectopic pregnancy
An ectopic pregnancy most often occurs in a fallopian tube (although it can locate in an ovary, the cervix, or even elsewhere in the abdominal cavity).

In some instances, surgery may be avoided and medications given to halt the growth of an ectopic pregnancy. Medications are used only when the fallopian tube has not ruptured, there is no active bleeding, and the embryo is small.

Eczema
See DERMATITIS.

Edema
Swelling in the body caused by a buildup of excess fluids. Edema can occur when increased pressure in the blood vessels disturbs the fluid exchange and forces more fluid out of the blood vessels and into the surrounding tissues. Edema can occur in different parts of the body and for various reasons, some of which are minor and others serious. A serious cause of edema is congestive heart failure (see HEART FAILURE, CONGESTIVE), which can cause persistent swelling in the lower extremities and fluid buildup in the lungs (see PULMONARY EDEMA). However, most cases of leg swelling are not serious, and the most common cause is increased pressure in the leg veins from damaged valves in the veins (see VASOSPASM and VARICOSE VEINS).

EEG
See ELECTROENCEPHALOGRAM.

Egg
The female reproductive cell; the medical term is ovum. Produced in the OVARY, the egg is the largest cell in the human body, big enough to be seen with the naked eye. All of the eggs a woman will ever produce are present in her body at birth. But the ovaries only release one egg a month

during a woman's reproductive years, a process called OVULATION. See CONCEPTION; REPRODUCTIVE SYSTEM, FEMALE.

Ego

The portion of the personality that exhibits reason and consciousness, processes thoughts and feelings, comprehends reality, and copes with life.

EKG

See ECG.

Electric shock treatment

See ECT.

Electrocardiogram

A recording of the electrical activity of the heart as a graph or series of waves on a strip of paper; commonly abbreviated ECG.

Electrocardiography

A testing method that records the electrical activity of the heart as a graph or series of waves on a strip of paper. See ECG.

Electrocautery

A surgical instrument that uses an electrical current to remove abnormal or diseased tissue or to control bleeding from small blood vessels.

Electrocautery is commonly used to remove skin lesions. It is also used to help control bleeding in surgery; it is one of the techniques that make bloodless surgery possible.

Electroconvulsive therapy

See ECT.

Electrodiagnostic studies

Tests that are used to diagnose diseases of the nerves and muscles. Electrodiagnostic studies record electrical activity in the body. They are used to evaluate symptoms such as numbness, tingling, pain, weakness, and muscle cramping. There are a number of possible electrodiagnostic tests, including ELECTROMYOGRAM (EMG), EVOKED RESPONSES, nerve conduction studies, which show how the body's electrical signals travel through the body's nervous system, and ELECTROENCEPHALOGRAM (EEG).

Electroencephalogram

Also known as an EEG, a neurological test in which the electrical activity of the brain is recorded and studied. The EEG is a useful tool in the diagnosis of medical problems, such as epilepsy, stroke, brain tumors, sleep disorders, and degenerative diseases.

Electrolysis

Removal of unwanted body hair through destruction of hair roots with an electric current. In electrolysis, a needle is inserted in the hair follicle, and an electric current is passed through it to destroy the hair at the root. Each hair is treated individually. The process is extremely time-consuming and can be painful. Because hair goes through dormant phases, many rounds of electrolysis must be performed to make even a small area of the body completely hair-free.

Electrolyte

A chemical substance capable of conducting electricity because it dissociates into electrically charged particles (ions) when dissolved or melted. Electrolytes are involved in metabolic activities and are essential to the normal function of all body cells, especially the heart's electrical system. The most important ions found in body fluids are those involving sodium, potassium, calcium, magnesium, chloride, bicarbonate, and phosphate. Electrolyte balance depends on adequate intake of water and electrolytes.

Electromyogram

Also known as an EMG, a test used to record the electrical activity of muscles. An EMG is most often performed when a person experiences numbness and weakness. Abnormal findings may indicate diagnoses such as ALS (amyotrophic lateral sclerosis), muscular dystrophy, myasthenia gravis, or peripheral nerve damage.

Electromyography

A diagnostic procedure, also referred to as EMG, that records and analyzes the electrical activity in muscles. EMG allows a physician to examine individual parts of the muscle and explore changes that indicate disorders or pathology of the muscle tissue and its associated nerve. The procedure is used to diagnose neuromuscular disease.

ELISA test

A blood test that detects the presence of specific antibodies or antigens in the bloodstream. Enzyme-linked immunosorbent assay (ELISA) testing is frequently used to diagnose Lyme disease and HIV (human immunodeficiency virus) infection.

Embolism

Blockage of a blood vessel by a blood clot, fat deposit, or other material that has lodged in the vessel after traveling through the bloodstream. The

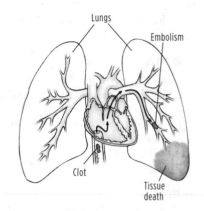

The danger of embolism

A pulmonary (lung) embolism often occurs when a blood clot in a deep vein breaks loose, travels through the bloodstream, and lodges in an artery supplying the lung.

medical importance of an embolism depends on the size of the blockage and the blood vessel it obstructs. Minor embolisms may produce no symptoms; major embolisms, such as those in the arteries of the heart or brain, can cause death by heart attack or stroke.

Embolisms particularly occur in arteries in the neck, lungs, brain, intestine, legs, arms, or kidneys. Occasionally embolisms occur in the veins and capillaries. Treatment depends on the location and size of the embolism and the condition of the person. Medications are used to break up blood clots in some cases and to prevent new ones from forming. Surgical removal of the embolism may be required.

Embolization, therapeutic

Injection of a material such as gel foam or polyvinyl chloride into an artery to cut off the blood supply. The procedure may be used to stop internal bleeding or to cut off the blood supply to a tumor.

Embolus

A mass of clotted blood, fat, calcium crystals, air bubbles, or other material that moves through the bloodstream until it lodges in a narrower blood vessel and blocks circulation. See EM-BOLISM and STROKE for additional information.

Embryo

A fertilized egg from the time of CON-CEPTION until the eighth week of PREGNANCY. Pregnancy begins with FERTILIZATION, the process in which the egg is united with a sperm. After fertilization, the egg (zygote) begins to divide into a cluster of cells, or blastocyst, which continues to divide as it moves down the fallopian tube toward the uterus. Five to eight days after fertilization, the blastocyst implants itself in the wall of the uterus and becomes a developing embryo. After 8 weeks the embryo is called a FETUS.

Embryo transfer

The implantation of an embryo or embryos into a woman's uterus, typically 3 to 6 days after in vitro fertilization (fertilization outside the body). The procedure is performed with a small tube that is placed through the vagina into the uterus while the woman reclines on an examination table.

Emergency

A medical crisis that threatens a person's life or limb(s) if appropriate care is not given within 2 hours. Medical emergencies are best identified according to these warning signs: fainting; shortness of breath or difficulty breathing; sudden dizziness, weakness, or change in vision; continuous bleeding; coughing up or vomiting blood; suicidal or homicidal urges; severe or persistent vomiting; high fever; pain or pressure in the chest or upper abdomen; confusion, lack of responsiveness, or unusual behavior; or sudden, severe pain anywhere in the body. An emergency physician is one trained especially to treat emergencies.

Emergency department

The department of a hospital that is continuously staffed 24 hours a day by specially trained personnel able to deal with any medical, traumatic, psychiatric, or environmental emergency.

Emergency medical technician (EMT)

A person trained to transport individuals to the hospital in an emergency; some emergency medical technicians, or EMTs, provide basic emergency first aid. EMTs have varying degrees of training. The highest level of EMT training is associated with a PARAMEDIC, who performs advanced medical procedures at the scene of an emergency or in the ambulance on the way to a hospital.

Emetics

Agents that cause vomiting. Emetics are used to induce vomiting when poisonous or toxic substances have been consumed. They may act directly on the gastrointestinal tract by irritating portions of it, or they may work indirectly, by affecting areas of the brain that control vomiting.

EMG

See ELECTROMYOGRAPHY.

Emphysema

A chronic lung disease characterized by destruction of the walls of the alveoli, or air sacs, in the lungs, resulting in overinflation of the air sacs. Emphysema occurs gradually, usually as a result of years of exposure to cigarette smoke. The disease process causes gradual irreversible damage that interferes with the normal exchange between oxygen taken from the air breathed in and the carbon dioxide in the blood. Less oxygen is transferred from the lungs into the bloodstream, and overexpansion of the chest makes it difficult for a person to breathe, causing shortness of breath (see BREATH, SHORTNESS OF).

Because the disease is irreversible, medical care is centered on helping a person to live more comfortably with the symptoms and to prevent progression of the disease. Advising and assisting a person with emphysema to quit smoking is the first and foremost element of treatment. Bronchodilators may be prescribed to relax and open air passages in the lungs and secondary bacterial infections of the lungs are treated with antibiotics.

Surgery can be performed to reduce the volume of the lungs. Lung transplantation is a major procedure that can be beneficial in some cases.

Employee assistance programs (EAPs)

A workplace-based, employer-funded treatment program for problems affecting a person's job performance, particularly a dependence on alcohol or drugs.

Empyema

A collection of pus in a body cavity, particularly in the space called the pleural space, which is located between the lung and the membrane that surrounds it. This form of empyema is usually caused by an infection that spreads from the lung. Empyema can also form between the outer and middle membranes covering the brain (when it is called subdural empyema). Subdural empyema is a medical emergency requiring immediate surgical draining of the pus surrounding the brain, as well as antibiotic therapy.

When empyema affects the area surrounding the lungs, the accumulation of fluid causes difficulty breathing, shortness of breath, and chest pain that worsens with deep inhalations. Other symptoms may include a dry cough, fever and chills, excessive sweating (especially at night), malaise, and weight loss.

Empyema may be diagnosed by physical examination and followup tests. Antibiotics are prescribed to treat the infection, and the fluid usually needs to be drained, either in a procedure called THORACENTESIS, or through surgery.

Emulsion

A suspension of small globules of one liquid in a second liquid with which the first will not mix. Examples of emulsions include oil in vinegar and water in oil. In pharmaceutical preparations, mixtures of oil and water are sometimes united by a third substance.

Enamel, dental

The hard, outer layer that covers and protects the teeth. Dental enamel is the hardest substance in the human body.

Encephalitis

An inflammation of the brain that may be due to many different causes, including injury to the head or brain or a complication of a viral, bacterial, or fungal infection. In rare cases, MEASLES can cause a very serious form of encephalitis.

There are several types of mosquito-borne encephalitis. Among them are arboviral encephalitis, WEST NILE VIRUS, eastern equine encephalitis, western equine encephalitis, St. Louis encephalitis, and La Crosse encephalitis.

The symptoms of encephalitis vary widely among people who have been bitten by infected mosquitoes. Most of these people do not contract the illness at all. Others have only flulike symptoms that include headache, lethargy, and fever that resolves within a few days. When the infection is severe, a person may have an intense headache, stiff neck, high fever, nausea, vomiting, aching muscles, chills, sensitivity to light, and mental confusion.

Encephalitis may cause seizures or localized paralysis. Symptoms may progress to unconsciousness and coma. These symptoms constitute a medical emergency, and the person should be treated in a hospital emergency department.

Diagnosis is made after the person's blood samples are evaluated for antibodies to the agent causing the infection. While there is no specific medical cure for mosquito-borne encephalitis, people usually recover fully from the infection with supportive care to treat symptoms and any complications such as a seizure.

Encephalitis due to other viral infections, including herpes simplex and varicella-zoster, can be treated with antiviral therapy. Mental retardation and high mortality are associated with some forms of encephalitis.

Encephalomyelitis

Inflammation of the brain and spinal cord that may occur as a complication of a viral infection. Encephalomyelitis is distinct from ENCEPHALITIS, which involves inflammation of the brain only. Both diseases can be serious and even life-threatening, especially in infants and older people. Many different viruses can cause encephalitis or encephalomyelitis, including herpes simplex, CHICKENPOX, measles, mumps, EPSTEIN-BARR VIRUS, HIV (human immunodeficiency virus), polio, rabies, and mosquito-borne viruses. The bacterium that causes Lyme disease, *Borrelia burgdorferi*, also can cause encephalitis or encephalomyelitis. Symptoms include fever, headache, nausea, vomiting, lethargy, weakness, seizures, stiff neck, memory impairment, and confusion. Diagnosis and treatment require hospitalization. Treatment includes antiviral drugs, if available for the infection; corticosteroids in some instances; and supportive care.

Encephalopathy

Any disorder of the brain that involves widespread dysfunction of brain activity. Encephalopathy is characterized by neurological symptoms, such as personality changes, behavior changes, and changes in consciousness. Signs include agitation, confusion, delirium, hallucinations, insomnia, nervousness, palpitations, unsteady gait, and abnormal eye movements. Symptoms may progress to unconsciousness and coma. Causes of encephalopathy include metabolic abnormalities, such as liver or kidney dysfunction, WERNICKE-KORSAKOFF SYNDROME (a brain disorder), lack of oxygen, toxins associated with metabolic abnormality, and diffuse brain damage. If the skin is jaundiced, liver disease may be responsible. Diagnosis usually requires tests, and hospitalization is usually required. Treatment of encephalopathy usually depends on the underlying cause.

Encopresis

Also known as soiling, a disorder in which children older than age 4 involuntarily pass feces into their clothing. Primary encopresis refers to the disorder in which the child has not yet achieved bowel control. Secondary encopresis occurs when a child who has previously established control loses it. Encopresis is most commonly caused by chronic constipation. Less commonly, it may be associated with an underlying medical condition such as an inadequate level of thyroid hormone or a weakness of the intestinal muscles. See also TOILET TRAINING.

Endarterectomy

A surgical procedure to remove the buildup of fat and cholesterol in an artery and restore normal blood flow. Endarterectomy is most commonly performed on the carotid artery, which supplies blood to the brain, and is known as CAROTID ENDARTERECTOMY.

Endemic

A disease or condition persistently found in a given population or geographical area.

Endocarditis

Inflammation of the endocardium (lining that covers the inside of the heart) and usually the heart valves. The most common cause of endocarditis is infection by bacteria, particularly varieties that normally reside in the mouth, respiratory tract, and intestinal system. The disease can also be caused by fungi. Endocarditis is a serious disease that is life-threatening.

Endocarditis most commonly affects people with underlying heart disease, particularly diseases or defects of the heart valves, heart disease present at birth (congenital), or a history of rheumatic fever. The disease also poses a risk for people who have had a heart valve replaced surgically. The symptoms of endocarditis may develop suddenly or slowly. They include fever, chills, weight loss, shortness of breath, fatigue, persistent cough, headache, and joint or chest pain.

Endocarditis is usually treated with antibiotics for at least 6 weeks. If damage to the heart valves is severe, surgery may also be required.

Endocrine system

A group of glands and organs that secrete hormones (chemical messengers) directly into the bloodstream to help regulate many essential body processes, including metabolism, growth, and sexual functioning. (By contrast, exocrine glands secrete substances through ducts into or onto organs).

Included in the system are the HY-POTHALAMUS and the PITUITARY GLAND in the brain; the thyroid gland, located in the neck; the PARATHYROID GLANDS, located behind the thyroid gland; the adrenal glands, which are on top of the kidneys and produce corticosteroid hormones, epinephrine, and aldosterone; and the PANCREAS.

In women, the ovaries secrete estrogen and progesterone, the sex hormones that regulate reproductive function; similarly in men, the testicles produce testosterone, the sex hormone that directs sexual and reproductive functions.

Endocrinology

The field of medical science that concentrates on the endocrine glands, including the structure and function of these glands and the hormones they secrete. The endocrine system is composed of the hypothalamus, pituitary gland, thyroid gland, parathyroid glands, thymus gland, adrenal glands, pancreas, ovaries in women, and testicles in men. An endocrinologist is a doctor trained in the diagnosis, treatment, and management of diseases and disorders of the endocrine glands.

End-of-life care

Care at the end of life that relieves symptoms and provides comfort but neither hastens nor postpones death. End-of-life care may include a medical decision to withdraw treatment or not to initiate a potentially ineffective treatment. End-of-life care may include stopping delivery of food and fluids by tube. In end-of-life care, medical ethicists think it is acceptable to give high doses of pain medication even if it potentially compromises respiration because the medical intention is clearly to relieve pain rather than to shorten life. See also HOSPICE care and ADVANCE DIRECTIVES.

Endometrial ablation

A surgical procedure used to treat abnormal bleeding from the uterus by eliminating tissue in the lining of the uterus. An alternative to HYSTERECTOMY, endometrial ablation is a relatively new approach to abnormal uterine bleeding, especially during menopause.

Surgery for uterine bleeding is always a treatment of last resort and, in most cases, the procedure is considered only when other treatments, such as HORMONE THERAPY, have failed. Some doctors are concerned about a possibility that endometrial ablation may promote cancer of the uterus by burying glandular tissue under scar tissue.

Endometrial biopsy

A procedure in which a tissue sample is taken from the lining (ENDOMETRIUM) of a woman's uterus to examine it under a microscope for conditions such as hyperplasia (tissue growth) or cancer. An endometrial biopsy may be recommended to evaluate abnormal vaginal bleeding, to screen for cancer of the uterine lining, or in an infertility evaluation.

Endometrial cancer

A malignant growth of the uterus. Endometrial cancer, which usually develops after menopause, is the most common reproductive cancer in women. If detected and treated in an early stage, it is most often curable.

Symptoms commonly include vaginal bleeding or spotting in a woman who has completed menopause or abnormal bleeding at any age, such as unusually heavy menstrual flow or bleeding between menstrual periods. Pain and discomfort are usually experienced only in advanced stages of the disease. After menopause, any vaginal bleeding other than that associated with HORMONE REPLACEMENT THERAPY must be considered abnormal and should be reported to the doctor as soon as possible.

Endometrial cancer is most common between the ages of 50 and 70 years old. The risk factors for endometrial cancer are related to increased exposure to the hormone estrogen. Women are also at risk if they have a history of infertility; POLYCYSTIC OVARIAN SYNDROME; ENDOMETRIAL HYPERPLASIA; or cancer of the ovaries, breast, or colon.

Diagnosis can be made at an early, curable stage with the help of an ENDOMETRIAL BIOPSY. Treatment includes a HYSTERECTOMY to remove the cancer and to find out whether it has spread to the lymph nodes or other organs. Some women with endometrial cancer require RADIATION THERAPY, too.

Endometrial hyperplasia

An overgrowth of the lining of the uterus. Thought to result from a relative excess of estrogen and sometimes considered a precancerous condition, this condition is easily treatable at all ages. Its most common symptom is abnormal vaginal bleeding.

Diagnosis is usually made by endometrial biopsy, which can help differentiate hyperplasia from endometrial cancer or polyps. A D AND C (dilation and curettage) may be done to obtain cells for microscopic examination or to eliminate the hyperplasia. If abnormal bleeding continues despite medical treatment and a D and C, however, a hysterectomy may be recommended.

Endometrial polyp

A spongy growth attached to the inner lining of the uterus (ENDOMETRIUM) by a stalk that protrudes into the uterine cavity and sometimes through the cervix and into the vagina. Symptoms may include cramping, irregular menstruation, and bleeding after intercourse.

A woman with symptoms of endometrial polyps will typically have a PAP SMEAR or a biopsy to rule out cancer. Once cancer has been ruled out, the doctor may recommend a D AND C (dilation and curettage) or HYSTEROSCOPY to examine the polyps and remove them. See also CERVICAL POLYPS.

Endometrioma

A cyst formed when endometrial tissue, which typically forms the lining of the uterus, becomes attached outside the uterus, usually to an ovary. Symptoms include pelvic pain, pain during intercourse, irregular or delayed menstrual periods, or a dull ache or feeling of pressure in the lower abdomen. Endometriomas, sometimes called chocolate cysts because of their color, are a form of ENDOMETRIOSIS and are treated with the same methods.

Endometriosis

A condition in which the type of tissue (endometrial) that normally lines the uterus is found outside the uterus, most often on the ovaries, fallopian tubes, the ligaments attached to the uterus, or the exterior of the uterus. Less often, endometriosis occurs on the surfaces of the bladder, bowel, or vagina. The tissue grows and bleeds during MENSTRUATION, The condition affects about 10 percent of women who are of childbearing age.

Endometriosis frequently causes pain, especially just before or during the first few days of the menstrual period. The symptoms of endometriosis often worsen over time, although some women have no symptoms. Endometriosis can also cause infertility.

The cause of endometriosis is unclear. Heredity probably plays a role, as a woman whose mother, sister, or daughter has endometriosis is more likely to develop it herself.

When endometriosis is suspected, based on symptoms and a pelvic examination, the doctor may perform a LAPAROSCOPY under general anesthesia to confirm the diagnosis. Mild cases often require no treatment.

Extensive endometriosis may require a laparotomy, a procedure in which a bigger incision than for a laparoscopy is made, giving access to a larger area for removal of endometrial tissue. If endometriosis returns after surgery and causes severe pain that is not controllable with medication, the doctor may recommend the surgical removal of the uterus (HYSTERECTOMY), the ovaries (OOPHORECTOMY), or both.

Endometritis

An inflammation of the endometrium, the lining of the uterus. Postpartum endometritis is a bacterial infection that typically develops in

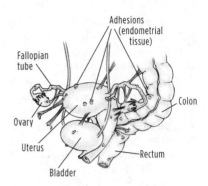

Tissue outside uterus

In endometriosis, bits of tissue from the lining of the uterus (endometrial tissue) escape from the uterus and attach on the ovaries, fallopian tubes, and other organs in the area.

a woman several days after giving birth. It is the most common infection seen just after childbirth. But it may also be seen after other procedures in which the uterine cavity has been penetrated, such as a D AND E, a D AND C, or a HYSTEROSCOPY. Symptoms include fever, tenderness of the uterus, and tachycardia (an accelerated heart rate). Treatment includes bed rest, fluids given by mouth and by intravenous drip, and antibiotics.

Endometrium

The tissue that lines the uterus. The endometrium is pink and velvety and consists of glandular tissue that undergoes cyclical monthly changes under the influence of hormones. After menstruation, it is thin, gradually becoming thicker until 1 week after ovulation. If conception does not occur, the endometrium sheds its surface during menstruation.

Endorphins

Hormones that are released by certain regions of the brain and function as chemical neurotransmitters to help control a person's response to pain and stress. Endorphins act as natural painkillers and can also help elevate a person's mood. Intense physical exercise can trigger the release of endorphins, producing a sense of well-being and suppressing sensations of pain.

Endoscopic retrograde cholangiopancreatography

See ERCP.

Endoscopy

A procedure in which interior parts of the body, such as the digestive tract, lungs, urinary system, and joints, are examined by using a slim, flexible, lighted tube called an endoscope. Endoscopy allows a doctor to view, photograph, and videotape the inside of the body without surgery. The procedure can detect abnormalities that do not appear on X rays. Causes of symptoms can be diagnosed, and tiny instruments may be passed through the endoscope to perform minor surgery or remove samples of tissue for analysis (see BIOPSY).

Endotracheal tube

A thin, flexible breathing tube inserted through the mouth or nose and into the windpipe (TRACHEA) past the vocal cords. An endotracheal tube is used to aid breathing during general anesthesia or after an injury.

End-stage renal disease

See KIDNEY FAILURE.

Enema

A liquid instilled from a tube or syringe into the rectum. Enemas are used for treatment of constipation or for medical diagnosis, such as a BARIUM ENEMA, a type of X-ray procedure of the lower gastrointestinal tract.

Enlarged prostate

See PROSTATE, ENLARGED.

ENT

Ear, nose, and throat physician or surgeon. See OTOLARYNGOLOGY.

Enteric fever

See TYPHOID FEVER.

Enteritis

See CROHN DISEASE.

Enterocele

A condition in which a portion of the intestines bulges into the top of the vagina. An enterocele can cause lower back pain and pressure in the pelvic area, although many women experience no symptoms. It is most common in women after menopause, particularly those who have given birth many times, are obese, or have conditions that cause chronic coughing, which puts pressure on abdominal muscles. Surgical repair is possible.

Enteroclysis

A fluoroscopic x-ray examination of the small intestine using a contrast medium.

Enteroclysis is the most effective method of examining the inside of the small intestine to diagnose polyps, ulcers, tumors, adhesions, and partial bowel obstruction.

Enterostomy

An operation in which a surgeon creates a connection between the small intestine and a stoma or opening in the abdominal wall, allowing for emptying of the feces into a bag attached to the skin. Sometimes referred to simply as an ostomy, an enterostomy may be necessary in severe cases of intestinal disorders, such as CROHN DISEASE, COLITIS, and cancer.

Entropion

Inward turning of the eyelid. Entropion usually affects the lower eyelid and causes the skin of the eyelid and the eyelashes to rub against the surface of the eye. The rubbing can lead to excess tearing, crusting of the eyelid, mucus discharge, the feeling that something is in the eye, irritation of the clear outer covering of the eye (cornea), and impaired vision. Scarring of the cornea can result, which may lead to some vision loss. Surgery to alleviate entropion is effective and should be performed before permanent damage occurs.

Enuresis

The medical term for involuntary BED-WETTING during sleep.

Enzyme

A protein that promotes or accelerates a specific chemical reaction. Most of the body's enzymes are manufactured in small quantities, and their function is to catalyze chemical reactions in cells. However, digestive enzymes are produced in large quantities to break down the fats, carbohydrates, and proteins in food into smaller chemical components that the body can absorb.

Ependymoma

The third most common type of childhood brain tumor. An ependymoma develops from cells of the ependyma (the membrane lining the ventricles and the central canal of the spinal cord). Symptoms of this tumor include headache, vomiting, and an unsteady gait. Ependymomas are graded based on how abnormal their cells appear under the microscope. Treatment options include surgery, radiation, and chemotherapy.

Ephedrine

A popular nonprescription decongestant that acts by releasing epinephrine from nerve cells to relieve nasal congestion. Derived from Ephedra, the scientific name for an Asian plant, the decongestant acts as a stimulant and is often abused for that reason. Ephedrine is also used in some weight-loss products because of its effect as a stimulant.

Epicondylitis

A painful condition caused by inflammation or minor tears of the tendons near the elbow, which are attached to muscles in the forearm. When the forearm muscles that flex the wrist are involved, the condition may be called GOLFER'S ELBOW. If the muscles that extend the wrist are involved, the condition is often termed TENNIS ELBOW. Elbow pain is caused by a movement that involves the combination of pressure on the wrist while it is being rotated. Treatment includes rest, cold packs, ultrasound, splinting, nonsteroidal anti-inflammatory drugs (NSAIDs), corticosteroid injections, and elbow stretching exercises.

Epidemic

An extensive outbreak of a disease, most commonly a contagious or infectious disease, that usually spreads rapidly within a community or region and affects a large number of people at the same time. Epidemics tend to occur suddenly and involve more cases of disease than could be anticipated. The cause of the rapid spread of a disease may be person-to-person contact (especially when overcrowding occurs) or contamination of the public drinking water or general food source.

Epidermal cyst

A closed sac filled with oily or fatty fluid and debris; also known as a sebaceous cyst. Epidermal cysts commonly develop on the face, neck, upper chest, and back. They are usually benign (not cancerous) and do not require treatment. However, in some cases, epidermal cysts grow large and painful or become infected. Treatment is with antibiotics and, as necessary, surgical incision and drainage or surgical excision (cutting out the cyst).

Epidermis

The outer layer of the SKIN. The epidermis itself has four layers, from the outside in: horny, granular, spiny, and basal layers. Cells in the basal layer divide constantly to form new cells, which push up toward the surface.

Epididymal cyst

See SPERMATOCELE.

Epididymis

A twisted or convoluted duct, attached to the back side of each testicle within the scrotum. The epididymis, about 20 feet long, connects the vas efferens (tube emerging from the testicle) with the vas deferens (a tube or duct leading into the urethra). See REPRODUCTIVE SYSTEM, MALE.

Epididymitis

Infection and inflammation of the epididymis, the tubular structure on the upper part of the testicle. If the testicle is also inflamed, the condition is known as epididymo-orchitis. Epididymitis is caused by bacteria from SEXUALLY TRANSMITTED DISEASES, such as gonorrhea, chlamydia, or infections of the urinary tract or prostate that infect the epididymis. Symptoms can include pain, usually quite severe and aggravated by bowel movements; rapid, painful swelling of the back of the scrotum and testicle; a temperature of up to 104°F; discharge from the penis; and pain during urination or ejaculation. Tests are performed to determine the bacterial cause of the infection, which is treated with appropriate antibiotics.

In epididymitis activity may need to be restricted because of the pain and a jockstrap should be worn. Pain medication can be prescribed to con-

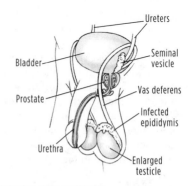

Infection of the epididymis

The epididymis, a structure on top of each testicle in which sperm mature, can become infected and inflamed. The infection can easily spread to a testicle, causing enlargement.

trol discomfort and fever; if pain is severe, the doctor may prescribe a local anesthetic.

Epidural abscess, spinal

An accumulation of pus, due to a bacterial infection, that collects in the space between the spinal bones and the outermost of the three membranes that cover the spinal cord.

When an abscess forms on the spine, it can cause muscle weakness in the legs and a lack of sensation in the lower body, in addition to the more general symptoms of fever, confusion, and sometimes delirium or seizures.

Treatment includes prompt surgical drainage of the abscess and antibiotics. Despite treatment, spinal cord injury may cause permanent weakness and loss of sensation.

Epilepsy

A neurological disorder characterized by two or more seizures. A SEIZURE is a sudden and transient episode of abnormal, uncontrolled electrical activity in the brain. Seizures may cause a series of involuntary muscle contractions or a temporary lapse in consciousness.

About half of all cases of epilepsy have no known cause. In other cases, seizures are linked to infection, trauma, or other medical problems. Epilepsy may also run in families. In children, seizures are frequently associated with CEREBRAL PALSY and other neurological abnormalities.

Types of seizures

There are more than 30 different types of seizures. Seizures are divided into two main categories: partial seizures, in which the abnormal impulses arise in just one part of the brain and during which the person remains conscious, and generalized seizures, which are caused by abnormal neuronal activity in multiple parts of the brain. Generalized seizures may cause convulsions, massive muscle spasms, falls, and loss of consciousness.

Different types of epilepsy

There are many different types of epilepsy. Absence epilepsy or petit mal is a type of epilepsy characterized by brief periods of inattention that last a few seconds; it tends to run in families. Childhood absence epilepsy usually disappears at puberty. Frontal lobe epilepsy is characterized by clusters of short seizures that have a sudden onset and termination. Lennox-Gastaut is a severe form of epilepsy that can cause atonic seizures, which in turn cause sudden falls also known as drop attacks.

Temporal lobe epilepsy (see EPILEPSY, TEMPORAL LOBE) is the most common type of epilepsy with partial seizures.

Diagnosis

Many different techniques are used to diagnose epilepsy. The history of the events (seizures) is the most important key to diagnosing epilepsy, but also helpful are blood tests; electroencephalogram (EEG) monitoring; and neurological, developmental, and behavioral tests. A number of brain imaging techniques are also used in evaluating a person with seizures, including CT SCANNING (computed tomography scanning), MRI (magnetic resonance imaging), and PET SCANNING (positron emission tomography scanning).

Treatment

Antiepileptic drugs are the first line of treatment. Most adults with epilepsy are able to work and live normal lives. Certain occupations in which a loss of consciousness could be catastrophic (for example, airplane pilot or bus driver) are usually off limits to people with epilepsy.

Status epilepticus, the occurrence of repeated or prolonged epileptic seizures, is a severe, life-threatening condition that must be treated as quickly as possible. The sooner medication is administered, the better the chance of recovery. A single medication can usually control the seizures of about 50 to 75 percent of people with epilepsy; for others, a combination of two or three drugs is needed.

First aid for a person known to have epilepsy who is having a seizure consists of making the person comfortable and not putting any object into his or her mouth near the tongue. A seizure in a person not already diagnosed with epilepsy is a medical emergency, and someone should call 911 or the local emergency number immediately.

Epilepsy, temporal lobe

Also known as TLE, the most common type of EPILEPSY with partial seizures. A SEIZURE is a sudden episode of uncontrolled electrical activity in the brain. TLE usually begins during childhood. Over time, repeated temporal lobe seizures can cause a brain structure known as the hippocampus to shrink. The hippocampus, which is part of the brain's limbic system, is essential to normal memory and learning. Multiple seizures over the years may cause significant damage to the hippocampus, so preventing seizures by early diagnosis and treatment is vital.

TLE is classified as a partial seizure because the seizures begin in a focal area or part of the brain, the temporal lobe. Temporal lobe seizures are frequently associated with auras. An aura is an unusual sensation that is a warning sign of an impending seizure. It may consist of a strange feeling, abnormal perceptions, or visual disturbances, such as seeing stars or flashes. When it precedes a generalized seizure, an aura followed by loss of consciousness represents the abnormal electrical impulses that start in a localized area of the brain and then spread more generally throughout the brain.

Antiepileptic drugs are the first line of treatment. When seizures cannot be adequately controlled with medications, doctors consider surgical alternatives, including temporal lobectomy.

Epinephrine

A hormone secreted in the brain by the adrenal medulla; also known as adrenaline. Epinephrine is secreted in response to a low blood sugar level, exercise, and stress, causing increased cardiac output and other physiological changes known as the "fight-or-flight response." Epinephrine can be produced synthetically for medical purposes.

Epinephrine is available both with and without prescription, by injection, and as an inhaler. Its chief use is to treat severe allergic reactions by opening the airways. In an inhaler, epinephrine is used to treat bronchospasm associated with asthma. It is also used to treat cardiac arrest and forms of heart block. Epinephrine is also available in eye drops to treat glaucoma.

Episcleritis

Inflammation of one of the outer layers of the eyeball. The episclera lies between the sclera (the white, fibrous, covering of the eye) and the conjunctiva (the outer mucous membrane). Episcleritis can cause mild pain and tenderness and increases light sensitivity and tearing. The blood vessels in the episclera become prominent, making the eye look pink or bright red. Episcleritis is common, usually mild, and occurs most frequently in young adults.

Rarely, episcleritis progresses to inflammation of the sclera (scleritis), which is more serious. Episcleritis usually runs its course without treatment in 2 weeks or longer, but the duration of the inflammation can be shortened with artificial tears, topical antihistamine, or corticosteroid eye drops.

Episiotomy

A procedure during childbirth in which an incision is made in the mother's perineum (the area between the vagina and the anus). The incision enlarges the vaginal opening and allows the baby to pass through it more easily to avoid tearing the vaginal skin during delivery. The incision is stitched closed after the birth.

An episiotomy sometimes is done to avoid pressure on the baby's head if the baby is premature, or when a baby is in distress and must be delivered immediately.

Epispadias

A congenital defect in which the upper wall of the urethra is missing. This condition occurs more often in males than in females. The opening of the urethra may be anywhere on the top surface of the penis in males born with epispadias; usually it appears as a groove or cleft without a covering. In females, the urethra may open into the clitoris or just above it. Epispadias may require surgery to repair the defect.

Epistaxis

See NOSEBLEED.

Epithelium

The layer of cells that covers the body and lines most of the structures within it. Epithelial cells thickly cover the skin; the layer may be only one cell deep in the delicate linings of body cavities, hollow organs, or structures such as blood vessels.

Epstein-Barr virus

One of the most common human viruses and a member of the herpes virus family. Epstein-Barr virus (EBV) was discovered in 1964. EBV affects people worldwide, infecting most people at some point in their lives. Most infections with EBV cause no symptoms.

Epstein-Barr is the virus that most often causes infectious mononucleosis, particularly when infection occurs for the first time in adolescence or young adulthood. (See also MONONUCLEOSIS, INFECTIOUS.) When the symptoms of mononucleosis have subsided, some cells of the body's immune system retain a lifelong dormant infection with EBV. Rarely, this dormant infection is believed to have a role in some cancers that are extremely uncommon in the United States: a cancer of the lymph glands in the jaw called BURKITT LYMPHOMA and a type of facial and oral cancer called nasopharyngeal carcinoma.

Transmission of EBV requires direct contact with an infected person's saliva. The virus is not normally transmitted through the air or via blood contact. The virus is often found in the saliva of healthy people, who may carry and spread EBV intermittently over a lifetime.

ERCP

An acronym for endoscopic retrograde cholangiopancreatography. The procedure combines the use of X rays and ENDOSCOPY to view the stomach, duodenum, bile ducts, and pancreas. ERCP is used to investigate the cause of symptoms such as jaundice (a yellowing of the skin and the whites of the eyes), upper abdominal pain, and unexplained weight loss. By using this procedure, doctors are able to diagnose problems in the liver, gallbladder, bile ducts, and pancreas. If a blockage in the bile duct is discovered during ERCP, the doctor may help alleviate the blockage by placing a tube called a stent in the bile duct. The stent creates a passageway for the bile to pass through.

Erectile dysfunction

Consistent inability to produce or maintain an erection of the penis sufficient to have sexual intercourse; also known as impotence. The cause can be either psychological or physical.

Treatment depends on the cause. Psychotherapy can help with psychological issues. Erectile dysfunction caused by medications can sometimes be resolved by changing to a different medication. Quitting smoking and abstaining from alcohol can also help. Prescription medications are available to help men produce and maintain erections. Vacuum devices that produce an erection can also be used. In some cases, surgery is performed to place an inflatable implant in the penis (see PENILE IMPLANT).

Erection

The rising and hardening of the penis due to blood accumulating in its tissues. During sexual stimulation, blood fills the erectile bodies of the penis, which are closed by exit valves in the veins to keep the blood in rather than let it flow out.

Erysipelas

An acute, red, raised, sharply demarcated rash caused by streptococcal bacteria (see STREPTOCOCCAL INFECTIONS). The rash can appear on the face and lower legs and occasionally on the arms.

The onset of erysipelas is ordinarily abrupt. The rash is hot to the touch, has clearly defined margins, and spreads quickly. Affected areas are painful, shiny, and swollen and can contain fluid-filled bumps. There may also be swelling of the eyelids, fever, chills, fatigue, nausea, and vomiting. In severe cases, abscesses (pusfilled sacs) develop. Left untreated, bacteria begin circulating in the bloodstream and can cause BACTEREMIA (the presence of bacteria in the bloodstream), which in turn leads to SEPSIS, a potentially fatal condition. Diagnosis of erysipelas is made by identifying the characteristic rash. Treatment is with penicillin.

Erythema infectiosum

See FIFTH DISEASE.

Erythema nodosum

An inflammatory skin condition that is characterized by tender, red bumps or swellings under the skin, most often on the shins. Although its exact cause remains unknown, half of all cases are associated with infection with *Coccidioides*, *Mycoplasma*, *Streptococcus*, or *Yersinia* organisms and diseases such as hepatitis B and tuberculosis.

Other symptoms of Erythema nodosum may include fever, joint aches, and a general feeling of illness. Doctors may prescribe nonsteroidal anti-inflammatory drugs to relieve pain and to control inflammation. Oral corticosteroids are prescribed in severe cases. Symptoms may last for up to 6 weeks.

Erythrocyte

A red blood cell. The erythrocyte is rich in hemoglobin, a protein that binds easily with oxygen and serves to transport it through the blood. Erythrocytes form in the bone marrow where they lose their nuclei before passing into the bloodstream, meaning that they cannot reproduce. Erythrocytes have a life span of about 120 days, after which they break down in the spleen and are destroyed. See BLOOD.

Erythrocyte sedimentation rate

See ESR.

Erythroderma

A skin condition characterized by redness and scaling over the entire body; also known as exfoliative dermatitis. Erythroderma usually occurs as a complication of another skin disease such as atopic dermatitis, psoriasis, or contact dermatitis. Less commonly, it is a symptom of a systemic disease such as leukemia or lymphoma.

In erythroderma, the continuous peeling and flaking of skin results in a loss of body protein. In serious cases, the loss of normal skin can result in severe heat loss and a drop in body temperature. Secondary infections may occur; severe cases of erythroderma can become life-threatening. Treatment of erythroderma includes diagnosing and treating the underlying primary disease, preventing secondary infection, stabilizing body temperature, and maintaining fluid balance.

Erythropoietin

A protein secreted by the kidney that stimulates formation of red blood cells in the bone marrow. Erythropoietin is used to increase the number of red blood cells in people with chronic kidney disease or those with other diseases that affect the ability of the bone marrow to make red blood cells. Erythropoietin is also used to counteract the tendency of some anticancer drugs to suppress bone marrow.

Escherichia coli

See E. COLI.

Esophageal atresia

A rare and severe birth defect in which an infant is born missing part of the esophagus (the muscular tube that connects the throat to the stomach). In esophageal atresia, there is no passageway to the baby's stomach.

A baby with esophageal atresia cannot be fed by mouth. Nourishment is given intravenously until the condition is surgically corrected. See GAS-TROSCOPY.

Esophageal dilation

Widening of the esophagus. The esophagus, part of the digestive tract, is a muscular tube that connects the throat to the stomach. Esophageal dilation may be performed to relieve blockage from noncancerous conditions that block the esophagus but cannot be removed.

Esophageal diverticulum

An outward bulge in the esophageal wall. There are three types of esophageal diverticula: the pharyngeal pouch, which must be surgically removed; the midesophageal diverticulum, which usually cause no symptoms and require no treatment; and the epiphrenic diverticulum, which

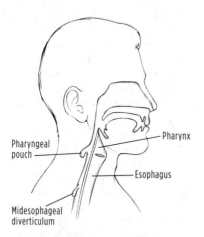

Pouches in the esophagus

Pouches, or diverticula, can form in several areas of the esophagus if the muscular wall of the esophagus bulges outward. A pharyngeal pouch forms at the back of the lower part of the throat (pharynx) if the action of the sphincter at the top of the esophagus becomes irregular.

are associated with disturbances in the sphincter between the stomach and esophagus.

Esophageal reflux

A condition in which acid from the stomach flows up into the esophagus, the muscular tube that connects the throat to the stomach. Esophageal reflux, which may affect about 15 million Americans, is also known as acid reflux, reflux, and gastroesophageal reflux disease (GERD). HEARTBURN is the most common symptom of esophageal reflux.

Normally, the muscle at the junction blocks the backflow of gastric acid from the stomach into the esophagus. If the lower esophageal sphincter is weak or defective, acid can wash up into the esophagus. In some cases, reflux is caused by a HIATAL HERNIA, in which part of the upper stomach protrudes into the chest through the opening in the diaphragm between the esophagus and the stomach.

Persistent esophageal reflux can lead to inflammation, ulceration, and formation of scar tissue that lead to ESOPHAGEAL STRICTURE (narrowing). Other potential complications include dysphagia (difficulty in swallowing), and bleeding.

Diagnosis of esophageal reflux is usually made through an upper GASTROINTESTINAL (GI) SERIES (an X-ray procedure also called a barium swallow), GASTROSCOPY and esophageal manometry.

In many cases, simple modifications in lifestyle can control esophageal reflux. Avoiding spicy or greasy foods, chocolate, coffee, and alcohol sometimes can help. Doctors recommend not smoking and losing weight for those who are overweight. Elevating the head of the bed 2 to 4 inches for sleeping or using an anti-reflux pillow can decrease heartburn at night.

When these measures prove insufficient, or if it is necessary to take antacids frequently, a doctor should be consulted. To manage reflux, doctors can prescribe drugs that reduce acid secretion, such as histamine blockers and proton pump inhibitors.

Esophageal stricture

A narrowing or obstruction of the esophagus (the tube that connects the throat and stomach) that may lead to dysphagia (see SWALLOWING DIFFICULTY). Esophageal stricture occurs as a result of the accumulation of scar tissue in the esophagus, as in persistent ESOPHAGEAL REFLUX. Scarring and narrowing can also be due to prolonged use of nonsteroidal anti-inflammatory drugs (NSAIDs), the antibiotic tetracycline, or potassium supplements.

To treat esophageal strictures, doctors perform ESOPHAGEAL DILATION to widen the passageway and permit easier swallowing. A laser may also be used to relieve blockages and destroy cancerous tissue. In some cases, more extensive surgery is required.

Esophageal varices

Large, swollen, varicose veins in the lower portion of the esophagus (the muscular tube that connects the throat to the stomach) that can erode and bleed. Esophageal varices are usually caused by portal hypertension (increased blood pressure in the portal vein, which carries blood from the intestines to the liver). Portal hypertension is usually due to liver disease.

Symptoms of esophageal varices include vomiting blood, black stools, and a dangerous drop in blood pressure. Varices may be diagnosed with a physical examination, taking a medical history, and tests, such as an upper GASTROINTESTINAL (GI) SERIES (an X-ray procedure also called a barium swallow) or GASTROSCOPY.

Esophageal varices are treated with the injection of a solution that shrinks and blocks off affected veins or by banding the veins. If veins burst, immediate medical attention is necessary, since this can be a life-threatening emergency.

Esophagectomy

Partial or total removal of the esophagus (the tube that connects the throat and stomach). An esophagectomy is usually performed to treat esophageal cancer (see ESOPHAGUS, CANCER OF THE). In some cases, an esophagectomy is performed to control severe recurrent bleeding caused by ESOPHAGEAL VARICES.

An esophagectomy is a major operation. In most cases, the stomach can be joined to the remaining part of the esophagus.

Following surgery, special coughing and breathing exercises must be practiced to keep the lungs clear. In some cases, CHEMOTHERAPY or RADIATION THERAPY are recommended, also.

Esophagitis

See ESOPHAGEAL REFLUX.

Esophagogastroscopy

See GASTROSCOPY.

Esophagogram

A series of X rays of the esophagus. An esophagogram is also known as a barium swallow or an upper GI series (see GASTROINTESTINAL [GI] SERIES).

Esophagoscopy

See GASTROSCOPY.

Esophagus

The muscular tube that passes from the throat (pharynx) to the stomach. When food is swallowed, the upper portion of the esophagus relaxes so the food can move into it. Then the food is automatically passed down to the stomach by rhythmic waves of muscular contractions (peristalsis). Gastroesophageal reflux disease (GERD; see ESOPHAGEAL REFLUX) is caused by a dysfunction of the sphincter valve; too much acid moves into the esophagus and causes heartburn. See also DIGESTIVE SYSTEM.

Esophagus, cancer of the

An uncommon cancer that can occur in any part of the esophagus (the tube that connects the throat and stomach). As a tumor grows, dysphagia (difficulty swallowing) is often the first symptom of cancer. Difficulty in swallowing requires a physician's attention. Other symptoms of cancer of the esophagus include coughing, hoarseness, choking on food, indigestion, heartburn, vomiting, and weight loss. Cancer of the esophagus most frequently appears in people age 55 or older. The diagnosis of cancer of the esophagus is based on a physical examination, medical history, and a number of tests, often including a GASTROINTESTINAL (GI) SERIES or a GASTROSCOPY.

Treatment depends on the size and location of the tumor and how advanced it is. An ESOPHAGECTOMY is usually performed to treat esophageal cancer.

When a tumor blocking the esophagus cannot be surgically removed, ESOPHAGEAL DILATION may be used.

Esotropia

A type of crossed eyes (strabismus), in which one or both eyes may turn inward toward the other. This can lead to diplopia (double vision) or AMBLYOPIA. See also STRABISMUS.

ESR

A medical test measuring the rate at which red blood cells settle through a column of liquid. The erythrocyte sedimentation rate (ESR) test is commonly performed to identify or monitor inflammatory diseases such as rheumatoid arthritis, rheumatic fever, or subacute bacterial endocarditis (heart valve inflammation). An elevated ESR usually indicates an acute inflammatory process occurring as a result of infection or other disease.

Estradiol

A hormone used to treat a lack of estrogen. Estradiol is chiefly produced in the ovaries, but also is produced in the placenta, testis, and adrenal cortex. When estrogen is lacking in a woman after menopause or removal of the ovaries, estradiol may be prescribed for hormone replacement therapy. It is also used to treat prostate cancer and osteoporosis, and it is used in some oral contraceptives.

Estriol

An estrogen hormone usually obtained from the urine of pregnant women. Pregnant women may be tested for estriol levels as part of a triple screen test, which measures the levels of estriol, AFP, and human chorionic gonadotropin, another hormone. The results of these tests can assess the risk of DOWN SYNDROME in a fetus.

Estrogen

The key female sex hormone produced primarily in the ovaries. Estrogen exists in several forms, including ESTRADIOL, estrone, and ESTRIOL. Estrogen is responsible for the development of women's sexual characteristics; it governs the monthly thickening of the endometrium that results in monthly periods; and it controls the quantity and quality of cervical and vaginal mucus necessary to transport sperm.

Estrogen replacement therapy

See HORMONE THERAPY.

Estrogen, conjugated

Female sex hormones used to treat symptoms of menopause. Conjugated estrogens are also used to treat vaginitis, osteoporosis, and breast and prostate cancer. While they are useful for treating symptoms of menopause, such as hot flashes and dizziness, the long-term use of estrogen is risky. Increased risk of heart disease, stroke, blood clots, high blood pressure, gallbladder disease, and endometrial cancer are all associated with the long-term use of conjugated estrogens. If a woman has no major risk factors for heart disease, a gynecologist may provide hormone replacement therapy for a brief period to relieve symptoms. See also HORMONE THERAPY.

Ethics, medical

The moral principles in the fields of medical treatment and research; a subset of the field of bioethics. Issues in medical ethics encompass a number of professional fields, including medicine, law, sociology, philosophy, and theology. Ethical issues affect physicians and patients as well as society.

Medical ethics have their roots in the HIPPOCRATIC OATH, which has the prime directive that physicians should "do no harm." The first formal professional code of medical ethics in the United States was established by the American Medical Association in 1847. Since the 1950s, innovations in medical technology have given rise to more complex ethical issues associated with medical research and practice.

Eustachian tube

The narrow channel connecting the middle ear with an area of the upper throat at the back of the nose. The basic functions of this tube are to replenish the air in the middle ear and to equalize any pressure changes that may occur with changes in altitude.

Infection in the tube can cause the eardrum membrane to suck in. The symptoms of this blockage are usually mild hearing impairment, ringing in the ears, and a feeling of fullness or pressure in the ears.

Euthanasia

Also known as physician-assisted suicide; formerly known as mercy killing. The intentional act of causing the painless death of a person with an incurable disease or condition. Many people involved in the "right-to-die" movement define euthanasia as the right of an individual, especially an individual who faces a possibly painful and prolonged death, to die in a dignified and controlled manner at a time of his or her choosing.

The medical profession does not consider the removal of artificial life support (even nutrition or hydration) to be euthanasia.

The arguments against euthanasia are centered on the "slippery slope" that doctors and policy makers will face in determining when euthanasia is acceptable. This position holds that physicians should not be placed in situations where it is acceptable for them to cause the ultimate harm of death. Physician-assisted suicide, within strict guidelines, is legal in the state of Oregon.

Evoked responses

Tests that assess the ability of information to travel to the brain. There are three commonly used evoked response tests: visual evoked response (VER), which assesses how well information travels from the eyes to the occipital lobes (visual cortex); brain stem auditory evoked response (BAER), which assesses neurological function and diagnoses nervous system abnormalities and hearing loss; and somatosensory evoked potential (SSEP), which assesses how information travels from the hands or feet through the spinal cord and to the brain.

Examination, physical

A thorough study of a person's state of health. The physical examination typically follows history-taking or medical interview. Examination usually includes inspection, palpation (direct feeling with the hand), percus-sion (striking parts of the body with short, sharp taps and feeling and listening to subsequent vibrations), and auscultation (listening with a stethoscope). If a person reports symptoms, the physical examination will help determine their cause and which tests may be helpful.

Excision

Surgical removal of an organ or tissue by cutting out diseased tissue. An excision is used to remove tissue that is abnormal or diseased, such as a breast lump.

Exercise

Increased energy expenditure due to muscular activity, usually resulting in movement of the body or its parts. Exercise involves one or more organs and structures of the body and is important for overall health. Regular exercise gives improved balance and coordination, improved sleep, and a longer life expectancy.

Exercise stress testing

See CARDIAC STRESS TESTING.

Exercise, aerobic

A form of physical EXERCISE that increases the heart rate and blood flow to deliver more oxygen to the working muscles. Aerobic exercise is physical exertion and repetitive motion of the large muscles, such as the leg muscles, that sustain increased heart, lung, and circulatory rates.

Exercise, anaerobic

Short-term EXERCISE that relies on anaerobic (meaning not requiring oxygen) metabolic processes for energy required to perform the activity. A good anaerobic exercise routine should include exercises that involve all the major muscle groups including the abdominals, legs, chest, back, shoulders, and arms. Anaerobic exercise can increase muscular strength and power; an example is weight lifting.

Exercise, resistance

Strength-building EXERCISE that requires the muscles to push against or resist the weight of an object or a force, such as gravity. Resistance exercise, which may also be called strength training, body building, body sculpting, and strengthening exercise, can also increase a person's endurance.

Exercise, strengthening

Physical activity that builds strength in the muscles. Strengthening exercises may also improve posture and balance. Exercises that strengthen muscles help support the joints, which can help reduce the symptoms of arthritis. Improved strength may help decrease the risk of injuries and improve a person's ability to perform many activities of daily life.

See also EXERCISE, ANAEROBIC; EXERCISE; and WEIGHT TRAINING.

Exercise, weight-bearing

Any physical activity that requires the body to support its weight, including many aerobic exercises (see EXERCISE, AEROBIC) as well as strengthening and resistance exercises (see EXERCISE, STRENGTHENING; EXERCISE, RESISTANCE). The principal benefit of weight-bearing exercise is that it strengthens the bones. When bones take on the weight of the body, the

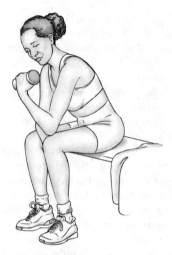

Strengthening muscles
Strengthening exercise increases metabolism and contributes to weight loss. A good strengthening workout, which often involves resistance exercise, involves all the major muscle groups.

process stimulates the bone tissue and increases the density and strength of the bones.

Exhibitionism

A mental illness characterized by highly arousing urges, fantasies, or actions involving the exposure of one's genitals to a stranger. Exhibitionism impairs the person's ability to function in a family, society, or work setting and usually causes significant distress.

Exocrine gland

A gland that releases substances through a duct or channel onto or into an organ or area of the body. For example, lacrimal ducts secrete tears onto the eye; the salivary glands secrete saliva into the mouth; sweat glands produce sweat on the skin;

pancreatic tissue secretes digestive enzymes that are carried through ducts into the intestine. Exocrine secretions may be controlled by hormones or by chemical neurotransmitters that function similarly to hormones. See ENDOCRINE SYSTEM.

Exophthalmos

Abnormal bulging of one or both eyes; also known as proptosis. The most common cause is a hyperactive thyroid gland (hyperthyroidism), which swells tissues in the eye socket and pushes the eyeball forward (see GRAVES DISEASE). The condition can also result from bleeding behind the eye (usually from injury), inflammation or infection of the eye socket, tumors, or blood vessel abnormalities that cause blood to back up behind the eye. A bulging eye requires prompt professional evaluation.

Treatment depends on the cause. Surgery is sometimes needed if the exophthalmos is causing damage such as pressure on the optic nerve. Control of hyperthyroidism with medication may improve exophthalmos from that cause. Inflammation of the eye socket is treated with corticosteroid medications, which reduce swelling, or with radiation to shrink the tissue.

Exotropia

A type of crossed eyes (strabismus), in which one or both eyes may turn outward. Exotropia may produce double vision or other types of vision impairment.

Expectorants

Drugs used to promote a productive cough and help people clear mucous secretions from their airways. Coughs are productive (produce phlegm) or nonproductive (dry and hacking). Expectorants are the treatment of choice to help thin the mucus and make it easier for the person to cough up. Guafenesin is among the most commonly prescribed expectorants and is found in several over-the-counter and prescription cough medicines. Although it is widely used, it is minimally effective, if at all.

Exploratory surgery

Any diagnostic procedure used to examine a portion of the body that is thought to be diseased. Exploratory surgery is an option when a medical problem exists and the exact cause, extent of disease, or treatment cannot be determined without direct examination.

Explosive disorder

A mental illness characterized by repeated episodes of serious violence against people or property that occur with little or no provocation. Relief follows the violent episode, and the individual usually expresses upset, remorse, regret, or embarrassment. Since explosive disorder is very rare, little is known about what causes it.

Extrapyramidal system

The portion of the central nervous system that affects electrical impulses sent from the BRAIN to the skeletal muscles, influencing large muscle movements such as walking. The system connects nerves in the CEREBRUM with the basal ganglia (structures deep within the brain that coordinate voluntary muscle movement) and parts of the brain stem.

Eye

The sensory organ of sight. The eyes focus light rays to perceive images and then convert these images into impulses that are transmitted to the brain.

The two spherical eyeballs lie within the skull, protruding through the eye sockets, but largely protected by bone. Inside the skull, the eyeballs are cushioned on all sides by fat. The EYELID protects the protruding portion of the eyes. The principal lacrimal glands, which produce and release TEARS, lie just inside the eye socket and drain onto an outer layer of the eye called the CONJUNCTIVA.

Behind the conjunctiva is the sclera, the white of the eye, which forms a tough outer layer over the eyeball. In the center front of the sclera, the CORNEA is a transparent, protruding structure that is the main focusing lens for the eye. The cornea is cushioned by the aqueous humor, a thick transparent fluid that fills an area in the front part of the eye. The iris, which is the colored part of the eye, lies behind the aqueous humor. It is a ring of muscle fibers surrounding the PUPIL, which is an opening through which light rays can pass.

Behind the iris is the crystalline LENS, which adjusts the focus of the light rays. The shape of the crystalline lens is altered by a circle of muscle, the ciliary body, which surrounds the lens. Behind the crystalline lens, the hollow of the eyeball is filled with a clear, gelatinous substance called the vitreous humor.

The RETINA lines the back of the eyeball. The pattern of light or image focused by the cornea and the crystalline lens falls on the retina. This complex structure is composed of nerve tissue containing light-sensitive cells called rods and cones. The rods and cones translate the image on the retina into a pattern of nerve impulses that travel to the brain via the optic nerve, which extends from the back of the eye. The area of the brain that controls sight, the visual cortex in the cerebrum, interprets the impulses. See VISION.

Eye drops

Liquid medicine used to treat conditions of the eye. Eye drops are used for chronic conditions such as glaucoma and dry eye, and they are also used for the short-term treatment of allergies and infections.

Eye injury

Physical damage to the eye or its surrounding tissue as a result of accident or mishap. Eye injuries may be caused by foreign objects (most commonly, contact lenses), blunt trauma, burns, or penetrating injuries, the most traumatic and dangerous type of damage.

A foreign object in the eye needs to be removed, but this should be done only by a medical professional if the object is touching the cornea or is embedded in the eye or surrounding tissue. After removing a foreign body, treatment includes applying antibiotic ointment if the cornea has been scratched.

A black eye usually indicates superficial damage to the tissues surrounding the eye and usually heals on its own within 2 weeks. Damage to the interior of the eye is more dangerous; for example, bleeding in the interior of the eye, tearing of the iris, dislocation of the lens, or detachment of the retina can all cause loss of vision. Ice packs are used to reduce swelling and bruising from blunt trauma. Damage to the surface or interior of the eye may require surgical repair.

An object that enters the eyeball or surrounding tissues is an emergency requiring the fastest possible treatment. First aid consists of placing a shield over the injured eye without touching the object, without trying to remove it, and without applying pressure to the object or the eye itself.

Eye tumors

Abnormal growth of tissue in the eyeball or its surrounding structures. Eye tumors can be benign, or noncancerous: that is, their growth is confined to a particular body structure and they do not metastasize or spread throughout the body. Some are malignant (cancerous): that is, they can spread and threaten life.

Among the types of tumors to affect the eye are retinoblastoma, a rare but dangerous cancer found in children and affecting the retina.

Treatment for retinoblastoma depends on the stage of the cancer and whether one or both eyes are involved. If the tumor is small and confined to the eye, treatments to preserve the eye may include radiation therapy (use of X rays to kill cancer cells), cryotherapy (use of extreme cold to kill cancer cells), thermotherapy (use of extreme heat to kill cancer cells), laser surgery (to destroy blood vessels that nourish the tumor), or chemotherapy (cancer-killing medications). If the tumor is large and the eye cannot be saved, it is usually removed surgically.

Another eye tumor is a melanoma, which usually occurs on the skin but can also appear on the eye and is the most common malignant eye tumor in adults. Melanoma is a particularly fast-growing and fast-spreading cancer, and it is often lethal. If the tumor is left untreated, it will eventually cause the retina to detach from the back of the eye, which results in distorted vision or blindness. Small melanomas are treated with radiation therapy or laser surgery. Large tumors may require removal of the eye to prevent spread of the cancer to the brain and other organs.

Orbital tumors can arise in the bones, muscles, and fat surrounding the eye, or they may develop in surrounding structures, such as the sinuses or brain cavity, and invade the eye socket (orbit). Orbital tumors appear in both children and adults, and most of these growths are benign.

Eye, examination of

A series of tests performed to measure the eyes' ability to see clearly and to screen for common eye diseases. If one sees normally, an eye examination every 3 to 5 years during adulthood until age 50 years is recommended. After that, the eyes should be examined more frequently. If one wears or needs glasses, examinations should be conducted at least every 2 years, or more often if recommended by an eye specialist. Contact lens wearers should be examined at least once a year.

During the examination, the sharpness of vision will be assessed. The most common test for visual acuity is performed using a Snellen chart, which shows letters arranged in lines of increasingly smaller size. Each row is designated by a number corresponding to the distance in feet from which a person with normal vision can read all the letters of the row. For example, the letters in the "40" row are large enough for a person with normal vision to read from 40 feet. By convention, vision is measured at a distance of 20 feet. If a person can read the "20" row, he or she is said to have 20/20 vision. Acuity is scored as a set of two numbers, such as 20/20. The first number represents the distance from the chart in feet, and the second number represents the smallest row of letters that a person can read from the testing distance. For example, if a person whose vision is less sharp can only read from 20 feet that which a person with normal vision can read from 60 feet, visual acuity would be scored as 20/60.

The eye specialist can also examine the eye with a slit lamp, a table-mounted microscope combined with a special light source.The eye specialist can look inside the eye with an instrument known as the ophthalmoscope. Finally, the pressure inside the eye is routinely tested to screen for glaucoma.

Eye, foreign body in

See EYE INJURY.

Eye, prosthetic

An artificial, cosmetic replacement for an eye lost to trauma or surgery; also known popularly as a glass eye. Although glass was used in the past to fashion prosthetic eyes, it is rarely used now. Prosthetic eyes achieve good cosmetic results in most cases, with a relatively small number of complications.

Eyelid

Two folds of skin that protect the surface of each EYE. The upper and lower eyelids close quickly as a reflex action to shield the eye against harsh light and foreign objects. They also secrete an oily component of tears. Their constant blinking action moves tears over the surface of the eyes to keep them moist and clean. The eyelashes along the edge of each eyelid are actually three to four rows of hairs that help sift out dust and other materials before they reach the eye.

Eyelid surgery

A procedure that tightens bagging or drooping eyelids by removing excess tissue; also called blepharoplasty. Typically, eyelid surgery is performed for cosmetic reasons; baggy eyelids make an individual look older and more tired than he or she feels.

Eyelid, drooping

Also known as ptosis or BLEPHAROPTOSIS, drooping of one or both upper eyelids can be an acquired or congenital condition. There are many different causes of drooping eyelids. Outpatient surgery under a local anesthetic is usually recommended to correct the problem.

Facial palsy

An abnormal neurological condition characterized by weakness or paralysis of the facial muscles. One common form of facial palsy is BELL

PALSY, a condition caused by damage to or dysfunction of the facial nerve. Other possible causes of facial palsy include strokes, tumors, and infections (such as SHINGLES). Any case of facial weakness, paralysis, or palsy calls for prompt and careful evaluation by a physician. Treatment of facial palsy depends on its underlying cause.

Factitious disorder

The intentional feigning or production of physical or psychological symptoms out of a deep-seated need to assume the sick role. The disorder may cause the person to seek unneeded medical tests and exploratory surgeries.

Factor IX deficiency

Hemophilia B, or Christmas disease, a genetically inherited bleeding disorder characterized by inadequate amounts of clotting factor IX in blood plasma. Factor IX, a protein also known as plasma thromboplastin component (PTC), is involved in blood coagulation (clotting). Hemophilia B occurs in only about 70,000 men worldwide at any given time and occurs a fifth as frequently as does hemophilia A (factor VIII deficiency). Factor IX deficiency affects males only; females who inherit the condition are carriers. Carriers are usually, but not always, symptom-free. People with factor IX deficiency may need supplementary factor IX or fresh frozen plasma if they have a bleeding injury or are undergoing surgery.

Factor VII deficiency

A bleeding disorder characterized by inadequate amounts of the plasma protein factor VII, an important clotting protein; also known as extrinsic factor deficiency. Factor VII deficiency may be either inherited or acquired via a vitamin K deficiency. Symptoms include bleeding into joints and muscles, excessive menstrual bleeding and bruising, and bleeding from the mucous membranes. Treatment with normal plasma, concentrates containing factor VII, or recombinant factor VII is generally effective for stopping bleeding episodes.

Factor VIII deficiency

A genetically inherited bleeding disorder characterized by inadequate amounts of clotting factor VIII in blood plasma. Factor VIII deficiency is the cause of the bleeding disorder known as hemophilia A (see HEMOPHILIA). Factor VIII, also known as antihemophilic factor (AHF), is a substance involved exclusively in blood coagulation (clotting). Factor VIII deficiency is inherited as a sex-linked recessive trait; only males can inherit the disorder. Females may carry the disorder and pass it on to their sons; their daughters can also be carriers. All daughters of affected males are carriers, but men cannot pass the disease on to their sons.

People with factor VIII deficiency may need treatment with factor VIII if they are actively bleeding or undergoing a surgical procedure. The condition has no cure and often requires counseling.

Fahrenheit scale

A scale used to measure temperature. In the Fahrenheit scale, the point at which water freezes is 32°, while the point at which it boils is 212°.

Failure to thrive

A lag in growth and development behind the expected rate for a child's age and sex. It most often affects children younger than age 5, especially those 2 and younger. Failure to thrive, also called FTT, refers to a cluster of symptoms rather than a specific disease. Among those symptoms are the failure to gain weight and length. Physical characteristics are often accompanied by developmental delays. For example, a failure to thrive may cause children to sit up, crawl, or walk later than their peers (see WALKING, DELAYED).

Frequently, failure to thrive is due to inadequate nutrition because the infant has difficulty feeding. Insufficient emotional stimulation can also cause failure to thrive. A lack of nurturing can lead to depression and loss of appetite in a child.

When a baby's growth does not reflect normal gains in weight, length, and development on standardized growth charts, a physical examination can help determine whether an underlying illness is responsible. The doctor will assess the child's nutritional needs by asking questions about his or her diet and medical history to determine if there are any illnesses that may be contributing to the problem.

Underlying diseases or disorders must be treated appropriately. Breastfeeding mothers may need to improve their diets to increase the quantity and quality of their milk. Enriched formulas or high-calorie diets may be prescribed. When physiological causes can be excluded, the doctor may refer parents to a social worker or mental health professional.

Fainting

Temporary loss of consciousness. Fainting occurs when there is an insufficient supply of blood and oxygen to the brain for a short period, which can happen if blood vessels in the body dilate (widen), causing blood (which carries vital oxygen) to drain away from the brain. Fainting may be characterized by a sudden pallor, or pale skin; nausea; sweating; loss of consciousness; and twitching or brief seizures.

By itself, fainting is not harmful, and, as a general rule, the person who has fainted will recover quickly with no lasting effects. Sometimes, however, a fainting spell is a signal of a serious condition, such as a heart condition.

Fainting can have many causes, among them standing at attention, rising quickly after lying down, wearing a too-tight collar, low blood pressure, abnormal heart rate or rhythm, severe pain or fright, alcohol or drug use, strenuous coughing, or hyperventilation (fast, shallow breathing).

Immediate first aid for fainting includes having the person lie down with legs elevated 6 to 12 inches. Assisting the person to a cooler environment may also be beneficial. Medical assistance should be sought at once if the person is having difficulty breathing, has chest pain, does not arouse promptly, or was injured by falling during the fainting spell. See also DIZZINESS; HYPOGLYCEMIA.

Fallopian tube

Either of two passages that extend from each ovary to the uterus; medically called the oviducts. Each tube

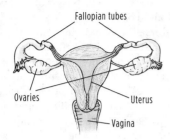

Passage of eggs
The fallopian tubes, about 4 or 5 inches long, extend from the ovaries into the cavity of the uterus.

fans out at the end closest to the ovary, and the open end has hairlike projections reaching toward the ovary. In a mature woman, the ovary releases an egg once a month (a process called ovulation), and the egg is waved into the fallopian tube by these projections. The egg travels along the tube toward the uterus, aided by muscular contractions. If sperm are present in the tube as a result of sexual intercourse, the egg can be fertilized, and the fertilized egg will continue to the uterus. See ECTOPIC PREGNANCY; REPRODUCTIVE SYSTEM, FEMALE.

Falls, in older people

The most common type of injury in older people. Falls are both more common and more serious for older people than for others and more frequently result in fractures.

Physiological changes associated with aging contribute to falls in older people. Typical examples include impaired vision or hearing, poor balance, slowing reflexes, loss of muscle strength and flexibility, DEMENTIA, chronic diseases such as

OSTEOARTHRITIS or diabetes mellitus (see DIABETES MELLITUS, TYPE 2), infection, and low blood pressure. Medications can cause dizziness and other changes that lead to falls.

A broken bone that results from a fall can be a critical injury for an older person. In hip fractures, hospitalization and surgery usually are required.

Even minor falls can lead to extensive injury in older people. If the head has been hit, dangerous bleeding can occur within the skull. The doctor may order imaging studies including X rays of bones, CT (computed tomography) SCANNING, or MRI (magnetic resonance imaging) to rule out a head injury.

Familial

Occurring more frequently among members of a family than would be expected by chance. The term is often used incorrectly to mean genetic.

Family medicine

Also known as family practice, the medical specialty that provides continuing and comprehensive care for a person or family. Its broad scope of care encompasses all organ systems and diseases and prevention of illness for people of any age and either sex. A family physician is a doctor who is educated and trained in family medicine or practice.

Family therapy

A form of psychological counseling that focuses on the entire family rather than an individual and is based on the belief that a person's emotional problems can best be understood and treated in the context of family behavior and communications.

Farmer's lung

A dust disease caused by inhalation of dust from moldy hay. Farmer's lung results from a reaction to exposure to a fungus known as *Thermoactinomyces vulgaris* (*T. vulgaris*) and occurs primarily in people who are sensitive to it. The symptoms may be acute, producing a flulike illness with a cough that resolves within a few days after exposure.

Farmer's lung causes abnormalities that appear on a chest X ray. Blood test results may reveal antibodies to *T. vulgaris*, and pulmonary function test results show restriction in lung function in the early phase of the disease and restriction combined with obstruction in the latter stage of the disease. Treatment consists of terminating a person's exposure to the moldy hay dust that causes the disease.

Farsightedness

A focusing (refractive) error of the eyes that makes it difficult to see close objects clearly; also known as HYPEROPIA. In most cases of farsight-

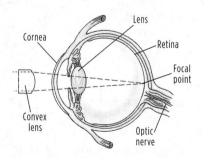

Correcting Farsightedness

When the eye is too short from front to back or the cornea is too flat, light rays focus behind the retina, causing difficulty seeing near objects.

edness, the eyeball is shorter from front to back.

Farsightedness is generally present at birth. Children often overcome mild farsightedness through the natural accommodation of the eye (changes in shape of the lens to see close objects). This ability diminishes with age, so glasses or contact lenses are commonly needed by farsighted adults. Farsighted people often have a narrower than normal angle between the iris and the interior surface of the cornea, which increases the risk for closed-angle glaucoma, a potentially sight-threatening disease. Regular testing for glaucoma is advised.

Fascia

Any fibrous connective tissues that lie under the skin, cover muscles or muscle groups, or enclose internal organs. Fascia surrounds many structures in the body to provide support and protection.

Fasciitis

A painful inflammation of the fibrous connective tissue, called fascia, that encloses the muscles. The condition often affects the tissues in the lower legs as a result of overuse or intense sports activities. Treatment usually involves rest, applying ice for pain relief, the use of special inserts into the heel portion of shoes, exercises to increase strength and flexibility of the foot, and corticosteroid injections. In severe cases, surgery may be necessary. See FASCIOTOMY.

Fasciotomy

Surgery involving an incision made into the fascia, or fibrous connective tissue, that encloses the muscles. The goal of the procedure is to relieve the pressure on the muscles that are causing pain. The surgery may be used to treat muscle swelling, often in the lower legs, from intense athletic activity. The procedure is generally not considered until it has been demonstrated that the symptoms of fasciitis will not respond to more conservative treatments, including orthotics (shoe inserts), cortisone injections, and physical therapy.

Fat, body

See ADIPOSE TISSUE.

Fatigue

Tiredness, lethargy, exhaustion, or lack of energy. Fatigue is usually a normal response to rigorous physical activity, stress, or a lack of sleep. However, it may also be a symptom of disorder such as DEPRESSION or EPSTEIN-BARR VIRUS.

Fats and oils

Fats are nutrients found in animal products and plant foods such as nuts, whole-grain cereals, seeds, avocados, and olives. Nutrition experts generally recommend that fats should constitute no more than 30 percent of an individual's total intake of calories each day. In addition, no more than 10 percent of daily calories should come from saturated fat. To lower the risk of heart disease and other health problems, doctors recommend that individuals reduce their total fat intake and replace some saturated fats with unsaturated fats. For individuals with atherosclerosis (arterial blockage from fat deposits), a diet even lower in fat content may be recommended.

No diet should be entirely fat-free. Fat is a source of stored energy for the body, and small quantities are needed for growth and repair. Fats or lipids also promote absorption of the fat-soluble vitamins A, D, E, and K in the intestines. However, fat contains more calories per unit than any other food.

Types of fats and oils

All fats and oils are mixtures of fatty acids: monounsaturated, polyunsaturated, and saturated. However, not all fats affect the body the same way. Certain fats are more healthful than others; fish oils and pure vegetable oils are healthier choices than animal fat, dairy fat, and hydrogenated oils. For example, some monounsaturated fats, such as olive oil and avocados, may even lower the risk of cardiovascular disease.

SATURATED FATS Fats that are solid at room temperature consist primarily of saturated fat. Common dietary sources of saturated fats include animal products such as meats, poultry, and dairy products, as well as coconut and palm oils. These fats (along with trans-fatty acids) are most responsible for high blood cholesterol levels and an increased risk of heart disease.

TRANS-FATTY ACIDS These fats are made in the hydrogenation process that solidifies liquid oils for use in preparation of many types of food products. Also known as trans-fats, trans-fatty acids are similar to saturated fats. They contribute to increased levels of harmful low-density lipoprotein (LDL) cholesterol, promote clogged arteries, and increase the risk of heart disease, so trans-fats should be avoided. Varying amounts of trans-fatty acids can be found in stick margarine, crackers, cookies, doughnuts, and deep-fried foods.

MONOUNSATURATED FATS
Monounsaturated fatty acids lower levels of harmful LDL cholesterol and have no negative effect on the helpful HDL (high-density lipoprotein) variety. Olive, canola, and avocado oils are good sources of monounsaturated fats, as are a variety of nuts: almonds, hazelnuts, macadamias, pecans, and pistachios.

POLYUNSATURATED FATS Found in corn, safflower, soybean, and sunflower oils, polyunsaturated fats lower total blood cholesterol even more than monounsaturated fats. However, they do so by lowering helpful, heart-protective HDL as well as harmful LDL cholesterol. Omega-3 fatty acids, another type of polyunsaturated fat, are found in deep-water fish such as salmon and tuna.

Fatty acids

Acids containing carbon, hydrogen, and oxygen that are found in fat. Some fatty acids cannot be manufactured by the body and must be consumed in food. These include linoleic, linolenic, and arachidonic acids, which are known as the essential fatty acids. Monounsaturated, polyunsaturated, and saturated fatty acids are different types of fats and oils found in food.

FDA

See FOOD AND DRUG ADMINISTRATION.

Febrile seizure

See SEIZURE, FEBRILE.

Fecal impaction

An accumulated hard mass of feces in the rectum. Fecal impaction results from constipation (infrequent bowel movements in which the feces are hard and dry). An enema may be needed to help a person with an impaction to have a bowel movement. If this proves unsuccessful, a physician may remove stool manually. Fecal impaction can be a symptom of a more serious disorder, especially when additional symptoms, such as weight loss, abdominal pain, or rectal bleeding, are present.

In many cases, only simple treatments, such as a change in diet or increasing fluid intake, is required. Because regular use of laxatives can make the colon inactive, they should be taken sparingly, if at all. Constipation that is due to an underlying problem, such as hemorrhoids or irritable bowel syndrome, requires appropriate treatment.

Fecal-occult blood test

A screening test to detect the presence of nonvisible (occult) blood in the feces. Blood in the feces can be a sign of serious disorders of the digestive system, including colitis, Crohn disease, and colorectal cancer (see COLON, CANCER OF THE; RECTUM, CANCER OF THE).

Feces

Excrement or stool discharged from the anus in a bowel movement. Feces are the solid waste that remains after food is broken down in the digestive tract (see DIGESTIVE SYSTEM). Feces that are an unusual color, contain blood, or are foul-smelling can be a symptom of a digestive disorder (see FECES, ABNORMAL; FECES, BLOOD IN THE).

Most people form and pass feces once a day. However, as many as three bowel movements a day or as few as three a week are considered normal. A change in the pattern of bowel movements can be the sign of a problem. See also BOWEL MOVE-MENTS, ABNORMAL.

Feces, abnormal

A sign of a disorder in the digestive system. There are many types of abnormal feces. Infrequent bowel movements that are hard and dry are the symptoms of CONSTIPATION. Three or more loose bowel movements a day are considered DIARRHEA. Chalk-colored feces may be a symptom of hepatitis (inflammation of the liver). Loose, greasy, strong-smelling feces that float may be due to malabsorption (impaired absorption of nutrients through the small intestine). Malabsorption can be a sign of such problems as CELIAC DISEASE (an inflammation of the small intestine due to an immune reaction to a protein found in grains), CROHN DISEASE, or PANCREATITIS (inflammation of the pancreas). Floating feces that are hard to flush are due to gas within the feces.

People who experience blood in the feces should seek immediate medical attention (see FECES, BLOOD IN THE).

Feces, blood in the

A sign of a possible gastrointestinal disorder. In many instances, blood in the feces is due to a minor problem, such as hemorrhoids. Sometimes, it is caused by a more serious disorder, such as COLITIS, CROHN DISEASE, or colorectal cancer (see COLON, CANCER OF THE; RECTUM, CANCER OF THE). Doctors recommend that anyone who experiences blood in the feces seek medical attention.

Blood in the feces may be visible, or it may be mixed in with the feces and not be visibly apparent. Therefore, doctors advise individuals older than age 50 to have a regular fecal-occult blood test to test for hidden traces of blood. Possible tests to determine the cause of blood in the feces include a GASTROINTESTINAL (GI) SERIES, GASTROS-COPY, proctoscopy, SIGMOIDOSCOPY, and COLONOSCOPY.

Feeding, infant

In a baby's first 4 to 6 months, either breast milk or formula can meet a child's nutritional needs. Cow's milk should not be given to babies younger than 1 year of age. Babies should be fed on demand. The younger and smaller an infant, the more frequently he or she needs to eat. Newborns do not take a great deal of formula or breast milk. Gradually, babies take larger amounts of breast milk or formula and go longer between feedings.

Although babies lose some weight after birth, most regain their birth weight by 2 weeks of age. In most cases, the baby correctly determines how much food he or she needs.

At around 4 to 6 months of age, solid foods are introduced. Most pediatricians recommend a single-grain cereal, such as rice cereal, as the first solid food. New foods—pureed table food or jarred baby foods—are slowly added, one at a time.

Fellatio

Oral stimulation of a man's penis with a partner's mouth and tongue. See ORAL SEX.

Female genital mutilation

The ritual cutting of parts of a girl's genitalia. A traditional practice in parts of Africa and Asia, female genital mutilation (FGM) marks a girl's achievement of womanhood. Two types of ritual cutting involve clitoridectomy, or removal of the CLITORIS. The immediate and long-term health consequences of this mutilation include excessive bleeding and shock at the time of circumcision, and the formation of abscesses, keloids (see KELOID), cysts, and scar tissue. Women who have undergone FGM often experience psychological trauma, recurrent urinary tract infections, dysmenorrhea (painful periods), chronic pelvic inflammatory disease, and painful sexual intercourse. The American Medical Association and the World Health Organization have condemned FGM as a form of child abuse and called on physicians not to perform the ritual.

Female sex hormones

See ESTROGEN.

Fertility

The biological capacity to reproduce.

Fertility drugs

See GNRH.

Fertilization

The union of an egg with a sperm. Fertilization produces the first cell of a zygote, with half of the genes from the mother and half from the father. The zygote becomes an embryo, which then develops into a fetus.

FESS

Functional endoscopic sinus surgery; a surgical treatment that uses endoscopes (lighted viewing devices of varying sizes for operating inside a cavity of the body) and is performed to promote sinus drainage. FESS may also be used to remove nasal polyps or to do a biopsy on a growth to see if cancer is present.

Most often FESS helps the sinuses drain more effectively. However, this procedure is reserved for people who do not obtain relief from nonsurgical treatment with medications.

Fetal alcohol syndrome

A group of birth defects that occur as a result of excessive alcohol consumed by a mother during pregnancy. The more a mother drinks during pregnancy, the more likely her baby is to develop fetal alcohol syndrome. Drinking heavily during the first trimester leads to the most severe problems. Babies have a 10 percent risk of developing the syndrome if their mothers drink more than an ounce of alcohol, or two drinks, a day; the risk doubles at two ounces of alcohol per day. Because of the concern that even small amounts of alcohol can cause neurological abnormalities, standard medical practice is to advise pregnant women to abstain altogether from alcohol throughout pregnancy.

In mild cases of fetal alcohol syndrome, the child's symptoms include irritability, difficulty in focusing attention, mild developmental delay, and sometimes hyperactivity. More severely affected babies may show developmental delay, hyperactivity, attention-deficit disorder, seizures, and severe mental retardation. Physical abnormalities associated with the syndrome include a small head, short upturned nose, narrowly spaced eyes, thin upper lip, clubfoot, characteristically creased palms, and cardiac defects. The syndrome is associated with higher-than-normal infant mortality.

The diagnosis of fetal alcohol syndrome is based on characteristic features in the child and a history of alcohol consumption by the mother during pregnancy. Newborns exposed to alcohol just before birth may show signs of withdrawal after delivery, including jitteriness, tremors, seizures, abnormal reflexes, disturbed sleep, decreased sucking, and low Apgar scores (a system for assessing the condition of newborns; see APGAR SCORE).

Fetal distress

Signs during labor that the well-being of a fetus may be compromised. Doctors and midwives often use fetal monitoring during labor to permit early detection of abnormalities that may endanger the fetus. The presence of more than one sign of fetal distress on the fetal monitoring tracing generally calls for taking a sample of the baby's blood from its scalp to test for pH level, which is a measure of acidity and alkalinity. A low pH level (less than 7.0) or other signs of distress call for immediate intervention, including cesarean section.

Fetal monitoring

Methods used by doctors to check a baby's heart rate and assess the baby's health before birth. There are two types of fetal monitoring: internal and external. No known risks are associated with external fetal monitoring. A minor risk of infection exists with internal fetal monitoring.

In external monitoring, a doctor presses a stethoscope or a handheld ultrasound device to a pregnant woman's abdomen to listen to a baby's heartbeat. To provide precise and continuous electronic monitor-

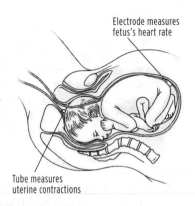

Electrode measures fetus's heart rate

Tube measures uterine contractions

Internal fetal monitoring
An electrode that measures the fetus's heart rate is attached to the fetus's scalp through the woman's vagina and cervix. Periodically, a thin tube is inserted through the vagina into the uterus to measure the mother's contractions.

ing, belts that measure the baby's heart rate and the length and frequency of contractions are placed around a woman's abdomen. The belts are connected to a machine that records and prints the information.

To internally monitor a fetus, an electrode is inserted through the mother's vagina and cervix. The electrode is attached to the baby's scalp to monitor the baby's heart rate. If a fetus has an abnormal heart rate, a blood sample may be taken from its scalp to check the oxygen supply. Internal fetal monitoring requires the rupturing of the amniotic sac, so it is usually done only when a woman is in labor.

Fetishism

A psychiatric disorder involving intense, repeated sexual urges or fantasies focused on nonhuman objects, most often articles of clothing.

Fetus

The product of conception, from the eighth week of pregnancy until birth. Before the eighth week, the fertilized egg is considered an embryo. A fetus in the eighth week is about 1 inch long. The fetus will grow rapidly and be ready to be born at about 40 weeks after conception.

Fever

Body temperature above the normal range, which is an orally taken body temperature of 98.6°F to 100°F in adults aged 18 to 40. Fever in children is measured at higher values because children have a slightly higher normal body temperature. A child is diagnosed with a fever when he or she has a temperature above 100.4°F when measured rectally, 100°F when measured orally or in the ear, or 99°F when measured under the arm. The body temperature rises in response to an attack on the body's immune system by agents such as bacteria or viruses.

Fever may last 24 hours or several weeks, depending on the cause. An elevated body temperature may be caused by any number of conditions or illnesses including common infectious diseases such as colds, flu, and gastroenteritis. Fever may also be caused by noninfectious disease including autoimmune disorders, inflammatory bowel disease, or some cancers.

Symptoms

The symptoms experienced when a person has fever include sweating, chills, shivering, headaches, aching muscles, loss of appetite, general weakness, fatigue, and possibly restlessness, dehydration, and rash. When fevers reach a very high level, symptoms may include confusion and other signs of mental dysfunction, extreme sleepiness, irritability, and seizures. In a small percentage of children, a rapid rise in fever may trigger seizures called febrile seizures. See SEIZURES, FEBRILE.

Most fevers are caused by bacterial or viral infections such as influenza, measles, or tonsillitis, but fever can also occur along with noninfectious conditions such as dehydration or tumors in the lymphatic system.

Diagnosis and Treatment

Most often the cause of fever is diagnosed by medical history, physical examination, and if needed a few simple tests. A medical history may include the time the fever began, immunization status, recent travel, exposure to people who are ill, and medications taken.

A physical examination may include observing the skin for signs of rash or infection and examining the person's lymph nodes, eyes, mouth, throat, and chest, too.

Diagnostic tests may be performed, including laboratory examinations of blood, urine, stool, or spinal fluid. X rays, scans, liver tests, and biopsies may be necessary to determine why a person has a fever.

When a fever is mild (below 102°F), it is generally treated by increased intake of fluids, which act as internal coolants and replenish vital salts; by restricting the person's diet to easily digestible foods; by bed rest and sleep to slow body functions and reduce the body's core temperature; and by taking medications that reduce fever. Adults may take NONSTEROIDAL ANTI-INFLAMMATORY DRUGS (NSAIDs), such as aspirin or ibuprofen.

Children may take acetaminophen or ibuprofen, which should lower the body temperature by about 2 degrees within 1 hour. Aspirin should not be taken by children younger than 18 years, as this medication is linked to Reye syndrome, a life-threatening neurologic disorder. Children with fever may be made more comfortable with tepid water sponge baths. Alcohol baths or rubs should never be used. Some health practitioners recommend using fever-reducing medication only when the child's fever is severe. A sustained body temperature of 106°F or above may result in brain damage.

A physician should be notified if milder fever persists for more than 24 hours or if associated symptoms become worse. Immediate medical attention is required for a fever of 105°F or higher or a fever accompanied by seizures, unconsciousness, a stiff neck, difficulty breathing, severe pain, swelling, blood in the stool, repeated vomiting, a discolored or foul-smelling discharge from the vagina or penis, or urinary tract symptoms.

When a fever is accompanied by severe headache and a stiff neck, meningitis may be the cause, and emergency attention is essential. Difficulty breathing associated with fever, or fever that is present with blood in the stool, urine, or mucus are considered medical emergencies.

Fever blister

A localized viral infection caused by the herpes simplex virus type 1. Fever blisters, also called cold sores, usually involve small areas of skin on the border of the lip, inside the mouth, on the gums or tongue, or on the inner surface of the cheeks. A primary infection is defined as the first time the virus infects the person. This usually occurs in childhood and may not even cause symptoms, although it often causes fever and blisters inside the mouth. Following the primary infection, the virus persists in the nerves near the affected skin in a dormant stage that is intermittently reactivated. Reactivation of the virus produces a fever blister and may be caused by factors including fever, emotional stress, poor nutrition, dental procedures, and sun exposure.

The first symptom of a fever blister is a sensation of tingling and itching in the affected skin. Swelling and redness in the area then occur, followed by the eruption of tiny blisters.

Fever blisters are diagnosed by examination and a medical history that explores factors that may have triggered the reactivation of the virus. Cells scraped from the infected area may be tested.

Fever blisters can be treated with antiviral medications, including acyclovir, which can reduce the amount of time symptoms last when taken early in the course of the illness.

Feverfew

An herbal remedy used for migraine, fever, and inflammation. Feverfew is a member of the chrysanthemum or sunflower family and has been used for centuries to reduce fever. It also may have a favorable effect on blood platelets, and it may be effective in the prevention and treatment of migraine headaches.

Fiber, dietary

Nondigestible substances found in plant foods such as fruits, vegetables, and grains. A diet high in fiber helps maintain proper bowel function and ·

prevents intestinal disorders ranging from constipation to irritable bowel syndrome. Certain types of fiber may also reduce the risk for cardiovascular disease, cancer, and diabetes. High-fiber foods include fruits and vegetables (especially with edible skins on), nuts, dried beans, and whole-grain breads and cereals. Although fiber itself provides no nutrients, the foods that contain it are rich in valuable vitamins and minerals.

Doctors recommend that people consume 20 to 35 grams of fiber each day. About one fourth of the total fiber consumed should be soluble fiber. However, many American adults consume much less than this. High-fiber foods are those that contain at least 2 grams of fiber per serving. Food choices should include 1 to 2 daily servings of good sources of soluble fiber.

Fibrillation

An extremely fast, chaotic heartbeat. Fibrillation reduces or eliminates the ability of the heart chamber to pump blood effectively, depending on what portion of the heart is affected. Fibrillation in the atrium (upper chamber) of the heart is known as atrial fibrillation. Fibrillation in the ventricle (lower chamber) is known as ventricular fibrillation, which is a life-threatening emergency that if not terminated abruptly can lead to death in minutes.

Fibroadenoma

A benign fibrous growth in the breast. Fibroadenomas are firm, solid lumps that contain no fluid and are usually freely movable when touched. See FIBROCYSTIC BREASTS.

Fibrocystic breasts

For symptom chart, see BREAST PAIN OR LUMPS, page xii.

Multiple painful, benign lumps and cysts in the breasts. Pain and lumpiness in the breasts occurs and increases toward the end of the menstrual cycle, when the cysts tend to enlarge. The size of the lumpy areas commonly fluctuates, and lumps may appear and disappear rapidly. Fibrocystic breasts are most common among women between the ages of 30 and 50 years and are rare in women after menopause. Symptoms usually subside after menopause.

A woman whose breasts contain fibrocystic lumps can be treated with needle aspiration, in which the lumps are drained. While fibrocystic breasts are not cancerous, there is a risk of breast cancer in women who have atypical cells lining the cysts. Women with fibrocystic breasts should examine their breasts carefully each month just after menstruation and inform their doctors of

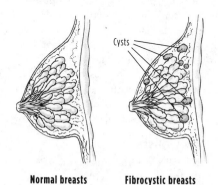

Normal breasts **Fibrocystic breasts**

Noncancerous, painful lumps
A fibrocystic breast contains small, benign cysts that give the breast a lumpy texture. The cysts tend to enlarge and become painful toward the end of the woman's menstrual cycle and can appear or disappear quickly.

any new lumps. To rule out cancer, the doctor may order a biopsy, in which tissue from the lump is examined microscopically. Mammography is also used to assess lumps, but is not always accurate in detecting cancer.

Fibroid, uterine

Benign growths in or on the uterus. Uterine fibroids, also known as myomas or leiomyomas, are the most common type of abnormal growth in a woman's pelvis. They occur in about 25 percent of women and are most common between the ages of 30 and 40 years. Among black women, fibroids are more common, occur at younger ages, and grow more rapidly. Most fibroids, even large ones, produce no symptoms, although some women experience pain in the abdomen and lower back, abdominal pressure, and more frequent urination. Changes in the amount, frequency, and duration of menstruation also may occur.

Fibroids vary in size from that of a pea to that of a grapefruit, sometimes growing so large they are mistaken for a pregnancy. They may become part of the inner or outer walls of the uterus, or they may hang from stems inside or outside it.

Diagnosis is based on clinical examination of the fibroids and, at times, on techniques such as ULTRASOUND SCANNING, LAPAROSCOPY, HYSTEROSCOPY, or HYSTEROSALPINGOGRAM. Treatment is not always necessary unless the fibroids cause excessive pain or bleeding, or if the doctor cannot distinguish the fibroid from a cancerous tumor. Very rarely, fibroids may become cancerous. When required, fibroids are removed surgically.

Fibroma

A benign or nonmalignant tumor composed largely of fibrous connective tissue. These smooth, usually painless, growths under the skin or in the bone are often caused by injury or infection. Doctors recommend medical evaluation of any unexplained lump or swelling.

Fibromyalgia

A common condition that produces stiffness and pain in the fibrous tissues deep in the muscles. Aching and fatigue along with a slight swelling of the muscles may also be symptoms. Fibromyalgia produces multiple tender areas in specific muscles, including those of the neck, shoulders, upper back, lower back, and hips. The cause is unknown, but it does not affect joints. Sleep disturbance, clinical depression, headache, and emotional stress may be associated with the condition.

Fibromyalgia is diagnosed on the basis of symptoms, especially persistent, widespread muscular pain, and the physician's discovery of tenderness in specific areas of muscle. Laboratory tests and X rays are normal but may be ordered to exclude conditions such as HYPOTHYROIDISM, lupus erythematosus, RHEUMATOID ARTHRITIS, and infections, all of which may mimic fibromyalgia. While there is no cure for the condition, it often improves on its own and does not damage the muscle tissue. Pain can sometimes be managed with aspirin or other NONSTEROIDAL ANTI-INFLAMMATORY DRUGS (NSAIDs) and by taking hot baths. If pain is severe, an injection of the anesthetic lidocaine or a corticosteroid is sometimes helpful. Massage, stretching, and range-of-motion exercises may also help relieve symptoms. A physician may treat fibromyalgia with medications that promote sleep and relax muscles or with antidepressant medications.

Fifth disease

A common infection of childhood caused by parvovirus B19; also called erythema infectiosum. Fifth disease is an illness that produces a mild fever and a redness of the skin formed by tiny red eruptions that may vary in intensity. This gives the person with the infection a "slapped cheek" appearance that may progress from a pale rosy hue to a bright red. Eventually, a lacy, netlike pattern of color develops on the skin of the face, arms, and trunk. Fifth disease gets its name from being one of the five common childhood infections that cause fever and a rash. The others are measles, mumps, chickenpox, and rubella (German measles).

Early in the illness before the rash appears, an infected person may have symptoms of a common cold and can spread the illness to others who are susceptible and come in contact with the infected secretions. Frequent hand washing is recommended to prevent spreading the infection. People who have been infected with parvovirus B19 develop immunity to the disease and cannot be reinfected.

Fifth disease is most often diagnosed by observation of the characteristic rash during physical examination by a doctor.

The illness is usually mild, and symptoms generally improve on their own in healthy children and adults within 10 days. During the course of the illness, fever, pain, or itching can be treated. Infected adults who develop joint symptoms may need to rest, restrict activities, and use aspirin or ibuprofen.

People who have certain medical conditions may develop acute, severe anemia from parvovirus B19 infection; symptoms include paleness, weakness, and fatigue. This group may include persons with sickle cell disease or other types of chronic anemia. In these cases, medical treatment is necessary.

Filling, dental

The restorative material used to fill a dental cavity caused by tooth decay or to replace part of a chipped or broken tooth. The fillings may be composed of silver amalgam or of tooth-colored materials, made of dental composite or ceramic.

Fistula

Abnormal passageway between two hollow organs or leading from a hollow organ to the outside of the body. A fistula is often caused by infection or injury, as when an abscess in the rectum bursts, thereby creating an opening between the anal canal and the surface of the skin. A fistula may also develop as a complication of surgery or may be congenital (present at birth).

Flail chest

A chest wound involving three or more ribs broken in two or more places, thus destabilizing a segment of the chest wall. Flail chest, which usually occurs after a severe crushing chest injury, is characterized by motion that is the reverse of

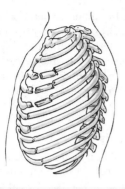

Unstable chest wall
When ribs are broken in several places on the same side of the chest (side view), a portion of the muscular chest wall will move independently of the rest of the wall.

normal—the loose chest segment moves inward when the person breathes in, outward when he or she breathes out; thus, the chest is not moving air effectively. Other symptoms include shortness of breath, extreme pain, and bluish skin. Flail chest is a medical emergency requiring immediate attention.

Flatulence

The expulsion of air from the digestive tract through the anus. Flatulence is also known as flatus. Lower intestinal gas is the result of bacterial fermentation of food residue in the colon. Approximately a half quart of gas is produced by the body each day. Management of flatulence depends on its cause. It is often helpful to eat fewer gas-producing foods or to exercise more to encourage passage of gas through the digestive tract. In some cases, medications are recommended or prescribed to relieve gas. If lactose intolerance is producing excess flatu-

lence, doctors suggest decreasing the intake of milk and dairy products or taking a supplement containing lactase, the enzyme that digests milk sugar. Flatulence is rarely a symptom of a serious disease. See also BOWEL MOVEMENTS, ABNORMAL; FECES, ABNORMAL.

Floaters

Small specks, threads, circles, cobwebs, clouds, or other shapes moving in a person's field of vision. Floaters are most easily seen against a plain background, like a blank wall or the sky. They are actually small clumps of material that form inside the clear jellylike fluid (vitreous) filling the cavity of the eye and cast shadows on the retina (the thin layer of light-sensitive tissue at the back of the eye). Floaters may be annoying, but they require no treatment. If a new floater appears suddenly, if the number of floaters increases, or if quick flashes of light also appear, these symptoms can signal damage to the retina (see RETINAL DETACHMENT), which requires prompt medical attention to prevent vision loss.

Floppy infant

A group of symptoms giving a child a floppy, loose-limbed appearance. All newborns are somewhat floppy because their muscles are still developing. However, infants who are especially limp should be examined by a physician promptly, since floppiness can be a sign of serious illness in infants.

Flu

A contagious disease caused by a virus. See INFLUENZA.

Fluorescein angiogram

A diagnostic test that uses a dye to analyze circulation in the eye. After eye drops that dilate the pupil are administered to the person being tested, pictures of the interior of the eye are taken with a special camera. Next, fluorescein dye is injected into a vein in the arm or hand, and more photographs are taken. The dye, which glows green under special light, outlines the blood vessels of the eye and allows the eye specialist to visualize them and to detect areas of leakage. The fluorescein angiogram is useful for diagnosing a number of eye diseases that affect the back (fundus) of the eye, including diabetic retinopathy (see RETINOPATHY, DIABETIC), damage from high blood pressure (HYPERTENSION), MACULAR DEGENERATION, optic disc edema, and retinitis pigmentosa, and for determining the effectiveness of treatment.

Fluoridation

The addition of fluoride to the public water supply as a way to decrease the incidence of tooth decay. Fluoridation has been endorsed by the American Dental Association since the first community fluoridation program began in 1945.

Fluoride

A naturally occurring mineral known to help prevent tooth decay. See also FLUOROSIS.

Fluoroquinolones

Antibiotics used to treat bacterial infections that affect many different parts of the body. First introduced in the United States in the 1980s, fluoroquinolones such as ciprofloxacin work by killing bacteria or preventing their growth. They are powerful antibacterials with broad-spectrum activity able to treat infections of bones and joints and infections in the respiratory, genital, and gastrointestinal tracts.

Fluorosis

A condition that changes the color and texture of the tooth enamel (see ENAMEL, DENTAL) as a result of excessive exposure to fluoride.

Folic acid

A water-soluble B vitamin essential to growth and cell repair. (See also VITAMIN B.) Adequate folic acid is required for a healthy pregnancy, DNA and RNA synthesis, and building red blood cells. A combination of folic acid and vitamins B6 and B12 can reduce the blood level of homocysteine, an amino acid that is associated with an increased risk of diseases related to the heart and blood vessels. However, it is not known if taking folic acid supplements reduces the chance of a heart attack.

Adults require at least 400 micrograms (0.4 milligrams) of folic acid daily. These minimal requirements double during pregnancy. Folic acid deficiency in pregnancy is associated with severe birth defects of the spine and brain known as neural tube defects, so folic acid is included in prenatal vitamin and mineral supplements.

In the United States, the most common dietary sources of folic acid are fortified commercial cereals, enriched breads, fruits, orange juice, and dried beans. Most folic acid in foods occurs as folate.

Follicle

A pouchlike depression or pore, such as the openings in the skin through which hair grows.

Follicle-stimulating hormone

See FSH.

Fontanelle

One of two soft areas on an infant's head where the skull bones have not yet joined. The fontanelle that is located at the top of an infant's head usually closes by 14 months. In most children, the fontanelle at the back of the head is closed at birth. In others, it closes by 3 or 4 months of age. Normal handling and washing of an infant does not harm the fontanelles. A baby's soft spot normally bulges when he or she is crying. However, a fontanelle that is firm and bulging when a baby is not crying can indicate that the brain is under pressure from HYDRO-CEPHALUS, an accumulation of fluid; an infection; or a tumor. A sunken fontanelle may indicate dehydration. It is important to consult a pediatrician in these cases.

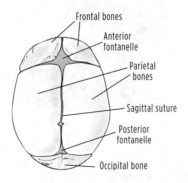

Soft spots
The skull is formed by several platelike bones that join at immovable joints called sutures. A fontanelle is a soft area on an infant's head where the bones of the skull have not yet fully joined.

Food additives

Chemicals added to food as preservatives, sweeteners, colorants, flavorings, or antioxidants. Thousands of food additives exist, and most are safe. Some, however, cause adverse reactions in susceptible individuals. Signs of a problem include headaches, hives, abdominal cramps, diarrhea, chest tightness, light-headedness, lowered blood pressure, and weakness. An allergist can help individuals identify food additives to which they are sensitive.

Food allergy

A specific response of the immune system to a specific food or food component to which a person is sensitized. Food allergies result when the immune system produces a large number of antibodies to attack the food that a person has ingested. This response releases histamine, which causes the symptoms of food allergies. Food allergens are generally proteins within the food that are not completely broken down by the digestive process. They may then be released from the gastrointestinal lining, enter the bloodstream, and cause allergic reactions throughout the body.

An allergic reaction to a food may begin at the first bite with an itching sensation in the mouth. ANAPHYLAXIS can occur when sensitized people eat peanuts, fish, eggs, or grains. The most common symptoms of food allergies include abdominal pain, diarrhea, nausea, and vomiting. Hives and swelling beneath the skin, or eczema (see DER-MATITIS) may also result from food allergies. There may be swelling of the lips, eyes, face, tongue, and throat. Nasal congestion and asthma may be symptoms of the allergy, and sometimes the affected person faints. If these symptoms are severe, or if anaphylaxis results, immediate emergency medical attention is essential and may be lifesaving.

Diagnosing a food allergy is generally aimed at pinpointing the specific food or food components that produce the allergic reaction and distinguishing a food allergy from food intolerance.

A skin scratch test, which involves introducing a small amount of food extract into the surface of the skin, may be used to identify a specific allergen. Blood tests called immunoassays that check for antibodies specific to certain foods can be useful for excluding possible food allergens.

Treatment of food allergies is based on learning which foods cause them so they can be avoided. In some cases, it is a simple matter of eliminating these foods from the diet.

Food and Drug Administration

Also known as the FDA, a regulatory government agency that is part of the US Department of Health and Human Services. The mission of the FDA is to protect the public health by helping safe and effective products reach the market in a timely manner and by monitoring products for continued safety once they are in use. The FDA regulates products ranging from medical devices and drugs to food ingredients and cosmetics.

Food Guide Pyramid

A chart developed by the US Department of Agriculture to illustrate the relative amounts of the different foods that should be consumed daily to achieve a balanced diet. The Food Guide Pyramid promotes balanced meals, moderation, and variety in food choices, with special emphasis given to grain products and vegetables. The pyramid image is used to represent relative amounts that individuals should consume from each food group. The revised pyramid published in 2005 is divided into vertical segments, with grains (bread, cereal, rice, pasta) and vegetables the segments with the most daily servings. The pyramid divides foods into five groups and indicates how many servings (newly stated in ounces or cups) from each group should be eaten daily.

Because women are generally smaller and require fewer calories than men,

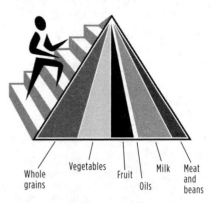

Dietary guidelines

The US Department of Agriculture created this new version of the Food Guide Pyramid recently to illustrate the types of foods that are needed daily for good health and to encourage people to be physically active each day.

smaller servings are usually more appropriate for them. One side of the new food pyramid shows a person climbing steps to remind people that exercise is another vital component of fitness, in addition to good nutrition.

Food intolerance

A response to food that may produce symptoms similar to those of a FOOD ALLERGY but does not involve the immune system or the production of antibodies in the body. Food intolerance is usually caused instead by a missing digestive enzyme, IRRITABLE BOWEL SYNDROME, emotional anxiety, or contamination of the food eaten. The symptoms generally experienced occur primarily in the gastrointestinal system and may include nausea, vomiting, abdominal pain, and diarrhea.

Food intolerance may be difficult to diagnose in part because a person may be sensitive to a substance or ingredient used in the preparation of the food rather than the food itself. Lactose-containing foods, wheat, certain vegetables, wine, monosodium glutamate (see MSG), sulfites, and salicylates fall into this category.

Food poisoning

An illness with vomiting, diarrhea, and abdominal pain that is caused by ingesting contaminated food or liquid. The contaminants can be bacterial or viral and can cause outcomes ranging from upset stomach to death. The signs of food poisoning vary according to their cause. In addition to vomiting, diarrhea, and pain, symptoms may include severe cramping, fever, and chills. Types of bacterial food poisoning include botulism, *Escherichia coli* (*E. coli*), *Campylobacter*,

listeriosis, and *Salmonella*. Toxins produced by staphylococcal infections can also cause food poisoning. In healthy adults, mild attacks often clear up spontaneously. However, food poisoning poses a special danger to very young children, older people, pregnant women and their fetuses, and anyone with a compromised immune system.

Diarrhea that persists for longer than 48 hours or is accompanied by other symptoms (such as fever, chills, or vomiting) requires medical attention.

Treatment varies according to the cause of the problem. Generally, doctors advise rest and drinking clear fluids until symptoms subside. Because diarrhea can quickly deplete body fluids and crucial body salts, oral rehydration fluid (see REHYDRATION FLUID, ORAL) may be required. Specially prepared commercial solutions containing water, salts, and glucose are available over-the-counter at pharmacies. In serious cases of dehydration, intravenous fluids are required.

Over-the-counter medications may relieve symptoms of diarrhea. In severe cases, the doctor may prescribe narcotic-like or antispasmodic drugs to slow intestinal activity and ease cramping. However, medications to reduce the contraction of the intestines should not be used in cases of bloody diarrhea.

To prevent food poisoning, all meats must be thoroughly cooked to destroy infectious organisms. Precooked and partially cooked foods also need to be completely reheated.

Food-drug interaction

An event in which foods and drugs consumed at about the same time alter the ability of the body to use one or the other; a side effect caused by the interplay of foods and drugs. Certain foods are known to interact with specific drugs in undesirable ways. For example, grapefruit juice and some drugs used to treat high blood pressure do not mix well; consuming calcium channel blockers and grapefruit juice may lead to headaches and light-headedness. A pharmacist should be consulted about any questions, and notes attached to a prescription drug will mention any known adverse interaction with food.

Foot

The mobile structure, beginning at the ankle, that supports and stabilizes the weight of the body and helps propel the body forward in walking or running.

Footdrop

An abnormal neuromuscular condition often caused by damage to the nerve that extends into the foot. In footdrop, there is an inability to flex the foot. Consequently, it catches on the ground when walking. Most cases of footdrop are caused by external pressure or trauma to the peroneal nerve or by pressure on the nerve as it exits the spinal column, as can occur with a herniated disk. Treatment depends on the underlying cause. A foot-drop splint can be used to keep the foot in a fixed position while walking.

Foramen

An opening, such as a hole in a bone through which a nerve passes.

Forceps delivery

A birth in which forceps (tonglike instruments) are used in the delivery of a baby. The forceps blades are placed on both sides of the baby's head; gently, the baby is pulled from the birth canal. Forceps are used during a prolonged labor or when a baby, far along in the birth canal, needs to be delivered quickly because of fetal distress.

Forensic medicine

The branch of medicine that applies medical knowledge to legal areas, chiefly to criminal cases. Forensic medicine is usually used to study injuries related to accidental trauma, chemicals, and violence, in order to establish the cause of a sudden or unexpected death.

Foreskin

The loose fold of skin that covers the tip (or glans) of the penis; also known as the prepuce. During the first months or years of a boy's life, the foreskin naturally separates from the tip of the penis. If the penis becomes erect, the foreskin moves back to expose the tip. The foreskin may be surgically removed in a procedure called circumcision. See CIRCUMCISION, MALE.

Formaldehyde

A gaseous compound that is a strong disinfectant. Formaldehyde is used in solution as a disinfectant and as a preservative and fixative for laboratory specimens. As a gas, formaldehyde is both toxic and carcinogenic (cancer-causing) if inhaled or absorbed through the skin. Inhaling formaldehyde can exacerbate ASTHMA.

Formulary

A list of approved pharmaceutical products; a collection of formulas for medicinal preparations.

Fracture

The medical name for a broken bone, referring to a break or crack in a bone or in cartilage. There are two basic types of fracture: a compound (open) fracture and a simple (closed) fracture. A compound or open fracture involves a broken bone that ruptures the skin, exposing the bone. This is a more serious fracture, which requires emergency medical attention, because it allows germs to reach the bone and cause infection. A simple or closed fracture is a broken bone that does not break through the skin and is not visible on the surface. The term single fracture indicates that one

break has occurred in a bone; multiple fractures means more than one break in the same bone. A fracture is called complete if the bone is broken straight through, and incomplete, or greenstick, if the break does not extend through the complete width of the bone shaft, sometimes involving bending or crushing of the bone. Greenstick fractures most commonly occur in young children whose bones are more pliable.

The usual symptoms of a bone fracture include intense localized pain, tenderness, swelling, and possibly a deformed appearance. When the skin has been ruptured in open or compound fractures, antibiotics may be administered to ward off potential infection. In many cases, the break in the bone leaves two bone segments that are separated by the fracture but remain in the proper anatomical relationship to each other. When the fractured bone or bones are not properly aligned, which is called a displaced fracture, treatment includes realignment of the sections of broken bone in a procedure medically termed reduction. This may be achieved by stretching, traction, or external manipulation.

In some cases, surgery may be necessary to realign and attach the bone segments in a procedure called open reduction in which screws, wires, or metal plates are used to join the sections of bone and hold them in place. The aligned bones' position is held in place by a plaster cast or a splint worn externally to hold the bones immobile. The newly created tissue contains minerals that harden into new bone. See also ARM, FRACTURED; LEG, FRACTURED; JAW, FRACTURED; HIP, FRACTURED; and RIB, FRACTURED.

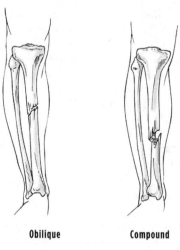

Obilique   **Compound**

Two types of bone fracture

An oblique bone fracture is an angled break across the bone, usually the result of a direct blow. In a compound fracture, the force of the break knocks apart the broken ends of the bone and layers of skin are penetrated.

Fragile X syndrome

An inherited genetic condition that is a leading cause of mental retardation. Fragile X syndrome results from an altered gene on the long arm of the X chromosome. Mothers are carriers of the condition, and their sons are at risk of being affected with the disorder, while their daughters are at risk for being carriers and are usually only mildly affected intellectually. A male with fragile X syndrome inherits it from his mother, who has a 50 percent chance of passing it on to her baby, since she has two X chromosomes.

Physical features associated with fragile X syndrome include a long, narrow face and prominent ears, jaw, and forehead. Enlarged testicles and loose finger joints are also seen in some cases. The physical features are more noticeable after puberty and are often less prominent in females.

Developmental delay is a common sign of fragile X syndrome in early childhood. Delayed speech and language skills and behavioral difficulties such as hyperactivity occur frequently. Some children with fragile X syndrome may also demonstrate autistic-like behavior, such as unusual hand gestures, repetitive speech, and refusal to interact with others.

DNA testing is used to diagnose fragile X syndrome. Laboratory analysis of blood cells will identify those with fragile X chromosomes for GENETIC COUNSELING. Fragile X syndrome does not have a cure. Medical care is recommended for related conditions.

Friedreich ataxia

Also known as spinocerebellar degeneration, an inherited disease characterized by progressive dysfunction of the cerebellum, spinal cord, and peripheral nerves. Friedreich ataxia is the most common form of inherited ataxia; hereditary ataxias are a group of diseases affecting the nervous system and consequent problems with balance, gait, movement, and speech.

In Friedreich ataxia, damage to structures in the cerebellum and spinal cord results in a gradual loss of coordination and balance. Symptoms generally begin in childhood or in the early teen years. One of the earliest symptoms is an unsteady gait that makes walking difficult. The ataxia gradually worsens and spreads to the arms and trunk. Later symptoms include muscle weakness, eye tremor, speech problems, clubfoot, hammer toes, flexion (involuntary bending) of the toes, foot inversion (turning in), and scoliosis (curving of the spine to one side). Severe scoliosis can affect breathing, and there may also be chest pain and heart palpitations. Most people with this disease eventually are confined to a wheelchair.

Diagnosis is made through careful physical examination, medical history, and tests such as ELECTROMYOGRAPHY and genetic testing. There is no cure. Physical therapy, braces, and surgery may be helpful in coping with orthopedic difficulties.

Frostbite

A condition occurring when areas of skin and underlying tissue freeze in cold weather. Frostbite is classified into four degrees of severity:

• *FIRST-DEGREE FROSTBITE*, or frostnip, is a superficial injury in which the skin turns white and is temporarily numb. No blistering is likely.

- *SECOND-DEGREE FROSTBITE* is deeper and more serious; outer skin layers are frozen and hard, while underlying tissue is still intact. Blistering is likely to occur.
- *THIRD- AND FOURTH-DEGREE FROSTBITE* freeze all layers of the skin and the underlying tissues. The skin becomes solid and hard and appears blue and white and blotchy. Skin may blister. If blood vessels freeze, gangrene (dead tissue) may appear and amputation may be necessary.

Frostbite usually occurs without pain in its later stages. Frostbite should not be treated until it is certain that the area will not refreeze. Any wet clothing should be removed. First aid measures include immersing affected areas for 20 to 30 minutes in water that is warm rather than hot or applying warm cloths to frostbitten areas such as the ears, nose, and cheeks. Affected areas should not be rubbed. Warming is complete when the skin is soft and sensation is restored. Warm fluids should be consumed.

Frozen shoulder

A painful condition, medically termed adhesive capsulitis, resulting in greatly restricted mobility of the shoulder joint. The pain may intensify at night.

Frozen shoulder may be the result of an injury to the shoulder or injury to another body part that prevents normal movement of the shoulder. Frozen shoulder has also been known to follow recovery from a heart attack and to occur following surgery for conditions not involving the shoulder. In many cases, the cause is unknown. One theory suggests the involvement of an autoimmune reaction, in which the body's defense system erroneously perceives a threat from its own tissues and begins to attack them. The tissues of the shoulder's joint capsule respond to the attack with a severe inflammatory reaction. Normally the tissue that encloses this joint capsule is loose and allows the shoulder a wide range of relatively unrestricted movements. When this tissue becomes inflamed, it sticks together and limits or prevents movement of the shoulder.

Frozen shoulder is diagnosed from symptoms, history, and physical examination. In general, routine X rays will not reveal the problem, but an arthrogram or MRI scanning can reveal scarring and contraction of the shoulder joint capsule.

Recovery from a frozen shoulder may take months. Anti-inflammatory medication is often prescribed to decrease the inflammation. Physical therapy, emphasizing stretching exercises, may be prescribed to regain movement in the shoulder. Injected cortisone with a long-acting anesthetic can help to control pain and inflammation to assist the person in stretching.

Fructose

A simple sugar or monosaccharide. Pure fructose naturally occurs in fruits, where it combines with glucose to form sucrose. Like other sugars, fructose is a carbohydrate that provides calories but few other nutrients.

FSH

Follicle-stimulating hormone. FSH is a hormone released by both women and men from the pituitary gland at the base of the brain. In women between puberty and menopause, the monthly menstrual cycle begins when FSH is released and transported by the blood to one of the ovaries. FSH stimulates the ovary to release a mature egg in the process called ovulation. FSH also signals the ovary to begin forming a follicle, which is a tiny cavity that holds and supports each egg. The female hormones estrogen and progesterone and a small amount of male hormones, called androgen hormones, are produced and secreted in response to stimulation of FSH. These hormones have a vital role in the reproductive cycle. In men, FSH stimulates the testicles to produce sperm.

Functional endoscopic sinus surgery

See FESS.

Functional improvement

The progress toward normalized activity in the musculoskeletal, neuromuscular, cardiovascular, or respiratory system of an individual who has been injured or debilitated by disease.

Fundoplication

Surgery that creates a new junction or valve between the esophagus and the stomach by wrapping the uppermost portion of the stomach (the fundus) around the lower end of the esophagus. Fundoplication is performed to treat gastroesophageal reflux disease (GERD), a common cause of severe heartburn.

Fungal infections

See MYCOSIS.

Fungi

A diverse group of organisms that obtain food by absorbing nutrients directly. With bacteria, they are responsible for the decay and decomposition of organic matter. Fungi may also cause mold-related illnesses in people who spend substantial amounts of time in water-damaged buildings. Some fungi are parasites on living organisms, including humans, and can cause serious infections and diseases.

Fungi also have beneficial medical uses. For example, antibiotics such as penicillin, which are now produced by nonfungal microorganisms, were originally derived from a fungus.

Furuncle

See BOIL.

G

G6PD deficiency

Glucose-6-phosphate dehydrogenase enzyme deficiency is a common inherited disorder that can cause anemia. G6PD deficiency is found more often among males, blacks, Italians, Greeks, Asians, and people of Mediterranean ancestry. Approximately 10 to 14 percent of black American males are affected.

Individuals with G6PD deficiency may not become anemic or have symptoms unless the red blood cells are exposed to certain chemical compounds or foods. Symptoms may include fatigue, pale skin color, shortness of breath, rapid heart rate, jaundice (yellow skin color), dark urine, and enlarged spleen. Treatment involves discontinuing the offending drug or compound, and recovery is usually complete. Blood transfusions are sometimes needed.

Gait training

A type of physical therapy used to help a person walk again after any orthopedic or neurological illness or when he or she has a chronic instability of gait.

Gallbladder

A pear-shaped organ of the DIGESTIVE SYSTEM, located just below the LIVER. The gallbladder stores and concentrates bile produced in the liver, then releases it into the duodenum, the first part of the small intestine. Bile is a substance necessary for digestion. Although the gallbladder has a useful role in digestion, it is not absolutely necessary because the liver can secrete bile directly into the duodenum. As a result, the gallbladder can be removed without harm when, for example, GALLSTONES form.

Gallbladder cancer

A rare cancer that originates in the gallbladder. Symptoms are typically intense abdominal pain and indigestion. An individual who experiences abdominal pain, unintentional weight loss, diminished appetite, fever, nausea, or jaundice (yellowing of the skin and the whites of the eyes) should contact a doctor. The only known cure is surgical removal of the gallbladder, if the cancer has not yet spread to other organs.

Gallium scan

A NUCLEAR MEDICINE scanning procedure involving the injection of radioactive gallium. Gallium is a rare bluish white metallic element that accumulates in areas of inflammation and certain tumors. A gallium scan is generally used to help diagnose Hodgkin disease and to locate abscesses, inflamed areas, and some types of tumors.

Gallstones

Hard masses made primarily of cholesterol that can develop in the GALLBLADDER where BILE is stored. Gallstones usually result from an imbalance in the chemical composition of bile. They range in size from a grain of sand to the size of a golf ball. Most are composed primarily of cho-

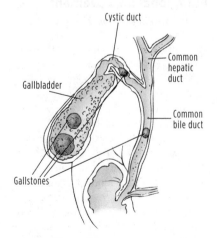

Where gallstones lodge
Gallstones travel out of the gallbladder and either pass out of the body unnoticed or lodge somewhere between the gallbladder and the small intestine.

lesterol, a fatlike substance that is excreted by the liver. Excess dietary cholesterol may be a factor in stone formation. A smaller proportion of stones are made up of bilirubin and calcium salts.

More than half of the individuals who have gallstones do not have symptoms. However, if a gallstone blocks the bile duct, it can cause BILIARY COLIC, or severe pain in the upper middle or right part of the abdomen. CHOLECYSTITIS, or inflammation of the gallbladder, may develop as the result of the blockage.

Pain from a gallstone may disappear on its own if the stone falls back into the gallbladder or is forced through the duct into the intestines. If the obstruction of the bile ducts persists and prevents bile from entering the intestines, increased pressure in the liver can result in jaundice (a yellowing of the skin and the whites of the eyes). Less frequently, pancreatitis (inflammation of the pancreas) occurs as a result of gallstones.

Gallstones may be diagnosed through ULTRASOUND SCANNING or ERCP (endoscopic retrograde cholangiopancreatography). If ERCP reveals a gallstone lodged in a duct, tiny instruments can be threaded down the endoscope to remove it. Less commonly, CHOLECYSTOGRAPHY and cholescintigraphy tests are performed.

The preferred surgical treatment of gallstones is laparoscopic CHOLECYSTECTOMY, which is a procedure to remove the gallbladder by using a fiberoptic viewing instrument.

Gambling, addictive

A pathological inability to suppress the impulse to gamble that results in severe personal, domestic, and vocational consequences, sometimes ending in financial ruin or divorce. Addictive gambling, which typically begins in adolescence, is considered an addiction because the attraction to the gambling behavior has the same characteristics as addiction to alcohol or a drug: loss of control, preoccupation, narrowing of interests, dishonesty, guilt, and repeated relapse.

Treatment options include individual and group psychotherapy, as well as self-help support groups such as Gamblers Anonymous, which is a TWELVE-STEP PROGRAM similar to Alcoholics Anonymous.

Gamete intrafallopian transfer

See GIFT.

Gamma globulin

A protein found in the blood that helps fight infection; also, a substance prepared from a mixture of proteins in the fluid portion of blood.

Gamma globulin can be used to quickly boost short-term immunity and improve the immune systems of people who have been exposed to serious infectious illnesses, including hepatitis A and measles. Gamma globulin medication is usually given by injection in a doctor's office.

Gamma knife radiosurgery

A technique developed in the 1990s that delivers a high dose of radiation to a precise target in the skull without cutting into the area. Gamma knife radiosurgery is used in neurological procedures, along with a local anesthetic, for treatment of malignant brain tumors, benign brain tumors, vascular abnormalities in the brain, and trigeminal neuralgia (a painful nerve disorder of the face).

Ganglion

A cyst that most commonly appears under the skin on the side of the wrist, hand, or the top part of the foot. They occur when a gel-like substance that leaks from a joint capsule accumulates and balloons out to form an external swelling or cyst. Ganglia are generally harmless and painless or only mildly painful, and they rarely impede movement of the wrist or foot. A doctor may determine that no treatment is necessary, or the decision may be made to aspirate or draw fluid from the cyst and sometimes to inject a corticosteroid drug. If these treatments are not successful, surgery may be considered.

Gangrene

A condition in which a tissue of the body dies because of blockage of arterial blood supply. Gangrene develops, most commonly in the extremities, when the blood supply to the affected body part is cut off due to infection, a blood clot in an artery, vascular disease such as arteriosclerosis, trauma due to accident or surgery, severe frostbite, or the vascular collapse that may accompany diabetes mellitus. Gangrene is most dangerous when it affects the intestines or stomach.

Symptoms may include blackened skin with underlying dead tissue of the muscle and bone, crinkling of the skin, swelling, pain or numbness in the affected area, fever, and possibly a discharge from open sores.

Gangrene is generally curable in the early stages. It is treated in a hospital setting with efforts to improve circulation to the impaired area and surgery to remove the dead tissue, sometimes by amputation when necessary. Antibiotics are given intra-venously in the early stages of gangrene to fight infection. Pain relievers and anti-coagulants to prevent blood clotting are also given. Bed rest is required until healing begins.

Gangrene can be fatal and, in severe cases, may necessitate amputation. Other possible complications of gangrene include blood poisoning, shock, and a blood-clotting disorder called disseminated intravascular coagulation.

Garlic

A plant used as a spice and as a medicinal herb to lower cholesterol levels and blood pressure.

Gastrectomy

Surgical removal of the stomach. A partial gastrectomy is the removal of part of the stomach, and a total gastrectomy is the removal of the entire stomach. A partial removal is most commonly performed to treat noncancerous stomach or duodenal ulcers, as well as stomach cancer that is low in the stomach near the duodenum. A total gastrectomy is required in some cases of stomach cancer and when ulcers that fail to respond to nonsurgical treatment bleed uncontrollably or perforate the stomach wall. The advent of new medical treatments for ulcer disease has made gastrectomy for ulcers far less common.

Gastric

Pertaining to, relating to, or originating in the stomach.

Gastric erosion

A superficial raw area in the mucous membrane that lines the stomach. Gastric erosion is a relatively common problem. The main symptom is bleeding of the affected area, although symptoms may not always be present. In rare severe cases, bloody vomiting may occur. Unlike a GASTRIC ULCER, there is no danger of gastric erosion penetrating or perforating the stomach lining. However, if internal bleeding persists, anemia will eventually result.

Gastric erosion is sometimes caused by the use of nonsteroidal anti-inflammatory drugs (NSAIDs), corticosteroid drugs, or the bacterium HELICOBACTER PYLORI. Gastric erosion also develops in people recovering from severe injuries or burns and in those under prolonged stress.

Treatment depends on the underlying cause. A physician may prescribe alternative drugs that are less irritating to the stomach lining or recommend taking drugs in combination with an antacid or acid-suppressing medication. See also GASTRIC ULCER.

Gastric lavage

See STOMACH PUMPING.

Gastric ulcer

A sore or wound in the mucous membrane lining the stomach. Gastric or stomach ulcers are a form of PEPTIC ULCER DISEASE. Gastric ulcers can develop anywhere in the stomach, but are most often located on the stomach's lesser curve or in the lower half of the stomach. The most common symptom of a gastric ulcer is upper abdominal pain that tends to be intermittent, burning, and gnawing and occurs a half hour to 2 hours after meals.

Evidence strongly suggests that in most cases the damage to the protective mucous lining of the duodenum is caused by bacterium HELICOBACTER PYLORI. Other factors that have a role are long-term use of nonsteroidal anti-inflammatory drugs (NSAIDs), heavy use of alcohol, and smoking.

Diagnosis is based on a variety of investigations, including blood tests, breath tests, an upper GASTROINTESTINAL (GI) SERIES (an X-ray procedure also called a BARIUM SWALLOW), or GASTROSCOPY (a visual method that can also take samples of tissue from the esophagus, stomach, and duodenum).

Medications have a vital role in treating gastric ulcers. Doctors prescribe drugs that reduce acid secretion, such as histamine blockers, proton pump inhibitors, or drugs that coat the lining of the duodenum and stomach with a protective layer to prevent acid from reaching the ulcer. A medical regimen called triple therapy (the use of three medications at once) can eradicate most cases due to *H. pylori* bacteria; the three medications are two ANTIBIOTICS and usually one of the PROTON PUMP INHIBITORS. Lifestyle modifications are also useful.

When a gastric ulcer fails to respond to treatment or if complications develop, surgery may become necessary. The most frequently performed surgery for gastric ulcers is a partial GASTRECTOMY, in which the lower part of the stomach is removed.

Gastritis

Inflammation of the mucous membrane lining the stomach. Gastritis may be sudden and acute, or chronic (persistent over a long period). In most cases, it exhibits no symptoms, but can cause indigestion, nausea, and vomiting. Gastritis is occasionally accompanied by GASTRIC EROSION, a superficial raw area in the mucous membrane that lines the stomach. Contributing factors can include bacteria, viruses, substances that damage the protective mucous lining of the stomach, the bacterium HELICOBACTER PYLORI, alcohol use, heavy smoking, heavy use of nonsteroidal anti-inflammatory drugs (NSAIDs), or side effects of other drugs.

Gastritis is diagnosed by physical examination, medical history, gastroscopy (visual examination of the esophagus, stomach, and duodenum through a lighted tube), or an upper GASTROINTESTINAL (GI) SERIES (an X-ray procedure also called a BARIUM SWALLOW).

Treatment of gastritis depends on its underlying cause. A physician may change a medication if it is causing side effects. Although no single medication has proven effectiveness against *H. pylori*, a medical regimen called triple therapy (the use of three medications at once) can eradicate most cases; see GASTRIC ULCER.

Gastroenteritis

Inflammation of the stomach and intestines as a result of infection. The symptoms of gastroenteritis include nausea, vomiting, diarrhea, severe cramping, weakness, and fever. Persistent diarrhea may also lead to DEHYDRATION, upsetting the body chemistry and depleting important body salts. Left untreated, dehydration can lead to shock.

Most frequently, gastroenteritis is caused by viruses, such as the adenovirus, coxsackievirus, and rotavirus. But it may be due to eating or drinking contaminated food or water; food poisoning may occur in a lone individual or as an epidemic when a number of people consume the same contaminated food. Changes in the bacterial population of the digestive tract due to taking antibiotics or traveling to a foreign country can also bring on gastroenteritis. See also DIARRHEA, E. COLI; DIARRHEA, TRAVELER'S.

Within 48 hours, most cases of gastroenteritis clear up without medical intervention. If symptoms persist, medical attention is necessary.

To treat gastroenteritis, physicians advise resting and drinking oral rehydration fluid. If gastroenteritis is caused by bacteria, antibiotics may be prescribed. No specific treatment exists for viral gastroenteritis. However, in severe cases, the doctor can prescribe drugs that slow intestinal activity and ease cramping, or antiemetic drugs to control violent vomiting.

Gastroenterology

The study of diseases, disorders, and conditions of the gastrointestinal tract, including the esophagus, stomach, small intestine, colon, liver, gallbladder, pancreas, and bile ducts. A gastroenterologist is a physician, usually board certified, who specializes in treating the gastrointestinal tract.

Gastroesophageal reflux disease (GERD)

See ESOPHAGEAL REFLUX.

Gastrointestinal (GI) series

A series of X rays using the contrast medium barium. An upper GI series uses X rays to diagnose problems in the esophagus, stomach, and duodenum (the first part of the small intestine into which the stomach empties). To prepare for the test, an individual drinks a chalky barium solution that coats and outlines the walls of the esophagus, stomach, and duodenum. Barium makes the linings of these organs show up more clearly on X rays. An upper GI series can detect problems such as a blockage, abnormal growth, ulcer, hernia, or accumulation of scar tissue. This series is also known as a barium swallow.

A lower GI series uses X rays to examine problems in the large intestine, which includes the rectum and colon. A lower GI series can reveal problems such as abnormal growths, ulcers, polyps, diverticula, and inflammation. This series is often called a barium enema, because the contrast medium is a thick liquid containing barium that is inserted anally to pass into the colon and rectum.

Gastrointestinal system

See DIGESTIVE SYSTEM.

Gastrointestinal tract

See DIGESTIVE SYSTEM; GALLBLADDER; STOMACH.

Gastrojejunostomy

A surgically created connection between the stomach and small intestine that is specifically designed to bypass the duodenum (the first part of the small intestine into which the stomach empties). A surgeon performs a gastrojejunostomy to prevent gastric acid from causing further irritation to a DUODENAL ULCER.

Gastroscopy

A procedure in which the linings of the esophagus, stomach, and duodenum are examined by using a slim, flexible, lighted tube called a gastroscope. Gastroscopy is a type of ENDOSCOPY that enables the physician to view, photograph, and videotape the inside of the body without surgery. A gastroscopy may be performed to help determine the cause of dysphagia (difficulty swallowing), nausea, vomiting, INDIGESTION, ESOPHAGEAL REFLUX (the backward flow of stomach acid into the esophagus), bleeding, abdominal pain, or chest pain. Gastroscopy may also be used in the emergency diagnosis and management of bleeding. Gastroscopy is more sensitive than X rays, so the physician can detect abnormalities that may not appear on radiographs.

Gastrostomy

A surgical procedure in which an external opening, or STOMA, is created in the stomach. The stoma provides a passageway through the abdominal wall for a temporary or permanent tube. The tube may be used for either feeding or drainage.

Gay

A slang term for homosexual. See HOMOSEXUALITY.

G-CSF

Granulocyte colony-stimulating factor; a chemical that fosters the development of the white blood cells known as granulocytes. This growth factor is used to treat people with leukopenia (a very low white blood cell count), particularly after bone marrow transplant or intensive chemotherapy for cancer.

Gender-identity disorder

Acting and presenting oneself as a member of the opposite sex, combined with strong feelings of discomfort in one's own physical gender, for a period of at least 2 years. This rare disorder appears in both children and adults.

Gene

The fundamental unit of genetic inheritance within a chromosome; a segment of DEOXYRIBONUCLEIC ACID (DNA) containing a sequence of biochemical information that determines a particular genetic trait. The sequence is called the genetic code. Each DNA molecule contains many genes and is located within the cell nucleus. Each gene contains the instructions to synthesize a specific protein that has a specific function. RIBONUCLEIC ACID (RNA) works as a messenger that carries the genetic instructions to a site in the outer cell where protein is manufactured.

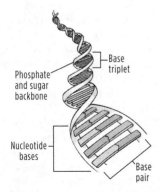

Phosphate and sugar backbone

Base triplet

Nucleotide bases

Base pair

Basic unit of heredity
Genes direct the function of all body organs and processes by regulating the production of many types of essential proteins.

Gene therapy

Changing the function of some genes in order to treat, cure, or prevent disease. Gene therapy is a largely experimental approach to the treatment of disease that involves replacing or counteracting a person's faulty gene. Potentially, it may be an alternative way to aid the production of proteins such as insulin and growth hormones. Gene therapy is intended to correct certain diseases at their most fundamental level and has been compared to the transplantation of a tiny organ.

Research into gene therapy has been limited to the targeting of specific cells known as somatic (body) cells. The recipient's genetic makeup is altered by the treatment, but the change is not passed along to subsequent generations.

General anesthesia

See ANESTHESIA, GENERAL.

Generic drug

A drug that is not protected by a trademark; the scientific name for a drug as opposed to its proprietary or brand name. Generic drugs contain identical active ingredients and amounts as the brand-name equivalents, but they are usually less expensive.

Genetic code

The biochemical language by which all known organisms transfer genetic information. DNA (DEOXYRIBONUCLEIC ACID) contains the genetic code to communicate the information or instructions that allow specific genes to function. A genetic code is present in all animals, plants, fungi, bacteria, and viruses.

Genetic counseling

A process in which individuals or families at risk for genetic disorders can learn about the disorders and the options for dealing with them. Genetic counseling can also help couples assess their risks of having children with genetic disorders.

Genetic disorders

Medical conditions caused by errors in genetic material. Some genetic disorders cause medical problems that are apparent at birth, while others do not show up until later in life. Some genetic disorders, such as CYSTIC FIBROSIS, can be so severe that they ultimately cause death, while others, like color blindness, produce mild symptoms. Genetic disorders can be rare or common.

Genetic engineering

Alteration of an organism's hereditary material to eliminate undesirable characteristics or to create desirable new ones. Examples of genetic engineering include selective breeding of plants and animals and the creation of hybrids by combining elements of different strains or species to create new ones. Genetic engineering is used to increase food production, to produce vaccines and other drugs, and to help eliminate industrial waste.

Hybridization, or crossbreeding, has been performed for at least 3,000 years. Hybrids featuring the most desirable qualities can be created from members of the same species with different characteristics or from members of different species. Mules, for example, are created by breeding female horses with male donkeys.

The newest method by which genetic engineering is implemented is RECOMBINANT DNA, or gene splicing. In this method, one or more genes of an organism are introduced into a second organism. If the DNA is incorporated into the second organism, recombined DNA is said to exist.

Genetic probe

Fluorescence in situ hybridization (FISH) testing. A test of DNA (DEOXYRIBONUCLEIC ACID) designed to identify the presence of genetic defects in a person or, usually, a fetus. In a genetic probe, a particular fragment of DNA is examined for genetic markers, specific base sequences (chemical configurations) that have been associated with a genetic defect. Genetic probes can be used to detect the presence of DOWN SYNDROME, CYSTIC FIBROSIS, TRISOMY 21 SYNDROME, and such chromosomal abnormalities as TURNER SYNDROME.

Genetic screening

Medically testing members of a population for individuals who have genes associated with a disease; a form of preventive medicine. Because many diseases are passed from generation to generation, genetic screening is used to detect disease by identifying persons who are at risk.

Various types of genetic screening are used, including prenatal screening such as AMNIOCENTESIS, newborn screening, and screening tests for individuals with genetic susceptibility to environmental hazards or with genes for a specific inherited illness such as Huntington disease.

Genetics

The branch of biology that is concerned with genes and heredity. Genetics involves the study of the origin of an individual's characteristics and the manner in which they are passed along to offspring. Medical genetics is the study of the relationship between heredity and disease.

Genital herpes

See HERPES, GENITAL; SEXUALLY TRANSMITTED DISEASES.

Genital ulceration

A lesion or sore on the external genitals, including the vulva, labia, penis, and anus. Genital ulcerations are caused by one of several infectious organisms, most of which are spread by sexual contact. They require medical attention to prevent the development of later complications and should not be self-treated.

The more common infections that can cause a genital ulceration include SEXUALLY TRANSMITTED DISEASES, LYMPHOGRANULOMA VENEREUM (LGV), CHANCROID, and SYPHILIS. See also CHANCRE.

Genital warts

Warts that develop in the genital area, including the urethra and the rectum, that are caused by HUMAN PAPILLOMAVIRUS (HPV). Genital warts are one of the most common of the SEXUALLY TRANSMITTED DISEASES. See also CONDYLOMA ACUMINATUM.

Genitalia

The male and female reproductive organs, both external and internal. The male genitalia include the penis, testicles, prostate gland, seminal vesicles, and system of ducts. The female genitalia include the ovaries, fallopian tubes, uterus, vagina, mons pubis, clitoris, and labia. See REPRODUCTIVE SYSTEM, FEMALE; REPRODUCTIVE SYSTEM, MALE.

Genotype

The entire genetic makeup of an individual.

Geriatric medicine

A medical specialty concerning the treatment of older people. A geriatrician is a physician specially trained in the care of older people.

Germ

Any tiny, living, disease-causing agent; the term often describes disease-producing microorganisms, such as bacteria and viruses.

Germ cell tumor

A tumor that develops in the reproductive tissues that become egg cells or sperm cells. Germ cell tumors are a type of ovarian cancer or testicular cancer.

Germ cell tumors sometimes can be identified through two blood tests: the alpha-fetoprotein (AFP) and the human chorionic gonadotropin (HCG) tests. They are usually treated with chemotherapy. They constitute one of the few groups of solid tumors that can be cured with chemotherapy even after the disease has metastasized (spread) to other organs. Certain combinations of drugs will cure up to 70 percent of patients with metastatic germ cell tumors.

German measles

See RUBELLA.

Gerontology

The scientific study of all aspects of the aging process, from clinical, biological, historical, mental, and sociological perspectives. A gerontologist is a physician who specializes in gerontology.

Gestation

Pregnancy; the period of time during which a fetus develops in the uterus, from conception to childbirth. The average time span for gestation is 266 days, or 38 weeks, from the date of fertilization. Since that date is rarely known, doctors traditionally measure gestation from the beginning of the mother's last menstrual period, calculating the baby's due date as 280 days, or 40 weeks, from that point. A pregnancy that results in a birth within 2 weeks of the predicted due date is called a term pregnancy.

Gestational diabetes

A form of diabetes that has its onset or is first diagnosed during pregnancy. In this condition, the pancreas is unable to produce enough insulin to counteract the hormones produced during pregnancy that increase the sugar level in the blood. Women who are older than 30 years, obese, have a family history of diabetes, or have had problems with a pregnancy before, such as a stillbirth or an unusually large baby, are considered to be at risk for gestational diabetes. About 5 percent of pregnant women develop this condition, usually between the 24th and 28th weeks of pregnancy.

Gestational diabetes is diagnosed with a GLUCOSE TOLERANCE TEST and initially treated with diet and exercise. For women whose blood sugar level remains high after 1 to 2 weeks of diet and exercise, insulin may be required. After delivery, women with gestational diabetes are at risk for developing diabetes in the future and should be monitored. Risk factors for diabetes that can be modified, such as obesity and a sedentary lifestyle, should be addressed.

Gestational trophoblastic disease

A group of pregnancy-related conditions in which abnormal growths develop inside the uterus from abnormal placental tissue. (See PLACENTA.) The conditions include a hydatidiform mole, a type of tumor, and the cancer choriocarcinoma, both of which involve trophoblasts, cells that make up one of the layers of the placenta. Symptoms include vaginal bleeding and excessive morning sickness early in pregnancy. The doctor may find that the uterus is larger than expected for the stage of the pregnancy, and there may be no detectable fetal heartbeat.

Gestational trophoblastic disease is usually treated by removing the contents of the uterus during a D AND C. If a woman has completed her childbearing years, a hysterectomy may be performed. After both procedures, the woman's blood is tested for human chorionic gonadotropin every 1 to 2 weeks until levels are normal, and thereafter at 3-month intervals for 6 to 12 months to make sure the tumor has been completely removed from the uterus. Choriocarcinoma is also treated with CHEMOTHERAPY, almost always successfully.

GI series

See GASTROINTESTINAL (GI) SERIES.

Giant cell arteritis

See ARTERITIS, GIANT CELL.

Giardiasis

A disease caused by the microscopic parasite called *Giardia lamblia* (*G. lamblia*) that lives in the small intestines of humans and animals. The cysts of the parasite in its infectious stage are passed out of the body in bowel movements. These cysts are environmentally resistant and can live outside a person or animal for long periods. *Giardia lamblia* exists throughout the world and is found in soil, food, water, and on contaminated surfaces. *Giardia lamblia* is one of the most common causes of waterborne illness in humans living in the United States. It is spread when a person accidentally ingests the parasite.

Transmission occurs by swallowing water containing cysts of the parasite or by eating uncooked, unwashed food that is contaminated.

People who become infected with giardiasis may have no symptoms, or they may have mild symptoms, which may include intermittent flatulence and watery diarrhea, mild abdominal cramps, and bloating. In more serious, acute infections, the symptoms can include severe and chronic diarrhea, abdominal cramps, and nausea. Associated symptoms may include fever, chills, malaise, and headaches.

Diagnosis is generally made by laboratory evaluation of a stool sample and blood tests.

The illness is treated with one of several prescription medications available. It is recommended that people who have acquired the infection without symptoms be treated to help prevent spreading it to others.

GIFT

Gamete intrafallopian transfer. GIFT is an ASSISTED REPRODUCTIVE TECHNOLOGY (ART) in which sperm and unfertilized eggs (gametes) are placed in a fallopian tube for normal fertilization. The advantages of this procedure over IN VITRO FERTILIZATION are that embryos develop in their natural environment and reach the uterus at the right time. GIFT is the only form of ART officially approved by the Roman Catholic Church because fertilization occurs within the body (in vivo).

Gingiva

The medical term for the gums. The tops of the teeth, or natural crowns, develop within the gingiva, grow outward from it, and are attached by the cementum, or tissue covering their roots. The gingiva has a rich supply of blood vessels that become red and inflamed if not properly cleansed and stimulated by flossing and using a rubber pick.

Gingivectomy

A minor surgical procedure to remove deep pockets of infected gum tissue or to surgically trim excess gum tissue that has grown over part of the natural crown in a tooth.

Gingivitis

See PERIODONTAL DISEASE.

Ginkgo biloba

Extracts from the leaves of the ginkgo tree used as an herbal medicine. Ginkgo biloba is used to treat many conditions. Its chief attributes include the claim—as yet clinically unproven—that it stabilizes tissue membranes, particularly in the brain, and enhances the use of oxygen and glucose. Its primary clinical use has been in the treatment of vascular problems, such as insufficient artery function in the brain caused by ATHEROSCLEROSIS (hardening of the arteries). By increasing cerebral blood flow, ginkgo biloba may reduce symptoms associated with aging, including short-term memory loss and depression.

Gland

An organ or collection of cells forming a structure that produces and releases chemical substances, principally hormones and enzymes. The substances are released into the system of the body by the glands for a variety of purposes. See also EXOCRINE GLAND.

Glands, swollen

A lay term that refers to enlarged lymph nodes, also called lymph glands. Swollen glands may be caused by an infection, an injury, a dental abscess, or reaction to a medication. When the swelling is gradual and painless, it may result from a tumor. (See also LYMPHOMA.)

Sore, swollen glands usually begin to improve within a few days. Lymph glands generally swell rapidly during the early stages of fighting infection and tend to take longer to return to their normal size. Medical attention is recommended if the glands do not decrease in size over a period of several weeks, if swollen glands are red and tender, if they are located behind the ears and occur with a scalp infection, or if they continue to swell for 2 to 3 weeks. If it appears that the swollen glands are the result of a bacterial infection, treatment usually consists of antibiotics.

Glass eye

See EYE, PROSTHETIC.

Glaucoma

An eye disease characterized by damage to the optic nerve and loss of vision. Often glaucoma is a result of high pressure in the eye.

Types

There are several major forms of glaucoma:

CHRONIC (OPEN-ANGLE) GLAUCOMA This is the most common form of the disease. It takes its name from the fact that the angle between the iris and cornea remains open and looks normal, although the drainage system in the front of the eye is blocked or fails to function properly. Pressure rises slowly in the eye, gradually affecting the optic nerve. The early stages of the disease are painless and produce no symptoms. Visual loss becomes apparent only as nerve damage progresses and blind spots appear in the field of vision. In most cases, chronic glaucoma affects both eyes.

ACUTE (ANGLE-CLOSURE) GLAUCOMA This form of the disease comes on very suddenly, causing significant pain and visual effects. The name comes from the fact that the angle between the iris and the cornea closes and prevents normal drainage of aqueous humor. Acute glaucoma usually affects only one eye. An attack of acute glaucoma occurs most commonly during conditions in which the pupil is dilated, such as in a darkened movie theater or as a result of stress. An acute glaucoma attack is an emergency that requires immediate attention. Untreated, the eye can be permanently damaged in as little as 1 or 2 days. Laser surgery is used to clear the blockage and restore normal flow of aqueous humor.

SECONDARY GLAUCOMA This form of the disease develops as a complication of other diseases or medical conditions. Secondary glaucoma is associated with advanced cataracts (cloudiness in the lens of the eye); eye surgery; inflammation of the eye (uveitis); certain eye tumors; traumatic eye injuries; diabetes mellitus, type 1 and type 2; and corticosteroid medications. In one form of the disease, pigmentary glaucoma, pigment flakes off the iris and blocks the trabecular meshwork.

CONGENITAL GLAUCOMA This form of the disease is present in newborns at birth. It results from abnormal development of the eyes that results in a drainage defect. Surgery to repair the faulty drainage may be effective, but cases of glaucoma at birth have a poor prognosis.

Risk factors and screening

Acute glaucoma is most common in older people and in people who are farsighted. Chronic glaucoma is most common among people older than 50 years with a family history of the disease; those who are of African or Asian descent; those with nearsightedness, previous eye injury, or diabetes mellitus; and those who have used corticosteroid medications for a long period. There are no effective measures for preventing glaucoma. Rather, the key is detecting the disease in its early stages and beginning treatment before visual impairment occurs.

The frequency of glaucoma testing depends on risk factors. People who have no risk factors and are younger than 45 years should be tested every 4 years. Testing every 1 to 2 years is recommended for people in the same age group who have risk factors. For people 45 years or older, testing every 2 years for those with no risk factors is advised; for those with risk factors, testing at least every year is best.

Treatment

With acute (angle-closure) glaucoma, treatment usually consists of surgery (iridotomy) to open the closed angle as soon as possible. Surgery is also the usual treatment for congenital glaucoma.

For chronic (open-angle) glaucoma, medicated eye drops are usually the first form of treatment. Various forms of medication are used to decrease pressure within the eye. If the medication fails to work or the side ef-

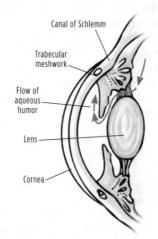

Open-angle glaucoma
While the exact cause of open-angle glaucoma is unknown, the flow of aqueous humor is obstructed somewhere at the level of the trabecular meshwork just before the canal of Schlemm.

fects are intolerable, laser surgery is an option. The third alternative is traditional surgery or trabeculectomy.

Glioblastoma multiforme

The fastest-growing and most malignant type of BRAIN TUMOR; a type of GLIOMA. Glioblastoma multiforme is a malignant tumor of nervous tissue, usually found in the cerebrum area of the brain. Symptoms can include seizures and signs of brain disturbance. The tumors are treated with surgery or surgery with radiation therapy.

Glioma

A brain tumor arising from the glial cells, which form the supporting tissues of the central nervous system. Gliomas are known by the names of the several cell types from which they develop. Like other brain tumors, gliomas can lead quickly to an increase in pressure inside the skull. Symptoms resulting from the pressure and the tumor can vary greatly, depending on the location and size of the growth. They may or may not include headache, vomiting, double vision, partial paralysis, loss of sensation, seizures, and personality changes.

Treatment is usually surgical removal of the tumor, often followed by radiation therapy. Success of the treatment depends on the location and accessibility of the tumor and the degree to which it has infiltrated various parts of the brain. Gliomas can vary greatly in their rate of growth and degree of malignancy.

Global warming

An average increase in the Earth's temperature, which in turn causes changes in climate. A warmer Earth may lead to changes in rainfall patterns and a rise in sea level and may have a wide range of effects on humans, wildlife, and plants.

Global warming could threaten human health through increases in heat-related mortality and illness resulting from expected increases in heat waves. See also HEAT EXHAUSTON; HEAT STROKE.

Glomerulonephritis

The group of kidney diseases characterized by inflammation and sometimes gradual and progressive destruction of the glomeruli (the filtering units of the kidneys). The damaged structures within the kidney may result in excessive leakage of protein into the urine and may affect the capacity of the kidneys to filter toxic waste products, water, and salt.

The damaged glomeruli associated with glomerulonephritis may also permit red blood cells and other substances to leak into the urine, making the urine a reddish or darker color. When large amounts of protein are lost in the urine, fluid retention and high blood cholesterol levels may result.

In mild cases, there may be no symptoms of glomerulonephritis. Symptoms that can develop include high blood pressure, swelling around the eyes, aching in the lower part of the back, reduced urination, and dark or reddish urine. If large amounts of protein are lost in the urine, generalized swelling may result, especially in the face, abdomen, lower legs, ankles, or feet.

Treatment generally includes diuretics (medications that aid in the excretion of salt and water) if there is swelling, high blood pressure medication, and dietary changes. It may be necessary for the person to take immunosuppressive medications to decrease the activity of the immune system. If glomerulonephritis results in a loss of the filtering function of the kidneys, resulting in KIDNEY FAILURE, medical treatment may include DIALYSIS or a KIDNEY TRANSPLANT.

Glomerulonephritis can have a number of causes, including STREP THROAT, particularly in young children. See also NEPHRITIS.

Glossectomy

Partial or complete surgical removal of the tongue to treat cancer of the tongue.

Glucagon

Substance used to treat severe hypoglycemia (low blood sugar level). Glucagon is a hormone that stimulates release of glucose from the liver and is an important part of the body's process of regulating blood sugar levels. Glucagon can be given by injection to reverse severe insulin-induced hypoglycemia.

Glucocorticoids

See CORTICOSTEROIDS.

Glucosamine-chondroitin

A popular nutritional supplement used to treat osteoarthritis. Both glucosamine and chondroitin are found naturally in the joints, where they are assumed to be involved in joint repair: glucosamine is thought to stimulate the formation of cartilage, and chondroitin is believed to stimulate cartilage repair and inhibit enzymes

involved in the breakdown of cartilage. The evidence is that these substances are safe and do reduce the symptoms of arthritis, especially pain.

Glucose metabolism

The chemical processes through which the body makes use of glucose. Glucose, a simple sugar or monosaccharide, is the body's chief source of energy. When consumed, CARBOHYDRATES are broken down by digestive juices into simple sugars. These simple sugars are absorbed from the intestines, where some are stored as glycogen while the rest enter the blood as glucose where they can be used by cells for energy and growth.

Complex carbohydrates (starches) provide more lasting sources of energy than simple carbohydrates (sugars) because they are absorbed and released into the blood more slowly. Simple sugar carbohydrates such as sucrose and lactose are rapidly broken down by the body and take only minutes to reach the bloodstream as glucose or galactose.

Following digestion, glucose passes into the bloodstream to be used by the brain, muscles, red blood cells, and fat tissue. However, in order for glucose to enter cells, the pancreas must release the hormone known as insulin. Specific insulin receptors on cells bind insulin, which signals the cell to increase the uptake of glucose into the cell and metabolize glucose.

Diabetes mellitus is a disorder of glucose metabolism. See DIABETES, MELLITUS, TYPE 1; DIABETES, MELLITUS, TYPE 2; and DIABETES, GESTATIONAL.

Glucose meter

A device that enables people to monitor their blood glucose levels on a regular basis. Glucose meters are generally used by people with type 1 diabetes and sometimes by people with type 2 diabetes who require insulin (see DIABETES MELLITUS, TYPE 1; DIABETES MELLITUS, TYPE 2). The person using the meter extracts a drop of blood, usually by pricking a fingertip, and places it on a specially coated strip. The strip is inserted into the glucose meter, which offers a digital reading of the blood sugar level in a matter of seconds.

Glucose meters, when used properly, are considered the most accurate means of self-monitoring of the blood sugar level.

Glucose tolerance test

A test of the body's ability to process glucose. The test involves ingesting a measured amount of glucose and monitoring subsequent levels of glucose in the blood over a period of hours. See GLUCOSE METABOLISM.

Gluten

A protein found in grains such as wheat, rye, and barley. Gluten gives bread dough its tough, elastic character. In CELIAC DISEASE, the lining of the small intestine is damaged by an allergic reaction to gluten.

Glycemic index

A ranking of food sources of carbohydrates based on their immediate effect on blood sugar levels. A high glycemic index indicates rapid absorption of glucose from that food, while a low glycemic index indicates a slow absorption of glucose. See GLUCOSE METABOLISM.

Glycogen

A carbohydrate made up of glucose. Glycogen is the principal form in which carbohydrate is stored in the body, the same way that starch is stored in plants. Glycogen is stored in the liver and the muscles and is readily broken down into glucose.

Glycosuria

The excretion of abnormally large amounts of glucose in the urine; also known as renal glycosuria. In pathologic glycosuria, large amounts of glucose appear in the urine for considerable periods. Pathologic glycosuria usually results from diabetes mellitus and occurs when the pancreas fails to produce sufficient INSULIN or the body is resistant to the insulin it makes (type 2 diabetes). This causes an abnormally high blood sugar level, leading to frequent or continuous elimination of glucose in the urine. When the blood sugar level is normal, glycosuria may be caused by the failure of certain cells in the kidneys to reabsorb glucose as urine is produced. The defect in itself is not harmful.

GM-CSF

Granulocyte-macrophage colony-stimulating factor; a chemical that stimulates the development of the white blood cells known as granulocytes and of macrophages in the bone marrow. White blood cells are found throughout the body and are important in the body's defense against invading microorganisms and other foreign matter. GM-CSF is used to treat people with leukopenia (a very low white blood cell count), particularly after bone marrow transplant or intensive chemotherapy for cancer.

GnRH

Gonadotropin-releasing hormone. GnRH is secreted by the hypothalamus. Release of GnRH signals the pituitary gland to secrete gonadotropic hormones, including FSH (follicle-stimulating hormone) and LH (luteinizing hormone) into the bloodstream. Gonadotropic hormones are essential for male and female fertility. They stimulate cell activity in a woman's ovaries and a man's testicles.

Women who are unable to conceive may be given synthetic GnRHs.

Synthetic GnRHs may also be used to treat endometriosis.

Goiter

A painless enlargement of the thyroid gland that causes a visible swelling in the neck. Some but not all goiters are associated with excess production of thyroid hormone, and most goiters are not malignant (cancerous). A goiter can be barely noticeable or as large as a grapefruit.

A small goiter that does not affect thyroid function usually requires no treatment. If the goiter does not shrink on its own, synthetic thyroid hormone medication may be prescribed to signal the pituitary to make less TSH (thyroid-stimulating hormone). Suppressing TSH levels has the effect of stabilizing the size of the thyroid gland and preventing further enlargement. If TSH therapy is ineffective and the goiter continues to grow, surgery may be considered.

Otherwise, treatment is generally directed at the specific cause of the goiter.

Gold compounds

Drugs used in the treatment of rheumatoid arthritis and other conditions. Gold compounds are given by injection to treat rheumatoid arthritis not adequately treated by other anti-inflammatory drugs. Gold sodium thiomalate is also used to treat psoriatic arthritis and Felty syndrome, a form of rheumatoid arthritis that includes splenomegaly (enlarged spleen) and leukopenia (reduced white blood cell count).

Gold compounds are thought to work by altering the immune system to reduce inflammation. Gold compounds are associated with serious side effects and must be taken only under close medical supervision.

Golfer's elbow

An overuse injury, most commonly caused by the repetitive force placed on the tendon that attaches to the inside part of the elbow joint during a golf swing. The part of the elbow joint involved in golfer's elbow is called the medial epicondyle, and the medical term for golfer's elbow is medial epicondylitis.

Symptoms of golfer's elbow may include tenderness and pain on the inside of the elbow. The pain may spread into the forearm. Any activity that involves flexing the wrist or gripping with the hand will engage the flexor muscles and increase the elbow pain. Self-help treatments include icing the sore area to decrease inflammation and relieve pain. An elbow strap or brace may help decrease symptoms. Exercises that help maintain muscle strength without overstressing the tendon may be helpful as the area heals and the pain lessens. Nonsteroidal anti-inflammatory drugs (NSAIDs) may be recommended to reduce inflammation. In some cases, cortisone

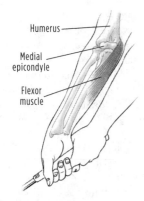

Humerus

Medial epicondyle

Flexor muscle

Strain on the inner elbow
The flexor muscles in the forearm attach to the inner knob (medial epicondyle) of the bone of the upper arm (humerus) at the elbow. Golfer's elbow is an inflammation or small tear in the tendon that attaches these muscles to the bone.

may be injected into the inflamed area to decrease inflammation and pain.

Gonadotropin hormones

The hormones regulating the levels of estrogen and progesterone in the body. The hypothalamus produces GnRH (gonadotropin-releasing hormone) in response to declining levels of estrogen at the end of the menstrual cycle. When estrogen levels are low, production of GnRH increases markedly. See GNRH.

Gonads

The sex glands—the ovary in the female and the testicle in the male—that produce reproductive cells and sex hormones. In a woman, the ovaries produce eggs and the female hormones estrogen and progesterone; in the male, the testicles produce sperm and the male hormone testosterone.

See REPRODUCTIVE SYSTEM, FEMALE; REPRODUCTIVE SYSTEM, MALE.

Gonioscopy

Ocular examination of the front portion (anterior chamber) of the eye. Gonioscopy is used primarily for viewing the angle between the iris (the colored part of the eye) and the cornea (the clear outer covering on the exposed part of the eye). This examination is important in diagnosing and managing GLAUCOMA.

Gonorrhea

One of the SEXUALLY TRANSMITTED DISEASES (STDs); caused by the bacterium *Neisseria gonorrhoeae*, which thrives in moist body areas including the vagina, penis, throat, eye, and rectum. Gonorrhea is one of the most common infectious bacterial diseases in the United States. It can affect anyone of any age, but is most common among sexually active adults between the ages of 20 and 30.

Many people carry the bacteria that cause gonorrhea without any symptoms; about 20 percent of infected men have no symptoms. When there are symptoms, they include inflammation of the urethra, which can result in a fluid discharge and painful urination in men.

Gonorrhea usually causes inflammation of the cervix in women, but most women do not experience symptoms and are unaware of the infection until complications occur.

When the infection occurs in the throat, it may cause a sore throat. Anal infections may not produce pain, or the person can have pain, itching, redness, and a discharge of pus or blood in the affected area.

Symptoms may be experienced at any time between 1 day and a few weeks after a person has become infected. Gonorrhea persists until it is treated; without treatment a person can have serious complications. In women, the infection can spread to the fallopian tubes and ovaries. If the infection spreads to the uterus or other internal sexual organs, it can cause PELVIC INFLAMMATORY DISEASE (PID), a major cause of infertility.

In men, the infection may spread up the urethra and into the prostate gland, seminal vesicles, and epididymis (the tube in which sperm mature), producing pain, chills, and fever. If the epididymis is scarred, infertility can result. If the eyes become infected and are untreated, gonorrhea can cause blindness.

The infection is detectable within 2 to 6 days after the bacteria invade the urethra. Once diagnosed, the infection is considered treatable, but gonorrhea is becoming more resistant to antibiotics such as penicillin and tetracycline.

To prevent reinfection and potential transmission to others, all sexual activity should be stopped until treatment is completed. Condoms offer protection from infection during sexual activity, and should be used to reduce the risk of acquiring an STD. Exposure to gonorrhea can be avoided also by limiting the number of sexual partners.

Gout

A form of arthritis that produces sudden and severe attacks of pain, swelling, and tenderness in joints. Gout most commonly affects the large joint of the big toe but also occurs in the knees, ankles, hands, and wrists. The attacks, which often resolve within 5 to 10 days, are usually interspersed with periods when there are no symptoms. The discomfort of gout is associated with excess amounts of uric acid in the blood, a condition called hyperuricemia.

Excess uric acid in the blood is the result of increased production of uric acid or the inability of the kidneys to excrete uric acid efficiently.

When extra uric acid circulates in the bloodstream, sharp, needlelike crystals may form in a joint and its surrounding tissues. These crystals cause the area to become painful and swollen.

Gout cannot be cured, but medication and dietary guidelines are the primary treatments. Medications may include NONSTEROIDAL ANTI-INFLAMMATORY DRUGS (NSAIDs) to help relieve pain and swelling. Uricosuric medications, which promote the excretion of uric acid in the urine, may be used to lower the uric

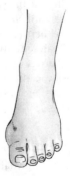

Swollen, painful joints
Although gout is a form of arthritis that can attack other joints, it almost always affects the joint at the base of the big toe.

acid level in the blood by increasing the amount of uric acid passed in the urine. Allopurinol can reduce the amount of uric acid in the blood.

Dietary guidelines are a useful adjunct to medication for controlling gout. Recommendations include reducing intake of foods containing purines (substances that occur naturally in the body as well as in certain foods), such as liver, brains, kidneys, sweetbreads, anchovies, herring, mackerel, seafood, beans, oatmeal, spinach, and cauliflower.

Grafting

Transplanting a portion of skin, bone, or other tissue from one part of the body to another. Grafting is used to replace diseased or injured tissue with healthy tissue from the same body.

Graft-versus-host disease

A rejection response that follows transplants (see TRANSPLANT SURGERY). After a bone marrow transplant, for example, graft-versus-host disease occurs because the donor's immune cells in the transplanted marrow make antibodies against the tissues of the person receiving the transplant. Treatment involves a careful balance of drugs that suppress the immune response but do not damage the new organ or tissue that was transplanted.

Gram stain

A widely used method for adding a color stain to normally colorless bacteria so they can be viewed and identified under a microscope. The bacteria are treated first with a dye called gentian violet and then with a solution of iodine, potassium, and water. Next, the bacteria are rinsed in alcohol, and a red dye is applied. The bacteria are then viewed under a microscope to see which color they have absorbed. If they are purple from the gentian violet, the bacteria are gram-positive. If they have absorbed the red dye, they are gram-negative. Gram-positive bacteria can usually be controlled with penicillin and similar antibiotics, while gram-negative bacteria resist these medications.

Grand mal seizure

An older term for a tonic-clonic SEIZURE. See EPILEPSY.

Granuloma

A diseased growth characterized by a mass of granulation tissue (tissue that develops in a wound during the healing process). Types of granuloma include granuloma annulare, granuloma inguinale, and pyogenic granuloma.

Graves disease

An autoimmune disease that affects the thyroid gland, skin, and eyes. Graves disease may also be referred to as diffuse toxic GOITER.

Graves disease is characterized by specific symptoms that may or may not occur in everyone with the disorder. The symptoms include an enlarged thyroid gland; bulging eyes; sudden weight loss; and warm, moist skin. It also causes red, thick, swollen skin on the shins and sometimes on the top of the feet.

Other symptoms include nervousness, irritability, sensitivity to heat, increased perspiration, thin skin, brittle hair, shakiness, weight loss despite increased appetite, increased heart rate, palpitations, irregular heart rhythm, elevated blood pressure, insomnia, confusion, an increase in bowel movements, weakened muscles in the upper arms and thighs, and light or irregular menstrual periods in women.

Graves disease occurs as a result of the immune system's abnormal attack on the thyroid gland, the tissue behind the eyes, and the skin of the lower legs. What produces this autoimmune response is not known.

Treatment for Graves disease varies depending on several factors including a person's overall health, medical history, and symptoms, as well as the degree of hyperthyroidism. Other considerations include the physician's judgment regarding the course of the disease and the person's tolerance for certain medications, procedures, and therapies.

Antithyroid medications, BETA BLOCKERS, radioactive iodine, or surgery may be used to treat Graves disease effectively.

People with Graves disease may also need treatment for the many symptoms and discomforts related to the disease.

Graves disease, eye

Swelling and bulging of the eyes caused by excessive production of thyroid hormones; also known as Graves ophthalmopathy. The thyroid gland, located to the front and sides of the windpipe (trachea) just above the breastbone (sternum), produces thyroid hormones that control important body processes, such as the rate of metabolism, body temperature, and muscle tone and vigor. In Graves disease, the thyroid gland becomes overly active (hyperthyroidism) and produces excessive levels of hormones. Treatment consists of medication to block the effects of thyroid hormones, destruction of a portion of the thyroid with radiation, or surgical removal of part of the thyroid.

Graves disease can cause the tissues behind the eyes to retain water, causing the tissues and muscles attached to the eyeball to swell and push the eye forward in the socket. The eyes look red and swollen, and they bulge prominently. The space between the lids may widen, drying the front portion of the eye. The eyes may tear excessively; become inflamed, uncomfortable, and sensitive to light; move only with difficulty; and cause blurred or double vision.

Control of the underlying Graves disease usually resolves eye symptoms; if it does not and the eyes remain swollen and bulging, a number of options are available. In cases of double vision, prisms can be added to glasses to align the eyes and help them converge on a single point. Double vision can also be treated with surgery that moves and reattaches the muscles controlling the eyeballs and brings them into better alignment. If the opening between the eyelids remains too wide and causes irritation, the eyelids can be repositioned surgically.

Gravida

In medicine, a pregnant woman. The term derives from gravid, meaning pregnant, while gravidity is the total number of normal and abnormal pregnancies a woman has had. A woman having her first pregnancy is a primigravida, while one who has had many pregnancies is a multigravida. Sometimes a Roman numeral follows the word to indicate a woman's number of pregnancies. For example, gravida I refers to a woman in her first pregnancy.

Groin strain

A pulled muscle that occurs suddenly during vigorous activity in a fall, twisting injury, or during a fast run. A groin strain causes pain in the area just below the crease between the lower abdomen and the thigh. What distinguishes a groin strain, or groin pull, is that the pain comes on suddenly. Pain in the groin area that develops gradually over several weeks, without a preceding single event, may be a symptom of a stress fracture in the hip and requires immediate attention from a physician, preferably one with expertise in sports medicine.

A groin strain may be treated for the first 48 hours with ice, nonsteroidal antiinflammatory drugs (NSAIDs), and gentle stretching exercises when symptoms allow. The upper leg may be wrapped with an elastic bandage to support the area during healing. In an older person, a groin strain may be more severe and take longer to heal. If pain persists, a doctor should be consulted.

Groin, lump in the

A raised swelling of variable size that may be tender. A lump in the groin may be due to any number of causes, including an infection, a hernia, an abscess, a mole, a localized response to irritation, and trauma to the area.

Any lump in the area of the groin should be medically evaluated and diagnosed by a physician.

Group A streptococcus infection

Disease resulting from a pathogenic bacterium. Group A streptococcal bacteria (group A strep) are also known as *Streptococcus pyogenes* and are frequently found in the mouth. Infections caused by this bacteria often involve the throat as in STREP THROAT, which is the most common bacterial throat infection and tends to affect children between the ages of 5 and 15 years. Consequences of strep throat include SCARLET FEVER, the kidney condition poststreptococcal GLOMERULONEPHRITIS, and acute RHEUMATIC FEVER, which affects the heart after a strep throat infection. A group A streptococcal infection may also cause skin conditions such as IMPETIGO.

In rare instances, group A strep may spread below the skin and cause serious soft tissue infections of the muscle. This severe invasion by the strep bacteria, sometimes called "flesh-eating disease," can cause a person to lose a limb or to develop liver and kidney abnormalities and may be even fatal. It is uncertain how or why these deep-tissue strep infections occur.

Streptococcal infections are contagious, and the bacteria are commonly passed from person to person via fluid droplets in coughs and sneezes. Streptococcal bacteria can also contaminate food, water, and milk.

The infections are usually diagnosed by bacterial culture of a swab taken from the throat or skin lesions and are treated with antibiotics.

Group therapy

A technique for dealing with emotional issues in which a professionally trained therapist meets with a group of people who have similar problems.

Growing pains

Arthritislike pains that occur, usually in the arms and legs of children 6 to 10 years old. The pains appear to be unrelated to growth but may be the result of fatigue, emotional difficulties, poor posture, or other problems. Children always outgrow growing pains. If a child experiences severe growing pains, or if pains are accompanied by swelling, a physician should be consulted to rule out other causes.

Growth

The process of developing to full size or to maturity. All living things gradually grow in size as they mature and develop. Growth is a term also used to characterize an abnormal development, such as a cancerous growth or tumor.

Growth hormone

A substance produced by the pituitary gland that is necessary for human growth; also known as human growth hormone, somatotropin, or somatotropic hormone.

When overproduction of growth hormone causes unusually TALL STATURE or ACROMEGALY, the syndrome may require surgery. Genetic engineering can now produce human growth hormone medications to treat children with deficiencies in growth hormone. Recently, growth hormone was approved for treatment of SHORT STATURE associated with Turner syndrome (a genetic disorder affecting girls and women with only one X chromosome) and for treatment of chronic kidney disease. The use of growth hormone in a normal but very short child is controversial

Risks of growth hormone therapy include generalized swelling, carpal tunnel syndrome, enlarged breasts in older men, and diabetes.

Growth, childhood

An important measure of a child's health; physical growth follows a similar pattern in most children. With some variation in the first year of life, girls and boys grow at the same rate. Boys are usually slightly larger, except briefly at PUBERTY. The rate of growth is fastest during embryonic and fetal development and remains fast during infancy until it slows at about age 2 or 3. The onset of puberty triggers another dramatic growth period that lasts until full adult height is reached in the late teens. Factors that influence growth usually can be categorized as either environmental or hereditary. Environmental factors may include nutrition and emotional welfare. Genetic traits, ethnicity, and hormones are considered hereditary influences. General health also influences growth. Slowed growth may indicate a number of illnesses or poor nutrition.

Guillain-Barré syndrome

Also known as GBS, a rare, potentially life-threatening, inflammatory disorder of the peripheral nerves. The onset of GBS is typically sudden and unexpected.

Guillain-Barré syndrome is characterized by progressive muscle weakness and paralysis. In fact, it is the most common cause of acute paralysis in young adults. A severe case of GBS is characterized by problems with breathing, blood pressure, and heart rate. The weakness and paralysis of GBS are caused by the loss of myelin, the sheath that normally coats nerve cells. Guillain-Barré syndrome is thought to be an autoimmune disorder (in which a person's own immune system reacts against his or her own tissues).

In moderate cases, the ability to walk is impaired. Severe cases that induce paralysis are a medical emergency, and immediate hospitalization is required to monitor the patient and in particular to watch for paralysis of the breathing muscles.

The diagnosis of GBS is based primarily on the symptoms and physical examination.

The doctor may also conduct tests, such as electromyography (see ELECTROMYOGRAM) or analysis of cerebrospinal fluid, to confirm the diagnosis and rule out other causes of symptoms.

There is no cure for GBS, and those who are diagnosed with it generally recover with or without treatment. However, early treatment can help prevent progression to complete paralysis and the need for a ventilator to assist with breathing. There are two primary treatments: plasmapheresis and intravenous immunoglobulins. Plasmapheresis is a blood-cleansing technique. Immunoglobulin, a substance naturally manufactured by the body's immune system, contains antibodies from blood donors.

Gum

The pink, soft tissue in the mouth that surrounds the teeth. The gum is medically called the gingiva. Healthy gums are firm and pale pink and do not bleed easily. If bacteria build up under the gums, a substance called plaque forms that can ultimately pull the gum away from the teeth. Careful, regular brushing and flossing are needed to avoid gum disease (see PERIODONTAL DISEASE).

Gynecology

The medical specialty focused on women's reproductive health, including diagnosis and treatment for the diseases and disorders that affect it. A gynecologist is a doctor who specializes in gynecology—the care of the female reproductive system—and diagnosis and treatment for the diseases and disorders that affect it.

Gynecomastia

Male breast enlargement. Gynecomastia results from an increase in the ratio of estrogen to testosterone, which may be due to an increase in estrogen or a decrease in androgen hormone levels. As men age and testosterone levels fall, gynecomastia may be a relatively normal finding.

Gynecomastia can be caused by certain medications; illnesses, such as chronic liver disease; or, rarely, tumors of the endocrine glands.

Treatment depends on the underlying cause. If a drug is responsible, an alternative medication may be tried. If there is no disease, swelling usually subsides without treatment in about 3 months.

H. pylori

Helicobacter pylori; a bacterium believed to cause duodenal ulcers, gastric ulcers, and gastritis. Infection with *H. pylori* sometimes has no symptoms. Other times symptoms are those of the diseases it causes, particularly upper abdominal pain. Other symptoms of ulcer disease include nausea, vomiting, loss of appetite, and weight loss. Gastritis may cause no symptoms, or at other times, indigestion, nausea, and vomiting.

Helicobacter pylori infection is usually acquired in childhood. Diagnosis is based on blood tests that can detect antibodies signifying exposure to *H. pylori*; a urea breath test, which detects the presence of bacteria; an upper GASTROINTESTINAL (GI) SERIES; or GASTROSCOPY; and a stool test to confirm the presence of *H. pylori*.

Although no single medication has proven effective against *H. pylori*, a 2-week medical regimen called triple therapy (the use of three medications at once) usually succeeds at eradicating this infection.

Haemophilus influenzae

A bacterium that is a common cause of respiratory infections. Strains of the bacteria commonly colonize the upper airways of adults and may colonize the lower respiratory tract of people with chronic BRONCHITIS.

Strains of the bacteria containing the type b polysaccharide capsule (Hib) tend to cause the most severe illness, including meningitis and epiglottitis, in children 3 to 5 years old.

Hair

Long, slender, threadlike filaments that grow from the skin. Made of a protein called keratin, hair on the head shields the scalp and head from temperature extremes and conserves heat. Hair also grows on the entire skin surface, where it helps prevent microbes or foreign matter from entering the skin.

What is commonly called hair is actually only the hair shaft, which protrudes above the surface of the skin. The root of the hair lies below the skin surface, originating in a structure called the hair follicle. The root of a new hair stimulates the development of a hair bulb, which brings keratin (a protein found in skin, hair, and nail cells) to the growing hair.

An individual hair on the head grows for 2 to 5 years and then re-

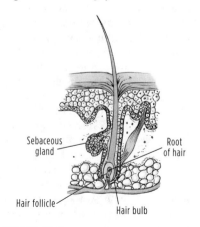

Sebaceous gland

Root of hair

Hair follicle

Hair bulb

Structure of hair
The visible hair shaft is composed of dead cells, pushed up through the skin by the living root of the hair deep in the dermis.

treats into a rest stage. When a hair falls out, a new hair grows behind it. Scalp hair grows at a rate of about one-half inch per month.

Hair removal

Excess hair (see HIRSUTISM) may be due to elevated androgen levels or an underlying endocrine disorder, which should be treated with appropriate medication. There are other causes. Hair can be removed for cosmetic reasons by shaving with a shaver or razor (which may cause problems such as skin irritation or infected hair follicles), using depilatories (chemical hair removers in the form of a cream or paste, which may cause skin irritation), waxing and tweezing (which can be painful and irritating to the skin), or ELECTROLYSIS and LASER SURGERY.

Hair transplant

A surgical procedure to remove small portions of hair-bearing scalp and relocate them to a bald area on the head of a person. Hair transplants are usually performed as COSMETIC SURGERY for the baldness that develops as a result of aging, hormonal changes, or from a family history of hair loss. Hair transplantation can also be used for baldness caused by traumatic injuries or burns. In almost all cases, hair transplantation requires a series of procedures.

It is normal for grafted hair to fall out about 6 weeks after surgery. Normal hair growth resumes approximately 5 or 6 weeks later and progresses at the usual rate of one-half inch per month.

An alternative technique to grafting involves relocating a section of scalp with hair to a bald spot. The sur-geon first removes a section of bald scalp. A hair-bearing flap of a matching shape is cut from an adjacent portion of the scalp. This incision does not completely free the flap from the underlying tissue. Rather, one end is left in its original position as the flap is shifted into the originally bald area and stitched in place.

In scalp reduction, a section of bald scalp is cut out; then, the adjacent hair-bearing scalp is loosened, brought up and forward, and stitched in place. The shape of the removed section of scalp varies with the pattern and degree of baldness. Scalp reduction can be used on the top or back of the head, but it cannot be used to create a frontal hairline.

Hallucination

False perceptions in any of the senses in a person who is awake, but the perceptions are not based on an external reality. Examples include hearing voices of the dead, feeling as if insects are crawling under the skin (formication), or seeing visions of people who are elsewhere.

Hallucinogenic drugs

Chemical substances that can alter a person's perception of reality and cause hallucinations and other alterations of the senses. Hallucinogenic substances occur naturally in plants, fungi, and animals; and they have been used throughout history in a wide variety of highly advanced and preliterate cultures.

Physical effects of hallucinogenic drugs include dilated pupils, elevated body temperature, increased heart rate and blood pressure, loss of appetite, sleeplessness, tremors, headache, nausea, sweating, heart palpitations, blurring of vision, memory loss, trembling, and itching. The psychological effects include hyperawareness of sensation, altered thinking and self-awareness, and hallucinations.

Hallux

The medical name for the big, or first, toe.

Hallux rigidus

A form of degenerative arthritis in the bottom joint of the big toe. Hallux rigidus causes a prominent outgrowth of bone at the back edge of the joint. It usually occurs in young adults; the joint may become fused or partially fused, and the toe loses some of its ability to bend at its juncture with the foot. With hallux rigidus, extending the toe is generally limited and painful, while the toe can flex more normally. Since extension of the big toe is necessary for walking properly, hallux rigidus may restrict a person's ability to walk normally. A splint for the toe is available, and its use can restrict toe motion and provide some relief. Nonsteroidal anti-inflammatory drugs (NSAIDs) and wearing a hard-soled shoe may be of some help. In severe cases, surgery may be necessary.

Hallux valgus

A deformity of the foot caused by an osteoarthritic degenerative condition in the joint of the big toe. It is characterized by the big toe moving inward toward the second toe and sometimes overlapping it or becoming positioned under it. With time, the condition becomes increasingly painful.

To diagnose hallux valgus, the doctor will perform a physical examination and order an X ray of the foot.

Orthotic devices, corrective footwear, and physical therapy may be prescribed to treat the condition. Medication may be recommended to control inflammation and pain. When more conservative treatments fail, surgery may be considered.

Halothane

See ANESTHESIA, INHALATION.

Hammer toe

A condition in which a toe becomes deformed in such a way that it bends downward or becomes clenched like a claw. It is painful and causes a reduction in the person's ability to move the toe, sometimes making it uncomfortable and difficult to walk and almost impossible to jog or participate in sports. It may be caused by poorly fitting shoes or by muscle and nerve damage as a result of diabetes mellitus. In some cases, corrective surgery is necessary.

Hamstring pull

An injury involving a strain in one or more of the three muscles located at the back of the thigh. The hamstring muscles run between the buttock and the knee, where they are connected to the bones of the lower leg. A hamstring pull often occurs following participation in strenuous sports or other activities involving the heavy use of leg muscles. The symptoms include a sharp pain in the back of the thigh, swelling and weakness in the upper leg, an inability to bend the leg, and discomfort and difficulty walking or sitting down. Treatment is centered on resting the leg as much as possible. In some cases, painkilling medication and physical therapy may be recommended.

Hand

The most flexible part of the skeleton, extending from the wrist to the tips of the fingers.

The framework of the hand is its bone structure. The hand begins where the two bones of the forearm (the radius and the ulna) join with four of the eight carpal bones that form the wrist.

Hand-foot-and-mouth disease

An illness caused by a virus (COX-SACKIEVIRUS) that primarily affects young children, occurs most commonly in the summer and early fall, and may be spread by the fecal-oral route.

Symptoms often appear to be those of a common cold with an associated rash that lasts for 7 to 10 days. The rash may appear as ulcers inside the mouth, on the inner cheeks, gums, and sides of the tongue. It may also appear as blisters or bumps on the hands, feet, and other parts of the body.

There is no specific treatment for the virus that causes hand-foot-and-mouth disease. Recommended practices for preventing infection include thorough hand washing with hot water and soap after using the rest room or handling soiled diapers; covering the mouth and nose when coughing or sneezing and instructing children to do this.

Hangover

The unpleasant symptoms that result from drinking an excessive amount of alcohol. Symptoms usually include nausea, headache, dizziness, irritability, thirst, and fatigue. There is no cure except time; the only treatment is over-the-counter pain medications, fluids to help offset dehydration, and rest.

Hansen disease

See LEPROSY.

Hardening of the arteries

See ATHEROSCLEROSIS.

Hashimoto thyroiditis

A slowly developing and persistent autoimmune disease caused by the action of certain antibodies that attack the tissues of the thyroid gland; also known as chronic lymphocytic or autoimmune thyroiditis. Hashimoto thyroiditis can eventually cause HY-POTHYROIDISM (underactivity of the thyroid gland). In Hashimoto thyroiditis, thyroid tissue is invaded by white blood cells called lymphocytes. The invasion produces inflammation, degeneration, and scarring of the tissue within the thyroid gland, gradually decreasing the gland's ability to produce and release hormones.

The initial inflammation is generally mild and causes few symptoms. People with Hashimoto thyroiditis may not be aware that they have it for many years.

Hashimoto thyroiditis may be detected early on by the presence of thyroid antibodies in blood, but it is usually discovered during a routine physical examination when a doctor notes an enlargement of the thyroid gland.

If there are other symptoms of the disease, blood tests may be performed to measure hormone levels. A low level of the thyroid hormone THYROX-INE and an elevated level of TSH (thyroid-stimulating hormone), along with the presence of thyroid antibodies, can confirm the diagnosis.

There is no cure for Hashimoto thyroiditis. Treatment primarily consists of compensating for low thyroid function. If hypothyroidism is present, oral thyroid hormone medication is generally prescribed.

Hay fever

A set of symptoms caused by the immune system's response to inhalation of tiny airborne pollens of certain seasonal plants; also called allergic rhinitis. Hay fever is caused by the body's antibodies reacting with the inhaled pollen, a reaction that causes HISTAMINE to be released. The histamine promotes an inflammatory response in the linings of the nose, sinuses, eyelids, and eyes. Inflammation in the sinuses causes congestion, and the nose begins to produce excess mucus. Inflamed mucous membranes result in an itchy sensation that occurs in the eyes, nose, throat, and the roof of the mouth. Other symptoms include eye irritation, a runny nose, and sneezing.

Hay fever is best controlled by avoidance of the pollens that produce symptoms. An allergist may prescribe antihistamines, decongestants, a corticosteroid nasal spray, or eye drops. Using over-the-counter nasal sprays and drops is usually not recommended as these products can cause nasal symptoms to worsen over the long-term. In severe and persistent cases, it may be necessary to consult an allergist.

While there is no cure for hay fever, a series of injections or allergy shots to desensitize an affected person to the specific pollen or pollens may be beneficial.

HCG

See HUMAN CHORIONIC GONADOTROPIN.

HDL

High-density lipoprotein. See CHOLESTEROL.

Head and neck cancer

A broad category of tumors that arise in the head and neck area, including tumors in the mouth, tongue, lips, gums, sinuses, salivary glands, throat, and larynx (voice box). Symptoms can include swelling or sores in the mouth that do not heal; pain, swelling, or obstruction of the nose; chronic sinus trouble that is unresponsive to antibiotics; paralysis of one side of the face; ear pain; pain when swallowing; bloody nasal discharges; persistent hoarseness; difficulty breathing; and double vision.

Head and neck cancers account for between 5 and 10 percent of all malignancies. Risk factors for head and neck cancers include being male, over 50, a smoker, and drinking alcohol. Oral cancers are sometimes discovered by dentists during routine examinations. Surgery is often the first choice for treatment, although radiation therapy is sometimes as effective and may better preserve the appearance and function of the affected area. Chemotherapy, usually with radiation, is sometimes used.

Head injuries

Any injury that results in damage to the brain or trauma to the head. Head injuries, also called traumatic brain injuries, are quite common.

The signs and symptoms of head injury may occur immediately or may develop slowly over several hours. Anyone who has received a hard bump on the head should be watched closely for a day because symptoms are sometimes delayed. The many possible symptoms of head injuries include: loss of consciousness; bleeding; slowed breathing; confusion; seizures; skull fracture; fluid drainage from the nose, mouth, or ears that is either clear or bloody; headache that may be severe; increased drowsiness; slurred speech; stiff neck; and swelling at the site of the injury.

There are two basic types of head injuries: closed head injuries, in which a head that is moving is stopped suddenly, as in a car crash, and penetrating head injuries, which happen when fast moving objects penetrate the skull.

The first step in treating head injuries is to provide emergency medical attention when appropriate. Anyone who has had a head injury, even a very mild one, should refrain from vigorous activity for 24 hours.

Head injuries can be prevented, par-

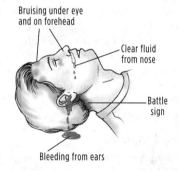

Bruising under eye and on forehead

Clear fluid from nose

Battle sign

Bleeding from ears

Signs of skull fracture
Bruising or deformity of the skull, discoloration under the eye, bleeding from the ear, bloody or clear fluid from the nose, a dark mark below the ear, and unequal pupils may be signs of injury.

ticularly by wearing a helmet when biking, in-line skating, snowboarding, or motorcycling and by wearing a seatbelt when in an automobile. See also CONCUSSION; WHIPLASH.

Headache

For symptom chart see HEADACHE, page xxii.

Pain in the head. About 7 of 10 people get headaches. A headache may be located in any part of the head and may even extend to the neck. The problem can be acute (short and isolated) or chronic (persistent or long-lasting). Most headaches are painful and annoying but can be easily relieved with aspirin or acetaminophen. However, in some cases head pain becomes severe and debilitating, and on rare occasions a headache is a symptom of a serious underlying medical problem.

It is important first to separate primary headaches from secondary headaches (those caused by another medical condition, such as a tumor). The most common primary headaches are tension headaches and migraines; other types include cluster headaches, sinus headaches, and rebound headaches.

Tension headaches are characterized by a feeling of dull pain that affects the entire head and are commonly triggered by stress, fatigue, depression, or anxiety. Migraine headaches are characterized by throbbing pain that commonly begins on one side of the head; they occur on a sporadic basis and may last several hours to several days. Their pain may become disabling. In addition, there may be other symptoms, such as nausea, vomiting, dizziness, chills, loss of appetite, irritability, fatigue, and sensitivity to light and sound. Some migraines are preceded by fatigue, depression, or an AURA. See also MIGRAINE.

Cluster headaches are rare and intensely painful; they are characterized by burning or boring pain that generally occurs at night, and they tend to occur in groups or clusters for a period of time (which can be as short as days or as long as months) and then disappear.

A sinus headache may develop when the sinuses become infected or inflamed. (See SINUSITIS.) Pain typically comes on quickly in the nasal area and worsens over time.

Rebound headaches may develop when a person takes medication for headaches more than two or three times a week. When analgesics are overused to treat headaches, the body adapts and grows dependent on them.

Doctors advise people who have chronic or severe headaches to seek prompt medical evaluation and treatment. Diagnosis of headache type is based on the nature of the pain, its frequency and duration, location, severity, and accompanying symptoms. Tests such as CT SCANNING (computed tomography scanning) and MRI (magnetic resonance imaging) may be performed to rule out any serious underlying causes of symptoms, such as a ruptured ANEURYSM, BRAIN TUMOR, or temporal arteritis (see ARTERITIS, GIANT CELL).

Home care for mild-to-moderate headaches includes rest, ice or heat packs, hot showers, massage, and over-the-counter pain relievers. To prevent rebound headaches, only the minimal necessary dose of medication should be taken.

Doctors treat chronic or severe headaches with two categories of medications: abortive (to relieve pain and other symptoms) and prophylactic (to prevent headaches from developing). Preventive medication is usually recommended only for people who have frequent attacks and for people in whom headaches are so severe that they prevent normal activity.

For sinus headaches, doctors recommend use of decongestants or antibiotics and in some cases draining the affected sinus. Because serious complications may develop, headaches resulting from temporal arteritis (a type of arterial inflammation) require careful medical evaluation and treatment with corticosteroid medications.

Health maintenance organization

See HMO.

Hearing

The ability to perceive and identify sound. All sources of sound send vibrations or sound waves through the air. These sound waves are funneled into the outer EAR opening and travel through the ear canal to the eardrum, causing this thin membrane to vibrate. These vibrations are passed through small bones in the middle ear to fluid in the inner ear. The vibrating movement of the fluid stimulates hairlike projections called hair cells to transform the sound wave vibrations into electrical nerve impulses and sends them to the hearing nerve in the inner ear. This nerve transmits the impulses to the brain. In the brain's hearing centers, the nerve impulses are identified and interpreted as individual sounds that are understandable to the person listening to them. Hearing is supplemented by vibrations conducted through the bones of the skull into the inner ear. A person hears his or her own voice via these vibrations within the skull.

Anything that interferes with the delicate hearing apparatus can contribute to HEARING LOSS, including infections or inflammation, physical trauma to the ear, disease, and abnormal ear structures.

Hearing aids

Electronic devices, consisting of four miniature components—a microphone, amplifier, receiver, and battery—that bring amplified sound to the ear of a person whose hearing is impaired. On most hearing aids, sound level controls are adjustable. Some hearing aids have directional microphones. For people with profound DEAFNESS whose auditory nerves are functional, a surgically implanted device may provide limited sound perception and serve as an aid to lip-reading or may even allow a person to understand while on the telephone (see COCHLEAR IMPLANT).

Purchasing a hearing aid is best done after a doctor's evaluation and medical recommendation.

Hearing loss

Partial or total loss of the ability to perceive and identify sound. There are four general categories of hearing loss: conductive hearing loss, sensorineural hearing loss, mixed hearing loss, and central hearing loss (see DEAFNESS). Each hearing loss can be distinguished from the other by the evaluation of hearing test results (see AUDIOMETRY).

Conductive hearing loss includes impairments to hearing caused by any interference with the structures and mechanisms that conduct sound waves from the external environment to the fluid in the inner ear. These hearing losses can usually be corrected by medical treatments or procedures, including surgery.

Sensorineural hearing loss can be caused by problems in the inner ear, problems with the nerve that transmits impulses from the inner ear to the brain, and problems with the brain's functioning. Aging is the most common cause of this kind of hearing loss.

Hearing tests

See AUDIOMETRY.

Heart

The hollow, muscular organ that pumps blood throughout the body. Lying in the chest midway between the sternum (breastbone) and the spine, the heart sits slightly left of center. At each beat its tip strikes the inner surface of the chest wall, sometimes producing visible movement and allowing it to be felt by hand. In an adult, the heart is a little larger than a clenched fist, weighing about 1 pound.

Structure and Function

The heart is a four-chambered organ composed of specialized muscle tissue called myocardium. The interior surfaces of the heart are lined with a smooth membrane called the endocardium; the entire heart is contained in a strong sac called the pericardium.

Each side of the heart is composed of an upper chamber called the atrium and a lower chamber called the ventricle. The right and left sides act as separate pumps. On the left side, blood rich in oxygen from the lungs is pumped from the atrium to the ventricle, then into the aorta to be transported throughout the body via arteries. On the right side, depleted blood that has traveled throughout the body discharging oxygen and other nutrients returns to the heart, via the vena cava, into the right atrium and then into the right ventricle. From there, it flows via the pulmonary artery into the lungs, where it is reoxygenated. This oxygen-rich blood is returned through the pulmonary veins into the left atrium. See CARDIOVASCULAR SYSTEM.

Each of the heart's four chambers has a one-way valve (see HEART VALVE) controlling blood flow in the right direction, to ensure the intricate sequence of the heartbeat.

Heart rate and cardiac output

There are two important measures of the activity and efficiency of the

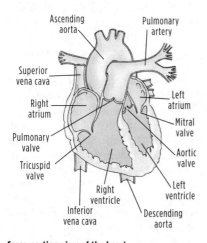

Cross-section view of the heart
The heart is a muscular organ that is approximately the shape and size of an average adult male fist.

Labels on diagram:
Ascending aorta
Pulmonary artery
Superior vena cava
Right atrium
Left atrium
Pulmonary valve
Mitral valve
Tricuspid valve
Aortic valve
Right ventricle
Left ventricle
Inferior vena cava
Descending aorta

function of the heart: heart rate and cardiac output. The heart rate is the number of times the heart beats per minute, and cardiac output is the volume of blood it pumps out with each contraction, multiplied by the number of beats per minute. At rest, the heart rate is usually 60 to 80 beats per minute, and the cardiac output is about 10 pints per minute.

Heart attack

For symptom chart see CHEST PAIN, page xiv.
A total or near-total blockage of one of the coronary arteries that supply the HEART with oxygen; known medically as myocardial infarction. In most cases, the blockage is caused by a blood clot that forms at a point in the artery narrowed by fatty deposits (plaque; see ATHEROSCLEROSIS). A spasm in an artery can also trigger a heart attack, although this is less common. Since the coronary arteries provide the heart muscle with its oxygen supply, tissue downstream from the blockage can die. The severity of the attack depends on the amount and location of affected heart tissue. Heart attack is one of the leading causes of sudden death and disability in the United States.

The pain accompanying a heart attack is often severe and sudden and classically described as comparable to someone "sitting on my chest." Typically, the pain begins in the chest, radiates through the upper body into the neck, arm, shoulder, or jaw, and does not go away with rest. The symptoms can vary tremendously, and in some people, a heart attack may occur with no pain, in which case it is called a silent heart attack.

If a heart attack is suspected, the

Warning: Heart attack symptoms

If a person has the symptoms below, someone should call 911 or the emergency services number for the area promptly. Symptoms vary from person to person; also, women are less apt to have the sharp pain in the chest that men commonly have.

- Pressure, fullness, squeezing, or pain in the center of the chest that lasts 5 minutes or more
- Pain that radiates from the chest to the shoulders, neck, or arm, particularly on the left side; in women, this may include the left jawbone
- Chest pain accompanied by lightheadedness, fainting, nausea, or shortness of breath

Other symptoms occur less frequently but also may indicate heart attack:

- Unusual pain in the chest, abdomen, or stomach
- Nausea or dizziness without chest pain (especially in women)
- Shortness of breath or difficulty breathing without chest pain (especially in women)
- Anxiety, fatigue, or weakness without an apparent cause
- Cold sweating, palpitations, or pallor

---

doctor typically requests an ELECTRO-CARDIOGRAM, which records the electrical activity of the heart and often shows evidence of the attack, and checks the level of chemical cardiac enzymes in the blood, which—if elevated—indicate damage to the heart muscle.

Since a heart attack is not an instantaneous event but develops over several hours, prompt emergency medical attention is critical for survival and limiting the damage. The initial treatment for a person who has had a heart attack can include medications that dissolve the blood clot, prevent new clots from forming and causing additional attacks, and reduce stress on the heart. These medications include beta blockers, angiotensin-converting enzyme (ACE) inhibitors, anticoagulants, nitrates, aspirin, and "clot-busters" (such as streptokinase, urokinase, and tissue plasminogen activator). Morphine is commonly given to reduce pain and anxiety.

Other treatments include BALLOON ANGIOPLASTY or BYPASS SURGERY.

For those who survive a heart attack, a number of complications can develop because of damage to the heart. Possible complications include HEART FAILURE, CONGESTIVE; cardiac arrhythmias, including VENTRICULAR FIBRILLATION; leakages between the two ventricles (lower chambers) of the heart; damage to the mitral valve between the upper and lower heart chambers; rupture of the ventricle; pericarditis (inflammation of the membrane that surrounds the heart); or the development of blood clots, which can travel through the bloodstream and lodge in other organs, where they can cause severe or life-threatening damage.

Heart block

A slowing of electrical impulses in their normal conduction pattern from the atria (upper chambers) of the heart to the ventricles (lower chambers). The delay in electrical communication between the top and bottom of the heart can slow the heartbeat to an abnormally low rate (bradycardia).

There are a number of possible causes for heart block: a lack of sufficient oxygen to the heart (cardiac ischemia) from coronary artery disease; myocarditis (inflammation of the heart muscle), rheumatic fever, heart surgery, electrolyte imbalances in the blood, aging, or heart medications (such as beta blockers and calcium channel blockers).

Heart block is graded by the severity of the blockage. Grades range from first-degree heart block, which usually produces no symptoms and requires no treatment; to second-degree heart block, which results in missed heartbeats; to third-degree heart block, in which no signals reach the ventricles from the atria, and the ventricles beat according to their own rhythm, which is insufficient to provide the body with enough blood. Third-degree heart block can cause dizziness, breathlessness, seizures, and loss of consciousness, and possibly lead to cardiac arrest (complete stoppage of the heart). An artificial PACEMAKER, which regulates heartbeat, is used to treat severe second-degree and third-degree heart block.

Heart disease, congenital

An abnormality or malformation of the heart or the blood vessels connected to the heart that is present at birth. The causes of congenital heart disease are unknown. Current research tentatively suggests that contributing factors may include genetic abnormalities (such as DOWN SYNDROME), certain medications taken during pregnancy, alcohol or drug abuse during pregnancy, and viral infections of the mother, particularly German measles (rubella). There are many types of congenital heart disease, including the following:

Ventricular septal defect

Ventricular septal defect is the most common form of congenital heart disease. It consists of an opening in the wall, or septum, dividing the ventricles (lower chambers) of the heart. As a result of this defect, an increased amount of blood under high pressure flows into the lungs. Symptoms depend on the size of the defect. Since as many as half of all ventricular septal defects close on their own during the first year of life, medication is used initially to alleviate symptoms. If the defect does not close, surgery to close the opening is performed.

Atrial septal defect

If an opening exists between the atria (upper chambers) of the heart, the disease is known as an atrial septal defect. Often there are few or no symptoms early in life. The defect can be repaired surgically, usually when the child is between 1 and 6 years of age.

Patent ductus arteriosus

In a newborn, the blood vessel known as the ductus arteriosus connects the pulmonary artery (the artery to the lungs) with the aorta, which carries blood to the rest of the body. Normally, the ductus arteriosus closes immediately after birth, but in premature newborns and some full-term infants the vessel remains open. Surgery is performed to close the vessel when the baby is 1 or 2 years old.

Coarctation of the aorta

Coarctation of the aorta refers to severe narrowing of the aorta, which is the main artery leading from the heart to the body, usually just past the point at which the artery that supplies the upper body branches off. This results in lower blood pressure in the lower body and higher blood pressure in the upper body, along with a number of other complications. Signs of the disease include cyanosis (a bluish tint to the skin) in the lower body, high blood pressure in only the upper body, and weak pulse in the groin along with strong pulse in the neck. Symptoms can include dizziness, headache, cramps in the legs with exercise, fainting, and nosebleeds. Surgery is the usual treatment.

Pulmonary stenosis

Stenosis (narrowing) of the valve leading to the artery that connects the heart to the lungs results in pulmonary stenosis. Symptoms depend on the degree of obstruction. If it is mild to moderate, there may be no symptoms. Severe obstruction produces cyanosis and heart failure. In the worst cases, congestive heart failure (see HEART FAILURE, CONGESTIVE) develops within a month of birth. Children with mild to moderate stenosis can live normal lives but require regular medical examinations. Severe stenosis requires surgical widening of the valve.

Aortic stenosis

In aortic stenosis, the narrowing occurs in the valve leading into the aorta. Unless the stenosis is severe, most children with aortic stenosis show no symptoms, and the problem is detected during a routine physical examination as a heart murmur. Children with mild to moderate stenosis require regular medical examinations to detect any worsening of the disease. Severe aortic stenosis can be repaired surgically.

Tetralogy of Fallot

Not one defect but four in combination ("tetra-" means four in Greek) and named after the French physician who first described them, tetralogy of Fallot consists of a large ventricular septal defect, pulmonary stenosis, enlargement of the right ventricle, and a rightward shift in the position of the aorta. Blood flow to the lungs is decreased, leading to an insufficient supply of oxygen to the body and cyanosis. Surgery is performed to correct the defects. Tetralogy of Fallot accordingly is what causes a "blue baby." Often more than one operation is needed.

Transposition of the great vessels

Another complex congenital heart disease, transposition of the great vessels refers to abnormal anatomy in which the aorta arises from the right ventricle and the pulmonary artery from the left—rather than the normal (opposite) arrangement. As a result, a portion of the blood circulates through the lungs without ever flowing to the rest of the body, while another portion of the blood circulates through the left side of the heart and into the body without passing through the lungs and picking up oxygen. This congenital heart disease produces bluish skin coloring and it usually causes death within the first year of life if not treated. Several surgical procedures are available.

Heart disease, ischemic

Disease caused by blood flow to the heart muscle that is insufficient to meet its oxygen needs. The shortfall in blood flow and oxygen supply occurs because of obstruction in one of the coronary arteries, the blood vessels that provide oxygen to the heart muscle. The obstruction can be caused by a buildup of fatty material (plaque; see ATHEROSCLEROSIS), a blood clot, or a spasm in the artery.

Minor episodes of ischemic heart disease usually cause little long-term damage to the heart, but more severe events that result in a HEART ATTACK do cause permanent damage or result in an abnormal heart rhythm (see ARRHYTHMIA, CARDIAC). Ischemia can also cause fainting or cardiac arrest.

The most common symptom of ischemic heart disease is pain or pressure (see ANGINA) that may radiate through the upper body into the neck, back, arms, shoulders, or jaw. In some cases there is no pain, in which case it is called silent ischemic heart disease.

Treatment for ischemic heart disease begins with medications that reduce the heart's need for oxygen by lowering the heart rate, reducing blood pressure, and relaxing the blood vessels. In more advanced cases, an invasive technique such as BALLOON ANGIOPLASTY or BYPASS SURGERY can improve the flow of blood to the heart muscle.

Heart failure, congestive

A serious, potentially life-threatening condition in which the heart cannot pump enough blood to meet the body's demand for oxygen. The name comes from the fact that the pumping failure often results in pulmonary edema (a buildup of fluid, or congestion, in the lungs). As the heart begins to fail, it works harder and harder to compensate, a response that worsens the disease over time. Congestive heart failure can occur at any age, but it is most common in people older than 70, in whom it is a leading cause of death and disability. Usually the disease is chronic, or long-term. Acute congestive heart failure can result from a coronary event such as a heart attack or cardiac arrhythmia (abnormal heart rhythm), which impair the heart's ability to pump blood. Acute heart failure constitutes a medical emergency.

Shortness of breath is one of the earliest symptoms of heart failure, resulting in fatigue even from ordinary activities and little or no tolerance for exercise. Edema (swelling) in the legs is another common symptom. Neck veins may bulge, and fluid buildup in the abdomen can cause bloating, pain, or nausea.

A doctor may detect other key signs, such as a heart murmur (a signal of valve problems), the sound of fluid in the lungs, fast or irregular heartbeat, swelling in the liver or abdomen, enlargement of the heart, and leg swelling. Several tests may be used in the diagnosis of congestive heart failure, including ELECTROCARDIOGRAM (to measure the heart's electrical activity), echocardiography (to visualize the heart via ultrasound), chest X ray, and radionuclide imaging tests.

The sooner congestive heart failure is detected, the less damage is done to the pumping function of the heart.

Although the disease cannot be cured, it can be managed successfully, particularly with early detection.

Medications are commonly used to relieve symptoms and to compensate for the effects of the disease. If coronary artery disease is the underlying cause of the congestive heart failure, BALLOON ANGIOPLASTY, bypass surgery, or heart valve surgery may be needed.

Heart murmur

An abnormal blowing, whooshing, or rasping sound in the heart that is detectable with a stethoscope. A heart murmur results from vibrations caused by abnormal blood flow patterns.

A heart murmur may or may not indicate heart disease. Tests such as an ECHOCARDIOGRAM are often performed after a heart murmur is detected to determine the cause and assess the need for treatment.

Heart rate

The number of heartbeats per minute; also known as pulse.

Heart transplant

A surgical procedure to remove an irreparably diseased heart and replace it with a healthy heart from a recently deceased person. Performed since 1967, heart transplants are now the third most common form of transplantation surgery, following only kidney and cornea transplants. Heart transplant surgery extends the lives of people who would otherwise die within a short time due to advanced heart disease.

The most common causes for heart transplant are severe ischemic heart disease (CORONARY ARTERY DISEASE), CARDIOMYOPATHY (impaired heart muscle function), heart disease present at birth (see HEART DISEASE, CONGENITAL), defective heart valves, and inability of the heart to meet the body's need for oxygen (heart failure).

In some cases, the heart is transplanted along with the lungs. This procedure is used primarily with persons who have abnormally high blood pressure in the lungs (HYPERTENSION, PULMONARY) or Eisenmenger complex, a congenital condition that combines pulmonary hypertension with a heart defect.

Donor hearts are taken from people who have consented to the use of their organs after death and who have died of an illness or accident that has left the heart intact and undamaged. The blood type of the donor and the recipient need to be the same to give the best chance of success. In addition, the size of the heart matters.

Most recipients of a donated heart live significantly longer than they would have without the transplant. But certain problems tend to develop over the long-term.

Heart valve

The structure at the exit of each of the four chambers of the HEART that allows blood to flow out, but prevents backflow. The mitral valve separates the left atrium of the heart from the left ventricle. The tricuspid valve divides the right atrium from the right ventricle. The pulmonary valve controls blood flow from the right ventricle into the pulmonary artery, which leads into the lungs. The aortic valve performs the same function between the left ventricle and the aorta, the artery that leads to the rest of the body.

The valves of the heart can be defective at birth (see HEART DISEASE, CONGENITAL), or they can become narrowed, a condition called stenosis (see STENOSIS, VALVULAR), or become unable to prevent backflow, called insufficiency or incompetence. The mitral valve and the aortic valve are the most common sites of disease, probably because they are under the greatest strain from the left ventricle. MITRAL VALVE PROLAPSE (MVP) is the most common valve disorder, usually an inherited structural defect in which the walls of the valve are thickened and elongated and cannot prevent backflow. AORTIC STENOSIS is an abnormal narrowing of the aortic valve, usually caused by deposits of calcium as a result of aging.

Heart valve surgery

An operation to repair or replace one of the four valves in the heart. In the normally functioning heart, the flaps of each of the four valves—pulmonary, mitral, aortic, and tricuspid—allow blood to flow in only one direction as it travels to and from the lungs and to and from the body. Stenosis (narrowing) of a valve limits normal blood flow, while regurgitation (leaking) lets blood flow in the wrong direction. Left untreated, severe valve problems can lead to life-threatening disease, such as heart failure.

Heart valve surgery is an open-heart procedure. That is, the chest is opened and the heart exposed, while a heart-lung machine takes over the function of oxygenating the blood and pumping it to the body. The procedure is performed under general anesthetic.

In recent years, a catheter-based procedure called VALVULOPLASTY has

replaced many heart valve surgical repairs. In addition, new minimally invasive techniques allow replacement of defective heart valves through a much smaller incision in the chest and heart, causing less pain and shortening recovery.

Heart, artificial

A mechanical device that substitutes for, or augments, the normal blood-pumping function of the heart. Still experimental, artificial hearts are generally seen as a temporary solution to prolong the life of a person with advanced heart disease who is waiting for a heart transplant and might otherwise die.

Heartburn

A burning sensation in the upper abdomen and chest. Also known as acid indigestion, heartburn is most common in older people and pregnant women. Heartburn is the most common symptom of ESOPHAGEAL REFLUX (the backward flow of acid from the stomach up into the esophagus). Simple modifications in lifestyle can control most cases of heartburn. Over-the-counter (OTC) antacids may also provide relief. If these measures prove insufficient, or if it is necessary to take antacids very frequently (more than 3 or 4 times a day), it is important to see a physician. He or she may recommend OTC H-2 blockers. If OTC products fail to offer relief, esophageal reflux may require treatment with prescription medication or, rarely, in severe cases with surgery.

Heart-lung machine

A device that takes over the functions of the heart and lungs during open-heart surgery. The heart-lung machine consists of a pump, which circulates the blood and substitutes for the heart, and an oxygenator, which, taking over for the lungs, removes carbon dioxide from the blood and adds oxygen. Because the heart-lung machine is keeping the person undergoing open heart surgery alive, the surgeon can stop the heart to work on it without causing bleeding.

Heart-lung transplant

A surgical procedure to remove a diseased heart and lungs and replace them with a healthy heart and lungs from a recently deceased donor. Heart-lung transplant is performed only on those who have both severely diseased lungs and advanced heart disease, are likely to die soon without the procedure, and have no other life-threatening diseases, such as diabetes mellitus. See HEART TRANSPLANT.

Heat cramps

A condition caused by prolonged activity in high temperatures that produces the sudden development of cramps in the skeletal muscles. Loss of water and salt (sodium chloride) through profuse perspiration obstructs the ability of the body to release heat, causing the muscles to cramp. A person who has heat cramps should stop exercising and move to a cool place. Tight clothing should be loosened, and the feet should be raised. Water and electrolyte solution, if available, should be given to the person. Cooling off and drinking water are important to help prevent heat stroke.

Heat exhaustion

A condition in which the body produces heat faster than it can sweat it off; overexposure to heat. Heat exhaustion is characterized by cool, moist, pale skin; headache; nausea and vomiting; weakness; and dizziness or fainting.

Risk factors for heat exhaustion include cardiovascular disease, high temperatures or humidity, sweat gland dysfunction, alcohol use, excessive exercise, and wearing too much clothing in hot weather. Heat exhaustion should be taken seriously. Once the signs of heat exhaustion appear, the person's condition can worsen rapidly. The person should be moved to the shade or a cooler area; take a tepid (medium cool) bath, if possible; and also drink a lot of cool water or an electrolyte replacement solution, slowly. If the person shows any signs of confusion or loses consciousness, medical attention must be sought.

Heat stroke

A condition caused by overexposure to heat in which the body stops sweating. Heat stroke is a life-threatening illness that can cause shock, brain damage, and death. The signs of heat stroke include extremely high body temperature, often as high as 106°F; red, hot, dry skin; progressive loss of consciousness; rapid pulse; confusion; and rapid, shallow breathing. Symptoms include weakness and fatigue, headache, dizziness, blurred vision, and vomiting.

All cases of heat stroke require emergency medical attention. First-aid measures include removing any tight or heavy clothing and applying cool sponges or towels soaked in cool water to the person's skin. Rubbing alcohol (isopropyl alcohol) should not be applied, and the person should not be given anything to eat or drink.

Heimlich maneuver

An emergency technique for dislodging an object stuck in the windpipe. The Heimlich maneuver is used to prevent suffocation when a person is CHOKING and unable to breathe, cough, or speak. It is advisable to learn how to perform the Heimlich maneuver in a first-aid course. Basically, the rescuer stands behind the person who is choking, clasps his or her hands over the person's mid-section, and pulls back to provide pressure that helps propel the food or other swallowed objects out of the person's mouth.

Helicobacter pylori

See H. PYLORI.

Helmets, sports

Protective covering worn during vigorous athletic activities to prevent head injuries. Helmets are the single most important piece of protective gear used in sports. Research has established that the wearing of helmets saves lives by reducing the risk of head injuries.

Hemangioma

A common tumor consisting of a proliferation of blood vessels that develops at or soon after birth. There are two primary types: capillary hemangiomas and cavernous hemangiomas. Capillary hemangiomas are slightly raised and bright red and are caused by blood vessels near the surface of the skin. Cavernous hemangiomas are blue and are caused by blood vessels that are located deeper in the skin.

Hemangiomas can occur anywhere on the face or body, including internal organs such as the liver. Usually a child has only one, but it is possible to have two or three hemangiomas. They usu-ally stop growing after the first year of life and then slowly begin to shrink and fade. Although a faint mark may remain, hemangiomas usually disappear on their own without treatment. However, it is impossible to predict how large a hemangioma might grow or if it will disappear completely.

Medical options include systemic corticosteroids and LASER SURGERY that destroys the blood vessels. However, both involve serious side effects.

Hemarthrosis

The presence of blood within a joint, usually the result of a moderately severe injury that causes bleeding into the joint. In hemarthrosis, the blood accumulates in the joint within a few hours of the injury, and the joint becomes swollen, stiff, and painful. The accumulation of blood suggests that one of the joint elements, for example, the ligament or joint capsule, has been damaged. Hemarthrosis may also occur spontaneously in people who have a blood clotting disorder, such as hemophilia, or people who are taking blood-thinning medication. Cells in the joint capsule will slowly absorb any remaining blood. A large hemarthrosis may require aspiration, in which a fine needle is used to draw the fluid out of the joint.

Hematemesis

See VOMITING BLOOD.

Hematocrit

The proportion or percentage of the blood's volume taken up by red blood cells; abbreviated Hct. Hematocrit is usually included as part of standard blood testing (see BLOOD TESTS), and it is useful for detecting and diagnosing a variety of diseases that affect or involve the blood. People with a low hematocrit level have anemia, while those with polycythemia have a high hematocrit level.

Hematology

The branch of medical science that studies blood and blood-forming tissues, such as the bone marrow, and the diseases that affect them. A hematologist is a physician who specializes in diagnosing and treating blood and diseases affecting the blood-forming tissues.

Hematoma

A collection of blood in a body part as a result of ruptured or injured blood vessels. The medical importance of a hematoma depends on its location and size. A small hematoma under a fingernail resulting from an injury will heal on its own within a few weeks. A hematoma on the outer surface of the brain, called an epidural hematoma, may lead to death if not treated.

Hematospermia

Blood in the semen. Hematospermia is occasionally associated with other symptoms, including pain with urination, ejaculation, or bowel movement; swelling or tenderness in the groin or scrotum; back pain; and fever. The condition may be a sign of prostate cancer or of infection, obstruction, or injury in the male reproductive tract. Treatment depends on the underlying cause, but although it looks alarming, hematospermia is most often a benign, self-limiting condition.

Hematuria

Blood in the urine. Small amounts of blood make urine look smoky or cloudy; large amounts turn it dark red or a tea-colored brown. Hematuria is abnormal and can be a sign of serious disease; it requires prompt attention from a physician. Depending on the cause, hematuria may be accompanied by other symptoms, such as pain on urination, aching in the abdomen or back, fever, frequent and urgent need to urinate, increased or decreased thirst, decreased appetite, nausea, vomiting, or diarrhea. Hematuria combined with pain in the side below the ribs may indicate problems such as a stone in the ureter (the tube connecting the kidney and bladder) or a kidney tumor. Infection, tumor, kidney stone, or blood vessels broken by the strain of urinating with an enlarged prostate are other possible causes.

A person seeking medical attention for hematuria will need a physical examination and a medical history. Diagnostic laboratory tests may be performed, including blood tests, analysis of the urine, and an examination of the bladder, kidneys, and lower abdomen by X ray, visual instrument (cystoscope), ultrasound, or CT (computed tomography) scan. In some cases, a sample of tissue, or a biopsy specimen, may be taken.

Treatment of hematuria depends on the underlying cause. Infections can be treated with antibiotics. Stones may pass on their own, or they may require removal (see CALCULUS, URINARY TRACT). Tumors are managed with surgery or medication, depending on their type and extent.

Hemianopia

Blindness in half of the normal visual field. Hemianopia may affect one eye or both eyes. Whenever partial or complete blindness develops in one or both eyes, it is important to seek prompt medical attention. There are many possible reasons for the loss of sight, including injuries, diabetic retinopathy (see RETINOPATHY, DIABETIC), MACULAR DEGENERATION, vitamin A (beta carotene) deficiency, retinitis pigmentosa, retinoblastoma, lead poisoning, glaucoma, trachoma, and progressive multifocal leukoencephalopathy (PML).

Hemicolectomy

Surgical removal of part of the colon. A hemicolectomy (see also COLECTOMY) is usually performed to remove colon tissue damaged by a blockage or to treat colon cancer, COLITIS, or DIVERTICULAR DISEASE. In hemicolectomy, the diseased segments of the colon are removed and the remaining healthy parts are joined together.

Hemiparesis

Weakness on one side of the body. Hemiparesis and HEMIPLEGIA (paralysis on one side of the body) commonly occur as a result of a STROKE.

Hemiplegia

PARALYSIS or weakness on one side of the body. Hemiplegia is one of the most common effects of a serious STROKE. Weakness without complete paralysis is called HEMIPARESIS.

Hemochromatosis

An inherited disorder in which the body absorbs too much iron from food. Symptoms include fatigue, abdominal pain, and JAUNDICE (a yellowing of the skin and the whites of the eyes). Skin color may change to gray or bronze. Left untreated, hemochromatosis can lead to serious health disorders, such as CIRRHOSIS (a severe liver disease), liver cancer, liver failure, diabetes, and heart problems. Women are less likely than men to acquire hemochromatosis because of blood loss through menstruation.

Diagnosis is based on blood tests that measure the level of iron in the body. In some cases, a LIVER BIOPSY is performed to measure the extent of liver damage. Treatment involves drawing blood to remove excess iron from the body.

Hemodialysis

A medical procedure that cleans and filters the blood by removing waste products, extra salt, and fluid from the blood through a dialysis machine.

Hemodialysis becomes necessary when the kidneys are impaired by disease or injury and are unable to excrete nitrogen-containing waste products and regulate pH and electrolyte concentration. In hemodialysis, the blood is passed through a dialysis machine, which filters the blood as kidneys normally do in healthy people, and then the blood is returned to the body.

Hemodialysis is generally performed three times a week in 2- to 4-hour sessions. The procedure is usually performed at an outpatient dialysis center. In some cases, the procedure may be done at home with help. Both the person being treated and his or her helper must receive special training.

Rapid changes in fluid and chemical balance may occur during treatment, producing muscle cramps and a sudden drop in blood pressure,

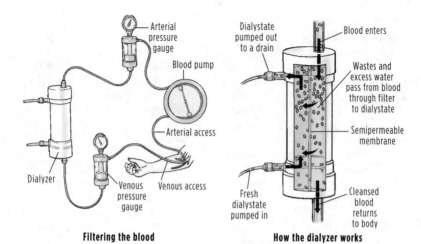

Filtering the blood

How the dialyzer works

Arterial pressure gauge

Blood pump

Arterial access

Dialyzer

Venous pressure gauge

Venous access

Dialystate pumped out to a drain

Blood enters

Wastes and excess water pass from blood through filter to dialystate

Semipermeable membrane

Fresh dialystate pumped in

Cleansed blood returns to body

Explaining Hemodialysis

During hemodialysis, blood is removed, filtered by a machine, and returned to the body as a treatment for kidney failure. This process requires a delivery system to circulate the blood, a site on the body to remove and return the blood, and a filtering mechanism (dialyzer) to clean the blood. Within the dialyzer is a semipermeable filter with tiny pores that permits wastes and excess water to pass from the blood into a cleansing fluid called dialysate, but prevents the blood and dialysate from mixing. An arterial pressure gauge and a venous pressure gauge are monitored to make sure the person's blood pressure does not rise or fall too drastically.

which may result in weakness, dizziness, or nausea. Side effects such as these should be reported to a doctor immediately. They can often be avoided if a proper diet and medication schedule are followed. See also DIALYSIS.

Hemodialyzer

See DIALYSIS MACHINE.

Hemoglobin

The pigment in BLOOD that transports oxygen. Hemoglobin is formed in bone marrow and is found in all red blood cells. Hemoglobin is a large, complex molecule consisting of a protein component (globin) and an iron-bearing component (heme). It makes up about 33 percent of a red blood cell.

Hemoglobinopathy

Inherited disorders involving abnormal hemoglobin molecules. Abnormal hemoglobin is generally less efficient than normal hemoglobin at carrying oxygen to the cells of the body. People with hemoglobinopathies may have mild to moderate anemia and occasional attacks of pain. The most common types of hemoglobinopathy are hemoglobin C disease, which involves the production of abnormal hemoglobin but may not require treatment; hemoglobin S-C disease, which produces mild to moderate anemia, occasional attacks of acute pain, and slightly shorter than normal life spans; hemoglobin E disease, which occurs chiefly in people of Southeast Asian ancestry; and SICKLE CELL ANEMIA.

Hemoglobinuria

The presence of hemoglobin in the urine without the simultaneous presence of red blood cells. Under normal circumstances, red blood cells break down after a life span of approximately 120 days. The breakdown process occurs largely in the spleen. Breakdown in the blood vessels releases free hemoglobin, which is then bound by another protein for reprocessing into new blood cells. If, however, the breakdown process in the blood vessels occurs faster than the protein binding, free hemoglobin appears in the urine and can be detected with a laboratory test. Hemoglobinuria can signal a variety of diseases, primarily hemolytic anemia, glomerulonephritis, SICKLE CELL ANEMIA, thalassemia, and malaria.

Treatment of the underlying infection often resolves the hemoglobinuria. Drugs that suppress the immune system can also be prescribed.

Hemolytic disease of the newborn

A disease most commonly caused by RH INCOMPATIBILITY, a situation in which the mother's blood develops antibodies in reaction to the blood of the fetus. The disease occurs when an Rh-negative mother is pregnant with an Rh-positive fetus; the fetus can develop anemia from the loss of red blood cells and JAUNDICE from its body's inability to process the destroyed cells, all of which may lead to a stillbirth. Giving blocking antibodies to an Rh-negative mother prevents her from developing antibodies to the fetus's blood in most cases. Blocking antibodies are usually given at the beginning of the third trimester and again within 72 hours of delivery.

AMNIOCENTESIS can detect Rh-factor problems in advance, and close monitoring of fetal development will enable the doctor to prepare for potential problems.

Hemolytic-uremic syndrome

A serious disease that involves the destruction of red blood cells, damage to the walls of the blood vessels, and failure of the kidneys. The disease is most likely to occur in children between the ages of 1 and 10 after a serious stomach and intestinal infection.

The cause of the infection is often ESCHERICHIA COLI (*E. coli*), a bacterium found in contaminated meat, dairy products, and fruit juice. Toxins produced by the bacteria in the intestinal system enter the bloodstream and destroy red blood cells, causing small, unusual bruises in the skin or hemorrhages in the mouth. The damaged red blood cells can clog the small passageways of the kidneys, forcing them to work harder and less effectively. Urine production falls. Fluid accumulating in the body raises the blood pressure and causes swelling, particularly of the hands and feet. The nervous system can be affected, leading to seizures, lethargy, and temporary blindness.

Once hemolytic-uremic syndrome begins, there is no cure. Treatment consists of supporting the child with fluids, salts, and blood transfusions as needed. In some cases, dialysis is required to augment the kidneys. Medication may be used to lower blood pressure and treat nervous system symptoms.

Hemophilia

An inherited disorder that causes the blood to clot ineffectively and can result in extensive bruising and bleeding. Because of the way in which it is inherited, hemophilia affects males almost exclusively. Individuals with hemophilia used to die at a young age, but with current treatments, the life span is nearly normal.

Hemophilia results from a deficiency in a protein required for clotting. The three different types of hemophilia result from deficiencies in three different proteins.

The genes that carry hemophilia A and B are sex-linked recessive genes transmitted on the X chromosome. Women have two X chromosomes. As a result, women with a hemophilia gene on one X chromosome are usually protected against the disease by the normal gene on the other. These women have no symptoms of hemophilia but are carriers of the disease, who can pass it on to their children. Men, however, have only one X chromosome, inherited from their mothers. If this X chromosome carries the hemophilia gene, the man is almost certain to have the disease, since there is no normal gene to counterbalance the hemophilia gene's effect.

The male children of a man with hemophilia cannot inherit hemophilia from him since he passes only his Y chromosome on to them, but his daughters inherit his X chromosome and become carriers. A woman can inherit hemophilia only if her father has the disease and her mother is a carrier. Since this happens very rarely, few women ever have hemophilia.

Not all cases of hemophilia are inherited. About 1 in 3 cases results from a spontaneous mutation in the gene in a person whose ancestors show no sign of the disease. The mutated gene is then passed on to subsequent generations.

In more severe cases of hemophilia, treatment for bleeding episodes consists of transfusing the person with the missing coagulation factor in concentrated form. People with particularly severe disease may need regular preventive transfusions.

People with hemophilia need to avoid situations such as contact sports and medications such as aspirin that make bleeding more likely. Immunization against HEPATITIS B is important because of regular exposure to blood products, which can transmit the infection.

Hemorrhage

A loss of a large amount of blood in a short time. The BLOOD LOSS may be due to internal bleeding, as from the intestine or stomach; external bleeding from an injury. If the volume of blood lost makes the heart unable to pump enough to the body, hypovolemic shock can occur, with symptoms that may include a rapid or weak pulse, pale skin, cool or moist skin, rapid breathing, anxiety, overall weakness, and low blood pressure. Emergency medical attention must be sought. If there is an external wound, sterile dressings and steady, firm, direct pressure should be applied to stop the bleeding.

Hemorrhage, cerebral

Also known as an intracerebral hemorrhage, a cause of STROKE in which blood vessels within the brain leak blood into the brain itself. A cerebral hemorrhage is a potentially life-threatening condition that requires immediate medical attention. Hemorrhage may be caused by trauma or by an abnormality such as an ANEURYSM (abnormal ballooning of a weakened area in the wall of an artery). It can also be associated with HYPERTENSION (high blood pressure). Blood irritates brain tissue and causes swelling or edema; blood can also form into a mass or HEMATOMA. Either condition puts further pressure on brain tissue.

Internal bleeding can occur anywhere in the brain. The extent of BRAIN DAMAGE depends on the location and the extent of tissue affected. Symptoms commonly include severe headache; nausea and vomiting; changes in consciousness, such as sleepiness, apathy, stupor, or loss of consciousness; vision changes; numbness or tingling; difficulty speaking or understanding speech; problems with swallowing; abnormal taste; loss of motor skills, coordination, or balance; and seizures.

Immediate medical attention is required to diagnose and treat a cerebral hemorrhage. Treatment varies but may include surgery. Possible medications include corticosteroids, diuretics, anticonvulsants, and analgesics. Rarely, blood products and intravenous fluids may be necessary. Outcomes vary widely. Even with prompt treatment, brain damage or death may occur.

Hemorrhage, intracerebral

See HEMORRHAGE, CEREBRAL.

Hemorrhage, intraventricular

Also known as IVH, bleeding from fragile blood vessels in the brain. Intraventricular hemorrhages are most common in premature infants born more than 8 weeks early. Symptoms of IVH include breathing problems, weak pulse, low blood pressure, paleness, seizures, and HYDROCEPHALUS (excessive accumulation of cerebrospinal fluid in the skull).

IVH is diagnosed and monitored in infants through ultrasound scanning. The goals of treatment are to prevent further bleeding and to keep the infant stable. Any related problems, such as infections or seizures, are dealt with appropriately. Treatment for hydrocephalus includes spinal taps to remove fluid and possibly surgery.

Hemorrhage, subarachnoid

Bleeding into the space between the brain and the arachnoid membrane (the middle membrane covering the brain). This is a life-threatening condition that can lead to STROKE, SEIZURE, BRAIN DAMAGE, or death. It may result in permanent brain damage caused by ischemia (loss of blood flow) or bleeding into the brain tissue. Most often, a subarachnoid hemorrhage is caused by a cerebral ANEURYSM that has ruptured or burst. However, it may also be a result of other blood vessel abnormalities (such as an ARTERIOVENOUS MALFORMATION) or trauma.

The primary symptom of a subarachnoid hemorrhage is the sudden onset of a severe headache. This may be accompanied by nausea, vomiting, fainting, a decreased level or loss of consciousness, breathing problems, difficulties with speech, trouble swallowing, confusion, irritability, vision problems, loss of movement or sensation, muscle aches, stiff neck, or a seizure.

Immediate medical attention is required to diagnose and treat a subarachnoid hemorrhage.

Treatment varies, but usually includes lifesaving interventions and supportive measures. Surgery is usually required to remove large hematomas or repair damage.

Hemorrhoidectomy

Surgical removal of HEMORRHOIDS, swollen or enlarged veins in the anal canal. Doctors use a number of different methods to remove painful or bleeding hemorrhoids.

Hemorrhoids

Swollen or enlarged veins in the anal canal. Hemorrhoids are a common problem in both men and women after age 50. Also known as piles, hemorrhoids can be internal or external. Internal hemorrhoids arise near the beginning of the anal canal and cannot be seen with the naked eye. External hemorrhoids are visible as a bulge under the skin outside the anus.

Hemorrhoids often cause no problems. However, bleeding is a common symptom.

The primary cause of hemorrhoids is persistent straining to move the bowels, often related to a diet low in fiber and consequent constipation. Pregnant women are prone to develop hemorrhoids that may persist until several weeks after childbirth.

Generally, hemorrhoids are not serious. However, rectal bleeding may be a sign of a serious underlying disease such as cancer. People who experience rectal bleeding should seek prompt medical attention even when they believe that bleeding is from hemorrhoids. Diagnosis is confirmed with a rectal examination and tests, such as SIGMOIDOSCOPY or COLONOSCOPY.

Often, the only treatment required for hemorrhoids is adding more fiber and fluid to the diet. Responding promptly to the urge to defecate is also important, as is good hygiene.

Hemothorax

Blood that has collected in the space between the chest wall and the lung, an area called the pleural cavity. Hemothorax may be caused by cancer, a pulmonary embolism, chest surgery, tuberculosis, or tissue death in the lung, but it is most commonly caused by trauma or injury to the chest. A large hemothorax can produce shock in a person who has experienced trauma, and it may also be associated with a collapsed lung. Respiratory failure can result if a large amount of blood gathers in the pleural cavity.

Symptoms of hemothorax include chest pain, shortness of breath, rapid heart rate, anxiety, restlessness, and temporary cessation of breathing. It can be diagnosed by a physical examination using a stethoscope, which will reveal a decrease in breathing sounds in the area where the hemothorax is present. Tests may be performed to confirm the diagnosis.

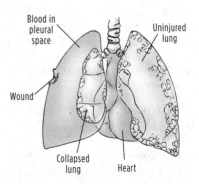

Bleeding into lung cavity
Hemothorax is mostly commonly caused by injury to the chest, as when a broken rib pierces lung tissue or an artery.

Treatment is based on stabilizing the condition of the affected person, stopping the bleeding, and removing the blood from the pleural cavity. Surgery may be necessary to treat the injury that has caused the hemothorax. Complications include shock, fibrosis, or scarring of the pleural cavity.

Hepatectomy, partial

The partial removal of the liver. A surgeon may perform this operation when cancer is contained within one lobe of the liver, in the absence of CIRRHOSIS (a severe liver disease), jaundice (a yellowing of the skin and the whites of the eyes), and ASCITES (an abnormal collection of fluid inside the abdominal cavity). Complete removal of a tumor usually offers the best survival rate from liver cancer.

Hepatectomy, total

See LIVER TRANSPLANT.

Hepatic

Pertaining to, relating to, or originating in the liver.

Hepatitis

Inflammation of the liver that can lead to swelling, tenderness, and permanent damage. When hepatitis harms the liver, it can no longer perform key functions at peak efficiency. Severe cases of hepatitis can lead to life-threatening liver failure. Even without symptoms, hepatitis may slowly be causing serious damage, such as scarring to the liver. Hepatitis is most commonly due to a virus, although certain drugs, poisons, or chemicals can also cause it. See HEPATITIS A, HEPATITIS B, HEPATITIS C, HEPATITIS D, and HEPATITIS E.

Excessive alcohol consumption can lead to alcoholic hepatitis. Severe alcoholic hepatitis is a life-threatening condition that requires hospitalization. See also LIVER DISEASE, ALCOHOLIC.

Symptoms

Acute hepatitis refers to liver inflammation and symptoms that are short-term. A mild case of acute hepatitis may cause no symptoms at all or vague flulike symptoms that last from several days to several weeks. On the other hand, sometimes (as in an acute attack of chronic hepatitis B with hepatitis D) symptoms are severe and debilitating. Such cases can lead to permanent liver damage, liver failure, and the need for a liver transplant.

Chronic hepatitis also can exhibit a range of symptoms, although sometimes no symptoms are apparent. Chronic active hepatitis is a continuing inflammation of the liver that damages liver cells. It can cause extreme weakness and disability and can lead to potentially life-threatening complications such as cirrhosis, liver cancer, and liver failure.

Diagnosis and treatment

A diagnosis of hepatitis is made by physical examination, medical history, and blood tests. When symptoms are not present, blood tests administered during the course of a routine physical examination may reveal elevated liver enzymes, which can be a sign of hepatitis.

Treatment of hepatitis depends on its cause and whether the disease is acute or chronic. In acute cases, doctors recommend bed rest, a balanced diet, and avoiding alcohol. Chronic cases may be treated with medication, depending on the underlying cause and the extent of the underlying liver damage.

Risk factors

Certain groups are at special risk of hepatitis. These include people who have sex with an infected person or multiple partners, infants born to infected mothers, IV drug users, people who get tattoos or body piercings with improperly sterilized equipment, people with hemophilia, and health care workers.

Hepatitis A

Inflammation of the liver due to infection with the hepatitis A virus (HAV). The infection is sudden and acute and does not cause chronic or long-lasting disease. Initially shed in the stool, this virus is spread through food or water contaminated by feces. It is frequently a childhood illness and can occur in nurseries and day care centers where diapers are frequently changed.

Infection with HAV usually passes in 6 to 8 weeks with no treatment other than bed rest, a balanced diet, and avoiding alcohol. However, a lack of energy and prolonged fatigue may last for weeks or months. In rare cases, severe hepatitis A results in liver failure.

Good personal hygiene and proper handling of food can effectively prevent the spread of hepatitis A. People who are infected with HAV should not prepare or handle food that is to be eaten by others.

Hepatitis B

Inflammation of the liver due to infection with the hepatitis B virus (HBV). The infection can be sudden and acute or chronic and long-lasting (defined as the persistence of the virus in the blood 6 months or more after the initial infection). In the United States, hepatitis B is most common in older adolescents and adults. In nine of ten affected people, the condition improves spontaneously; only a few develop chronic HBV infection. Of these, about half have active symptoms in addition to carrying the virus.

In some cases, severe, acute flare-ups of HBV are triggered by infection with hepatitis D virus (see HEPATITIS D). Hepatitis B is highly infectious during the 6- to 12-week incubation period (the time between initial exposure to the virus and the development of symptoms). Even after acute symptoms disappear, some individuals with HBV develop chronic disease while others (who may have no symptoms) become lifelong HBV carriers.

The virus can also be passed from an infected mother to her infant during childbirth.

Treatment of acute cases consists primarily of bed rest, a balanced diet, and avoiding alcohol. Infants born to infected mothers should receive hepatitis B immune globulin within 12 hours of birth. Drugs have had some success in treating chronic hepatitis B. If HBV destroys a major portion of the liver and prevents it from functioning properly, a liver transplant may be considered.

Because a vaccine for hepatitis B exists, HBV is preventable. It is routinely given to children in the United States (see VACCINATION) and should also be given to adults who are at risk for infection.

Hepatitis C

Inflammation of the liver due to infection with the hepatitis C virus (HCV). Hepatitis C is more likely than any other type of viral hepatitis to lead to chronic hepatitis (meaning that the virus persists in the blood 6 months or more after the initial infection). Nearly nine of ten people who contract hepatitis C retain evidence of it indefinitely and are carriers of the virus. Hepatitis C most frequently occurs in intravenous (IV) drug users who share needles; people who get tattoos or body piercings with poorly sterilized equipment; health care workers; and those with bleeding disorders such as hemophilia. It is not common for hepatitis C to spread through sexual activity with an infected person or from an infected mother to an infant.

Because this form of hepatitis often has few acute symptoms, it is often detected through abnormal levels of liver enzymes obtained during the course of routine blood tests.

The only cure for chronic infection with HCV is a complicated year-long regimen of interferon injections and ribavarin capsules. In many people, interferon causes devastating, flulike side effects (including fever, chills, and body aches) and severe depression. Many find that they cannot tolerate the regimen. Treatment is not universally successful, and in many cases, the infection returns.

Eventually, if hepatitis C destroys a major portion of the liver, a liver transplant may be required. Hepatitis C is currently the most common reason for liver transplants in the United States. Because there is no vaccine against hepatitis C, prevention is key.

Hepatitis D

A liver infection that occurs only in people who are already infected with the hepatitis B virus (HBV); also known as delta hepatitis and abbreviated HDV. Like HEPATITIS B, this infection is spread primarily through contact with infected blood and through sexual activity.

Infection with HDV affects the body in two ways. It may occur simultaneously with acute hepatitis B, in a condition called coinfection. The likelihood of recovery from coinfection is excellent. However, HDV infection can also develop when HBV infection enters a chronic stage, in a condition known as superinfection. Superinfection with chronic HDV is a more serious disease than either chronic hepatitis B or C. It is more likely to lead to severe acute hepatitis, which can result in liver failure.

Even when symptoms are not present, a person with chronic HDV is a carrier of the virus. Treatment options are limited. Supportive care including a balanced diet and avoiding alcohol may help alleviate symptoms. If HDV infection destroys a major portion of the liver and prevents it from functioning properly, a liver transplant may be considered. However, even when a transplant is successful, cirrhosis may recur.

Hepatitis E

Inflammation of the liver due to infection with the hepatitis E virus (HEV). This virus is also known as epidemic non-A, non-B hepatitis; it is transmitted through the intestinal tract. No outbreaks of HEV have occurred in the United States. The disease occurs mainly in areas with poor sanitation.

Hepatitis E is an acute, short-lived

disease. In most cases, hepatitis E is mild and disappears within a few weeks with no lasting effects. However, although it does not become a chronic disease, a severe case of hepatitis E may destroy so many cells that it causes liver failure. Pregnant women are more at risk of this complication with HEV than with other types of hepatitis.

There is no vaccine for HEV. When traveling, the best way to prevent infection with hepatitis E is to use only sterilized water and beverages.

Hepatitis, nonalcoholic steatohepatitis

See NONALCOHOLIC STEATOHEPATITIS.

Hepatitis, viral

Inflammation of the liver that is caused by viral infection. There are many viruses currently known to cause liver inflammation, including HEPATITIS A, HEPATITIS B, HEPATITIS C, HEPATITIS D, HEPATITIS E, hepatitis F, hepatitis G, the EPSTEIN-BARR VIRUS (EBV), and CYTOMEGALOVIRUS.

Hepatoma

A tumor originating from liver cells that is usually malignant. Common symptoms of a malignant hepatoma (hepatocellular carcinoma) include bloating, abdominal pain, fever, weight loss, nausea, and decreased appetite. In advanced stages of the disease, symptoms can include AS-CITES (swelling of the abdomen from fluid), jaundice (yellowing of the skin and the whites of the eyes), and swollen legs. Liver cancer is not common in the United States, although it may be the most common cancer worldwide. It is not generally diagnosed early and often reaches an ad-

vanced stage before symptoms develop and a person seeks medical care. Diagnosis of liver cancer usually requires a biopsy. Early-stage hepatomas can be removed surgically, or destroyed by injecting alcohol, using cryotherapy (freezing), or by embolization, in which a substance is injected into the artery supplying blood to the tumor to block the blood flow. Current treatments of advanced liver cancer are not very effective; the primary goal is the relief of symptoms. Some patients can be treated with liver transplantation.

Hepatomegaly

Swelling or enlargement of the liver. Among the causes of hepatomegaly are liver congestion due to heart failure, obstruction of the veins that drain the liver, a cyst or tumor, or a fatty liver due to alcoholic liver disease (see LIVER DISEASE, ALCOHOLIC), or metastatic liver disease, in which cancer from another part of the body spreads to the liver. A physical examination, medical history, and various laboratory and imaging tests can detect the underlying cause of hepatomegaly. The treatment of an enlarged liver is determined directly by its cause.

Herbal medicine

The use of leaves, flowers, fruits, stems, bark, and roots of plants to prevent, relieve, and treat illness. Herbal medicine has a significant role in Chinese medicine and ayurveda.

In the United States, herbal remedies are not classified as drugs but as foods or dietary supplements. As a result, the Food and Drug Administration (FDA) does not regulate herbal remedies or oversee the research that would establish their effectiveness and safety. However, the FDA does restrict the claims that manufacturers of herbal remedies can make in labeling their products.

Heredity

The genetic transmission of characteristics or traits from one generation to the next; the genetic makeup of an individual, derived from ancestors.

Hermaphroditism

A genetic abnormality in which a person is born with both male and female sex organs. The cause of this abnormality is not well understood.

When a baby is born with hermaphroditism, a pediatric endocrinologist, a specialist in the hormonal problems of infancy, should be consulted. The correct assignment of the baby's sex can be made only after thorough testing and evaluation. This process is critical because the baby's future life and emotional health are at stake.

Hernia

Protrusion of an organ or tissue through a weak spot in a muscle or other tissue that normally contains it. The muscles and connective tissues are ordinarily firm enough to hold organs in place. However, when muscles grow slack due to disease or injury, tissue may bulge through the weak point. Although hernias can occur anywhere in the body, they are most common in the abdominal wall. Herniation may also occur internally where it cannot be detected by external examination.

Most abdominal hernias are diagnosed by a physical examination. A truss can be worn to keep a hernia in place. However, surgery is generally the best treatment. (See HERNIOR-RHAPHY.) Without surgery, hernias generally grow worse and develop complications (see INTESTINE, OBSTRUCTION OF), which require immediate medical attention.

Herniated disk

See SLIPPED DISK.

Herniorrhaphy

An operation in which a HERNIA (a protrusion of soft tissue through other tissue, usually muscle, that normally contains it) is surgically corrected.

Herpangina

An acute infectious disorder characterized by fever and ulcerated blisters on mucous membranes inside the mouth. Herpangina is most commonly caused by a COXSACKIEVIRUS, but may also be caused by other intestinal viruses. The disorder tends to occur in infants and children, spreading rapidly within a group.

Symptoms include a sudden onset of fever with sore throat, headache, and loss of appetite. Often pain is experienced in the areas of the neck, abdomen, and extremities. There may be vomiting and seizures in infants. Within a few days of initial symptoms, small grayish, blistering sores with red borders appear inside the mouth on the soft palate, uvula, or tongue and on the tonsils.

Herpangina is diagnosed by a clinical history of symptoms and observation of the characteristic sores in the mouth. Blood tests may be used if it is necessary to diagnose the cause of infection. There are no medications to treat this viral disorder, so treatment is recommended to alleviate symptoms.

Herpes B virus

A member of the herpes group of viruses that is carried by rhesus and other Asiatic macaque monkeys. Herpes B virus is also referred to as *Herpesvirus simiae* and can cause serious disease, including ENCEPHALITIS.

Herpes B virus is believed to be transmitted to humans by exposure to the contaminated saliva of an infected primate that may occur when a person is bitten or scratched by a monkey. Symptoms generally occur within 1 month of exposure and may include blistered lesions on the skin and pain and numbness at the site of the bite or scratch. The infection may progress to encephalitis. The antiviral medication acyclovir has been successful in treating early stages of mild infections. Because of the potential seriousness of the infection, preventive guidelines must be strictly followed by people who regularly handle macaque monkeys.

Herpes gestationis

An itchy rash that develops in the second or third trimester of pregnancy and usually disappears by 3 months after childbirth. The rash consists of fluid-filled blisters that can occur anywhere on the skin. The cause of herpes gestationis is not known. (It is not related to genital herpes.)

Herpes keratitis

Painful inflammation and ulceration of the outer surface (cornea) of the eye because of infection with the herpes virus. Most herpes infections of the eye are caused by type 1 herpes simplex virus, the type of herpes virus that causes fever blisters and cold sores. Prompt treatment with antiviral drugs (eye drops or pills) can prevent the infection from penetrating more deeply into the eye surface, where it is difficult to control and more likely to result in permanent damage.

Herpes zoster

See SHINGLES.

Herpes, genital

One of the SEXUALLY TRANSMITTED DISEASES (STDs); typically caused by the herpes simplex virus type 2 (HSV-2). Genital herpes is a chronic, lifelong, viral infection that affects millions of people. Genital herpes is spread from person to person via sexual activities.

An infected person can spread genital herpes when he or she has symptoms and also when there are no visible symptoms.

A woman who is pregnant and who has an HSV-2 infection can spread the infection to her newborn during childbirth. This is the single greatest danger of genital herpes because the virus may infect the infant's skin, mouth, lungs, eyes, brain, or other vital organs. For this reason, a CESAREAN SECTION is generally performed if a woman has an outbreak of genital herpes when her baby is due.

Most people who are infected with HSV-2 have no symptoms. When there are associated symptoms, they are usually mild and may include itching and burning sensations or tiny, red, painful blisters in the genital area, swollen glands in the groin, headaches, fever, and general malaise. Some people with genital herpes acquire a FEVER BLISTER near the mouth.

For women, the infection may spread into the vagina and up to the cervix, which may increase the risk of cervical cancer. For this reason, women with the infection should have a PAP SMEAR every 1 to 2 years to screen for this cancer. Women who are pregnant and who experience symptoms of genital herpes should seek a medical evaluation immediately.

Genital herpes is diagnosed by taking a sexual history and a clinical history of symptoms and by performing a physical examination during which the characteristic blisters or ulcers on the genitals can be observed. There is no cure for genital herpes, but when recurring episodes cause disturbing symptoms, the infection can be treated with oral or topical antiviral medications. When HSV-2 infection spreads into the bloodstream causing widespread infection, intravenous antiviral medication may be necessary.

As with all STDs, genital herpes can be prevented by approaching sexual relationships responsibly. See SAFE SEX.

Herpes, orolabial

An acute viral infection caused by the herpes simplex virus type 1 and characterized by blisters in or around the mouth and lips. Orolabial herpes may or may not be related to genital herpes (see HERPES, GENITAL).

The infection tends to recur, often in association with emotional or physical stress, fever, menstruation, gastrointestinal disturbances, infection, the common cold, fatigue, or sun exposure. Symptoms usually last about 2 weeks, during which time the infection is contagious. Orolabial herpes may be contagious without symptoms as well.

Orolabial herpes may be diagnosed by a doctor after he or she physically examines the characteristic lesions inside the mouth and on the lips. Oral or topical antiviral medications such as acyclovir can help prevent spread of the infection.

Heterosexuality

Enduring erotic, emotional, romantic, or sexual attraction to members of the opposite sex. Most men and women are heterosexual. Heterosexuality, like the other sexual orientations, is an inborn predisposition.

HGE

See HUMAN GRANULOCYTIC EHRLICHIOSIS.

Hiatal hernia

Protrusion of part of the stomach upward into the chest through an opening in the diaphragm.

Hiatal hernias are very common and are not fundamentally dangerous. In many cases, there are no symptoms at all. However, hiatal hernia is associated with ESOPHAGEAL REFLUX (the backward flow of acid from the stomach up into the esophagus).

Diagnosis of a hiatal hernia is made by obtaining an accurate medical history and tests, such as an upper GASTROINTESTINAL (GI) SERIES (an X-ray procedure also called a BARIUM SWALLOW) and GASTROSCOPY (visual examination of the esophagus, stomach, and duodenum with a lighted tube called a gastroscope). In many cases, simple lifestyle modifications control symptoms. Antacids are often helpful, although prolonged heavy use can disrupt body chemistry. Stronger prescription medications are also available to reduce secretion of acids. However, if symptoms persist or complications occur, surgery may be necessary. See HERNIORRHAPHY.

Hib vaccine

The vaccine that induces antibodies that help prevent infection with *Haemophilus influenzae* type b (see IMMUNIZATION).

Hiccup

An involuntary contraction of the diaphragm, followed by the closing of the epiglottis over the vocal cords, producing a characteristic sound.

HIDA scan

Hepatobiliary iminodiacetic acid scan. A HIDA scan assesses the excretory system of the liver after injection with the radionuclide iminodiacetic acid (IDA). A HIDA scan is an imaging procedure used in NUCLEAR MEDICINE to examine the liver, gallbladder, and duodenum.

High blood pressure

A popular name for the medical term HYPERTENSION.

Hip

The joint that connects the bone of the upper leg to the pelvis and largely supports the weight of the upper body. The hip is a stable ball-and-socket joint. The round end of the upper thighbone (femur) fits into a rounded hollow in the pelvis called the acetabulum. The acetabulum is a deep cavity enclosing about two thirds of the head of the femur.

Three strong ligaments attach the femur to the pelvis and contribute to the joint's stability. Because the hip is a ball-and-socket joint like the shoulder, it allows a limited range of movement. The hip is the most commonly replaced joint in the body. See JOINT REPLACEMENT, HIP.

Hip replacement

See JOINT REPLACEMENT, HIP.

Hip, congenital dislocation of

A birth defect caused by incomplete development of the hip joint. Newborns with hip dislocation are usually fitted with a brace that positions the top of the femur (thighbone) in the hip socket. The brace is usually worn for 6 to 8 weeks. Failure to treat congenital hip dislocation can lead to permanent hip disability.

Hip, fractured

A serious injury involving a broken bone of the hip. Hip fractures are almost always surgically repaired. Traction may be used to repair a broken hip bone, but only when surgery is inadvisable. The lengthy confinement to bed involved in traction poses several serious risks, including pneumonia.

If the bone is still properly aligned after it has broken, a surgical procedure that involves inserting metal screws into the bone to hold it firmly together while it heals may be recommended. This approach to treating a fractured hip is called open reduction with internal fixation and is usually appropriate for younger people.

Hippocratic oath

An oath of professional conduct attributed to Hippocrates, an influential Greek physician of the fifth century BC. The oath outlines the nature of a doctor's role in society at the time. In general, when taking the oath, physicians swear to practice medicine to the best of their ability and for the benefit of patients and, above all, not to do harm.

Hirsutism

Excess facial and body hair in women. Hirsutism is not a disease, and the underlying cause is not usually a serious disorder. The principal problems associated with hirsutism are aesthetic. See HAIR REMOVAL.

If a woman experiences a sudden increase in hair growth or if hirsutism cannot be controlled by standard cosmetic approaches, an evaluation by an endocrinologist is recommended.

Oral contraceptives that contain the hormones estrogen and progestin may prove effective for controlling hirsutism by suppressing androgen hormone levels.

Histamine

A chemical that is released by mast cells in the immune system and can act as an irritating stimulant. Histamine is considered responsible for most of the swelling and itching symptoms of HAY FEVER and other allergies. The mast cells lining the skin and the respiratory and gastrointestinal tracts release histamine when an ALLERGEN enters the body. The function of histamine is to combat the allergen, which the body perceives as harmful.

When the entire system becomes overwhelmed by an excessive release of histamine, the life-threatening medical emergency known as ANAPHYLAXIS occurs. Antihistamine drugs are a type of medication that combats the effects of histamine.

Histamine₂ blockers

A class of drugs used to treat conditions in which the stomach produces too much hydrochloric acid; histamine$_2$ (H$_2$) receptor antagonists. H$_2$ blockers are used to treat stomach ulcers (gastric ulcers and duodenal ulcers), as well as other stomach disorders caused by excess stomach acid, such as heartburn caused by acid that moves back into the esophagus.

Histocompatibility antigens

Substances that help the body identify tissue as its own or as foreign. Histocompatibility antigens also help determine whether tissue or organ transplants will be accepted or rejected. Histocompatibility means "tissue compatibility."

Histoplasmosis

A disease primarily affecting the lungs that is caused by the fungus *Histoplasma capsulatum*. Histoplasmosis occurs when soil that is contaminated with bird or bat droppings, which contain histoplasmosis spores, is disturbed and the airborne spores are inhaled.

Acute histoplasmosis causes a flu-like syndrome and affects the lungs, causing malaise, fever, chest pains, respiratory symptoms, and a dry cough. A chest X ray may reveal a characteristic pattern of the disease. In its chronic form, histoplasmosis bears a clinical resemblance to tuberculosis; this form may remain dormant or become more severe over months or years.

Chronic histoplasmosis can result in permanent lung damage. A form of the disease in which organs in addition to the lungs are affected is called disseminated histoplasmosis. This form can be fatal if untreated.

Mild disease tends to improve on its own without treatment. Severe cases of acute histoplasmosis and cases of chronic or disseminated histoplasmosis are treated with antifungal medications.

Histrionic personality disorder

A mental disorder marked by a constant pattern of excessive emotions and attention-seeking behavior that usually begins in early adulthood. Treatment consists of behavioral therapy.

HIV

Human immunodeficiency virus; a virus that attacks the body's immune system and leads to associated infections and malignant tumors. HIV is the virus that leads to acquired immunodeficiency syndrome, which is known as AIDS.

HIV infection is caused by one of two related retroviruses, HIV-1 and HIV-2, that produce a wide range of conditions varying from the presence of contagious infection with no apparent symptoms to disorders that are severely disabling and eventually fatal.

HIV transmission requires contact with body fluids containing infected cells or infected plasma. These fluids include blood, semen, vaginal secretions, and breast milk.

The greatest risk of being infected with HIV is through genital intercourse, particularly penile-anal intercourse. Sexual practices that do not involve exposure to bodily fluids are considered safe and do not generally spread HIV infection. HIV infection may be spread by contact with lesions caused by other SEXUALLY TRANSMITTED DISEASES (STDs).

HIV-infected cells in blood can be transferred during a blood transfusion, so as a result, all blood donors are now screened for risk factors and the blood tested for the presence of the virus.

Symptoms

The symptoms that develop during the initial acute HIV infection are nonspecific and include sore throat, myalgias, fever, and rash. About 50 to 70 percent of infected people develop symptoms, usually 3 to 6 weeks after infection. Symptoms usually resolve in 2 to 3 weeks, followed by a chronic phase in which the body's immune system is able to contain the virus.

The final stage is marked by a failing immune system. People usually have fatigue, pain, weight loss, and diarrhea. Finally, the patients develop opportunistic infections, cancers, and neurological symptoms.

Diagnosis and treatment

An HIV diagnosis can be made by evaluating the results of blood tests that look for the presence of antibodies to HIV, or immunological abnormalities, and a decline in helper T cells.

There is no cure for HIV infection. The first line of defense against the infection is to prevent its spread. Those who have HIV should inform their sex partners and anyone with whom they have shared needles and syringes; all of these people should be tested for HIV.

A severely weakened immune system is indicated by the T-cell count of an infected person going below 200. At this point, anti-HIV therapy is generally initiated. Antiretroviral medications are the basis of treatment for HIV and have been shown to prolong life and reduce the progression to AIDS. The major emphasis of treatment is finding effective combinations of antiviral medication that the person can tolerate indefinitely. Also, major emphasis is placed on the prevention of opportunistic infections that can prove fatal to a person whose immune system is already compromised.

Risks and prevention

The practice of safe sex reduces possible exposure to the HIV virus that can cause AIDS. Safe sex is defined as avoiding any behavior that may expose a person or his or her partner to bodily fluids.

It is possible to become infected with HIV by performing oral sex. Since blood, semen, preseminal fluid, and vaginal fluid are all possible carriers of the virus, the cells in the mucous lining of the mouth can transmit HIV to the lymph nodes or the bloodstream. The use of a DENTAL DAM may offer some protection during oral-genital or oral-anal activities. Also, using a latex condom during oral, vaginal, or anal sex as a barrier can help prevent risk of infection.

Paraphernalia involved in illegal drug use can spread HIV infection, as any reused materials—including syringes, water, bottle caps, or spoons used to dissolve drugs in water or heat drug solutions—may carry the blood-borne virus.

The risks of HIV infection associated with sexual contact are increased when a person has an STD. Medical treatment of other STDs can be an effective approach to reducing the risk of HIV infection.

Hives

Pink, itchy, round swellings that can occur anywhere on the body; also known as urticaria. Each individual hive usually disappears in 24 hours or less. Hives develop when natural chemicals including histamine are released in the skin. Most commonly, this occurs in response to an allergic reaction to a food, medication, pollen, or infections. Less frequently, hives are due to nonallergic causes such as autoimmune disease.

The best treatment for hives is to find the cause and eliminate it. Hives are usually treated with over-the-counter antihistamines. For persistent or severe cases, it is important to consult a doctor. Prescription medications may be necessary to control the problem. Emergency medical care is required when hives are accompanied by breathing problems or swelling in the throat.

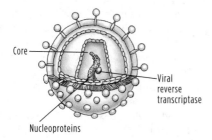

Core

Viral reverse transcriptase

Nucleoproteins

The HIV virus

HIV, the deadly virus responsible for developing AIDS, is composed of an inner core with genetic information and a protective outer shell of proteins (nucleoproteins).

HME

See HUMAN MONOCYTIC EHRLICHIOSIS.

HMO

The abbreviation for a health mainte-nance organization, or a managed care plan that provides medical ser-vices to members on a prepaid basis. Medical care is usually coordinated by one primary care doctor, who makes referrals as necessary to spe-cialists within the HMO.

HNPCC

See COLON CANCER.

Hoarseness

An abnormal harshness or distortion in the voice. Hoarseness, medically termed dysphonia, can make the voice sound breathy, strained, or rasping. It can also result in changes in volume or in pitch, ranging from high to low.

The most common causes of hoarseness include swelling due to inflammation (see LARYNGITIS), usu-ally from a viral infection, and irrita-tion due to vocal abuse.

When hoarseness lasts longer than a few days, it is often caused by pro-longed overuse or abuse of the voice. Excessive or improper use of the voice can result in VOCAL CORD NODULES (small, benign growths on the vocal cords) sometimes called singers' nodes, which cause hoarseness. Vocal abuse may also cause extensive swelling and the development of a POLYP.

Smokers experiencing hoarseness are often referred to an otolaryngol-ogist (ear, nose, and throat special-ist), since smoking is the leading cause of throat cancer. Other causes of hoarseness include allergies, thy-roid problems, neurological disor-ders, and physical trauma to the voice box.

Most hoarseness resolves on its own. But medical attention is required if hoarseness persists for more than 2 weeks, does not seem to be caused by an infection, or is accompanied by persistent throat pain, coughing up of blood, difficulty swallowing, or a lump in the neck.

Treatment will depend on the cause of hoarseness. Possible treatment op-tions include resting the voice or modifying voice use, speech exer-cises, or surgery.

Hodgkin disease

A type of LYMPHOMA; cancer of the lymphatic tissue. Hodgkin disease is an uncommon lymphoma, account-ing for less than 1 percent of all cases of cancer in the United States. All other lymphomas are called non-Hodgkin lymphomas. Hodgkin dis-ease is commonly characterized by painless enlarged lymph nodes (see LYMPH NODE) in the neck, underarm, or groin; weight loss; recurrent fevers; night sweats; and anemia. There are no benign forms of the disease. Because Hodgkin disease de-velops in lymphatic tissue, which is present throughout the body, it spreads easily and progressively from one group of lymph nodes to the next. Eventually, it can spread to almost every part of the body. Diag-nosis depends on a biopsy of part or all of a lymph node.

Treatment is based on the extent of the disease. Early-stage Hodgkin disease can be cured with radiation therapy; even advanced disease can be cured with various chemotherapy regimens. Individuals whose disease recurs after treatment with chemotherapy may still be cured with a bone marrow transplant.

Holistic medicine

Any approach to healing that addresses the whole person, including the mind, body, and spirit. Holistic medicine integrates both traditional and alternative therapies to prevent and treat disease, but its hallmark is its emphasis on promoting health and wellness.

Holter monitor

A portable device for recording and analyzing the electrical activity of the heart over an extended period, usually 24 to 48 hours. Holter monitoring is also known as ambulatory ELECTROCARDIOGRAPHY, since it allows continuous recording of the electrical activity of the heart, even as the person being monitored goes

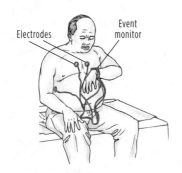

Electrodes

Event monitor

Monitoring the heart at home
The Holter monitor, which records heart activity over a period of 24 hours or more, is lightweight and painless. While wearing the device, the person can follow a normal routine. He or she is asked to keep a diary of activities and is taught how to use an event monitor (wristwatch style) to record symptoms.

about his or her daily tasks. The Holter monitor is particularly useful for detecting heart problems such as an arrhythmia (irregular heartbeat) that can come or go and may escape detection in the standard electrocardiogram. Holter monitors are often used to see if dizziness might be related to an arrhythmia. The monitor is also used to assess the effectiveness of medications used to control heart rhythm.

Home pregnancy tests

Kits that can be purchased without a prescription to help diagnose pregnancy. Home tests are similar to the pregnancy tests performed by doctors, but the results may not be as accurate. Several different types of home pregnancy testing kits are available; they all involve the detection of a hormone called HCG (HUMAN CHORIONIC GONADOTROPIN) in the woman's urine. HCG is produced in large quantities by the developing placenta during the first few weeks of pregnancy and is evident in the woman's urine. See also PREGNANCY TESTS.

Homeopathy

A system of medicine developed in Germany based on the belief that disease is cured by a substance that creates symptoms similar to those experienced by the person being treated. The three principles that govern homeopathic medicine are the law of similars, the single medicine, and the minimum dose. According to the law of similars, "like cures like," which means that an illness can be treated by giving persons small doses of substances that produce effects similar to those of the illness itself.

Homocysteine

An amino acid found in the blood. At high levels, homocysteine is associated with increased risk of heart attack and stroke. Homocysteine levels can usually be kept within normal limits through a diet that includes adequate amounts of folic acid and B-complex vitamins.

Homosexuality

Enduring erotic, emotional, romantic, or sexual attraction to members of the same sex. Homosexual men are commonly called gay and homosexual women, either gay or lesbian. Homosexuality appears in all cultures and societies, socioeconomic and educational levels, and religious and ethnic groups. It is generally thought that about one of every ten persons is homosexual.

Hookworm infestation

A condition that occurs when one or two species of nematodes, or roundworms, enter the human body.

Adult hookworms are parasites that live in the small intestine of humans where they attach to the intestinal wall. Blood is lost at the site of this intestinal attachment, and this is the cause of anemia in people who have a hookworm infestation. The hookworms' eggs are passed in the stool, and given a favorable environment including moisture, shade, and warmth, they will hatch within 1 to 2 days, releasing larvae. The larvae grow in the feces or soil, becoming filariform larvae, which are infective, after 5 to 10 days. In this infectious stage, the larvae can survive 3 to 4 weeks under favorable conditions and will penetrate the skin of a human host or carrier when they come into contact with it.

In addition to iron deficiency anemia, hookworm infestation may produce skin irritation with itching, respiratory symptoms, heart problems, and gastrointestinal disturbances.

Hookworm infestation is diagnosed by evaluation of a stool specimen and the finding of hookworm eggs. Medications including mebendazole, pyrantel pamoate (also called pyrantel embonate), and albendazole are generally used to treat a hookworm infestation.

Hormone therapy

A treatment in which a woman's declining hormone levels are supplemented with additional hormones. The treatment, also known as estrogen therapy and formerly known as hormone replacement therapy, is used to address the short-term symptoms of menopause, such as hot flashes, night sweats, and sleep disturbance, and for its potential benefits such as reducing the risk of OSTEOPOROSIS.

Hormone therapy for a woman with an intact uterus consists of estrogen combined with progestin, a synthetic form of another important female hormone, progesterone. Since estrogen increases the risk of uterine cancer, progestin—which lowers the risk of cancer of the endometrium—is usually prescribed along with estrogen to help prevent uterine cancer. Estrogen alone is usually prescribed for a woman who has had a hysterectomy.

Like all medications, hormone therapy has drawbacks. Estrogen may cause bloating, nausea, breast tenderness, and headaches. The use of estrogen alone can cause the lining of the uterus to overgrow and can increase the risk of endometrial cancer. Taking a preparation of hormone therapy that includes progestin protects the uterine lining from excessive growth by inducing menstruation. Women report various other side effects from taking progestin, including water retention, bloating, irritability, mood swings, and anxiety. Women who take hormone therapy almost double their risk for developing gallstones and increase their risk of breast cancer by 10 to 30 percent. Recent studies have shown that hormone therapy also increases the risk of heart disease.

When weighing the risks of heart disease and breast cancer against the benefits of hormone therapy, each woman should review her health history and discuss the question with her doctor.

The most common form of hormone therapy is a pill taken either every day or for 25 days each month. Progestins can be taken in combination with estrogen daily or for 10 to 14 days each month. In women taking the daily combined hormone pills, irregular bleeding is common during the first few months, but most women stop bleeding after 1 year. As an alternative to pills, adhesive transdermal patches (skin patches) containing time-release hormones can be placed on a woman's buttock. Estrogen can be supplied in a cream for vaginal dryness.

Hormone therapy effectively reduces hot flashes. However, if treatment is stopped abruptly, the symptoms may return after a few months.

Hormone therapies, alternative

The use of natural alternatives to hormone replacement therapy for symptoms associated with menopause. Some plant compounds can produce estrogenlike and progestinlike effects in humans and are used to treat menopausal symptoms by women who do not wish to take traditional hormone therapy.

Herbal and nutritional remedies used in menopause include Native American black cohosh, a hormone stabilizer; chasteberry, used for severe symptoms; Siberian ginseng for energy; dong quai, to maximize effects of other herbs; and soy isoflavones to reduce symptoms. However, there are few studies to advise physicians about the safety and effectiveness of these preparations.

Hormones

Chemicals produced by glands in the ENDOCRINE SYSTEM and released directly into the bloodstream to perform specific functions elsewhere throughout the body. Hormones balance each other in the bloodstream and control many vital functions of the body. Interference or disturbance in a person's hormonal equilibrium can affect normal growth and overall health and may even endanger survival.

The endocrine glands involved in the production and release of hormones include the hypothalamus, pituitary gland, thyroid gland, parathyroid glands, adrenal glands, pancreas, ovaries in women, and testicles in men.

Hormones produced by the hypothalamus include CRH (corticotropin-releasing hormone); ACTH (adrenocorticotropic hormone); GNRH (gonadotropin-releasing hormone); TRH (thyro-tropin-releasing hormone); TSH (thyroid-stimulating hormone); ADH (antidiuretic hormone); and oxytocin, which stimulates contraction of the uterus in preparation for labor.

The hormones produced by the pituitary gland, which is considered the control center of the endocrine system of glands, include GROWTH HORMONE; TSH; ACTH; FSH (follicle-stimulating hormone); LH (luteinizing hormone); and PROLACTIN (which stimulates the formation of milk in a nursing mother). Hormones produced by the thyroid regulate all aspects of cell metabolism. They include THYROXINE, triiodothyronine, calcitonin. PARATHYROID HORMONE is released by the parathyroid glands, located just behind the thyroid.

The hormones produced and released by the pancreas are INSULIN and GLUCAGON.

The adrenal cortex (the outer layer of the adrenal glands) produces ALDOSTERONE. The adrenal medulla (the inner layer of the adrenal glands) produces and releases EPINEPHRINE. Other adrenal hormones are NOREPINEPHRINE and CORTISOL, which help maintain blood pressure and reduce inflammation.

The testicles produce ANDROGENS such as TESTOSTERONE. The ovaries produce ESTROGEN and PROGESTERONE. The placenta also produces progesterone during pregnancy.

The mucous membrane of the small intestines secretes hormones during digestion to control the movement of various structures involved in digesting food. These hormones also stimulate digestive juices and liver bile, as well as certain secretions of the pancreas. Gastrin is a hormone secreted by the stomach that also has a role in digestion.

Hospice

A facility or a program that provides a combination of housing, medical care, and personal services for people with terminal diseases. In hospice programs, the emphasis shifts from finding a cure to maximizing the quality of remaining life. Most patients accepted in hospice programs have a condition such that their expected life span is 6 months or less.

Hot flashes

A symptom of MENOPAUSE or PERIMENOPAUSE in which a woman experiences fluctuations in body temperature. During a hot flash, the skin, particularly on the head, neck, and upper chest, becomes uncomfortably warm and perspires. The heart may race or skip beats, and the woman may feel dizzy. Hot flashes can last from 1 to 5 minutes and may be followed by chills. Some women get chills before a hot flash.

Hot flashes can be treated with HORMONE REPLACEMENT THERAPY. If other factors prohibit a woman from having hormone replacement therapy, her doctor may prescribe clonidine, a medication for high blood pressure that can reduce hot flashes.

HPV

The virus that causes common warts. See HUMAN PAPILLOMAVIRUS.

HRT

See HORMONE REPLACEMENT THERAPY.

Human chorionic gonadotropin

A hormone produced in the early weeks of pregnancy by the placenta. Human chorionic gonadotropin, or HCG, stimulates the ovaries to produce the hormones ESTROGEN and PROGESTERONE for the first 10 to 12 weeks of pregnancy. The hormones are needed so that the endometrium (the uterine lining in which the embryo grows) can be properly nourished. After about 12 weeks, the PLACENTA becomes the major source of progesterone, a hormone essential to the maintenance of the pregnancy and prevention of miscarriage. Human chorionic gonadotropin also stimulates the male fetus's testicles to produce TESTOSTERONE, which stimulates the development of the fetus's sex organs. The tests used to confirm a pregnancy all involve detecting HCG in the woman's urine or blood.

Human Genome Project

An international collaboration in which the entire genetic blueprint of a human being has been mapped. Since its inception in 1990, the goals of the Human Genome Project have been to identify all the genes present in the nucleus of a human cell; to establish where those genes are located on the chromosomes in the nucleus, using gene mapping; and to determine the genetic information encoded by the order of DNA's (see DEOXYRIBONUCLEIC ACID) chemical subunits.

Human granulocytic ehrlichiosis

An infection in humans that is transmitted by the black-legged tick (*Ixodes scapularis*) and the western black-legged tick (*Ixodes pacificus*) in the United States. Human granulocytic ehrlichiosis (HGE) is an illness that resembles ROCKY MOUNTAIN SPOTTED FEVER. Unlike Rocky Mountain spotted fever, which is caused by bacteria of the *Rickettsia* genus, HGE is caused by bacteria of the *Ehrlichia* genus.

A person with the infection may have no symptoms, but most people have a sudden fever, chills, headache, muscle pain, and malaise that occur about 12 days after a person has been bitten by the infected tick. Other symptoms may include abdominal pain, vomiting, and diarrhea. Clots throughout the blood vessels and coma may result.

Specific blood tests and polymerase chain reaction analysis are used to establish a diagnosis of HGE early on. Diagnostic tests may also reveal blood abnormalities, including a deficiency of white blood cells and platelets, and abnormal liver function.

In many cases, when there is a suspicion of HGE, treatment will begin before diagnosis is confirmed by test results. Quick action may prevent serious complications of the infection, including a viral or a fungal SUPERINFECTION, and even death. Antibiotics such as tetracycline, doxycycline, or chloramphenicol may be given.

Human immunodeficiency virus

See HIV.

Human monocytic ehrlichiosis

A disease caused by bacteria in the *Ehrlichia* genus that is carried and transmitted to humans by ticks, probably the dog tick or Lone Star tick. For many people, exposure to the bacteria does not cause symptoms. Other people who are infected may have mild symptoms including fever, severe headaches, malaise, muscle pains, chills, and a rash. Nausea, vomiting, confusion, and joint pain may also occur. Symptoms usually improve on their own without treatment.

In some instances, however, particularly among people who are older and those with weakened immune systems, symptoms are severe and the infection is life-threatening. Immediate antibiotic treatment at the first suspicion of HME infection is essential to prevent death.

The initial diagnosis is based on a person's symptoms and routine laboratory test results that may show a low white blood cell count, a low platelet count, and elevated liver enzyme levels. Diagnosis can be confirmed with a polymerase chain reaction analysis or an immunofluorescent assay.

Treatment consists of antibiotic therapy and supportive care. The symptoms of HME infection usually subside within 1 or 2 days after treatment begins.

Human papillomavirus

The virus that causes warts. Human papillomavirus (HPV) infects only the topmost layer of the skin and is responsible for the appearance of skin growths called warts that may appear anywhere on the outer surface of the body.

There are 70 different types of HPV, each of which causes the eruption of warts in a distinct area of the body. There are 25 different types of human papillomavirus responsible for producing warts on the skin of the

sex organs and anus; these are called GENITAL WARTS. At least five of the HPV types that cause genital warts have been linked to cervical cancer (see CERVIX, CANCER OF) and less commonly to SQUAMOUS CELL CARCINOMA of the penis, vagina, anus, and vulva. Infections with the human papillomaviruses that produce genital warts are considered SEXUALLY TRANSMITTED DISEASES, as they are transmitted via sexual contact.

All the virus types in the HPV group are spread by direct contact with infected sites on the skin where warts have appeared or by contact with a surface that has been contaminated by contact with warts.

Symptoms

The singular symptom of HPV infection of the skin is the appearance of warts; however, it is possible to have the infection without any symptoms, especially when it occurs in the genital area. When warts occur, their appearance varies depending on the specific type of human papillomavirus that caused them and their location on the body.

The common skin warts are painless, usually no larger than $1/4$ inch, rounded, firm, and smooth or roughly abraded.

Genital warts are painless and tend to occur as clusters of up to 10 small, pink growths with rough surfaces.

Diagnosis and treatment

Warts are diagnosed by a doctor's physical examination of the affected skin. When genital warts are discovered on the exterior areas of a woman's genitals, a Pap smear is done to test for cervical cancer, and in some cases, a biopsy of cervical tissue may be performed. There are now DNA tests to detect an HPV infection in women without symptoms; these tests are done on cells scraped from the cervix.

About half of all common warts disappear without treatment within a period of 6 months to 1 year. Others may persist for 2 years or longer. Over-the-counter topical treatments may be recommended by a physician to dissolve the wart's cells slowly. These chemicals cannot be used by people who have diabetes mellitus (type 1 or type 2), poor circulation, or signs of infection on the skin where the warts are located. Over-the-counter remedies should not be used for warts located on the face, genitals, or anus. These warts should be examined by a doctor who may prescribe a medication for a person to use at home. Sometimes, the doctor may remove warts in the office.

Huntington chorea

Also known as Huntington disease, a progressive brain disease involving degeneration of nerve cells in the cerebrum. "Chorea" is from the Greek word for "dance" and refers to the involuntary, uncontrollable movements characteristic of the disease. These include facial grimacing and quick jerking and flinging movements of the body. The other primary characteristics of Huntington chorea are progressive mental deterioration, including the loss of cognitive functions, such as judgment and speech, and personality changes. Diagnosis is made by genetic testing, MRI (magnetic resonance imaging) findings of wasting (atrophy) in a specific part of the brain, and clinical examination. Medication may

lessen the symptoms of Huntington chorea, but there is no treatment for the mental deterioration. Most affected people eventually require institutional care.

Hydatidiform mole

An abnormal pregnancy, also called a molar pregnancy, which probably results from the fertilization of a so-called empty egg, an egg without chromosomes. In this condition, the fertilized egg degenerates and the placenta grows into a mass of tissue resembling a cluster of grapes. When a woman has a hydatidiform mole, the uterus expands much faster than it would during a normal pregnancy. Fetal movement and a heartbeat are absent. Some women may have vaginal bleeding or expel grapelike clusters of tissue from the vagina, or they may have severe nausea and vomiting, high blood pressure, and a fast heart rate.

A hydatidiform mole produces unusually large amounts of a hormone called HCG (HUMAN CHORIONIC GONADOTROPIN), which can be detected by testing a woman's blood or urine. ULTRASOUND SCANNING can be used to visually detect a hydatidiform mole, which appears as an abnormal placenta and no fetus. A doctor can remove a hydatidiform mole by suctioning out the contents of the uterus.

Hydramnios

An excessive amount of AMNIOTIC FLUID surrounding the fetus. This condition occurs in the middle or late stages of pregnancy and is usually harmless. In most cases, the uterus swells to a size only slightly larger than normal and the woman experiences either no symptoms or a gradual onset of breathlessness, indigestion, and tension in her abdominal muscles. In some cases, swelling is pronounced; symptoms, including nausea, may begin suddenly, and there is risk of premature labor.

Hydramnios occurs more commonly in women with diabetes mellitus (see DIABETES MELLITUS, TYPE 1; DIABETES MELLITUS, TYPE 2), in those carrying multiple fetuses, or when the fetus has a malformation of the spine, gastrointestinal system, or brain. Pregnancies in which RH INCOMPATIBILITY is a problem are also associated with hydramnios.

Diagnosis is based on a combination of a physical examination and ultrasound to rule out fetal malformations. Most cases require no treatment, but in severe cases the doctor may order bed rest and close monitoring.

Hydrocele

Accumulation of fluid in a male's scrotum, the protective pouch of skin

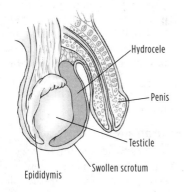

Fluid in the scrotum
The testicle is cushioned in a thin layer of fluid within the scrotum. Excess fluid can accumulate, causing swelling.

that contains the testicles. Hydrocele at birth results from incomplete closure of the canal that links the scrotum with the abdomen during development of the fetus. This kind of hydrocele is sometimes accompanied by a loop of intestine protruding into the scrotum (HERNIA). Hydrocele can also occur in adults. Hydrocele without hernia in newborns often repairs itself within the first year of life. In adults and newborns with a hernia, hydrocele can be repaired surgically. Sometimes a hydrocele found in an adult without symptoms may require no treatment.

Hydrocephalus

A disorder characterized by the presence of excessive fluid in the brain. If the circulation or absorption of cerebrospinal fluid (CSF) is blocked or excessive fluid is produced, excess fluid accumulates and puts pressure on the brain. The pressure forces the brain against the bones of the skull, damaging or destroying brain tissue.

Symptoms vary, depending on the age at which hydrocephalus develops and the cause of the obstruction. In newborns, hydrocephalus is often a genetic birth defect. The head will be abnormally enlarged, and there may be bulging at the soft spots of the head (fontanelles). Other symptoms include spastic muscles, irritability, temper tantrums, delayed development, slow growth, lethargy, difficulty feeding, loss of bladder control, and decreased mental function. Older children may have headaches, vomiting, crossed eyes, loss of coordination, and confusion. Hydrocephalus can develop in adults, after either a head injury or an infection.

Treatment of hydrocephalus depends on the time of onset and its cause. Surgery to remove the obstruction is the primary treatment whenever possible. Untreated hydrocephalus has a poor prognosis.

Hydrochloric acid

A strong acid produced by the stomach that helps to break down food into chemical components usable by the body. Hydrochloric acid, or HCl, also kills bacteria and other microorganisms that may accidentally be ingested with food.

Hydrocortisone

See CORTICOSTEROIDS.

Hydronephrosis

Dilation or widening of the ureter, kidney, or kidneys caused by total or partial blockage of the urinary tract. As the urine backs up, pressure inside the kidney increases, distending the collecting system. Hydronephrosis may produce no symptoms, but sometimes continuing or intermittent pain in the abdomen or flank (side of the torso, below the ribs) can be symptoms of an obstruction. The condition is usually diagnosed by ultrasound scanning. Hydronephrosis can also occur before birth and is sometimes diagnosed in the fetus.

Treatment is aimed at resolving the underlying cause. Medication can be used to combat an infection if there is one, and surgery may be needed to remove tumors or stones or to repair anatomical defects. Prompt treatment is necessary because persistent hydronephrosis can severely and permanently damage the kidney. Persistent hydronephrosis in both kidneys leads to kidney failure, which can be life-threatening.

Hydrops

An abnormal accumulation of fluid in fetal tissues. This condition can be detected by ultrasound and can include scalp edema (accumulation of fluid), ASCITES (abdominal edema), and fluid in the lungs. Fetal hydrops can lead to serious birth defects, including severely impaired intellectual or motor abilities. Termination of the pregnancy may be an option.

Hymen

A thin membrane stretching across the opening of the vagina, just inside the inner lips (labia minora). The hymen has a small hole in the center that allows menstrual blood and other discharges to flow out. See REPRODUCTIVE SYSTEM, FEMALE.

Hyperactivity

A state of excessive muscular activity characterized by constant fidgeting or moving, wandering, incessant talking, easy distractibility, or difficulty with quiet behavior such as reading. See ATTENTION DEFICIT/HYPERACTIVITY DISORDER.

Hyperaldosteronism

See ALDOSTERONISM.

Hyperalimentation

See PARENTERAL NUTRITION.

Hyperbaric injuries

See DECOMPRESSION SICKNESS.

Hyperbaric oxygen treatment

A system of increasing the oxygen supply to the tissues by providing oxygen at a higher-than-normal atmospheric pressure. Hyperbaric oxygen treatment is used to treat people with gas GANGRENE, carbon monoxide poisoning (see POISONING, CARBON MONOXIDE), DECOMPRESSION SICKNESS, and smoke inhalation (see INHALATION, SMOKE).

Hypercholesterolemia

An abnormally high level of the waxy fat known as CHOLESTEROL in the blood. Hypercholesterolemia is a key factor in hardening of the arteries (see ATHEROSCLEROSIS); increases the risk of angina, heart attack, and stroke; and poses a significant threat to health.

Cholesterol in the blood is measured in terms of milligrams (mg) of cholesterol per deciliter (dL) of blood. Hypercholesterolemia is defined as a blood cholesterol level of 240 mg/dL or higher. Total cholesterol levels less than 200 mg/dL are considered desirable, and those between 200 mg/dL and 239 mg/dL are borderline high.

Diets high in fat, especially from animal products or from saturated fats, are a leading cause of hypercholesterolemia.

Hypercholesterolemia can also result from certain inherited conditions. The most widespread genetically based cholesterol disorder is familial hypercholesterolemia. Persons with this condition may have a blood cholesterol level over 500 mg/dL, develop visible waxy plaques (xanthomas) under the skin, and develop atherosclerosis before puberty. Men with this disorder can have heart attacks as early as their 20s; in women, heart attacks may occur about 10 years later.

Regular screening of blood cholesterol levels should begin in men at age 35 and women at age 45. Screening at 5-year intervals is advised unless a person's cholesterol level is abnormally elevated, in which case more frequent screening is warranted.

If hypercholesterolemia is discovered, initial treatment consists of changes in diet to reduce the amount of cholesterol and saturated fat, combined with increased exercise. Should these measures fail to control the condition, medications are used to reduce the cholesterol level. The most widely prescribed drugs are the statins, which reduce both total cholesterol and LDL levels. Other medications used include bile sequestrants, fibrates, ezetimbe, and nictotinic acid. Aspirin use may also be advised to reduce the risk of blood clots that can form in arteries clogged with plaque and cause a heart attack or stroke. In addition, people with high cholesterol levels should control their blood pressure and stop smoking.

Hyperemesis

Excessive vomiting that can result in severe dehydration and weight loss. Symptoms of hyperemesis may include a rapid pulse, a drop in blood pressure, dry mucous membranes in the mouth and elsewhere, a loss of skin elasticity, and confusion. Forceful vomiting can lead to RETINAL HEMORRHAGE, which impairs vision, or to rips in the digestive tract, which cause the vomiting of blood. HYPEREMESIS GRAVIDARUM is excessive vomiting during pregnancy.

Hyperemesis gravidarum

Persistent intractable vomiting, usually beginning in early pregnancy, leading to weight loss and dehydration. This condition is uncommon and is associated with obesity and carrying twins. Hospitalization may be necessary to restore normal metabolic balance and prevent serious liver damage.

Hyperglycemia

High blood sugar. Hyperglycemia may be caused by INSULIN RESISTANCE, by an insufficient supply of insulin from the pancreas, or by other factors involving the inability of the body to respond to insulin. Factors that contribute to hyperglycemia include overeating, inactivity, illness, stress, certain medications, and hormone disorders. Hyperglycemia may be mild or severe. The symptoms can vary and may include extreme thirst, frequent urination, fatigue, blurred vision, and unexplained weight loss.

See also DIABETES MELLITUS, TYPE 1; DIABETES MELLITUS, TYPE 2; ACROMEGALY; HEMOCHROMATOSIS; CUSHING SYNDROME; and HYPERTHYROIDISM.

Hypernephroma

See RENAL CELL CARCINOMA.

Hyperopia

See FARSIGHTEDNESS.

Hyperosmolar hypoglycemic nonketotic syndrome

A complication of diabetes mellitus that results from extremely high glucose (blood sugar) levels without the presence of ketones, a by-product of fat metabolism; abbreviated as HHNS. Sometimes wrongly called diabetic coma, HHNS is characterized by decreased consciousness, extreme DEHYDRATION, and very high blood glucose levels (often over 600 mg/dL). Symptoms may include increased thirst, increased urination, nausea, lethargy, confusion, and seizures. HHNS is usually seen in people who have not yet been diagnosed with diabetes or those who have neglected their diabetes.

Preventive measures include good control of diabetes and recognition of early signs of dehydration. Once a person has HHNS, the goal of treatment is to correct dehydration through intravenous therapy while treating the high glucose levels with short-acting insulin. More than half the people who experience HHNS die as a result.

Hyperparathyroidism

A disorder in which overactive parathyroid glands, located on the back of the thyroid gland in the neck, produce excessive parathyroid hormone. The excessive hormone in turn stimulates the release of calcium from the bones and produces an elevated calcium level in the bloodstream. Hyperparathyroidism can lead to bone-weakening diseases such as OSTEOPOROSIS and osteomalacia. It is associated with kidney failure, which makes the body resistant to the activity of the parathyroid hormone. Excess calcium excreted into the urine by the kidneys may cause kidney stones.

The condition is most frequently caused by an ADENOMA, a benign (not cancerous) tumor of the parathyroid glands. Enlargement of the parathyroid glands is the next most common cause. Only rarely does the disorder result from cancer of the parathyroid glands.

Hyperparathyroidism may cause no symptoms, or the symptoms may be minor or severe. Mild symptoms include body aches and pains, depression, and muscle weakness. When hyperparathyroidism is more severe, abdominal pain, nausea, vomiting, fatigue, increased thirst, frequent urination, confusion, and impaired memory may be experienced. Thinning of the bones may occur without apparent symptoms and can increase the risk of fractures. Kidney stones may develop as a result of increased calcium and phosphorus excretion in the urine. Excess parathyroid hormone also increases the risk of developing peptic ulcers, high blood pressure, and pancreatitis.

In a person who does not have symptoms, hyperparathyroidism is usually detected during a routine blood test that reveals elevated calcium in the bloodstream.

A diagnosis of hyperparathyroidism may be confirmed by a complete medical history, physical examination, DIAGNOSTIC IMAGING (including X rays of the bones), and blood tests.

A bone density scan may be needed. Urine tests can reveal possible kidney damage. Abdominal X rays, CT (computed tomography) scans, or ultrasound may be used to detect kidney stones.

Although surgery is the only cure for hyperparathyroidism, most doctors recommend surgery only for those with moderate or severe symptoms.

Hyperplasia

An abnormal increase in the number of normal cells in an organ that results in the organ becoming larger than normal. Hyperplasia is not necessarily a cancerous condition, although it may sometimes become cancerous.

Hyperplasia, endometrial

See ENDOMETRIAL HYPERPLASIA.

Hypersensitivity

An excessive or abnormal reaction of the immune system to a specific stimulating or provoking agent or antigen.

Hypersplenism

Increased activity by the spleen. Hypersplenism usually results from another malady, such as liver disease (for example, CIRRHOSIS), certain blood diseases (including leukemia and ANEMIA), or infectious or parasitic diseases (such as tuberculosis or malaria). Symptoms include enlargement of the spleen, pain in the upper left side of the abdomen next to the stomach, and premature feelings of fullness after meals because of the spleen's pressure on the stomach. Most people with hypersplenism require treatment for the underlying disorder. In some cases, the spleen is removed surgically.

Hypertension

The medical term for high blood pressure. High BLOOD PRESSURE and hypertension are interchangeable terms used to describe blood traveling through the arteries at a pressure that is consistently too high to maintain good health. Although hypertension often causes no symptoms, it is dangerous. Left untreated, the disease can lead to severe and possibly life-threatening damage to the heart, kidneys, and arteries.

Hypertension is among the most common chronic diseases affecting people in the United States. Blood pressure is measured in millimeters of mercury (mm Hg) and given as two numbers that are written like a fraction, such as 125/75 mm Hg. The first, larger number, representing the blood pressure when the heart is contracting, is called the systolic pressure. The second, smaller number, representing the pressure between beats when the heart is relaxed, is called the diastolic pressure

Blood pressure lower than 120/80 mm Hg is considered normal. A person with readings of 120-139/80-89 mm Hg is considered to have PREHYPERTENSION. Blood pressure that is consistently over 140/90 mm Hg indicates stage 1 hypertension. Blood pressure above 160/100 mm Hg is stage 2 hypertension.

When a cause cannot be established, a person is considered to have essential hypertension. Essential hypertension occurs in approximately 19 of every 20 people with the disease. The remaining 1 of 20 has an identifiable cause of his or her hypertension, such as medications (for example, oral contraceptives and nasal decongestants), certain kidney diseases (such as glomerular nephritis), and diseases of the adrenal glands (for example, CUSHING SYNDROME). Hypertension with an identifiable cause is called secondary hypertension.

Malignant hypertension is a form of hypertension in which blood pressure suddenly rises to extremely high levels. It is more likely to occur in people who already have hypertension, particularly as a result of kidney disease, and is a life-threatening med-ical emergency that requires hospitalization and treatment to prevent or minimize damage to the heart, kidneys, brain, and blood vessels.

Some people with advanced hypertension may have symptoms such as nosebleeds or headaches. However, most people with advanced hypertension do not have any symptoms, which is why regular blood pressure checks are so important to early detection and treatment.

Increasing age, obesity, a sedentary lifestyle, a diet high in salt, excessive use of alcohol, diabetes mellitus, smoking, and gout are principal risk factors for hypertension.

Left untreated, hypertension causes damage to various parts of the body or target organs, including the heart, brain, kidney, and eyes. The damage can lead to disability or death. See also CORONARY ARTERY DISEASE; ATHEROSCLEROSIS; ANGINA; CARDIOMYOPATHY; and HEART FAILURE, CONGESTIVE.

When a doctor determines that a person has consistently high blood pressure, he or she next determines whether the disease is essential or secondary. This requires a review of a person's medical history and laboratory tests to look for kidney disease or other potential causes. If hypertension is secondary, treatment is directed at the underlying cause. In addition, tests will be ordered to check for damage to target organs such as the heart and to look for atherosclerosis. If hypertension is essential, initial treatment consists of lifestyle changes. These include a low-salt diet, weight loss if necessary, and increased physical activity. If these fail to control the blood pressure, then medications are prescribed. See ANTIHYPERTENSIVES.

Hypertension, pulmonary

A serious disease in which blood pressure in the arterial network supplying the lungs with blood (pulmonary arteries) is abnormally high. The condition arises because the blood vessels in the lungs have narrowed, restricting blood flow. As a consequence, the condition may affect the heart and lead to a condition known as COR PULMONALE.

There are two kinds of pulmonary hypertension. Primary pulmonary hypertension has no known cause and is very rare. Secondary pulmonary hypertension arises as a result of another condition or disease. Symptoms include bluish skin, chest pain, coughing (sometimes with blood), swollen neck veins, dizziness, fainting, enlarged liver, shortness of breath, swollen ankles or feet, swollen abdomen, and fatigue. Pulmonary hypertension is often difficult to diagnose because symptoms may come on slowly and vary greatly among individuals.

There is no cure for pulmonary hypertension, but treatment may be beneficial. Lifestyle changes are important. These include avoiding strenuous physical activity, alternating short periods of regular exercise with rest, eating a healthy diet, and restricting salt intake. Supplemental oxygen may also be recommended. A number of medications are also available.

Hypertensive hemorrhage

Bleeding caused by hypertension (high blood pressure). Hypertensive hemorrhage typically occurs in the blood vessels of the brain, is also known as cerebral hemorrhage, and can destroy the affected brain tissue.

The severity of the hemorrhage and the symptoms it causes depend on the location and extent of the bleeding. Symptoms can come on suddenly or gradually. They include rapid loss of function on one side of the body, changes in vision, numbness, tingling, difficulty speaking or swallowing, difficulty reading or writing, loss of coordination or balance, seizure, headache, nausea or vomiting, and change in consciousness, such as extreme apathy or sleepiness. Surgery to remove the hematoma (swollen area in which blood has accumulated) is performed if the damage is likely to cause death or major disability. Medications are also used to control blood pressure, reduce swelling in the brain, stop seizures, and reduce pain.

Hyperthyroidism

A condition produced by excess thyroid hormone in the bloodstream, which leads to overactivity of the metabolism of the body. The three most common causes of hyperthyroidism are GRAVES DISEASE; toxic multinodular GOITER, in which several nodules on a diffusely enlarged thyroid gland become overactive; and toxic ADENOMA, in which a benign nodular growth secretes excess hormone. THYROIDITIS can cause temporary hyperthyroidism, as does taking too much oral thyroid hormone medication. Rarely, hyperthyroidism is caused by excess thyroid hormone secreted from abnormal tissue growth in a woman's ovaries.

The symptoms of hyperthyroidism can vary from person to person. They can include nervousness, irritability, increased perspiration, thinning of the skin, brittle hair, shakiness, increased heart rate, palpitations, elevated blood pressure, diarrhea, increased appetite, unexplained weight loss, insomnia, confusion, irregular menstrual periods, and muscle weakness.

A complete medical history, physical examination, DIAGNOSTIC IMAGING for hyperthyroidism or THYROID SCANNING, and blood tests are generally used to diagnose the disorder.

The goal of treating hyperthyroidism is to restore thyroid hormone to normal levels. Treatment options include antithyroid medications to lower the level of thyroid hormones in the blood, radioactive iodine taken as a pill or liquid to destroy thyroid cells and slow production of thyroid hormones, and surgery to remove an overactive nodule or nodules or larger areas of thyroid tissue.

Hypertrophy

Enlargement or overgrowth of a body part or organ due to an increase in the size of its cells. Organs such as the heart, liver, and muscles are prone to hypertrophy, a condition that can cause medical problems. Treatment is aimed at the underlying cause.

Hyperventilation

Excessive, rapid, deep breathing that leads to reduced carbon dioxide in the blood. Hyperventilation usually occurs in people who are anxious or tense, but it may be a symptom of specific disorders, including ASTHMA, CROUP, severe pain, CHRONIC OBSTRUCTIVE PULMONARY DISEASE (COPD), pneumonia, pleurisy, and other diseases.

If symptoms persist for more than 15 minutes despite breathing into a paper bag, or if the person complains of chest pain, medical help should be sought. If no medical problem is found, relaxation techniques are often helpful.

Hyphema

Bleeding within the front portion (anterior chamber) of the eye. A hyphema can be caused by a blunt or penetrating injury to the eye or certain medical conditions, including severe inflammation of the iris (the colored portion of the eye), an abnormal blood vessel, or cancer of the eye. A hyphema carries a risk of acute GLAUCOMA, which causes pressure inside the eyeball to rise suddenly and damages the optic nerve. Hyphemas need prompt evaluation by an eye specialist to determine the causes of the bleeding and assess its severity. Emergency treatment is indicated if severe pain or nausea and vomiting are present.

In mild cases, a hyphema resolves on its own within a few days. With more pronounced bleeding, bed rest, patching of both eyes, limitation of

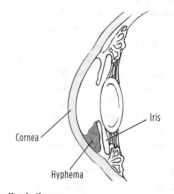

Bleeding in the eye

Hyphema, or bleeding between the cornea and the iris, usually as the result of injury, makes the eye appear filled with blood and causes pain and blurred vision. Immediate medical treatment is necessary.

movement, and sedatives are often prescribed. If pressure within the eye increases, an eye specialist may remove the blood surgically.

Hypnosis

A sleeplike mental state in which the individual is unusually open to suggestion and may behave, think, or perceive in uncharacteristic or seemingly impossible ways. Under hypnosis, consciousness is reoriented from the outside world to mental, sensory, and physiological experiences. Hypnosis is usually induced by a hypnotist.

Hypnosis has been used medically for pain control; to treat anxiety, posttraumatic stress, conversion disorders, and morning sickness in pregnancy; and to help people remember forgotten actions, stop smoking, control overeating, overcome abnormal fears (phobias), and resolve insomnia. It is not used to replace anesthesia during surgical procedures.

Hypnotic drugs

Drugs used to decrease the time needed to fall sleep. Hypnotic drugs prescribed to treat insomnia, or sleeplessness, include BENZODIAZEPINES, novel nonbenzodiazepine hypnotic drugs, ANTIDEPRESSANTS at low doses, the hormone MELATONIN, and chloral hydrate.

Nonprescription hypnotic agents are also available to induce sleep; most of them contain antihistamines.

Hypoaldosteronism

A condition resulting from a deficiency of the hormone ALDOSTERONE, which is normally produced by the adrenal cortex (the outer layer of the adrenal glands). Hypoaldosteronism produces biochemical changes in the body that result in a low level of sodium in the blood combined with an increased level of potassium. The condition is often associated with kidney disease, or it can be the result of a hereditary defect in an enzyme involved in aldosterone production. Symptoms include general weakness and an increased risk of serious heart rhythm abnormalities, which can be fatal. Administering fludrocortisone, a synthetic mineralocorticoid, is the most common treatment because oral aldosterone cannot be properly absorbed by the body.

Hypochondriasis

A persistent and abnormal preoccupation with physical health combined with the fear that one is suffering from a grave or major undetected illness, even though medical evidence to support that worry is lacking.

Hypogammaglobulinemia

An antibody deficiency that involves low levels of gamma globulin in the bloodstream and is characterized by both an immune system disorder and an autoimmune disorder. Gamma globulin is a class of immunoglobulin, IgG, that includes four kinds of antibodies. Normally, these antibodies enter tissue spaces and coat antigens, which makes the antigens readily absorbed by other cells involved in the immune system. In hypogammaglobulinemia (HGG), this function is disrupted. There is a depressed antibody response, and some of the antibodies that are produced attack the body's own tissues.

Infections experienced by people with hypogammaglobulinemia frequently involve the respiratory tract (recurrent ear infections, chronic sinusitis, recurrent pneumonia, and BRONCHIECTASIS) and the gastrointestinal system (diarrhea caused by the poor absorption of protein, fat, and certain sugars). People with hypogammaglobulinemia may be particularly predisposed to infection caused by exposure to certain bacteria or parasites. There is also an increased frequency of autoimmune disorders, such as rheumatoid arthritis or pernicious anemia and of autoimmune neurological disorders, such as GUILLAIN-BARRÉ SYNDROME.

The diagnosis can be confirmed by blood tests that reveal a low level of immunoglobulins in the bloodstream. People who have been completely immunized against polio, measles, diphtheria, and tetanus have extremely low or absent antibodies to the microorganisms that cause these diseases.

The goal of treatment is to prevent new infections and stop the development of chronic lung disease. An individual who has hypogammaglobulinemia can almost always benefit from injections of GAMMA GLOBULIN, a component extracted from human plasma.

In the presence of bacterial infections, long-term treatment with broad-spectrum antibiotics is generally required. If bronchiectasis occurs, physical therapy and POSTURAL DRAINAGE, involving physical therapy of the lungs, are generally necessary to remove pus from the airways and lungs.

Hypoglycemia

Low blood sugar. Hypoglycemia occurs when the blood level of glucose becomes too low to supply the need for fuel in the body. In people who take insulin, hypoglycemia is sometimes referred to as an insulin reaction because it is a response to excessive insulin in the bloodstream. It is generally defined as a blood sugar level lower than 60 milligrams per deciliter (mg/dL). It most commonly occurs in people with type 1 diabetes (see DIABETES MELLITUS, TYPE 1. But sometimes hypoglycemia may occur in people with type 2 diabetes (see DIABETES MELLITUS, TYPE 2) if they take certain diabetes medications or insulin.

Symptoms of hypoglycemia include nervousness, shakiness, fatigue, increased perspiration, sensation of cold, hunger, confusion, and irritability. The most immediate treatment is to eat something such as a glucose tablet or drink fruit juice to quickly raise the blood sugar level. If untreated, hypoglycemia can lead to seizures, unconsciousness, and even death.

Medical help is essential if a person with hypoglycemia loses consciousness or is unable to swallow. GLUCAGON can be injected to quickly raise blood sugar.

Hypogonadism

A condition produced by a decrease or total lack of the secretion of hormones from the testicles (see TESTICLE) in men and boys and the ovaries (see OVARY) in women and girls. Hypogonadism can be from a deficiency of two hormones from the PITUITARY GLAND—FSH (follicle-stimulating hormone) and LH (luteinizing hormone)—or from the failure of the testes or ovaries to make hormones.

Failure of the testes or ovaries to produce the sex hormones because of a lack of the hormones that stimulate them may be caused by CRANIO-PHARYNGIOMA (a brain tumor that develops near the pituitary), a tumor in the area of the hypothalamus, Kallmann syndrome (a hereditary absence of the front part of the pituitary gland), rare chromosomal defects, and head injuries. Hypogonadism may also be associated with alcoholism and other chronic illnesses, including kidney disease and SICKLE CELL ANEMIA.

Diseases of one or both testicles, including MUMPS, may interfere with production of the male hormone TESTOSTERONE and lead to hypogonadism. Other elements that may temporarily or permanently impair the synthesis of testosterone and result in hypogonadism include physical trauma to the testicles and certain medications and therapies.

The signs of hypogonadism depend on the stage of life in which the condition originates. In males, if the appropriate sex hormones are not released during early fetal development, the external genitals may be affected, leading to a condition in which the sex of the newborn is not obvious.

If a deficiency of the male hormone androgen occurs at puberty, the physical changes characteristic of this phase do not take place. When hypogonadism occurs during adulthood, male sexual potency and fertility are decreased.

The treatment of hypogonadism is generally based on its cause. A complete evaluation by an endocrinologist (a specialist in the hormone-producing glands) can determine the source of the disturbance and the appropriate course of treatment. The male sex hormone testosterone or GNRH (gonadotropin-releasing hormone) may be administered. Females may be treated with estrogen and progesterone. Prompt treatment at the onset of the disorder causing the abnormalities is usually successful.

Hypoparathyroidism

A condition caused by a deficiency of PARATHYROID HORMONE in the blood as the result of damaged or absent parathyroid glands, which are located on the thyroid gland in the neck. Symptoms of hypoparathyroidism include numbness, tingling, and muscle cramps and twitching; seizures can also occur. Insufficient levels of parathyroid hormone can cause hypocalcemia (low levels of calcium in the blood). Hypoparathyroidism may be treated with vitamin D and calcium supplements.

Hypophysectomy

The surgical removal of the hypophysis (pituitary gland). Hypophysectomy is usually performed to slow the growth of some cancers such as breast, ovarian, and prostate cancer. It is also used to eradicate pituitary tumors, which cause the majority of disorders of the pituitary gland. It can be used to treat disorders such as CUSHING SYNDROME and ACROMEGALY. Hypophysectomy is also sometimes performed to treat a prolactinoma or a CRANIOPHARYNGIOMA.

Hypopituitarism

A disorder resulting from a deficiency in one or more of the pituitary hormones. Hypopituitarism can be caused by a tumor on the pituitary gland, inflammation of the gland, or a head injury that damages the pituitary gland.

The effects of hypopituitarism depend on which of the pituitary hormones are deficient. A life-threatening inability of the body to respond properly to physical stresses, including injury and illness, is caused by deficiency of the pituitary hormone that controls adrenal function. Impairment of the growth hormone results in problems with physical development, including unusually SHORT STATURE. Loss of sex hormones can cause absent menstrual periods in women and a loss of fertility and sex drive in men. Hormone replacement therapy can help to overcome these problems.

Hypopituitarism is diagnosed by blood and urine tests to measure hormone levels. When warranted, DIAGNOSTIC IMAGING, including MRI (magnetic resonance imaging), may be performed, too.

Hypoplasia

The failure of an organ to develop completely and reach its normal adult size; also refers to the lack of complete development of tissue in the body.

Hypoplastic left heart syndrome

A serious congenital disease (present at birth) in which severe malformation of the chambers, valves, and blood vessels on the left side of the heart prevents blood from being pumped efficiently into the rest of the body. Such infants are treated by HEART TRANSPLANT or the Norwood procedure, a series of three open-heart surgeries performed from infancy through the toddler years.

Hypospadias

A developmental abnormality in males in which the urethra opens on the underside of the penis. Surgery to correct the birth defect is usually successful.

Hypotension

For symptom chart see DIZZINESS, page xx.

Low blood pressure. Physicians define hypotension as blood pressure below 90/60 millimeters of mercury (mm Hg) (see BLOOD PRESSURE for details on how blood pressure is measured). Many normal people may have low blood pressure, particularly young, slender women. However, hypotension can indicate problems with the heart or nervous system, such as HYPOTHYROIDISM (an underactive thyroid), diabetes mellitus, heart disease, HYPOGLYCEMIA (low blood sugar), liver disease, or ANEMIA. Hypotension can also result from the overdosing of medication to control blood pressure, high or low body temperature, substantial blood loss, allergic reaction (for example, to a bee sting), severe blood infection, or dehydration. Temporary hypotension can result from heavy menstrual bleeding, unusually hot weather, overheating (for example, from too much time in a hot tub, a sauna, or the sun), or sudden emotional shock.

Symptoms of hypotension include dizziness or light-headedness, fainting, blurry vision, lack of concentration, cold and clammy skin, nausea or stomach upset, muscle weakness, weak and rapid pulse, headache, and fast and shallow breathing. If blood pressure falls so low that the oxygen supply to the brain and other organs is insufficient, the person may lose consciousness or go into shock.

Treatment of hypotension depends on the underlying cause. If hypotension results from another disorder, treatment of that problem may resolve the hypotension.

Hypothalamus

A structure located near the center of the base of the BRAIN. The hypothalamus directs the workings of the AUTONOMIC NERVOUS SYSTEM, which regulates vital, involuntary functions such as blood pressure, sleep, body temperature, appetite, and thirst. The hypothalamus also directs the hormonal activities of the ENDOCRINE SYSTEM (hormonal system) by stimulating and inhibiting production of hormones by the pituitary gland. The hypothalamus also controls the SYMPATHETIC NERVOUS SYSTEM, which prepares the body for a response to stress—the so-called fight-or-flight mechanism.

Hypothermia

A condition in which the body temperature drops below 95°F. Hypothermia is usually caused by prolonged exposure to cold and occurs when more heat is lost than the body can generate. The onset of symptoms of hypothermia is usually slow and includes a gradual loss of mental and physical ability. The person with hypothermia may be entirely unaware of the condition. Other symptoms include apathy, lethargy, confusion, large pupils, drowsiness, loss of coordination, weakness, slow pulse, dizziness, slurred speech, and uncontrollable shivering.

Emergency treatment includes getting the person out of the cold and into warm, dry clothing. If it is not possible to get indoors, the person's head should be covered, and the person should be insulated from the cold ground. Warm drinks not containing alcohol may be given, unless the person is vomiting. The person's arms or legs should not be massaged. Emergency medical assistance should be sought.

Hypothyroidism

A condition resulting from a deficiency of the thyroid hormone THYROXINE, which regulates the metabolism of the body. When this hormone is decreased to abnormally low levels, there is a slowing of the metabolism. The decrease in energy production disrupts many vital functions, including heart rate and ability to regulate temperature.

Hypothyroidism may be caused by complications of thyroid surgery; treatments for HYPERTHYROIDISM (over-activity of the thyroid gland), including radioactive iodine therapy; autoimmune disorders that make antibodies which attack the thyroid gland; or a congenital defect in the gland. Transient episodes of hypothyroidism are generally caused by inflammation of the tissue or viral infections of the thyroid gland.

Symptoms of hypothyroidism differ among individuals, depending on the severity of thyroxine deficiency. The symptoms of a mild insufficiency may include sensitivity to cold temperatures, dry skin, constipation, and forgetfulness. Symptoms of more severe hypothyroidism also include chronic fatigue, muscle stiffness and cramping, poor appetite combined with weight gain, hair loss, hoarseness, decreased heart rate, and depression. Untreated, advanced hypothyroidism may produce myxedema.

When hypothyroidism is a possibility, a doctor evaluates the person's medical history and conducts a physical examination that includes feeling the thyroid gland, which may be enlarged. Blood samples are taken to measure the levels of thyroid hormones and TSH in the bloodstream.

Chronic forms of hypothyroidism are lifelong disorders that are usually treated with synthetic forms of thyroxine. Once thyroid hormone replacement therapy is started, the symptoms usually resolve quickly.

Hypotonia

Decreased muscle tone, especially in infants and usually indicating the presence of genetic, muscle, or central nervous system disorders. Infants who are hypotonic feel floppy when held, and when at rest, they lie with their limbs loosely extended, unlike infants with normal muscle tone, who tend to flex their elbows and knees. Hypotonic infants often display poor or no control of their heads. Hypotonia can be a symptom of DOWN SYNDROME, MYASTHENIA GRAVIS, PRADER-WILLI SYNDROME, Werdnig-Hoffmann disease, MARFAN SYNDROME, MUSCULAR DYSTROPHY, TAY-SACHS DISEASE, trisomy 13 syndrome, and congenital hypothyroidism.

Hypoxia

An inadequate supply of oxygen to the tissues. A lack of oxygen causes changes in breathing and neurologic symptoms that range from headaches and confusion to, rarely, a loss of consciousness. Hypoxia can be acute and severe, as when a person has an airway obstruction. Chronic hypoxia, which may be due to the effects of emphysema or another lung disease, causes persistent fatigue and mental sluggishness and gradual damage to internal organs such as the heart. Cerebral hypoxia, in which circulatory failure deprives the brain of oxygen, causes irreversible brain damage after 4 to 6 minutes.

Hysterectomy

A surgical procedure in which a woman's uterus is removed. Hysterectomy is the second most common major surgical procedure performed on women in the United States. Indications for a hysterectomy include treatment of fibroid tumors, excessive bleeding, ENDOMETRIOSIS, prolapse of the uterus, or the need to remove a cancerous growth.

There are different types of hysterectomies. In a subtotal hysterectomy, only the body of the uterus is removed, leaving the cervix. In a total hysterectomy, the entire uterus and the cervix are removed. Radical hysterectomies involve removal of the uterus, cervix, surrounding tissue, lymph glands, part of the vagina, and sometimes the fallopian tubes and ovaries.

In an abdominal hysterectomy, an incision is made into the abdomen, either horizontally along the upper pubic hairline or vertically between the navel and pubic hair. In a vaginal hysterectomy, the labia and vulva are retracted to give access to the vagina. An incision is made in the front wall of the vagina, through which the bladder is moved aside to expose the uterus. Under some conditions, a laparoscopically assisted vaginal hysterectomy is performed. If the woman's ovaries are also removed, her estrogen supply will be severely reduced, and so-called surgical menopause will begin.

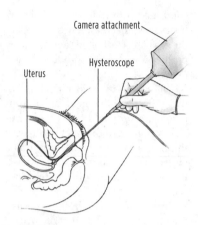

Hysteria

An emotional disorder in which the person develops one or more dramatic physical symptoms, such as blindness, paralysis, altered consciousness, or abdominal pain; the symptoms are not due to organic or physical disease but can be traced to unconscious psychological reasons. The various types of hysteria are recognized as separate disorders: CONVERSION DISORDER (in which physical symptoms mimic a major disease but lack physical basis), DISSOCIATIVE DISORDERS (in which consciousness is altered, as in amnesia), FACTITIOUS DISORDER (in which the person feigns the symptoms of disease out of a psychological need to be sick), and SOMATIZATION DISORDER (in which the individual is preoccupied with physical symptoms at times of stress).

Hysterosalpingogram

An X-ray procedure (also called an HSG) used to visualize the uterus and fallopian tubes. A hysterosalpingogram may be done for either infertility or recurrent miscarriages.

Hysteroscopy

A surgical procedure usually done by a gynecologist in which a hysteroscope (a thin, telescopelike instru-

Viewing the uterus
A hysteroscopy allows the doctor to look inside the uterus to evaluate problems and treat some conditions.

ment) is inserted through a woman's vagina and into the uterus to allow the doctor to view and treat a condition in the uterus. Hysteroscopy is useful for evaluating abnormalities in the uterus and can also be used to confirm the results of other tests.

Iatrogenic

Any undesirable condition occurring as a result of a treatment or medicine.

ICD

Implantable cardioverter defibrillator. See DEFIBRILLATOR.

Idiopathic

Of unknown cause. An idiopathic disease is one that develops for no apparent reason or cause.

Idiopathic thrombocytopenic purpura

See ITP.

Ileal pouch-anal anastomosis

A surgical procedure in which the colon and rectum are removed and part of the ileum (the lowest part of the small intestine) is used to construct an internal pouch in which waste collects. Ileal pouch-anal anastomosis is performed to treat large-bowel disease such as ulcerative colitis. This procedure ensures a high degree of continence and an acceptably low number of daily bowel movements. The operation is done in a hospital under general anesthesia.

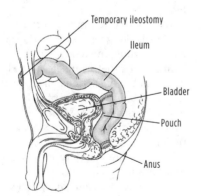

Removal of the colon

Ileal pouch-anal anastomosis is major surgery usually done in two operations. In the first procedure, the colon and rectum are removed. The surgeon constructs a pouch from part of the ileum, as shown here, and attaches the pouch directly to the anus.

Ileitis

See CROHN DISEASE.

Ileostomy

A surgical procedure in which a stoma, an artificial opening, is created in the abdominal wall to allow the discharge of feces into a device attached to the skin.

An ileostomy is generally done in conjunction with another surgical procedure being performed to treat a serious digestive disorder such as colon cancer (see COLON, CANCER OF THE), colitis, or diverticular disease. The operation is done in a hospital under general anesthesia. Ileostomies can be temporary or permanent.

Ileum

The final and longest portion of the small intestine; an important part of the digestive system. Together, the duodenum, the jejunum, and the ileum compose the small intestine. The ileum, about 12 feet in length, passes from the jejunum to the large intestine, or colon.

The function of the ileum is to absorb nutrients from food that has been broken down in the stomach and the first parts of the small intestine.

Ileus, paralytic

A serious condition in which the muscles of the small intestine become paralyzed and fail to function normally. Paralytic ileus may develop following abdominal surgery or in people who are otherwise severely ill. (See also PSEUDO-OBSTRUCTION.) It can be caused by inflammatory conditions such as a perforated ulcer, acute diverticulitis, or acute cholecystitis.

In paralytic ileus, a person is unable to pass gas or propel intestinal contents and have a bowel movement. Retained gas distends the abdomen and intestines. Fever, vomiting, and persistent abdominal pain may occur. Even if pain lessens, treatment is required to prevent potentially life-threatening complications.

Paralytic ileus is treated by decompressing the intestine by means of a tube passed into the mouth, through the stomach, and into the intestine to suck out accumulated air and fluid.

Immune globulins

Proteins obtained from human plasma; passive immunizing agents. Immune globulins are used to protect immunocompromised people against hepatitis A and B, measles, pertussis (whooping cough), poliomyelitis, varicella (chickenpox), human rabies, and tetanus. They are also given to people who are not immunocompromised: for example, immune globulins are recommended for newborn babies exposed to chickenpox and for mothers who contract chickenpox shortly before or after delivery. The immunity provided by immune globulins starts immediately, but it lasts for only a few months.

Immune system

The complex set of mechanisms by which the body prevents or fights infection by disease-causing microorganisms such as bacteria, viruses, and fungi.

The body has many natural, or innate, protections against infection. These mechanisms are called the nonspecific immune system because they respond to any invading organism in the same way. Some of them are physical barriers, like the skin, or chemical defenses, such as stomach acids. See also INFLAMMATION.

Another natural mechanism is a type of white blood cell called a killer cell, which chemically destroys disease organisms and cancer cells. Interferon, part of a natural immune response, is a type of specialized protein that the body produces to defend against viruses. The interferons prevent the virus from multiplying in the body.

If the nonspecific immune system fails to destroy disease organisms, the body utilizes a different system that can recognize specific organisms and develop a specialized defense. The basic functional cell in this defense is the lymphocyte, a type of white blood cell. There are two types of lymphocytes that are involved in adaptive immune response: B cells, which are important in antibody defenses, and T cells, which perform in cellular defenses.

An antibody is a protein produced by B cells designed to combat a specific invading microbe. T cells are lymphocytes that complete their development in the thymus, an organ of the lymphatic system located in the upper chest. See ALLERGIES; IMMUNIZATION; and IMMUNE SYSTEM DISORDERS.

If the immune system mistakenly identifies the body's own cells or tissues as harmful and attacks them, the result is one of the autoimmune disorders such as lupus (see LUPUS ERYTHAMETOSUS, SYSTEMATIC); RHEUMATOID ARTHRITIS; SARCOIDOSIS.

Immune system disorders

Disorders caused by problems with the body's mechanisms for protecting itself against viruses, bacteria, and other foreign substances. Immune system disorders result in conditions in which some portion of the immune response is weak or absent. In one form of immune system disorders, called autoimmune disorders, the immune system mistakenly identifies the body's own normal cells or tissues as foreign and attacks these cells and tissues as though they were antigens. Multiple interacting factors may contribute to the development of autoimmune diseases, including genetic predisposition, immunologic

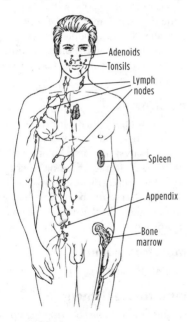

Immune system

The lymphatic system, composed of clusters of lymph nodes connected by lymphatic vessels, carries disease-fighting white blood cells (lymphocytes) throughout the body. The thymus maintains lymphocytes while the spleen contains white blood cells. The tonsils and the appendix are made of lymphoid tissue. White blood cells are produced in the soft marrow of the bones.

abnormalities, and even microbial infections.

Many diseases and conditions are known or believed to be associated with immune deficiency disorders. They include: Addison disease, ankylosing spondylitis, HEPATITIS, celiac sprue, crest syndrome, CROHN DISEASE, discoid lupus, fibromyalgia, Graves disease, GUILLAIN-BARRÉ SYNDROME, Hashimoto thyroiditis, hemolytic anemia, idiopathic pulmonary fibrosis, insulin-dependent diabetes (see DIABETES MELLITUS, TYPE 1), juvenile rheumatoid arthritis, lupus (see LUPUS ERYTHEMATOSUS, SYSTEMIC), multiple sclerosis, psoriasis, Raynaud phenomenon, Reiter syndrome, rheumatic fever, rheumatoid arthritis, sarcoidosis, scleroderma, Sjögren syndrome, ulcerative colitis (see COLITIS), vasculitis, and vitiligo. A major infectious disease of the immune system is AIDS.

Immunity

The body's ability to defend itself against potentially harmful foreign substances and cells called antigens. Immunity invokes the immune response, which includes both nonspecific and specific components. It initially activates nonspecific immune responses followed by highly specific responses that are exactly matched to the specific threats presented. See IMMUNE SYSTEM.

Immunization

The process of inducing the immune system to produce protective antibodies to create immunity as a preventive measure against particular infectious diseases. Active immunization is accomplished when a person receives a vaccination that introduces antigens into the body that prompt the body's immune system to create antibodies directed against the antigen (see ANTIGEN). The antibodies are generally administered as a vaccine that consists of a suspension of whole or partial bacteria or viruses that have been inactivated or treated to prevent them from causing disease in the person being immunized. Passive immunization occurs when an individual is given antibodies to provide immediate protection against an antigen or an infective organism such as bacteria. Immunizations given routinely in the United States include vaccines against measles, mumps, and rubella; against tetanus, diphtheria, and pertussis, called the DTaP vaccine (see DTaP VACCINATION); against hemophilus influenza B (hib); against chickenpox with varicella vaccine; against hepatitis B for those at risk of exposure; against influenza A, for those at high risk of serious consequences from flu.

Immunoassay

Any one of several techniques for identifying and measuring chemical substances by using the specific binding interaction between an antigen and its corresponding antibodies. Immunoassays are diagnostic tools that can quantify the body's response to infection. Immunoassay is also the technique for evaluating urine drug screens.

Immunology

The branch of science concerned with the study of the immune system and the various aspects of immunity and immune responses. The science is concerned with the specific responses made by lymphocytes (one type of white blood cells) to foreign substances and the interactions between antigens and antibodies. The study of immunity involves investigating the responses of lymphocytes that are beneficial in preventing infections and the treatment of infections caused by microorganisms. A physician trained in the medical specialty of the immune system's normal functions and possible disorders is called an immunologist.

Immunotherapy, allergen

A process of exposing the body to small, injected amounts of a particular allergen in gradually increasing doses until the body builds up immunity to the allergen. See DESENSITIZATION, ALLERGY.

Impairment

Damage, injury, or deterioration that affects the structure or function of normal physical or psychological abilities. The degree of impairment is variable. Impairment also implies an increased risk for being involved in an accident because of a medical condition.

Imperforate anus

See ANUS, IMPERFORATE.

Imperforate hymen

A solid membrane covering the opening of the vagina. If this condition is noticed in infancy or childhood, a doctor can remedy this by cutting an opening in the central part of the membrane.

Impetigo

A contagious, superficial skin infection. Impetigo is caused by *Staphylo-*

coccus and *Streptococcus* bacteria, and most commonly occurs on unexposed areas of the arms, legs, and face.

The infection appears as groups of lesions that vary in size and form. The skin elevations may take the form of pea-sized, pus-filled, inflammatory pustules, or they may be larger and circular, resembling ringworm. The infection develops quickly into yellowish, circular lesions that become crusted over.

A clinical examination of the characteristic lesions is the basis for diagnosis. Cases of impetigo in which there are a limited number of lesions can be treated topically with the prescription ointment mupirocin, which is applied three times a day to affected areas. If there is no improvement after using this medication or if there are more than a few lesions, an oral antibiotic may be prescribed.

Impingement syndrome

A painful condition of the shoulder. Impingement syndrome is caused by repeated overhead movement of the arm, abnormal anatomy of the shoulder, or a combination of the two. Symptoms of impingement syndrome may include pain, stiffness, and a pinched feeling when the arm is raised. If bursitis (inflammation of the bursa in the shoulder) is involved, there may be pain at rest or during sleep.

Impingement syndrome is diagnosed by physical examination and X rays. Preliminary treatments may include applying ice to the painful area, gentle massage, heat therapy, and physical therapy. Pain-relieving medications, including aspirin, ibuprofen, or other nonsteroidal anti-inflammatory drugs (NSAIDs), may be recommended. If the problem persists, cortisone injections or, in rare cases, surgery may be recommended. Left untreated, impingement syndrome can lead to ROTATOR CUFF DISEASE.

Implant

Any material placed inside the body to repair or replace damaged tissues or organs, deliver drugs or hormones, or improve appearance. Implants include artificial joints, screws, and pins to hold broken bones together; synthetic lenses used to replace lenses affected by cataracts (see CATARACT SURGERY); patches for strengthening hernia repairs; pacemakers (see PACEMAKER) to control heartbeat; and artificial heart valves. In a procedure called BRACHYTHERAPY, radioactive seeds are implanted in the prostate gland for treatment of prostate cancer.

Implantable bone conduction hearing device

See COCHLEAR IMPLANT.

Implants, dental

An artificial tooth root that is surgically anchored into the jaw, or placed over it, to replace a permanent tooth, a dental bridge (see BRIDGE, DENTAL), or full dentures.

Impotence

The inability to produce or maintain an erection of the penis. See ERECTILE DYSFUNCTION.

In situ

The earliest stage of cancer, in which the disease has not spread beyond its original site or layer of cells. In situ cancer also is known as stage 0 cancer. Surgical removal of cancer in situ has a very high likelihood of curing the cancer. Cancers known to have an in situ stage are those affecting the anus, bladder, breast, cervix, colon, endometrium (lining of the uterus), esophagus, lung, rectum, stomach, and skin (melanoma).

In vitro fertilization

A method of assisted reproductive technology for treating infertility. In vitro fertilization (IVF) involves several steps leading to the fertilization of one or more of a woman's eggs outside her body. An egg or eggs are removed, fertilized in the laboratory, and reinserted into the woman's uterus or fallopian tube.

A 2-week program of intensive preparation generally precedes IVF. Daily injections of hormone medications are usually given to a woman to stimulate the development of multiple eggs. The optimal time to retrieve the eggs is just before ovulation when the eggs are mature enough to be fertilized. There are two methods for recovering eggs from a woman's body; the most commonly used is ultrasound-guided needle aspiration egg recovery, which is performed on an outpatient basis in a procedure called transvaginal oocyte retrieval.

After removal, the eggs are placed in a fluid medium in a laboratory. Semen from a woman's male partner is placed with the eggs for about 18 hours. After this, the eggs are removed and placed into a special growth medium, a nutrient mixture that imitates the environment of the fallopian tubes. At this time, the eggs divide and develop into preimplantation embryos, or pre-embryos. After

approximately 40 hours, the pre-embryos are examined to see whether they are ready to be implanted in the uterus of the woman from whom the eggs were retrieved or to the uterus of another recipient if a surrogate mother is the carrier.

In vivo

Occurring in the living body.

Incest

Sexual contact between family members so closely related that marriage between them is legally or culturally barred. It most often occurs between older male relatives and minor-aged girls, and in most cultures is considered a form of child abuse.

Incompetent cervix

Abnormal weakness in a woman's cervix that can result in a miscarriage. If the cervix is weak, after the 12th or 14th week of pregnancy the weight of the developing fetus and the amniotic fluid around it can force the cervix open, allowing the fetus and placenta to drop down prematurely, resulting in a miscarriage. To help hold the baby in, a stitch may be placed at the opening of the cervix to hold it together firmly (see CERCLAGE, CERVICAL). The stitch is removed at the start of labor or around the 37th or 38th week of pregnancy, so the woman can deliver the baby.

Incontinence, fecal

The inability to retain feces in the rectum and control defecation. Fecal incontinence is less common than urinary incontinence. Temporary fecal incontinence can occur at any age during bouts of severe diarrhea. Chronic inability to control the bowel occurs more frequently in older people because the efficiency of muscle sphincters declines with age. It is also found in people with nervous system disease or damage, such as stroke, multiple sclerosis, or diabetes. Fecal incontinence also can occur if the anal sphincter muscles are damaged by childbirth, trauma, cancer of the rectum, or surgery. Fecal impaction (accumulation of hard feces in the rectum) can cause incontinence when fluid and new feces pass around the impacted mass.

Treatment of fecal incontinence varies according to its cause. Diagnosis of the cause is made by a complete physical examination and tests that may include a lower gastrointestinal (GI) series (an X-ray procedure also called a barium enema); a sigmoidoscopy or colonoscopy; and manometry. If impaction is the cause, an enema or manual removal of the mass is necessary.

Incontinence, urinary

Inability to control the bladder. Incontinence is not used to describe the normal lack of control in newborns and toddlers; the term applies only to individuals who are old enough to have voluntary control.

Lack of bladder control affects 10 to 20 percent of people older than 65, and it is twice as common in women as in men. The amount of urine lost involuntarily can range from a few drops to complete emptying of the bladder. Temporary urinary incontinence can result from urinary tract infections, infection in the vagina, severe constipation, or the side effects of medications. The incontinence disappears when the underlying condition resolves or the medication is changed. Persistent urinary incontinence continues and often worsens over time.

In stress incontinence, the most common variety, sudden physical pressure on the abdomen, such as laughing or sneezing, causes urine to leak. Stress incontinence is caused by the stretching of pelvic muscles during childbirth, weight gain, and certain surgeries. The muscle that holds urine in the bladder (urinary sphincter) is too weak to retain urine during physical stress. Stress incontinence is more common in women and often worsens after menopause. In urge incontinence, the interval between the desire to urinate and the loss of urine is so short that the person may not be able to get to the bathroom in time. Urge incontinence is usually caused by infection of the bladder, nerve damage or disease (such as stroke or Parkinson disease), alcohol, and certain medications.

In overflow incontinence, the bladder is full; yet, the person cannot urinate or produces only a small amount of urine because the bladder muscles are weak or there is an obstruction. Eventually the pressure from the full bladder increases, and small amounts of urine leak out. Overflow incontinence is rare in women. Diabetes, an enlarged prostate gland, or blockage because of tumors or stones are possible causes. Overflow incontinence requires prompt treatment because the backup of urine can produce permanent kidney damage.

Determining the cause of urinary incontinence requires a physical examination, a medical history, and laboratory tests including urinalysis and a urine culture (to check for infection). Other tests include CYSTOSCOPY, cystometrics (an instrument that measures fill-up pressures in the bladder and ureters), X rays with contrast dyes, and studies of urine flow, retention, and loss.

For temporary incontinence, treatment consists of identifying the cause, such as an infection, and treating it, usually with antibiotics. For persistent incontinence, therapies include Kegel exercises to strengthen pelvic muscles; restricting fluids and following a voiding schedule; biofeedback to retrain the bladder for better control; medications; or surgery.

Incubation period

The period of time that begins when a person is first exposed to an infection and ends with that person's first signs or symptoms of infection. The incubation period is the process of disease development.

Indigestion

General discomfort in the upper abdomen. Nausea, heartburn, upper abdominal pain, gas, belching, a sour taste of acid, or an uncomfortable feeling of fullness or bloating after a meal may all occur with indigestion. Often, indigestion worsens during times of stress. Indigestion that becomes more frequent, persistent, or intense or occurs for no apparent reason requires medical attention. Treatment varies according to the cause of indigestion. See also ESOPHAGEAL REFLUX.

Induction of labor

The use of artificial methods to start labor intentionally. In general, induction is indicated when continuation of the pregnancy represents a significant risk to the mother, fetus, or both. This is especially true if the pregnancy has gone beyond term; the mother has developed an illness due to the pregnancy, such as preeclampsia (high blood pressure brought on by pregnancy); the fetus is endangered or has died; or the mother has a preexisting health condition that makes induction safer than continuing the pregnancy.

Labor can be induced by giving the woman oxytocin, a hormone that signals the uterus to contract. If a woman's cervix has undergone the changes that normally occur before delivery (a thinning, softening, and widening process referred to as ripening), the doctor may rupture the membranes surrounding the fetus to help begin labor.

Infarction

An area of tissue that dies because of blockage of the artery supplying it with blood. The usual cause of an infarction is a blood clot, which can form at the site of the blockage (a thrombus) or develop elsewhere in the body, then travel through the bloodstream until it lodges in a blood vessel (an embolus). Infarction in the heart (technically, myocardial infarction) is known as a heart attack.

Infection

The invasion and multiplication of infectious microorganisms in body tissues. A common symptom of infection is fever.

When the body's defense system is effective, the infection may remain localized and temporary, producing only mild, treatable symptoms. If the infection persists and spreads, it can progress to an acute or chronic disease. Local infections can also develop into body-wide infections affecting many organs.

Infections are commonly caused by bacteria or viruses and are often diagnosed by laboratory evaluation of blood samples. Once diagnosed, many infections can be treated with medication, often antibiotics. See also COLD, COMMON; INFECTIOUS DISEASE; INFLUENZA; PNEUMONIA; SEXUALLY TRANSMITTED DISEASES; VACCINATION.

Infection, congenital

Infection that affects an unborn fetus at any time during a pregnancy up through and including the time of delivery. Congenital infections exist at birth and are generally caused by viruses such as cytomegalovirus (CMV), herpes viruses, German measles, parvovirus, chickenpox, and enteroviruses.

Diagnosis can be difficult. An obstetrician may suspect an infection in a pregnant woman based on her symptoms and blood tests or based on physical findings in the fetus as evaluated by ultrasound scanning. A pediatrician may diagnose a congenital infection in a newborn based on signs, physical findings, and blood tests. Medical complications of congenital infections are related to the type of infection involved. Cytomegalovirus infections can cause brain damage in which the brain does not grow properly and the head is smaller than normal, a condition called microcephaly.

It is important that complications associated with congenital infections be identified as early as possible to allow interventional therapy such as surgery to begin immediately.

Infectious disease

An illness caused by an organism, such as bacteria, that enters the body, then grows and multiplies in the cells, tissues, or cavities of the body. Infectious disease may be spread by direct or indirect contact with an infected person or by a common vehicle such as food or water. It may also be airborne or vector-borne, which usually means transmitted by insects.

The organisms that cause infectious disease are called pathogens. Depending on the interaction between the pathogen and its human host, infection can be silent or without symptoms, or it can be overt, which means signs and symptoms of infectious disease occur in the infected person.

Infectious disease can be acute, a disease of short duration that may or may not have symptoms, and is contagious only for a short time. Infection may also be chronic, which refers to a longer duration caused by the continual reproduction of pathogens. Infectious diseases continue to cause many deaths. Leading causes of death in the United States include the infectious diseases AIDS, PNEUMONIA, and INFLUENZA.

Infectious mononucleosis

See MONONUCLEOSIS, INFECTIOUS.

Infertility

The inability of a man and woman of reproductive age to produce offspring after unprotected sexual intercourse. A couple should seek help for infertility if the woman is younger than 35 years and has not become pregnant after having unprotected intercourse for 1 year. If the woman is older, but still of childbearing age, most experts recommend that help be sought after no more than 6 months of unprotected sexual intercourse.

Causes of infertility

Four general conditions interfere with a couple's ability to conceive a child: the inability of a man to produce healthy sperm or a woman to produce healthy eggs; the inability of gametes (sperm and eggs) to get close enough to allow fertilization to occur; the inability of a fertilized egg to become successfully attached to the lining of a woman's uterus; and the inability to carry a pregnancy to its full term.

The root of female infertility is often the failure of a woman's fertility hormones to properly transmit chemical signals to control regular ovulation. Problems involving female hormone disorders are often successfully treated with fertility drugs.

Another major cause of female infertility is ENDOMETRIOSIS.

Commonly identified causes of male infertility are VARICOCELE and PROSTATITIS.

Sexually transmitted diseases (STDs) are a leading cause of infertility in both men and women. In the United States, chlamydia and gonorrhea are the two major infections that most often lead to infertility. STDs can cause pelvic inflammatory disease (PID) in women, and a single episode of the disease can often cause infertility.

The inability of a woman's ovaries to produce mature eggs (anovulation) causes female infertility. Certain severe illnesses, being overweight, being under-weight, and extreme physical exercise regimens can contribute to anovulation.

A pregnancy that develops outside the uterus, called an ECTOPIC PREGNANCY, usually occurs in a fallopian tube. The surgical treatment of this complication may damage the affected tube, resulting in infertility.

The fertility of men and women whose mothers took the medication diethylstilbestrol (DES) may be affected as a result of their exposure to DES in the uterus. Some daughters of women who took DES have abnormal fallopian tubes or misshapen uteruses or vaginas. Men born to mothers who took DES during pregnancy can have missing reproductive system ducts.

Genetic factors can have a role in male infertility, in some cases involving defects of a man's Y chromosome that produce abnormalities in the development of the sperm-producing system. Other factors linked to male infertility include undescended testicles, disorders of the hypothalamus or pituitary gland, testicular damage from diseases such as mumps, chemotherapy or radiation treatments for testicular cancer, and severe trauma to the testicles. See INFERTILITY TREATMENTS.

Fertility testing

Comprehensive testing may be required to explore the reason or reasons why a couple is unable to conceive. Usually the first step is obtaining a semen specimen from the male partner to rule out a low sperm count or sperm abnormalities before beginning the more extensive testing of the woman partner.

Both partners may have thyroid gland function tests and blood screening tests to check blood type, to measure cell count and cholesterol levels, and to determine whether viral infections are present. The woman's blood may be tested for levels of progesterone, a hormone that increases in the bloodstream after ovulation, to determine that ovulation has occurred. A man's blood may be tested for chromosome irregularities and the levels of hormones that stimulate the function of the testicles. High levels of gonadotropic hormones are an indication that the testicles are no longer producing sperm, an untreatable condition. If excess numbers of certain antibodies against sperm are detected in a man's blood, treatment may be possible.

X rays of a woman's uterus and fallopian tubes may reveal anatomical irregularities that prevent conception. A woman's cervical mucus may be cultured to rule out the presence of fertility-diminishing infections, including gonorrhea and chlamydia.

Tests of the fallopian tubes may involve the use of a hysterosalpingogram, a procedure that verifies that the fallopian tubes are open. Another diagnostic technique that may be used is laparoscopy, the insertion of a special viewing telescope into the abdomen so that the internal pelvic organs can be inspected. An endometrial biopsy may be performed, in which tissue from the uterine lining is removed and examined under a microscope for indications of ovulation and to assess the ability of the uterine lining to support pregnancy.

A woman's cervical mucus may be tested during her most fertile day, usually at the midpoint in her menstrual cycle. A postcoital test of the cervical mucus may reveal the vitality and motility of a man's sperm in his partner's cervical environment. The ovaries and uterine lining may be evaluated by ultrasound examination during the middle of the menstrual cycle to monitor the follicle development and to confirm that an egg has been released from the follicle.

Infertility treatments

Nonmedical or medical therapy for individuals who are unable or have a diminished capacity to conceive. When a specific disease or disorder that causes infertility is diagnosed, a physician may treat the underlying disorder. Some conditions are treatable only with assisted reproductive technology (ART).

When the cause of infertility is not a disease or functional problem, the solution may lie in coordinating sexual activity with the woman's most fertile period.

When a woman's cervical mucus produces antibodies to her partner's sperm, infertility treatments that bypass the cervix, such as in vitro fertilization (IVF), may be tried. When a couple's infertility involves a man's low sperm count, a specialized form of IVF involving a procedure called ICSI (intracytoplasmic sperm injection) may be implemented to place individual sperm into each of several eggs that have been removed from a woman's ovaries.

Fertility drugs are used to treat women who are having difficulty conceiving because of irregular or absent ovulation. Surgical procedures are sometimes necessary to treat female infertility. Treatable conditions include endometriosis, fibroids (noncancerous tumors), blockage in the fallopian tubes, or an abnormally shaped uterus that cannot support a pregnancy to term.

Inflammation

Redness, swelling, heat, and pain in a tissue that comes from the body's protective response to chemicals, or physical injury, or to INFECTION. See also C-REACTIVE PROTEIN; FEVER; INFECTIOUS DISEASE.

Inflammatory bowel disease

A general term used to refer jointly to chronic ulcerative colitis and Crohn disease. Both diseases cause recurrent bouts of intestinal inflammation that include diarrhea, fever, and abdominal pain. Both diseases damage the digestive tract, can cause complications in other parts of the body, and can increase the risk of colon cancer. Treatment usually involves the use of medications that reduce inflammation.

Influenza

An acute, contagious infection caused by a virus that primarily affects the respiratory tract, but may also affect the musculoskeletal, gastrointestinal, and nervous systems. Influenza, which is also called flu, occurs in outbreaks with variable severity in the United States, usually during the winter months. Infection with an influenza virus does not give a person lasting immunity, so people are susceptible to episodes of influenza throughout their lives. A person with influenza may experience some or all of the following symptoms: moderate to high fever (temperature between 101°F and 103°F; chills; sore throat; cough; runny nose; general aching in the muscles; headache; loss of appetite; fatigue and weakness; diarrhea; burning of the eyes; and dizziness. If there is fever, it generally subsides within 2 or 3 days. Symptoms may last only 24 hours or as long as 2 weeks. Influenza is contagious as long as the person has symptoms.

Influenza is diagnosed by an evaluation of symptoms, the taking of a medical history, and a thorough physical examination. Blood tests and chest X rays may be performed. A sample of coughed-up mucus, called a sputum culture, may be ordered to check for bacteria. Laboratory testing to identify the specific flu virus may be done if there is risk of a serious influenza epidemic.

Treatment of influenza is usually based on easing the symptoms and preventing complications. The body can become so weakened by the flu that it cannot summon defenses against secondary bacterial infections. Physicians generally recommend reduced activity for the duration of severe symptoms and for at least 2 days after the fever has subsided. Prescription antiviral medications are effective in reducing the severity of symptoms only if taken during the first 48 hours of infection. Also, the newer antiviral medications, such as oseltamivir phosphate and zanamivir, are effective and work against influenza A and B.

Most people fully recover from influenza. Others may develop serious, even life-threatening complications, such as pneumonia. Medical attention is extremely important if fever and coughing get worse, or if blood or thick and foul-smelling mucus are coughed up. Other dangerous symptoms that require immediate help include chest pain and shortness of breath.

Since the influenza viruses are often spread through direct contact, frequent hand washing during a known outbreak or flu season may be helpful in avoiding infection. The influenza vaccine is considered highly effective for preventing the flu or diminishing its severity.

Informed consent for surgery or treatment

A consent form a person signs before undergoing a surgical procedure and some diagnostic treatments or tests. Health care professionals are required to provide a careful explanation to the person of what to expect, potential benefits and risks, and any alternative options to the surgery or treatment. The person is asked to sign a form that states that he or she understands the procedure or test and the risks involved.

Ingrown toenail

A toenail that grows into the surrounding skin or tissue of the toe. Symptoms include pain, swelling, redness, and the discharge of pus. Home care includes soaking the affected foot in warm water and placing a small piece of clean cotton under the corner of the nail to lift it up. A doctor may prescribe antibiotics to control any infection. If the problem worsens, minor surgery may be necessary to remove part of the toenail. Prevention consists of trimming toenails straight across, wearing shoes that fit properly, and keeping the feet clean and dry. Doctors advise those who have diabetes mellitus to seek prompt treatment for ingrown toenails or other foot sores because they are more prone to infections, which are difficult to treat, because of a reduced blood supply.

Inguinal

Having to do with the groin. An inguinal HERNIA, or rupture, occurs in the lower abdomen when the intestine or its covering, the omentum, protrudes through the inguinal canal.

Inhalants

Breathable chemicals that produce psychoactive, or mind-altering, effects. Using these drugs is also known as glue sniffing, huffing, and solvent abuse. Inhalants are not usually thought of as drugs since they are produced for very different purposes.

There are three principal categories of inhalants: solvents, such as paint thinners, gasoline, model glue, and correction fluid; gases, such as aerosols; propellants; spray paints; and cyclohexyl nitrite (generally available).

Inhalants have effects like anesthetics and slow the body down. At low doses they may make the user feel stimulated. At higher doses they lead to a loss of inhibition. A high enough dose will cause a loss of consciousness. Even one-time use of inhalants carries a risk of sudden death from heart failure or from suffocation.

Most inhalant users are between 7 and 17 years of age. Besides intoxication, signs of use include a rash around the nose and mouth and the smell of paint or solvents on skin, clothes, or hair.

Inhalation, smoke

Excessive breathing of smoke during a fire. The inhalation of smoke can cause serious lung damage. Many people who die from fires have both smoke inhalation and burns. Smoke inhalation injury happens because smoke contains toxic fuel by-products and sometimes contains fine solid particles, all of which can injure the lungs. Smoke inhalation symptoms include irritated eyes, gasping for breath, and coughing up black sputum.

Emergency treatment for smoke inhalation includes moving the person to a smoke-free area a safe distance from the fire and keeping as low to the ground as possible. The air at floor level is less toxic. If the person has not inhaled too much smoke, long, deep breaths of fresh air may help stop the coughing and clear the lungs. Artificial respiration should be started if the person is not breathing. Emergency medical assistance must be obtained by dialing 911 or the emergency number for your area.

Inhaler

Device used to deliver medication in an aerosol form that can be inhaled by people with asthma or other respiratory diseases.

Injectable contraceptives

See CONTRACEPTION, HORMONAL METHODS.

Injection

The act of forcing a drug or other substance physically into the body by syringe or catheter. Drugs may be injected under or through the skin or into a body cavity, a vein, or the tissues.

Inoculation

The introduction into the body of microorganisms, such as bacteria or viruses, that have been modified or killed, for the purpose of stimulating resistance to specific diseases. Inoculation is usually accomplished by injection and may also be referred to as immunization or vaccination. Over a period of years, inoculations have significantly decreased the number of deaths caused by serious illnesses, including smallpox, diphtheria, poliomyelitis, tetanus, and certain types of meningitis. In some cases, repeated inoculations, or booster shots, are required at certain intervals (see also ANTIBODY; IMMUNIZATION).

Inoperable

A condition or disease state that most probably will not be improved or cured by using a surgical procedure. The term is often used to describe very advanced cancer or cancer situated in tissue that is not surgically accessible. People with inoperable tumors can be treated with other therapies, such as radiation, chemotherapy, or hormones.

Insemination, artificial

A procedure in which sperm (from the woman's partner or from a donor) is inserted with a syringe into a woman's vagina, cervix, or uterus during ovulation to try to impregnate her. In the procedure, the man's semen is introduced with a syringe into the woman's cervix or, less often, into her vagina or uterus, as close to the time of ovulation as possible. The chance of becoming pregnant increases with subsequent attempts. By the sixth try, artificial insemination results in pregnancy in eight of ten women who have no infertility risk factors, such as having problems ovulating.

Insoluble fiber

See FIBER, DIETARY.

Insomnia

Difficulty getting to sleep or remaining asleep. Insomnia is a very common problem that can be short and self-limiting or may persist for years. Its causes range from stress and depression to physical pain (such as the chronic discomfort of arthritis) and sleep disorders, such as restless leg syndrome. Symptoms include difficulty falling asleep, waking frequently during the night, waking abnormally early in the morning and being unable to return to sleep, feeling tired during the day, and feeling restless and anxious as bedtime approaches. It is important to diagnose and treat the underlying cause of insomnia. In some cases, sleeping pills are helpful, although they should be used on a temporary basis only. Regular use can make a person dependent on sleeping pills. Good sleep hygiene is the best way to cope with insomnia. This means getting up at a regular time every morning, even on weekends; trying not to nap during the day; avoiding caffeine, alcoholic beverages, nicotine, and strenuous exercise for 4 to 6 hours before bedtime; avoiding heavy meals before retiring; and minimizing noise, light, and extreme temperatures in the bedroom. If sleeplessness persists, professional help should be sought.

Insulin

A hormone found in animals and humans; also an antidiabetic drug. Defective secretion of insulin by the pancreas is the cause of diabetes mellitus (see DIABETES MELLITUS, TYPE 1; DIABETES MELLITUS, TYPE 2). All people with type 1 diabetes and many with type 2 must have insulin injections to control their blood glucose level.

Insulin is secreted by the pancreas in response to high levels of blood sugar. It helps the body convert food to energy and to store energy for later use. Insulin works by processing sugar or glucose into body cells to make fat, sugar, and protein. Insulin has a role in the process by which stored fat, sugar, and protein are used for energy between meals. Without insulin, glucose cannot get into body cells, and the cells cannot work properly.

Various types of insulin are available for people who are required to use it because diet, exercise, and oral medication do not adequately control their blood sugar levels or because they had bad reactions to oral medications. Because insulin is destroyed by stomach acid, it cannot be taken orally. However, recently insulin that can be inhaled has become available.

Insulin pump

An appliance for delivering insulin to people with type 1 diabetes (see DIABETES MELLITUS, TYPE 1). The pump steadily injects insulin into the body in a pattern that is similar to the way the pancreas normally releases insulin into the bloodstream of a person who does not have diabetes.

Insulin resistance

A condition in which the body does not respond properly to the activity of insulin even though the pancreas produces sufficient amounts. To maintain a normal blood level of glucose (sugar) in insulin-resistant people, the pancreas needs to release abnormally large amounts of insulin into the bloodstream to compensate for insulin resistance. The elevated levels of insulin may damage the blood vessels and increase the risk of heart disease even if the blood sugar level remains normal.

Insulin resistance is common in people with type 2 diabetes (see DIABETES MELLITUS, TYPE 2). Being overweight—particularly with central obesity, or an apple-shaped torso—is associated with insulin resistance because fat cells do not respond well to insulin. Insulin resistance is associated with high blood pressure and high levels of fat in the blood. Aging is another factor that contributes to insulin resistance.

Recent research has demonstrated that in many cases exercising regularly to build muscle and reduce fat can help control insulin resistance even if the activity does not result in weight loss.

Insulinlike growth factor

A peptide hormone made by most tissues of the body and believed to be secreted by the liver and released into the bloodstream. Insulinlike growth factor I (IGF-I) is involved in various biological activities in the cells. These activities include mitosis (normal cell division) and may be similar to the action of insulin. IGF-I is important to human survival because it regulates normal growth. It is mainly active in adults; the main growth factor in fetuses is insulinlike growth factor II.

Insulinoma

A tumor of the beta cells that is found in the islets of Langerhans of the pancreas; also known as an insuloma or islet cell adenoma. An insulinoma is usually benign (not cancerous) but may be malignant (cancerous). In some cases, there is more than one tumor.

Symptoms that may indicate an insulinoma include increased perspiration, rapid heartbeat, hunger, dizziness, headache, clouded vision, confusion, shakiness, seizures, and loss of consciousness. Severe hypoglycemia as a result of an insulinoma can cause coma.

If an insulinoma is suspected, MRI (magnetic resonance imaging) may be performed to determine the location of the tumor or tumors in the pancreas. Blood tests may be evaluated for levels of insulin in the bloodstream.

Surgery is the most common treatment. Usually only part of the pancreas is removed so that enough tissue is left to provide sufficient enzymes to avoid malabsorption.

If the tumor cannot be found during surgery, the medication diazoxide, which inhibits the release of insulin, may be prescribed as an alternative treatment. Diazoxide must be taken along with a diuretic to prevent excess salt retention.

Integrative medicine

A blend of conventional medical practice with selected proven alternative therapies. Integrative medicine incorporates holistic medicine, with its emphasis on person-centered care, and high-tech conventional medicine, with its focus on the cure of disease.

Intelligence tests

Question-and-answer devices used to measure the general intelligence of individuals. The most commonly used measurement of intelligence is the intelligence quotient, or IQ, which compares a person's intelligence with the average for his or her age. In most intelligence tests, an average score for a given age group is 100; an individual score between 90 and 109 is statistically average. Superior intelligence falls in the 120 to 140 range, with genius beginning at 140. Individuals with IQ scores from 80 to 89 are considered slow learners, and below 80 they are deficient in ways that usually cause school problems. Individuals with IQ scores below 70 are considered mentally retarded.

Controversy has arisen over the accuracy of intelligence testing, particularly the proven influence of education and social and cultural background on test scores.

Intensive care

See CRITICAL CARE.

Intensive care unit

The area of a hospital in which critical care is provided for people with life-threatening conditions. Types of intensive care units (ICUs) include medical, surgical, neurological, pediatric, neonatal (newborn), coronary care unit (CCU), and special burn units. All intensive care units are staffed by nurses and physicians who have specialized training in critical care.

Intercourse, painful

Pain felt by a woman during arousal or during or after sexual intercourse; also called dyspareunia. The pain may occur at the vaginal opening, in the vagina, or deeper in the pelvic cavity. Pain can arise from such problems as insufficient lubrication during sex; vaginismus (tightening of the muscles of the pelvic floor); infections of the organs and tissues of the reproductive system; endometriosis

(a condition where the lining of the uterus grows outside the uterus); or scar tissue from infections, childbirth, or surgery. Pain can also be caused by infections in the bladder or urethra.

When a woman reports feeling pain during intercourse, a doctor will take a thorough history and perform a pelvic examination to help diagnose the cause of her pain. For undiagnosed persistent pain, a laparoscopy may be done to determine the cause of the pain. If no physical cause is found, a woman may need counseling to address any emotional issues.

Interferons

Substances produced by cells in the body to help fight infections and tumors. Interferons have been made synthetically since the late 1980s using recombinant DNA technology to treat diseases including leukemias, cancer of the skin and the cervix, Kaposi sarcoma, multiple sclerosis, and chronic viral hepatitis (hepatitis B and C). Naturally produced interferons are proteins secreted by cells in response to many triggers, or inducers, including viruses, parasites, and the proliferation of cells, both normal and malignant. Three major classes of interferons have been identified—alpha, beta, and gamma—all of them useful in the fight against infectious disease.

Interleukins

A large group of hormonelike substances produced by white blood cells. Interleukins are part of the immune system and stimulate the body to fight infection and disease. They have become important in fighting some cancers.

Intermediate care facility (ICF)

A type of nursing facility that provides food, lodging, and custodial care for people who are too ill or frail to care for themselves independently. ICFs provide regular (but not around-the-clock) nursing care.

Intern

A resident in the first year of hospital training after medical school. An intern is able to practice medicine only under the supervision of an attending physician. Today interns are more frequently referred to as first-year residents.

Internal medicine

The branch of medicine concerned with the physiologic and pathologic characteristics of the internal organs of the body. Practitioners of internal medicine are known as internists; they specialize in the diagnosis and treatment of disorders of the internal organs, and they often provide a person's primary care.

Interstitial fibrosis of the lung

A disease in which the lung tissue becomes damaged by a known or unknown cause that produces inflammation of the lungs' air sac walls, which ultimately scars the interstitium (the tissue between the air sacs of the lungs). Interstitial fibrosis of the lung causes the tissue of the lung or lungs themselves to thicken and become stiff, which makes breathing difficult.

Interstitial radiation therapy

See BRACHYTHERAPY.

Intervention

A technique to encourage someone addicted to alcohol or drugs to enter treatment by telling that person to either recognize the disease or face its consequences, such as divorce or job loss. An intervention, in which the person is confronted with the abuse by loved ones, can help break down denial, which is the first step toward effective treatment.

Intestine

The portion of the digestive system between the stomach and the anus, where absorption of nutrients into the bloodstream takes place. The intestine is in fact a long section of coiled tubing that has two parts—the small intestine and the large intestine, or colon—with different functions.

The small intestine lies between the pyloric sphincter at the exit from the stomach and the first part of the large intestine. Within the length of the small intestine, the chemical breakdown of food is completed and the usable components are absorbed into the bloodstream.

When digestive materials finally reach the first part of the large intestine called the cecum (a large pouch from which the appendix extends), nutrient absorption is complete. The undigested material that remains is composed of water, fibrous waste, and sloughed-off cells and mucus from the rest of the digestive tract. The function of the large intestine is to convert these waste materials into a form that can leave the body.

Intestine, obstruction of

A partial or complete blockage of the intestines that prevents the passage of the contents of the intestines. Obstruction of the intestine can be due to a number of causes. Symptoms vary according to where the blockage occurs and may include severe abdominal pain, cramping, and distension. Abdominal distension due to obstruction is a medical emergency. Profuse vomiting and cessation of passing gas and feces are also signs. High-pitched borborygmi (loud, rumbling, gurgling noises produced by the intestines) may indicate obstruction early on.

Intestinal obstruction is diagnosed by physical examination, X rays, and imaging studies, such as a lower gastrointestinal (GI) series (an X-ray procedure that uses a contrast medium). If the doctor suspects obstruction, hospitalization is necessary to find its cause and location. Often, surgery is needed to provide a diagnosis and to remove the obstruction.

Intestine, tumors of

Abnormal growths in the small or large intestine that may be benign (noncancerous) or malignant (cancerous).

Tumors of the small intestine

Tumors of the small intestine grow slowly and are extremely rare. Although most are benign and without symptoms, 10 percent are malignant. Symptoms of a malignant tumor include fatigue, paleness, weight loss, abdominal pain, diarrhea, and blood in the feces. The tumors are generally diagnosed when a gastrointestinal (GI) series (a type of X-ray procedure) or colonoscopy is performed to determine the cause of the symptoms. If a tumor grows large enough, intestinal

blockage can occur (see INTESTINE, OBSTRUCTION OF). Surgery is usually required to remove a malignant tumor or prevent obstruction. If tumors are too numerous or widespread for surgical removal, doctors may recommend chemotherapy or radiation therapy.

Tumors of the large intestine

Benign tumors are more common than malignant growths in the large intestine. Most of these are polyps or abnormal tissue growths that arise from the intestinal wall and protrude into it. However, because polyps may become cancerous over time, doctors recommend their removal. See also COLON, CANCER OF THE; and RECTUM, CANCER OF THE.

Polyps are usually removed in a procedure called a colonoscopy (the viewing of the entire colon with a lighted tube). For large growths, a more extensive operation called a laparotomy is necessary to identify and remove tumors. Tissues from abnormal growths are removed and examined under a microscope to find out whether they are cancerous. Surgery may be necessary to remove a malignant tumor (see COLECTOMY).

Warning signs of cancerous tumors in the large intestine include blood in the stool and a sudden change in bowel habits.

Intoeing

An abnormality in which the leg or foot is slightly rotated, forcing the toes and foot to point inward. Many babies are born with feet that turn in. Intoeing is usually not a serious problem, often correcting itself by about age 7. Severe cases may require surgery.

Intracavitary therapy

Treatment directed into a body cavity. The advantage to this method is that very high doses of radiation can be delivered directly to a tumor site while sparing surrounding tissue.

Intracerebral hemorrhage

See HEMORRHAGE, CEREBRAL.

Intracorneal ring

A small semicircle of plastic surgically implanted within the clear, surface layer (cornea) of the eye to treat nearsightedness. The ring spreads the cornea's layers apart, flattening its overall curve and reducing its focusing power. In most cases, this reduction decreases or eliminates nearsightedness by refocusing light onto the RETINA, rather than in front of it.

The advantage to intracorneal ring surgery is that the central cornea is not touched, reducing the risk of central scarring. Also, the rings can be removed if necessary. The surgery can vastly improve vision in some cases of nearsightedness. The disadvantages of intracorneal ring surgery are greater discomfort during recovery, the risk of insufficient correction, and possible changes in vision, including glare and halos around light sources.

Intractable

Unstoppable. An intractable condition is one that cannot be cured or relieved, such as intractable diarrhea or intractable pain.

Intraductal papilloma

A small benign tumor growing in the cells lining a breast duct. Symptoms include a discharge from the nipple; the discharge may be clear and sticky, greenish yellow, or bloody. A discharge is normal in women who have recently been pregnant, but other women experiencing a nipple discharge should see their doctors right away. Because the symptoms of intraductal papilloma can resemble those of breast cancer, diagnosis will include a biopsy of the papilloma, a mammogram, and laboratory testing of the discharge.

Intraocular lens implant

See CATARACT SURGERY.

Intraocular pressure

The force exerted by the fluid inside the eye pressing out against the eyeball. Normal intraocular pressure is between 10 and 21 millimeters of mercury. If intraocular pressure is abnormally high, it can result in a higher risk for developing glaucoma, a disease that damages the optic nerve and can lead to blindness.

Intrauterine device

A contraceptive device, usually made of plastic, that is placed inside the uterus for long periods. It interferes with the fertilization of eggs and the ability of fertilized eggs to attach to the wall of the uterus. See IUD; CONTRACEPTION, OTHER METHODS.

Intrauterine growth retardation

Stunting of fetal development. Newborns weighing less than 5 pounds and measuring less than 18 inches in length are considered to have intrauterine growth retardation (IUGR).

This condition is usually caused by problems limiting the ability of the placenta to deliver nutrients to the fetus. Intrauterine growth retardation is associated with severe preeclampsia, high blood pressure, hemorrhage, placenta previa, heart disease, diabetes mellitus, malnutrition, and drug and alcohol abuse during pregnancy.

Babies born with IUGR have many more medical and developmental problems and have three times the risk of dying in infancy as babies born at normal weights. The risk for IUGR can be decreased with regular prenatal care, including ultrasound scans.

Intravenous pyelography

An X ray of the structures of the urinary system after the injection of an intravenous contrast medium containing iodine into a vein. The contrast medium allows the kidneys, ureters, and bladder, which are normally not observable on X rays, to be visible for testing. The X rays are taken to locate tumors, anatomical abnormalities, kidney and ureteral stones, and obstructions in the urinary tract.

A contrast medium is injected into an arm vein. People who have had an allergic reaction to the iodine contrast medium in the past or who have a shellfish allergy should mention that fact to the physician or X-ray technician.

Intubation

An emergency medical procedure that involves inserting a tube through a person's mouth or nose into the trachea to allow the lungs to be manu-ally or mechanically inflated. It also can be used to allow air to flow past a partial blockage of the throat, voice box, or windpipe. Intubation is common during general anesthesia and is also used as emergency treatment for people experiencing acute respiratory failure.

Intussusception

A rare disorder in which part of an intestine retracts within itself, much as a telescope retracts. Intussusception most often occurs in the small intestine of babies 4 to 6 months old. Babies scream in pain when muscular contractions occur in the telescoped portion of the intestine. Afterward, they often become limp and pale, vomit, and pass bloody, mucous-filled stools. Babies who experience these symptoms require prompt medical attention. Diagnosis is made through a lower gastrointestinal (GI) series (an X-ray procedure also called a barium enema). The enema may force the telescoped portion back into place. If not, corrective surgery is recommended.

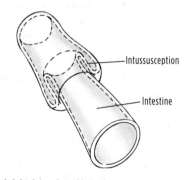

Painful telescoping of intestine
Intussusception affects babies only a few months old, comes on suddenly, and causes extreme pain.

Iodine

A chemical element that is an important mineral in the human body. It is concentrated in the thyroid gland and is essential to the formation of the thyroid hormones, especially the hormone thyroxine. Thyroid hormones maintain normal metabolism in the cells. The principal dietary source of iodine is seafood and iodized salt.

Radioactive iodine may be used as a medical treatment for hyperthyroidism (overactivity of the thyroid gland) or for thyroid tremors. Because iodine is essential to the thyroid hormones, the thyroid gland takes it in readily. The radioactive iodine becomes concentrated in the thyroid where it acts on the glandular tissue. Since the radioactive iodine concentrates in the thyroid, the overactivity of the cells can be controlled without exposing other areas of the body to radiation.

Ipecac

A substance that when ingested induces vomiting; it is used to remove harmful or poisonous substances from the stomach and is commonly known as syrup of ipecac. Ipecac is available without prescription from any pharmacy.

Ipecac can be used by adults and given to children older than 6 months. The syrup should be stored at room temperature and will last several years. It should be taken with water.

Although ipecac is the safest way to induce vomiting, it should not be used by people who are unconscious or drowsy, by people with heart conditions, or by women during the third trimester of pregnancy. At one time doctors recommended that all parents keep ipecac on hand for emergency use, but then research focused on the possible dangers of vomiting poisons into the esophagus, windpipe, and mouth.

Ipecac should not be used in every poisoning emergency. Before using ipecac, it is important to consult with a doctor or a specialist at a poison center.

IQ

Intelligence quotient, one measure of intelligence. See INTELLIGENCE TESTS.

Iridectomy

A surgical operation to remove a portion of the colored portion of the eye (iris). Iridectomy is usually performed to alleviate the buildup of fluid in the eye in cases of angle-closure glaucoma. It is also occasionally done to create an artificial pupil (opening in the iris).

Iridotomy

A laser procedure in which a tiny hole is placed in the colored portion of the eye (iris). This is most often performed for angle-closure glaucoma.

Iron

An element essential to life. Iron is present in the adult body chiefly in the form of hemoglobin in the red blood cells, but also in muscles and other iron stores. Iron is essential to the transfer of oxygen from the lungs to the body tissues. If body cells do not receive adequate iron, the result is iron-deficiency ANEMIA, which causes a person to feel weak and tired. The best dietary sources of iron are liver, lean red meat, poultry, fish, shellfish, and kidney. Iron is often added to enriched breads, cereals, wine, molasses, and dried fruits. Oral iron supplements are available without a prescription but should only be taken when recommended by a doctor.

Iron-deficiency anemia

See ANEMIA, IRON-DEFICIENCY.

Irradiation

Exposure to radiation. Medical irradiation is used for diagnostic or therapeutic purposes and may involve X rays or radioactive isotopes. See also NUCLEAR MEDICINE; RADIATION; and RADIATION THERAPY.

Irrigation, wound

To flush an area of the body with a stream of liquid for the purpose of cleansing or medicating the area. Wound irrigation may be accomplished with clean, warm water, or with a disinfectant such as hydrogen peroxide. See also PUNCTURE WOUNDS.

Irritable bladder

Another name for urge incontinence, which refers to the involuntary loss of urine immediately after the need to urinate is felt. See INCONTINENCE, URINARY for details.

Irritable bowel syndrome

For symptom charts, see CONSTIPATION, page xvi, and see DIARRHEA, page xviii.

A condition characterized by a combination of symptoms, including abdominal pain, indigestion, bloating, diarrhea, and constipation, with no clear cause. The most common disorder of the digestive tract, irritable bowel syndrome (IBS) is a functional disorder that affects the muscles of the intestine and can be brought on or aggravated by emotional stress.

The symptoms of IBS are similar to those of many other gastrointestinal disorders. A sudden change in bowel habits after years of regularity can be a symptom of IBS or of a serious digestive disorder, such as colon cancer (see COLON, CANCER OF THE). As a result, the diagnosis of IBS is made by eliminating other possible causes of symptoms. To rule out other underlying problems, the doctor may order a number of tests including imaging procedures, such as ultrasound or CT (computed tomography) scanning, SIGMOIDOSCOPY, barium X rays of the gastrointestinal tract, and stool analysis. When chronic symptoms include abdominal discomfort, problems with passing stools, and emotional stress, and tests do not reveal the presence of any other disease, the diagnosis is most likely IBS.

Although IBS has no cure, symptoms can be managed. Patients may be advised to reduce stress, stop smoking, adopt a high-fiber diet, limit consumption of gas-producing foods and dairy products, and use glycerin suppositories or enemas in severe cases. For diarrhea, doctors advise resting and drinking clear fluids until symptoms subside. Watery diarrhea can cause dehydration and loss of crucial body salts, which may be restored with oral rehydration fluid (see REHYDRATION FLUID, ORAL). Medications, such as antispasmodic drugs, mild sedatives, and tranquilizers, are recommended in some cases of IBS. Laxatives other than fiber should be used only cautiously and infrequently.

Irritable colon

See IRRITABLE BOWEL SYNDROME.

Ischemia

A temporary shortage of oxygen in a part of the body caused by impaired blood flow. The usual cause of ischemia is a buildup on the artery walls of fatty material known as plaque; the plaque narrows the artery and slows blood flow. If a blood clot forms at the site of the narrowing, the oxygen supply may be completely interrupted, leading to the death of the affected tissue.

Cardiac ischemia, or ischemia that affects the heart, can be treated with medication, such as beta blockers to decrease the workload on the heart and aspirin to prevent blood clots. Surgery may also be used.

See CAROTID ENDARTERECTOMY; BALLOON ANGIOPLASTY.

Isolation

A method of preventing the transmission of infection in hospitals to the hospital staff, visitors, and other patients. Isolation procedures are generally used for the care of patients in acute-care hospital settings when serious symptoms come on suddenly. Isolations may be necessary for patients who have highly contagious or dangerous infections such as an infected wound. See also NOSOCOMIAL INFECTIONS; QUARANTINE.

Isopropyl alcohol

A transparent, volatile, colorless liquid with disinfectant properties (see DISINFECTANTS); also called rubbing alcohol. Isopropyl alcohol is used as a solvent and disinfectant and as an antiseptic (see ANTISEPTICS) when applied to the skin. Rubbing alcohol, available over-the-counter, is a combination of 68 to 72 percent isopropyl alcohol and water.

Isopropyl alcohol is poisonous if a person ingests it. It should not be used as a bathing solution to cool children with a high fever. Symptoms of an overdose include labored breathing, lack of coordination, nausea and vomiting, low blood pressure, dizziness, and unconsciousness. If a person is suspected of drinking isopropyl alcohol, a poison center or hospital emergency department should be contacted immediately.

Itching

See PRURITUS.

ITP

Idiopathic thrombocytopenic purpura; a condition of unknown cause in which the blood has an insufficient number of platelets and the person bruises excessively. Platelets are tiny cells that help the blood form clots. When these blood cells are deficient, a person bruises easily and bleeds for a long time after being injured. While the cause is not known, it is known that people have ITP as the result of an autoimmune disorder. An acute form of ITP affects children, mainly from 2 to 4, and the chronic form appears in adults, usually between 20 and 50 years old.

ITP is generally diagnosed by evaluating a medical history, by a physical examination that may reveal a bleeding tendency, and by a blood test. The presence of antibodies against platelets may help establish the diagnosis.

Treatment of children with ITP is aimed at managing the symptoms. Most children recover completely with no treatment because the disease usually resolves on its own.

In adults, ITP treatment is directed at increasing the platelet count by taking oral prednisone, a corticosteroid, for a month or longer. About 80 percent of people will respond to treatment, and the platelet count will usually return to normal. If there is no response to prednisone therapy, surgical removal of the spleen may be necessary. Alternative therapies include high-dose intravenous immunoglobulin, danazol, and immunosuppressive drugs.

IUD

Intrauterine device. IUDs are small, usually plastic, devices containing copper or hormones that are placed in the uterus to interfere with ovulation and conception and to prevent

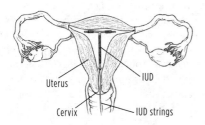

A T-shaped IUD
An intrauterine device, inserted into the uterus by a doctor, changes the environment of the uterus so that sperm are unable to reach the fallopian tubes or so that fertilized eggs cannot implant in the uterus. Strings attached to the bottom of the device extend through the cervix down into the vagina; the woman wearing the device can locate the strings with her finger.

pregnancy. The copper IUD releases a small amount of copper that affects the lining of the uterus and inhibits fertilized eggs from implanting. The hormonal IUD releases small amounts of the hormone progesterone into the uterus. The hormone thickens cervical mucus, creating a barrier to sperm entering the uterus. It also affects the uterine lining in ways that prevent implantation of a fertilized egg. A hormonal IUD must be replaced every year; the copper version can be kept in place for up to 12 years.

The IUD is a highly effective method of contraception and is one of the safest. However, it is not recommended for women who have had a pelvic infection, an ectopic pregnancy, severe pain during menstruation, abnormal vaginal bleeding, or those who have multiple sexual partners (because of the risk of sexually transmitted diseases). See also CONTRACEPTION, OTHER METHODS.

IVF

See IN VITRO FERTILIZATION.

IVP

See INTRAVENOUS PYELOGRAPHY.

Jaundice

A yellowing of the skin and the whites of the eyes. Jaundice is a symptom of many liver disorders, including cirrhosis, hepatitis, and liver cancer. Also known as icterus, jaundice is usually a sign of a blockage of the bile ducts from the liver or disease within the liver. It is due to an excess of bilirubin (a normal byproduct of the breakdown of hemoglobin from aging red blood cells) in the bloodstream.

Jaw

Usually refers to the lower jaw, called the mandible, the only movable bone in the face.

Jaw, dislocated

The displacement of the bones of the jaw's temporomandibular joint, which causes soft-tissue damage to the joint capsule and to the ligaments. Muscles connected to the joint may be strained, resulting in painful muscle spasms in the area of the jaw. When the jaw is dislocated, it is often impossible to close the mouth. The condition may be treated by manipulating the joint back into proper position, sometimes with the use of an anesthetic. Once the jaw has been properly realigned, a bandage may be used to hold it in place. A person whose jaw has been dislocated repeatedly should consult with a maxillofacial surgeon for possible treatment.

Jaw, fractured

A completely or partially broken lower jaw bone, or mandible. An inability to close the mouth or align the teeth properly, as well as a lower jaw that hangs without support, may all indicate a broken jaw. Other symptoms include severe pain in the area; swelling of associated muscles, tendons, and ligaments; or an apparent deformity of the jaw in complete breaks, which may cause the bone segments to separate. Other symptoms include tenderness with light contact and possibly a movable upper jaw, bleeding at the base of the teeth near the fracture site, and numbness. If a broken jaw is suspected, the person should seek immediate medical attention. Using a bandage to immobilize the jaw is the first step in first aid. Diagnosis is made on the basis of a physical examination, special X rays, and possibly a CT (computed tomography) scan. Surgery is often necessary to realign the segments of jaw bone and allow healing. In many cases, the jaw must be wired to the opposing jaw or otherwise immobilized for up to 8 weeks.

Jet lag

A groggy, dragging, "out-of-sync" feeling that is caused by lost sleep when a person crosses time zones during air travel. Jet lag is most frequent when a person flies eastward, thus subtracting hours from his or her day. To minimize jet lag, doctors recommend resetting the body's clock to the sleep-wake pattern of one's destination several days before departure; drinking plenty of fluids, avoiding the dehydrating effects of alcohol; eating lightly; and exercising regularly, but not late in the evening.

Jock itch

A fungal infection of the groin; also known as *tinea cruris*. Jock itch is characterized by itching of the groin and a scaly red skin rash with sharply defined borders. Usually the genitals are not involved, but there may be itching and discomfort around the anus. Often the rash spreads in a circle, leaving normal-appearing skin in the center. The diagnosis is made through appearance of the skin and possibly a skin scraping or fungal culture.

Most cases respond well to treatment with over-the-counter antifungal creams or powders such as clotrimazole or miconazole. It is also essential to keep the skin clean and dry.

Joint

The juncture of two bones. Some joints are fixed and immovable, but most have varying ranges of movement. The seven types of joints are the ball and socket (for example, the hip); hinge (for example, the elbow); ellipsoidal (for example, the radius); saddle (at the base of the thumb); pivot (the neck); gliding (for example, the foot); and fixed (the skull).

All movable joints have ligaments holding the bones together (external ligaments). Ligaments are made of tough connective tissue with very lit-

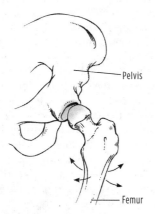

Ball-and-socket joint
A ball-and-socket joint, as in the hip, gives a person the greatest range of movement of all joint structures.

tle elasticity. Some complex joints have internal ligaments that run between bones inside the joint to stabilize it. The entire joint is enclosed in a fibrous capsule that prevents the ends of the bones from dislocating. The capsule is strengthened with an inner layer of ligaments referred to as capsular ligaments. The lining of the joint capsule, called the synovial membrane, is lubricated by a secretion called synovial fluid. The synovial fluid enables the ends of the bone to slide smoothly in the joint. The ends of the bones themselves are covered with a layer of smooth, hard connective tissue called the articular cartilage, which provides a good sliding surface. Some joints have additional disks of cartilage (menisci) that are attached just loosely enough to act as shock absorbers.

Joint aspiration

A procedure that involves the withdrawal of synovial fluid, the fluid that lubricates the surfaces of the bones and provides nutrients to the cartilage inside a joint. Fluid obtained from joint aspiration or arthrocentesis may be used as a diagnostic tool; an analysis of the fluid can help establish the cause of swelling in a joint, distinguish between different forms of arthritis, and detect the presence of blood in the joint, indicating trauma or fracture. The procedure can also help diagnose septic arthritis and joint diseases associated with the presence of crystals in the joint.

Joint injection

A procedure to inject medication into an affected joint for the relief of inflammation, pain, and swelling. The corticosteroids, also known as glucocorticoids, which include cortisone, are often used for joint injections. The injections may be used to treat the joint pain caused by osteoarthritis and rheumatoid arthritis; bursitis of the shoulder, hip, or knee; frozen shoulder; tennis elbow; golfer's elbow; plantar fasciitis; carpal tunnel syndrome; and some forms of backache. Joint injections may decrease the time it takes to recover from an injury and are a source of pain relief. But no more than three or four injections are generally given within a year in one area of the body.

Joint replacement

A prosthetic device made of metal or a combination of metal with plastic or porcelain, which is used to replace an arthritic or damaged joint that has been removed. A joint is generally removed and replaced with a prosthesis because it is no longer functional, because of extreme pain, immobility, or both. Hip joint replacements and knee joint replacements (see JOINT RE-PLACEMENT, HIP and JOINT REPLACE-MENT, KNEE) are the most common.

Joint replacement, hip

A surgical procedure performed to replace the ball-and-socket joint of the hip with a specially designed prosthesis. A prosthetic hip joint replacement is implanted after removal of the diseased bone tissue and cartilage from the natural hip joint. Conditions that may lead to the need for this procedure include degenerative osteoarthritis, rheumatoid arthritis, injury, bone tumors, and avascular necrosis of the femoral head (insufficient blood supply leading to death of bone tissue). Before surgery the extent of damage to a joint is diagnosed and evaluated by a physical examination, by X rays, and possibly by certain laboratory tests.

The structure of a hip joint replacement includes a metal ball attached to a metal stem that is fitted into the thighbone, and held there, usually with plastic bone cement. A polyethylene socket is implanted into the pelvis to replace the damaged socket and to receive the prosthetic, ball-shaped head of the thighbone, forming a complete ball-and-socket joint.

Full recovery usually takes from 3 to 6 months. Exercise and physical therapy are important elements of total recovery.

Joint replacement, knee

A surgical procedure to replace the knee joint with a specially designed prosthetic joint. The surface of the knee joint may be worn away by osteoarthritis, fractures, rheumatoid arthritis, or gout, making walking and normal daily activities difficult and painful.

What is called a knee joint replacement is actually a resurfacing of the knee joint. There are several techniques for performing the procedure. The thighbone (femur) is covered with a metal sheath, and plastic is placed on the shin bone (tibia), using acrylic cement. Usually, the undersurface of the kneecap is also replaced with a plastic surface so that it fits smoothly with the metal-covered thighbone. The smooth, nonsticking surfaces replace the irregular arthritic surfaces so that the knee's movement and function are restored. As with hip replacement surgery, physical therapy is an essential part of the recovery process. The success rate of the surgery is high.

Jugular vein

The large vein that returns oxygen-poor blood from much of the head and neck toward the heart. The name "jugular" comes from the Latin word for throat.

Jumper's knee

An irritation, sprain, or overuse of the large tendon that lies just below the kneecap. This tendon, called the patellar tendon, allows the knee joint to straighten and extend. Jumper's knee, medically termed patellar tendinitis, is caused by repeated pressure on the knee's tendon during activities that require frequent jumping, such as basketball, net ball, volleyball, and long jumping. The resulting irritation causes symptoms of pain, swelling, and inflammation of the tendon.

Self-care for the condition includes resting the overused tendon, icing to decrease swelling, and later, when swelling and pain are decreased, applications of heat to promote healing. A doctor may recommend nonsteroidal anti-inflammatory drugs (NSAIDs) to control the inflammation, the use of knee braces to support the knee, and physical therapy.

Cortisone injections into the tendon sheaths may be recommended. Surgery may be needed if all other treatments have failed.

Juvenile rheumatoid arthritis

A disease that can cause chronic inflammation of a child's joints and internal organs. Also known as JRA, juvenile rheumatoid arthritis most commonly begins between ages 2 and 5 or 9 and 12.

There are three types of juvenile rheumatoid arthritis. The most common form is pauciarticular JRA, in which joint inflammation occurs in four or fewer joints (usually the knees, ankles, or elbows). The second most common form is polyarticular, which affects five or more joints, including small joints in the fingers and hands.

Least common is systemic JRA, the most serious type, which affects the internal organs as well as the joints. Between one third and one half of those with polyarticular or systemic JRA will develop a residual joint deformity and functional limitations. Although juvenile rheumatoid arthritis is a potentially disabling disease, most children who have had appropriate treatment recover from it completely, particularly those with pauciarticular JRA. The exact cause of JRA remains unknown. Researchers believe that JRA is an autoimmune disorder triggered by viral infections in susceptible children.

An early warning sign of juvenile rheumatoid arthritis is joint stiffness in the morning. Other symptoms include a fever with no apparent cause, persistent joint stiffness, swelling, and pain. The skin over swollen joints may appear red and feel hot. A child's appetite may also be affected, leading to weight loss or gain.

Symptoms vary according to the type of JRA. Juvenile rheumatoid arthritis is not uniformly painful. Children may experience periods of remission, in which symptoms recede and they feel much better. At other times there will be flare-ups when pain, stiffness, and inflammation are at their worst.

Juvenile rheumatoid arthritis can be difficult to diagnose. A doctor should be consulted if a child develops a limp or consistently favors one hand, arm, or leg over another. To make a diagnosis, the doctor will examine the child and take a medical history and may order X rays and blood tests.

Treatment varies according to the type of JRA but is generally directed toward reducing inflammation. Nonsteroidal anti-inflammatory drugs (NSAIDs), corticosteroids, gold therapy, or methotrexate may be prescribed to control symptoms. However, aspirin should never be given to children because of the risk of developing Reye syndrome, which may be fatal.

When swollen or acutely painful, the joint needs to be rested. However, when symptoms are in remission, regular exercise is recommended. All children with JRA should see an ophthalmologist at least annually.

K

Kaposi sarcoma

A cancerous tumor primarily of the skin that may also involve intestines, lymph glands, lungs, heart, spleen, and adrenal glands.

In the United States, Kaposi sarcoma occurs almost exclusively in people with AIDS (acquired immunodeficiency syndrome), but the number of new cases has started to decline with recent advances in the treatment of AIDS. The tumors chiefly arise in the skin, where they appear as irregular, slightly raised spots, ranging in color from purple to brown. Treatment can also include chemotherapy or radiation therapy to individual skin lesions.

Karyotyping

Chromosome analysis. Medical diagnostic tests used to identify chromosomal abnormalities as the cause of malformation or disease. Karyotyping can be conducted on samples of blood, bone marrow, amniotic fluid, or placental tissue. Cells are stained, viewed under a microscope, and then photographed to provide a karyotype showing the arrangement of the chromosomes, which sometimes can indicate the presence of abnormalities.

Chromosome analysis is usually used to evaluate suspected genetic abnormalities, detect chromosome abnormalities before birth, evaluate a couple with a history of miscarriages, or identify the chromosome present in a type of leukemia. Abnormal results may indicate Down syndrome, trisomy 18 syndrome, Turner syndrome, Klinefelter syndrome, leukemia, and other disorders.

Diagnostic prenatal testing is reserved for women who are at high risk for having a fetus with a genetic abnormality. Diagnostic testing is considered invasive; the two diagnostic testing procedures, amniocentesis and chorionic villus sampling, involve a risk of miscarriage.

Kawasaki disease

A rare but serious childhood disease of unknown origin that causes inflammation of blood vessels. Also called mucocutaneous lymph node syndrome, it is accompanied by fever, swollen lymph glands, and a skin rash.

Kawasaki disease is most common in boys between ages 6 months and 5 years. Children of Japanese or Korean ancestry are more frequently affected. Symptoms include a high fever that persists for 5 days or longer and does not respond to antibiotics; a measles-like rash that may be particularly severe in the diaper area of infants; reddened and swollen hands and soles of the feet; red, cracked lips; reddened eyes; swollen lymph glands in the neck (see GLANDS, SWOLLEN); and irritability, apathy, or crankiness. An affected child may complain of stomach pain, headache, or joint pain. Without treatment, a child may appear to improve after 2 weeks. However, internally, the disease begins to affect the heart. Coronary arteries may grow inflamed, and the child can develop a fast, irregular heartbeat (see ARRHYTHMIA, CARDIAC). A life-threatening aneurysm can occur.

Treatment consists of large doses of intravenous gamma globulin, a blood product containing human antibodies. The child will also be given aspirin for 8 weeks, in high doses for the first 2 weeks to inhibit clot formation in damaged blood vessels. (However, as a general rule, aspirin is not given to children without a doctor's advice because of the danger of developing Reye syndrome, which is potentially fatal.) The outlook for complete recovery is good when Kawasaki disease is diagnosed and treated early.

Kegel exercises

Exercises done by women to strengthen the pelvic floor muscles that control urine flow and support the bladder, uterus, vagina, and rectum. Kegel exercises (also called pelvic floor exercises) involve repeated tensing, holding, and releasing of the muscles. If done correctly and regularly, Kegel exercises may help a woman have a more comfortable childbirth, overcome urinary incontinence (lack of bladder control; see INCONTINENCE, URINARY), and increase sexual satisfaction. Kegel exercises can be done anywhere.

Keloid

A raised scar that extends beyond the original site of injury or that occurs around the incision line after surgery. Keloids are the result of an abnormal healing response and are caused by an excess buildup of collagen. Most keloids occur on the chest or on the earlobe after ear piercing. They may occur after an injury, surgical incision, or burn. Although harmless, keloids can be unsightly, and some are itchy or tender.

Keloids can be treated with corticosteroid injections directly into the keloid and cryosurgery (freezing with liquid nitrogen). Surgical removal can present a problem because a new surgical incision may create a new scar that in turn can lead to another keloid.

Keratoacanthoma

A papule (small superficial bump on the skin) or nodule (solid mass of tissue) with a central crater that appears on sun-damaged skin. The papules or nodules may disappear on their own. Keratoacanthomas should be treated by a dermatologist because, although they are benign (not cancerous), they closely resemble tumors of squamous cell carcinoma.

Keratoconjunctivitis

Inflammation of the clear outer covering of the eye (cornea) and of the membrane lining the eyelids and covering the eye surface (conjunctiva). It can lead to visual impairment from scarring of the cornea. Keratoconjunctivitis can be caused by infection of the eyes with a virus that also causes headache and swelling of the lymph nodes. It can also be caused by autoimmune disease or allergies. Vernal keratoconjunctivitis involves the development of large bumps on the lining of the upper eyelid, itching, burning, foreign body sensation, excessive tearing and mucus production, and blurred vision. Depending on severity, the disease is treated with topical corticosteroids.

Atopic keratoconjunctivitis largely affects people with atopic dermatitis (eczema), an allergic skin disease. Symptoms include itching, burning, foreign body sensation, excessive tearing and mucus production, and blurred vision. The disease is treated with antihistamine and other allergy medications.

Keratoconus

A disease that involves a progressive, gradual thinning of the clear outer covering of the eye (cornea) and changes its shape from a dome to a cone; also known as conical cornea. The change in the cornea's shape causes nearsightedness (blurring of distant objects) and astigmatism (tilting and distortion of the field of view), which can range from mild to severe. Most cases of keratoconus begin in adolescence or early adulthood and progress over a 10- to 20-year period. Keratoconus has a number of possible causes, including an inherited abnormality of the cornea, certain eye diseases (for example, retinitis pigmentosa and vernal keratoconjunctivitis), and some systemic diseases, such as Down syndrome. Treatment depends on the severity of the disease. Eyeglasses can correct nearsightedness and astigmatism in the early stages. In more severe cases, rigid contact lenses are used to flatten the surface of the cornea and provide improved vision. If vision remains badly impaired even with contact lenses, the person may need to undergo a corneal transplant. See KERATOPLASTY, PENETRATING.

Keratoplasty, conductive

A medical procedure that uses radiofrequency energy to heat and reshape the cornea, the clear front surface of the eye, and thereby correct hyperopia (farsightedness). Conductive keratoplasty (CK) is considered innovative because it is less invasive than the other procedures used to correct vision by reshaping the cornea with lasers. People who undergo the procedure may no longer need to wear glasses or contact lenses to see clearly.

During CK, the heat from a radiofrequency energy device is used to shrink the cornea at specific treatment spots, creating a band of tightening. This band of tightening steepens the cornea and allows light to focus precisely on the retina. The entire procedure takes about 5 minutes. CK is not recommended for women who are pregnant or nursing, nor is it recommended for people with a tendency to form scars or with severe dry eye, thin corneas, or keratoconus. In addition, CK is not recommended for people with any disease that affects the body's ability to heal, such as AIDS (acquired immunodeficiency syndrome) or systemic lupus erythematosus (see LUPUS ERYTHEMATOSUS, SYSTEMIC).

Keratoplasty, penetrating

Surgery to replace the clear outer covering of the eye (cornea). The donor cornea is taken from a recently deceased person who has agreed to donate his or her eyes after death. Penetrating keratoplasty is performed in people who have had diseases or injuries that scar their own corneas and leave them with little or no vision. Penetrating keratoplasty is highly successful in restoring or improving sight.

Keratosis

A skin growth caused by the overproduction of keratin, a protein found in skin, hair, and nails. An actinic keratosis is a precancerous growth that occurs in sun-exposed areas of the body.

Kerion

A tender, swollen mass of dandruff-like scales, broken stubbles of hair, and pustules (small pus-filled blisters) caused by a fungal infection of the scalp. Fever and enlarged lymph nodes in the neck and scalp may occur. It is often the result of a tinea infection of the hair follicles and is treated with oral antifungal medication.

Ketoacidosis

An emergency medical condition usually occurring in people with type 1 diabetes (see DIABETES MELLITUS, TYPE 1) but that can also occur in people with type 2 diabetes (see DIABETES MELLITUS, TYPE 2). It starts when the blood sugar level becomes too elevated. As glucose accumulates in the blood, the cells become less able to utilize it. These cells begin to use stored fat for energy, causing the production and release of acids called ketone bodies. Glucose and ketones accumulate in the blood, making it more acidic.

Ketoacidosis occurs when diabetes is undiagnosed, untreated, or inadequately controlled, sometimes as a result of stress from an injury or illness. Bouts of diarrhea or vomiting that cause dehydration can lead to ketoacidosis.

Over the course of a few hours, a person with ketoacidosis typically experiences an unquenchable thirst and frequent urination. This may be followed by weakness, sleepiness, nausea, and vomiting, which may cause dehydration, as well as stomach pain. Other signs may include flushing of the face, dry skin and mouth, a weak but rapid pulse, low blood pressure, and a sweet odor on the breath. In more advanced ketoacidosis, deep and rapid breathing occurs. If a person with diabetes shows these signs and does not receive insulin and fluids immediately, ketoacidosis can result in the loss of consciousness and ultimately death.

The first line of emergency treatment for ketoacidosis is to restore hydration by replacing fluid and electrolyte losses. This is generally accomplished by giving liquids containing isotonic saline and potassium intravenously. Insulin therapy is administered. Complete recovery from ketoacidosis is usually rapid when immediate medical treatment is given.

Ketosis

An abnormal accumulation of ketones in the body caused by a deficiency or the inefficient use of carbohydrates. Ketones are a by-product of the metabolism of fatty acids. Ketosis occurs when glucose is unavailable for use as a source of energy, and the body instead uses fats, resulting in fatty acids being released into the blood where they are converted to ketones. See GLUCOSE METABOLISM.

Kidney

The major organ of the urinary tract, in which blood is filtered and waste products and excess fluid are excreted as urine. The two kidneys are located in the back of the abdominal cavity on either side of the spine, at about waist level. The right kidney is positioned under the liver; the left kidney, which sits slightly higher, is near the spleen.

Blood enters the kidneys through the renal arteries. Inside the kidneys, the arteries subdivide until they are a network of tiny vessels called arterioles. An individual arteriole carries blood into the smallest functioning unit of the kidney called a nephron. A nephron consists of a structure called a glomerulus and an elongated structure called a tubule. Within the glomerulus, the blood is filtered and then released into a tubule. The tubule, which is surrounded by capillaries, reabsorbs some essential chemical components and allows others to flow back into the center of the kidney, called the medulla. In the medulla, which is a holding area, fluid containing wastes pools before passing out of the kidney into a ureter (the tube leading from the kidneys to the bladder). Waste materials are eventually excreted in the waste liquid called urine.

Kidney biopsy

The taking of a tiny sample of kidney tissue to help determine the cause of protein or blood in the urine or to monitor the effectiveness of treatments for kidney disorders. A kidney biopsy is done by administering a local anesthesia and then inserting a sterile, narrow, hollow needle into a kidney to extract tissue, which is then examined by a pathologist under a microscope. A kidney biopsy is considered the most accurate assessment of abnormalities in kidney tissue.

Kidney cancer

A cancer that originates in the kidney. Symptoms may include pain on one side of the back, blood in the urine, a mass in the abdomen or side, high blood pressure, and fever. Some people with kidney cancer also experience loss of appetite, nausea and vomiting, constipation, weakness, and fatigue.

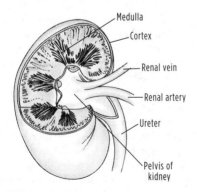

Medulla
Cortex
Renal vein
Renal artery
Ureter
Pelvis of kidney

Anatomy of the kidney
Blood enters a kidney through the renal vein and passes into a nephron, where wastes are filtered out. The waste pools in the medulla until it leaves the kidney via the ureter.

Diagnosis of kidney cancer may include blood tests, ultrasound, urinalysis, CT (computed tomography) scanning and MRI (magnetic resonance imaging), and an IVP (intravenous pyelogram, or X rays of the kidney). Many tumors found in the kidney are benign (noncancerous); surgical biopsy is the only way to distinguish benign from malignant tumors. Kidney cancer is usually treated with surgery, radiation therapy, biological therapy, chemotherapy, or hormone therapy. Kidney cancer occurs twice as often in men as in women.

Kidney cyst

A common, usually benign (noncancerous) lesion on the kidney. Kidney cysts are hollow, round growths that contain a watery fluid.

Kidney cysts usually cause no symptoms but may sometimes cause blood in the urine, back pain, or abdominal pain if the cyst is unusually large. Kidney cysts are most commonly discovered in the course of ultrasound scanning or CT scanning (computed tomography scanning) performed in connection with other conditions.

Treatment is not usually required. If a cyst becomes infected, antibiotics will be prescribed. See also POLYCYSTIC KIDNEY DISEASE.

Kidney failure

The inability of the kidneys to perform their normal function of filtering waste products from the blood. Kidney failure may be caused by infection, injury, exposure to toxins, kidney disease, and other diseases such as diabetes, systemic lupus erythematosus, or sickle cell anemia. Structural disorders obstructing the flow of urine from the kidneys may be associated with kidney failure.

Kidney failure may be acute or chronic. The acute form results in a sudden loss of kidney function. Acute kidney failure is potentially life-threatening and may require hospitalization and constant monitoring. Chronic kidney failure involves the slow, progressive destruction of kidney function as a result of kidney disease. End-stage renal disease is chronic, irreversible kidney failure. It requires either dialysis or a kidney transplant for survival.

Kidney function tests

Diagnostic evaluations performed to determine the level of a person's kidney function. Kidney function tests involve taking blood and urine for analysis in a laboratory to determine the levels of substances that measure the ability of the kidneys to filter the blood properly.

Substances being measured include blood urea nitrogen (BUN), which measures the amount of urea in the blood, and creatinine, which is a waste product of the normal breakdown of muscle during activity. Elevated levels of these substances in a urine sample indicate compromised kidney function, as does the presence of protein in the urine.

Creatinine clearance is a calculated value that describes the kidney's ability to filter and remove creatinine from the blood. It is a common way to look at the kidney's ability to clean waste from the blood stream.

Kidney imaging

Diagnostic scanning performed to detect anatomic abnormalities in the kidneys, including a tumor, mass, cyst, or kidney stone. It may also be performed to pinpoint the location of a kidney during a kidney biopsy or to examine the blood vessels that supply blood to the kidneys. Specific types of kidney imaging include ultrasound scanning, angiography, CT scanning (computed tomography scanning), and intravenous pyelography.

Kidney stones

Also known as renal calculi; stones composed of abnormal chemical deposits that form inside the urinary tract. Kidney stones are hard and range in size from a grain of sand or larger than a marble. When they are very small, they pass out of the kidneys through the ureters (two narrow tubes, each connecting a kidney and the bladder) in the urine. If they are large, they may remain in the kidneys or travel into a ureter where they become trapped, causing a variety of symptoms that include extreme back pain or pain in the side, blocked urine flow, and bleeding. Other symptoms include nausea and vomiting, as well as blood in the urine.

Anyone with kidney stones, even very small ones that do not cause symptoms, should be examined by a doctor. A physician will take a general medical history and ask about changes in urine color and if there is a family tendency for kidney stones or gout.

If a kidney stone is not too large, pain medication may be prescribed until the stone is passed. This may take hours, days, or weeks. Smaller stones are usually flushed out through urination and should be saved and brought to a doctor for chemical analysis. If the stone is large and causing intolerable pain, infection, or heavy bleeding, it may be nec-essary to break up the stone in a procedure called LITHOTRIPSY.

Drinking 2 to 4.25 quarts of water daily reduces the risk of recurrence. To prevent stones, it is important to determine what type of stone the person has—calcium, struvite, uric acid, or cystine. Thiazide diuretic medications are prescribed to help prevent calcium stones. Uric acid stones may be treated with allopurinol.

Kidney transplant

A surgical procedure in which a healthy kidney is taken from one person (see NEPHRECTOMY) and placed in another person with end-stage renal disease (see KIDNEY FAILURE). Kidneys for organ donation may also be taken from deceased donors, but the chances of success are greater when a live donor is used. A kidney transplant restores sufficient kidney function so the person does not need dialysis.

Kidney, polycystic

See POLYCYSTIC KIDNEY DISEASE.

Kilocalorie

A measurement of energy used in nutrition. A kilocalorie (kcal) represents the amount of energy necessary to raise the temperature of 1 kilogram of water by 1 degree Celsius (centigrade). In popular, nonscientific usage, a kilocalorie is usually called a calorie.

Kleptomania

A rare mental illness characterized by a compulsive, uncontrollable desire to steal.

Klumpke paralysis

Paralysis of the forearm resulting from injury to the lower brachial plexus. Klumpke paralysis is present from birth, most often with breech deliveries. It is often associated with other problems, such as Horner syndrome.

Knee

The hinge joint between the thighbone (femur) and the shin (tibia). This powerful joint joins the two longest bones in the body and helps bear much of the weight of the upper body. The kneecap (patella) is a disk of bone that lies in front of the knee joint. The kneecap is cushioned above and below by an upper and a lower bursa (sac of synovial fluid).

Knee replacement

See JOINT REPLACEMENT, KNEE.

Knock-knees

Knees that touch due to an inward curving of the legs. Knock-knees help children maintain balance as they learn to walk and are normal between the ages of 2 and 6. In rare cases, knock-knees are the result of a more serious underlying condition, such as rickets (a vitamin D deficiency that causes bones to soften), a fracture, infection, tumor, or juvenile rheumatoid arthritis.

In most cases, knock-knees correct themselves over time and require no treatment. If knock-knees persist after age 10, children are usually referred to a pediatric orthopedist for possible treatment, including braces (see BRACE, ORTHOPEDIC), corrective shoes, or corrective surgery.

Korsakoff psychosis

A condition marked by extreme confusion, mental impairment, memory loss, and symptoms of nerve damage. Also known as alcohol-induced persisting amnesic disorder, Korsakoff psychosis usually is caused by alcoholism but may also be a result of a brain tumor, a head injury, starvation, or a minor stroke. The loss of memory and intellect cannot usually be reversed.

Kyphosis

An abnormal and excessive outward curvature of the vertebrae in the upper spine. It is usually painless unless severe, but can result in chronic fatigue in the back muscles. Kyphosis produces humpback, hunchback, or rounding of the shoulders and can occur in several different age groups. Kyphosis is diagnosed by physical examination, X rays, and in some cases, laboratory tests. Treatment generally emphasizes the use of orthotic braces and exercise routines to strengthen the muscles and ligaments associated with the spine and upper back. Medication may be prescribed to treat related conditions such as osteoporosis. When kyphosis is severe, it may be treated by a surgical procedure involving spinal fusion.

Labia

The lips of the vaginal opening that protect the female's external genitalia. The outer, thicker folds, which have hair and sweat glands, are called the labia majora. The thinner, inner folds, called the labia minora, form the hood over the clitoris. See REPRODUCTIVE SYSTEM, FEMALE.

Labor

A series of physiological changes in a woman that allow for the delivery of a fetus through her birth canal. Changes in hormone levels appear to cause the start of labor, although the exact cause is unclear. The duration of labor varies for each woman and each birth.

Definitive signs of the beginning of labor include experiencing contractions that progressively become stronger and more regular, mucus tinged with blood passing from the woman's body (referred to as a bloody show), or a clear fluid flowing from her vagina. Doctors ask women to call when contractions are 4 to 5 minutes apart and have continued for an hour or more, if there is more than a small amount of vaginal bleeding, and when a woman's water breaks.

Labor proceeds in three specific steps with distinct physiological characteristics:

- Stage one, usually the longest for most women, is when a woman's cervix dilates (opens) and effaces (thins), to permit the baby to pass through the cervix and into the birth canal.

- Birth occurs during stage two, when the woman will be asked to bear down and push during contractions to assist in the delivery of her baby. Before the pushing the doctor will first confirm that the cervix has dilated fully. This stage ends when the baby is delivered.

- In stage three, the afterbirth (the placenta and membranes surrounding the fetus) are delivered.

Labyrinthitis

An inflammation of the inner ear's system of fluid-filled tubes and sacs called the labyrinth. The symptoms of labyrinthitis depend on the severity and extent of the inflammation. Hearing loss or ringing in the ears may result if the inflammation affects the cochlea (hearing organ of the inner ear). Difficulty with balance, dizziness, and nausea may be experienced if the inflammation reaches the vestibular system (group of organs in the inner ear responsible for balance control and eye movements). It is important to seek medical attention promptly if these symptoms are experienced, because they can also be symptoms of a more serious condition such as stroke.

Labyrinthitis is caused either by bacterial or viral infections. Bacterial infection of the labyrinth may also be caused by bacterial meningitis (in-

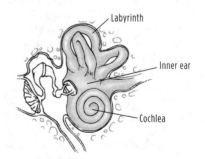

Site of labyrinthitis
The labyrinth is a region of convoluted passages in the inner ear including the cochlea (the principal organ of hearing) and the vestibular system (a group of organs concerned with balance). Labyrinthitis is an inflammation of any of these organs.

flammation of the protective sheath covering the brain). Rupturing of the membranes between the middle ear and the inner ear may also cause bacteria to infect the labyrinth.

Bacterial labyrinthitis is treated with antibiotics. The only treatment for the viral form, which is by far the most common, is bed rest, mild tranquilizers, and medication to relieve dizziness. Remaining as still as possible in dim lighting may help ease dizziness and nausea.

Laceration

Wound in which the skin is opened or cut. Lacerations usually bleed heavily, and deep cuts can bleed severely. Cuts that are less than $1/4$ inch deep and $1/2$ inch long, with smooth edges not over any joint, can usually be treated at home without stitches by cleaning the wound thoroughly, applying antibiotic ointment, closing the wound with butterfly bandages, and applying a sterile dressing.

Lacrimal apparatus

A body system associated with the production and drainage of tears. The tear-forming system, which includes the lacrimal glands, the eyelid margins, the conjunctival sac, and the tear drainage system, keeps the eye moist and free of dust and other irritants.

Lacrimal gland

Any one of four tear-producing glands that lubricate and drain the eye.

Lactase deficiency

A shortage of the enzyme lactase, which breaks down lactose (the predominant sugar in milk and other dairy products) so it can be absorbed

by the body. See also LACTOSE INTOLERANCE.

Lactation

The production and secretion of milk from the breasts after childbirth. The first 2 weeks following birth are crucial for establishing the milk supply, and therefore nursing must be initiated at that time.

Lactic acid

A compound that forms in body cells as an end product of the metabolism of glucose. Lactic acid levels are normally raised during exercise, and lactic acid can accumulate in the muscles and cause cramps following strenuous exercise.

Lactobacillus

Bacteria used as a food supplement to help control diarrhea. *Lactobacillus* (Lactinex) is a harmless bacterium that occurs naturally in unpasteurized whole milk and yogurt. Lactobacilli produce lactic acid from the breakdown of carbohydrates responsible for making milk go sour. The bacteria are used commercially to prepare cheese and yogurt. Doctors have used lactobacilli for years to help control certain kinds of diarrhea, especially that caused when oral antibiotics destroy the bacteria normally found in the intestine.

Lactose intolerance

The inability to digest lactose, the predominant sugar found in milk and other dairy products. Lactose intolerance is due to a shortage of the enzyme lactase, which breaks down lactose so it can be absorbed by the body. The symptoms of lactose intolerance develop 30 minutes to 2 hours after consuming dairy products. They include nausea, bloating, gas, and diarrhea. The severity of symptoms and the amount of lactose that can be consumed before developing symptoms differs among individuals. A diagnosis of lactose intolerance is suggested by the appearance of characteristic symptoms after ingesting lactose and the resolution of symptoms by a lactose-free diet. Tests such as the lactose intolerance test and the hydrogen breath test or measuring stool acidity can be used to confirm a diagnosis. Lactose intolerance is treated by eliminating or reducing the amount of dairy foods in the diet. Many people can continue to enjoy dairy products if they consume them in small amounts or along with other foods. Others can take advantage of products such as lactose-reduced milk or tablets that help digest lactose. Because milk and dairy products are a rich source of calcium, doctors recommend that people who are lactose-intolerant take calcium supplements and consume other foods that are high in calcium but low in lactose.

Laminectomy

The surgical removal of one or more pieces of bone from a vertebra. The purpose of a laminectomy is to relieve the pain caused by pressure on a nerve being compressed by bones in the spine from arthritis, trauma, or a cancerous tumor.

Lance

To pierce or cut an abscess or boil in order to release accumulated pus. Abscesses and boils (called furuncles) should never be lanced by a person at home; this can result in the spread of infection, which is usually caused by bacteria. Doctors lance lesions in sterile surroundings, inserting a drain if the infection is large or deep.

Lancet

A small, pointed, two-edged surgical knife.

Laparoscopic surgery

An operation performed under general anesthesia with the use of a fiberoptic device called a laparoscope (a viewing tube), which projects images onto a television monitor while the surgeon manipulates surgical instruments within the body. When patient safety allows it, laparoscopic surgery is preferred over more invasive open procedures because of the smaller incision, reduced postoperative pain, and quicker recovery.

Examples of how surgeons use the laparoscope include diagnosing infertility in women, removing a gallbladder, repairing hernias, removing a lung nodule, antireflux surgery, and voluntary sterilization in women (tubal ligation).

Laparoscopy

A diagnostic and surgical procedure performed under general anesthesia in which the abdomen is examined and sometimes treated, using a laparoscope, a fiberoptic viewing tube that transmits images to the surgeon on a screen. The laparoscope also enables a surgeon to perform various surgical functions.

Laparotomy, exploratory

An open diagnostic operation within the abdomen. An exploratory laparotomy is performed when noninvasive tests fail to reveal the cause of symptoms, such as inflammation, abdominal distension, pain, vomiting, and fever. Intestinal obstructions, ruptured ulcers, cancer, ovarian cysts, and ectopic pregnancies are commonly diagnosed by laparotomy. When operable tumors, obstructions, or other problems are discovered during a laparotomy, the surgeon removes or otherwise treats them during the procedure.

Larva migrans

An infestation with the larvae of roundworms that move through the tissues of the human body. Roundworm parasites live in the small intestines of both dogs and cats and are transmitted to humans most commonly by dogs, their natural host. The infestation is carried in the feces of cats and dogs. The infection is generally contracted by accidental oral contact with embryonated eggs, or larvae.

The symptoms of visceral larva migrans can include loss of appetite, rash, wheezing, cough, abdominal pain, and neurologic problems. Severe infection with seizures, encephalitis, and heart failure can also occur.

Treatment is based on medications that kill parasitic worms, as well as treatment of associated conditions and symptoms. See also ROUNDWORMS and TOXOCARIASIS.

Laryngeal papilloma

A tumor on the larynx (voice box) that is usually benign and resembles a wart. Laryngeal papillomas are believed to be caused by a virus. They usually develop in groups and may cause difficulty breathing, in addition to hoarseness. Rarely, papillomas will grow large very quickly. In these instances, they may obstruct breathing and should be treated as soon as possi-

ble to prevent total blockage of the air supply. In recent years, laser treatment has yielded more satisfactory results than traditional surgical procedures for removing laryngeal papillomas.

Laryngectomy

Surgical removal of all or part of the larynx (voice box) to treat cancer of the larynx. The procedure may involve complete or partial removal of the larynx and surrounding structures, depending on the location, size, and stage of the tumor, as well as the person's age and health. Radiation therapy may be given in combination with the surgery. Generally, laryngectomy is the only possible treatment for cancer of the larynx if the tumor is large or if previous radiation therapy has failed.

If only part of the larynx (voice box) is removed, the person's ability to speak is preserved, but the voice may be weak and hoarse. Patients recovering from a partial laryngectomy can usually speak within a few weeks after surgery. After a total laryngectomy, normal speech is not possible, but various new ways of communicating can be learned, usually from a speech pathologist.

Laryngitis

An inflammation of the mucous membrane of the larynx (voice box). Symptoms of laryngitis include hoarseness, gradual loss of voice, and throat discomfort. If a virus is the cause, the laryngitis will go away within a few days without treatment. If hoarseness lasts more than a week, a physician should be consulted. Children with a sharp barking cough may have croup.

Symptoms of severe croup require

urgent medical evaluation by a doctor; these include rapid breathing, shortness of breath, turning blue, and visible working of the chest and throat muscles in order to breathe. For laryngitis caused by bacteria, antibiotics may be prescribed, but antibiotics cannot treat disease caused by viruses. If allergies are the cause of laryngitis, antihistamines or corticosteroids may be prescribed.

Laryngomalacia

The most common problem of the larynx (voice box) in infancy. As a result of soft or deformed cartilage or muscular weakness, portions of the upper part of the larynx collapse into the airway, causing a partial obstruction. The baby will make a wheezing or hoarse breathing sound known as stridor and may have some degree of difficulty breathing. The disease appears in the first few weeks of life and typically goes away in the first few months. Only rarely is treatment needed to keep open the child's airway.

Laryngoscopy

An examination of the larynx (voice box) that includes the use of a slender, flexible medical instrument called a laryngoscope, which is threaded through the nose and down the back of the throat to the larynx. The laryngoscope is used to look for ulceration or inflammation of the vocal cords, to collect tissue samples to diagnose or exclude cancer, to locate and remove polyps or other growths, to photograph the vocal cords, or to evaluate the severity of a malignant tumor that has already been diagnosed. Laryngoscopy is performed in a hospital or outpatient surgery clinic by a surgeon.

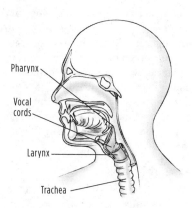

The voice box
The larynx is the organ of the respiratory system that generates sound for speech. The larynx, located at the top of the trachea, is constructed of linking pieces of cartilage.

Larynx

The organ in the throat responsible for voice production; commonly called the voice box. The larynx is a structure of the respiratory system, lying between the pharynx (throat) and the trachea (windpipe).

The larynx is constructed of cartilage lined with mucous membrane. The most prominent piece of cartilage is the thyroid cartilage (Adam's apple), which lies at the upper, outer part of the throat. It is connected to the trachea by cartilage.

Larynx, cancer of

A cancer that develops in and around the larynx (voice box). This cancer can be detected at an early stage if changes in the voice occur. Symptoms usually include hoarseness, pain, and difficulty swallowing. If untreated, as the cancer grows within the larynx, it may eventually cause discomfort in the ears or spitting up blood.

Diagnosis of cancer of the larynx usually includes an examination of the area using a laryngoscope. A biopsy may be performed during the examination. Cancer of the larynx can be treated with radiation therapy, chemotherapy, surgical removal of the tumor, or partial or complete removal of the larynx.

The two principal risk factors for cancer of the larynx are smoking and alcohol abuse.

Laser

A medical instrument that produces a very thin, powerful beam of light. The term "laser" stands for light amplification by stimulated emission of radiation. There are several types of lasers, each of which has a specific use. The color of the laser used is directly related to the surgery being performed and to the tissue being treated. See LASER SURGERY.

Laser in situ keratomileusis

See LASIK.

Laser resurfacing

A technique for removing fine wrinkles, scars, damaged skin, and uneven pigmentation from the face with a laser light source. Laser resurfacing, or laser peel, can be performed on the entire face or a specific portion, such as around the mouth or eyes. See LASER SURGERY.

Mild swelling, soreness, itchiness, and oozing in the treated area are normal reactions during the first 48 to 72 hours after the procedure. They can be controlled with ice packs and oral pain medications prescribed by the surgeon. For the 6 months following laser resurfacing, the new skin must be carefully protected from the sun with a hat, sunblock with a sun protection factor (SPF) of 30 or higher, and good-quality sunglasses.

Possible complications from laser resurfacing include burns caused by the heat from the laser, scarring, new skin that is either lighter or darker than the surrounding areas, and outbreaks of herpes simplex virus infections (see COLD SORE).

Laser surgery

The use of a concentrated, pulsating beam of light to perform surgical procedures such as shrinking, destroying, or removing tumors or lesions; cutting, burning, sculpting, or vaporizing tissue; and sealing blood vessels. Because laser wavelengths can be adjusted to focus selectively, lasers are uniquely suitable to many forms of dermatologic or plastic surgery. At high intensity, the concentrated beam of light released by a laser can destroy cells on which it is focused and cut through tissues without causing bleeding. Laser surgery is also used to relieve the pressure of glaucoma and to treat diseases and disorders of the eyes such as retinal detachment, macular degeneration, and the blurred vision that occurs after cataract surgery. It is used by ophthalmologists to correct common eye problems such as nearsightedness, farsightedness, and astigmatism through refractive surgery. Lasers can be used to break up kidney stones and pulverize gallstones. In gynecology, they are used to vaporize fibroid tumors, destroy precancerous lesions, and remove the excess tissue of endometriosis.

LASIK

Laser in situ keratomileusis; a surgical procedure that uses a laser to reshape the clear outer layer of the eye (cornea) in order to permanently correct vision problems. LASIK is used for people who are highly motivated to stop wearing glasses or contact lenses and who have nearsightedness (difficulty seeing distant objects), farsightedness (difficulty seeing close objects), or astigmatism (tilted and distorted vision caused by an abnormally shaped cornea).

LASIK has generally good results, with most people able to see well enough after surgery to stop wearing contacts or glasses. In people with particularly severe nearsightedness or farsightedness, vision is usually improved, but glasses or contacts may still be needed. The improvement appears within the first few days after the surgery, but often vision continues to improve for up to 6 months.

Possible complications after LASIK include overcorrection or undercorrection of vision requiring repeated surgery (or enhancement), scarring or misshaping of the cornea, infection in the cornea, loss of sharpness in vision, difficulty with night vision because of the appearance of halos or starbursts around bright lights, sensitivity to light, dry eye, and problems with the flap. Most complications resolve soon after surgery, but they can be permanent.

Lateral

The side of the body; the outer side of the body, the outer side of a body part, or a position or structure that lies away from the midline of the body. The lateral or outside part of a knee, for example, is that side farther from the other knee. The opposite of lateral is medial.

Lavage, gastric

See STOMACH PUMPING.

Laxatives

Foods or drugs that stimulate a person's bowels. Laxatives may be taken orally to help produce bowel movements, or they may be used rectally as enemas or suppositories to generate bowel movements in a short time. Laxatives should be used only to provide short-term relief, unless directed otherwise by a doctor. Most laxatives are available without prescription.

There are several types of laxatives, including bulk-forming oral laxatives (for example, psyllium and malt soup extract), which work by absorbing liquid to form a soft, bulky stool that is easier to pass; hyperosmotic laxatives (for example, glycerin and sorbitol), which draw water into the bowel from surrounding tissues to produce a soft stool and increased bowel action; stimulant laxatives (for example, bisacodyl and castor oil), which stimulate muscle contractions that move the stool mass through the intestines; and stool softeners, or emollients (for example, docusate), which encourage bowel movements by drawing water into the stool to prevent dry, hard stool.

Lazy eye

See AMBLYOPIA.

LDL

Low-density lipoprotein. See CHOLESTEROL.

Lead poisoning

Poisoning from overexposure to lead. Exposure to excessive amounts of lead is most common in young children. Symptoms of lead poisoning include poor appetite, vomiting, fatigue, weakness, abdominal pain, irritability, and seizures. Severe exposure can cause permanent brain damage or even death. People are exposed to lead from many sources, particularly through cracked paint chips and dust. Other sources of lead include drinking water, food, and soil that have been contaminated. Airborne lead enters the body through inhaling or swallowing lead dust or particles; lead can leach into drinking water from pipes; and it can be deposited on floors and other surfaces.

Treatment for lead poisoning should always begin with the advice of a poison center professional or a doctor. The first step is to eliminate the sources of exposure to lead. In some cases of lead poisoning, chelation therapy may be used to help remove lead from the body.

Learning disabilities

A group of lifelong disorders that affect the ability to master basic skills such as reading, writing, doing mathematics, following instructions, and paying attention. Learning disabilities are among the leading reasons for failure in school. Learning disabilities appear to be caused by a malfunction in the way a child's brain receives, processes, and communicates information. Most disabilities occur in children of average or above-average intelligence. Typically, achievement in a certain area lags behind what is expected based on the child's full intelligence. In some cases, learning disabilities may also be related to hearing or vision problems, poor motivation, emotional difficulties, or mental retardation.

Types of learning disabilities

Common learning disabilities diagnosed in children include:

DYSLEXIA A reading disability involving spatial impairment. In reading, a person may see words, letters, and numbers reversed. Dyslexia is not caused by a problem with vision but with how the brain processes visual information.

DYSGRAPHIA Children with dysgraphia have trouble forming letters and writing within a designated space.

LANGUAGE PROBLEMS A disability in which children have problems speaking or comprehending words or sentences.

DYSCALCULIA Inability to grasp basic mathematical concepts or perform calculations appropriate to one's age.

PROBLEMS WITH TIME AND PLACE Not understanding the concept of time; confusing yesterday with tomorrow or today. The concept of direction is also confusing.

MEMORY PROBLEMS Difficulty remembering even very recent events.

SENSORY INTEGRATION DYSFUNCTION Having difficulty interpreting sensory input such as the meaning of symbols or the rules of a game.

ATTENTION DEFICIT/HYPERACTIVITY DISORDER Inability to maintain attention and avoid being distracted. Some children also experience hyperactivity, a syndrome in which the child may be continuously overactive, fidgety, often impulsive, and likely to sleep less than their peers do (see ATTENTION DEFICIT/HYPERACTIVITY DISORDER).

Diagnosis and treatment

Federal law requires that all schools test and provide help for children who have learning disabilities at no direct cost to parents. Diagnostic and remedial services are available to all children with learning disabilities from birth to age 21. A child suspected of having learning disabilities should be evaluated comprehensively by an expert. Eye and ear examinations are recommended to rule out physical causes of learning problems.

If a learning disability is diagnosed, recommendations will be made concerning appropriate school placement and support services. A child may require special education services or speech therapy.

LEEP

Loop electrosurgical excision procedure; also known as LLETZ, or large loop excision of transformation zone. A procedure for diagnosing and treating abnormalities of the cervix. Using a colposcope (a small viewing tube), the doctor removes any apparent abnormal tissue from the cervix with a thin wire loop that sends out low-voltage, high-frequency radio waves. The tissue is then examined under a microscope for cancerous cells.

Leg ulcer

A slow-healing, open sore on the leg, often accompanied by swelling. Leg ulcers are typically caused by insufficient arterial blood supply or by inadequate drainage through the veins. This often painful and disabling condition is a common problem for older people. It is frequently associated with varicose veins, circulation problems, trauma, bacterial infection, long-term immobility, and diabetes mellitus, type 2.

Leg ulcers, especially the nonvenous kinds, tend to resist treatment. Treatment for venous ulcers includes elevation of the leg two or three times daily. Elastic support and compression hosiery are also helpful. However, even when ulcers heal, they frequently recur, so surgery may be needed.

Leg, fractured

A break or crack in one of the bones of the leg. This occurs when a bone cannot withstand the physical force exerted on it. The shin (tibia) is one of the most frequently fractured bones.

A fractured leg is diagnosed by physical examination and the evaluation of X rays. The lower bone of the leg (tibia) may be broken straight across, which is called a transverse fracture, or on an angle, which is called an oblique fracture. A crush or comminuted fracture is one in which a section of the leg bone shatters into many pieces.

As is true for fractured bones in other areas of the body, treatment emphasizes properly aligning the broken bone segments, followed by applying a cast or splint to immobilize the bone and allow it to heal. Some fractures require that the surgeon insert pins to hold the parts of a bone together until healing takes place.

The thighbone is difficult to immobilize in a cast because of the large muscles surrounding it. These muscles tend to pull the ends of the broken bone fragments over each other. To prevent this from happening when a bone of the thigh is broken, a system of weights, called traction, may be necessary to maintain the broken bone segments in alignment so they can heal properly. Tibial fractures usually require a long leg cast for 4 to 6 weeks. See also FRACTURE.

Legg-Calvé-Perthes disease

See OSTEOCHONDROSIS.

Legionnaires disease

An infection caused by the bacterium *Legionella pneumophila* that may cause pneumonia. The *Legionella* bacterium, which is common in the environment, is found predominantly in warm, stagnant water, including in some plumbing systems, hot water tanks, cooling towers, condensers of large air-conditioning systems, humidifiers, showers, and whirlpool spas. In nature, it can be found in creeks and ponds and in soil at excavation sites.

Symptoms generally occur 2 to 10 days following exposure to the bacteria, which sometimes cause a mild respiratory illness. People with mild infections usually recover within 2 to 5 days without treatment. In some cases, people infected with the bacteria do not develop any illness at all. Symptoms of legionnaires disease can include muscle aches, diarrhea, fatigue, loss of appetite, headache, and abdominal pain. In the more severe form of legionnaires disease, the person may develop a cough that is either dry or produces sputum, followed by a high fever with a temperature of 102°F to 105°F, shaking, chills, disorientation, and extreme lethargy. These symptoms may progress to a severe pneumonia.

Pneumonia associated with legionnaires disease may be suspected with the presence of shadowy areas on chest X rays and confirmed by a blood test, urine test, or sputum test.

Laboratory tests that reveal improper kidney function may be included among diagnostic tools. Antibiotics are effective in treating the disease.

Leiomyoma

A noncancerous tumor of the smooth muscles that control the movements of the internal organs. Leiomyomas can occur in the bladder, breast, esophagus, and very commonly inside the uterus, as fibroid tumors. Cancerous tumors of the smooth muscle (leiomyosarcomas) are very rare, developing most often in the uterus, the rear area of the abdominal cavity, or the walls of the blood vessels.

Leishmaniasis

A parasitic infection spread by the bite of certain types of phlebotomine sand flies. Leishmaniasis, also called kala-azar, occurs most commonly in rural areas of countries ranging from Central America to western Asia; the infection is rare in the United States, but residents in rural Texas have developed a form of the infection. Also, US troops in the second Gulf War in the 2000s reportedly contracted this infection. The parasite attacks the body's phagocytes, the "hunter-killer" cells in the immune system.

There are two types of leishmaniasis: cutaneous and visceral. Cutaneous leishmaniasis, the more common form, causes one or more skin sores that may change in size and appearance over time and may or may not be painful. Some people experience swollen glands (see GLANDS, SWOLLEN) near the areas of the sores, under the arm, or in the groin. The skin sores usually heal over time without treatment, but healing may take months or years and leave scars.

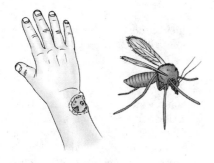

Typical wound　　　**Sand fly**

Skin infection
Cutaneous leishmaniasis causes one or more skin lesions with a raised rim. The sores can be treated with medication. The infection is transmitted by a bite from a sand fly, but the sores may not appear until months after the bite.

Diagnosis may be made by examining cells from the skin sores under a microscope to detect the parasite. Treatment is based on antiprotozoal medications.

Visceral leishmaniasis affects some of the body's internal organs, especially the spleen and liver, which may be enlarged by the infection. The bone marrow may also be affected. The infection can produce swollen glands and is detected by abnormal results on blood tests. A person who becomes ill with visceral leishmaniasis may require hospitalization and intensive supportive care, in addition to antiprotozoal medication. Untreated, the visceral infection can cause death.

Lens

The transparent structure within the pupil of the eye that helps focus incoming light; also called the crystalline lens. Light entering the eye is bent (focused) first by the cornea, which directs the light through the pupil (the opening in the black center of the eye). The light then passes through the crystalline lens, which bends it into final focus.

Lens dislocation

Any condition in which the lens is out of its normal place behind the iris (the colored portion of the eye). Lens dislocation can be present at birth; it may develop as the result of diseases such as syphilis or Marfan syndrome that weaken the fibers holding the lens in place; or it can result from injury to the eye. Treatment depends on the position of the dislocated lens and its effect on vision. If vision is affected, the lens can be removed surgically. A synthetic lens is implanted in the normal lens position and takes over its function.

Lens implant

See CATARACT SURGERY.

Leprosy

A chronic infectious disease caused by the bacterium called *Mycobacterium leprae*, which affects the peripheral nerves, skin, and mucous membranes. Leprosy is also known as Hansen disease and affects about 10 million people worldwide, most commonly in Asia and Africa, but also in Mexico, South and Central America, and the Pacific islands.

The infection is believed to be transmitted by contact with respiratory or nasal droplets from an infected person. A milder tuberculoid form of leprosy is believed to be noncontagious.

Tuberculoid leprosy produces a rash and inflammation of peripheral nerves. Lepromatous leprosy causes symptoms including many severe ulcerations of the skin all over the body, inflammation of the eyes, and loss of body hair such as eyelashes and eyebrows. This type of leprosy may progress to include fever, anemia, glaucoma, loss of interior and exterior tissue of the nose, impotence and sterility, arthritis in the large joints, and severe inflammatory disorders of the nerves, kidneys, and lymph system.

Leprosy is diagnosed by physical examination and by biopsy. For more severe cases, antimicrobial, antibiotic, and corticosteroid medications have been shown to be an effective cure. Surgical procedures may be used to correct functional disabilities associated with leprosy.

Leptin

A hormone produced by fat cells that is involved in appetite control and the regulation of body weight.

Lesbianism

Sexual attraction and relations between women. See HOMOSEXUALITY. As with male homosexuality, lesbianism is not a lifestyle choice but an inborn predisposition. Homosexuality is not considered a disorder.

Lesion

A wound, injury, or other pathologic alteration of an organ or tissue. Skin lesions include sores, rashes, and boils. Lesions can be benign or malignant (cancerous).

Leukemia

A malignant, or cancerous, disease that affects the blood-forming cells found in the bone marrow and the lymphatic system. Leukemia results in an abnormally high number of abnormal white blood cells (blasts). The blasts are cells that would normally develop into white blood cells but with leukemia stop short in their development. High concentrations of blasts in the bone marrow, lymph nodes, and bloodstream can impair the function of these tissues. Some types of leukemia may also affect the liver, spleen, or brain. In addition, overproduction of the blasts can crowd out normal cells in the bone marrow and decrease the number of red blood cells, platelets, and normal white blood cells formed by the bone marrow. This can lead to fatigue, weakness, increased bleeding and bruising from slow blood clotting, and a decreased ability to fight infection. Leukemia worsens over time and may result in death if left untreated.

Leukemia is classified according to two key characteristics. The first is the speed with which symptoms develop. In acute leukemia, symptoms begin very rapidly. People with acute leukemia almost always seek medical attention because they feel ill and quickly become sicker. Almost all childhood leukemias are acute. In chronic leukemia, the number of blasts (immature cells) is lower and increases slowly. As a result, in the early stages, many people with chronic leukemia may not realize they are ill. The second way of classifying leukemia pertains to the type of blast. The abnormality can arise in either of the two main types of white blood cells: lymphoid or myeloid. If the leukemia affects the lymphoid cells, it is known as lymphocytic or lymphoblastic. If it affects the myeloid cells, it is known as myeloid or myelogenous.

There are four principal types of leukemia: acute lymphoblastic leukemia, the most common type of leukemia in children; acute myelogenous leukemia, found in both children and adults; chronic lymphocytic leukemia, primarily a disease of people older than 65; and chronic myeloid leukemia, also primarily an adult disease.

Leukemia's symptoms vary somewhat between the different forms of the disease. Common symptoms include fever and chills; fatigue and weakness; frequent infections and poor wound healing; unusual bruising or bleeding; loss of appetite or weight; swelling or tenderness in the spleen (upper left abdomen), liver (upper right abdomen), or lymph nodes (such as in the neck, armpits, or groin); tiny red spots under the skin (called petechiae and caused by pinpoint hemorrhages); swollen or bleeding gums; sweating, especially at night; and pain in the bones or joints.

Treatment varies with the type of leukemia and the extent of the disease. For details on treatment and outcome, see entries on the four principal types of leukemia: LEUKEMIA, ACUTE LYMPHOBLASTIC; LEUKEMIA, ACUTE MYELOGENOUS; LEUKEMIA, CHRONIC LYMPHOCYTIC; and LEUKEMIA, CHRONIC MYELOID.

Leukemia, acute lymphoblastic

A rapidly developing cancer of the blood-forming tissues, particularly the bone marrow, that causes overproduction of immature white blood cells known as lymphoblasts. Untreated, acute lymphoblastic leukemia leads to death within months, usually from infection or bleeding.

Acute lymphoblastic leukemia develops quickly and progresses rapidly. Malaise (overall weakness), pallid skin, and fatigue are key signs of the disease. Weight loss and bone and joint pain may also occur. In children, the lymphoblasts often accumulate inside the brain and spinal cord and lead to seizures, blurred vision, and other nervous system symptoms.

A complete blood cell count, a blood smear, and a small sample (biopsy) of bone marrow and bone are used to establish the diagnosis. Imaging studies, such as X rays, ultrasound scans, CT (computed tomography) scans, and MRI (magnetic resonance imaging), are useful to determine if the leukemia is affecting the lymph nodes and internal organs.

The goal of treatment in acute lymphocytic leukemia is remission, which means that the blood and bone marrow return to normal. The primary treatment is chemotherapy. Among children, eight of ten cases now result in a cure. Among adults, however, only two or three of ten survive 5 years or longer.

Leukemia, acute myelogenous

A rapidly progressing cancer that causes overproduction of immature white blood cells known as blasts. If the leukemia were not present, the blasts would go on to develop into the white blood cells known as granulocytes. The blasts multiply rapidly and replace the granulocytes, crowding out normal cells and causing the bone marrow to fail and the number of normal blood cells to decrease. Untreated, acute myelogenous leukemia leads to death within 3 to 4 months, sometimes in a matter of weeks, usually from infection or bleeding.

Malaise (overall weakness), pallid

skin, and fatigue are key symptoms of the disease. Swelling and bleeding of the gums is also characteristic of this type of leukemia, as are weight loss and bone and joint pain. Lymph nodes in the groin, armpit, and neck may become enlarged. The blasts often accumulate inside the brain and spinal cord and lead to neurological symptoms such as seizures and blurred vision.

A complete blood cell count, a blood smear, and a biopsy of bone marrow and bone are needed to confirm diagnosis. Imaging studies, such as X rays, ultrasound scans, CT (computed tomography) scans, and MRI (magnetic resonance imaging), may be used to see whether the leukemia is affecting the lymph nodes and internal organs.

The goal of treatment in acute myelogenous leukemia is remission, which means that the blood and bone marrow return to normal. The primary type of treatment is CHEMOTHERAPY, which results in remission of the leukemia in 70 to 80 percent of cases, with survival over the long-term achieved by 20 to 30 percent.

An alternative treatment is a bone marrow transplant (see BONE MARROW TRANSPLANT, ALLOGENEIC; BONE MARROW TRANSPLANT, AUTOLOGOUS), a difficult therapy that allows the administration of large doses of chemotherapy drugs combined with radiation to eliminate the cancer.

Leukemia, chronic lymphocytic

A cancer that involves proliferation of the white blood cells known as lymphocytes. Unlike normal lymphocytes, which are involved in maintaining the body's immunity against invading microorganisms and other foreign invaders, the cancerous cells have little immune function and tend to accumulate in the bone marrow, bloodstream, spleen, and lymph nodes.

Chronic lymphocytic leukemia develops slowly and insidiously. Most cases are discovered through routine blood testing before any symptoms appear. As the disease progresses, symptoms such as fatigue may develop. Later symptoms include unusual bruising, pallid skin, jaundice (yellowish color of the skin and whites of the eyes), infection, bone tenderness and pain, weight loss, and swollen lymph nodes. The spleen and sometimes the liver also enlarge. In advanced disease, cancerous lymphocytes may invade the testicles or ovaries, digestive system, skin, and kidneys.

Diagnosis of chronic lymphocytic leukemia is confirmed through tests, including a complete blood cell count, a blood smear, and a biopsy of bone marrow and bone. Imaging studies, such as X rays, ultrasound scans, CT (computed tomography) scans, and MRI (magnetic resonance imaging), may be used to see whether the leukemia is affecting the lymph nodes and internal organs.

Treatment of chronic lymphocytic leukemia depends on the course of the disease, which varies markedly from person to person. The basic treatment for chronic lymphocytic leukemia is CHEMOTHERAPY, which may be combined with radiation and the removal of the spleen. Corticosteroid drugs such as prednisone are often combined with the chemotherapy to suppress the formation of abnormal lymphocytes. Chronic leukemia is only rarely cured. Rather, treatment aims to control symptoms.

Leukemia, chronic myeloid

A cancer characterized by an abnormal increase in white blood cells arising from rapid, malignant growth of blood-forming cells in the bone marrow. Once it is detected, chronic myeloid leukemia tends to remain in a long-lasting (chronic) phase that may last up to several years, followed by a sudden acute attack known as a blast crisis, when the number of immature white blood cells (blasts) increases rapidly. The blast crisis is very difficult to treat and can result in death.

The earliest signs of chronic myeloid leukemia are fatigue, shortness of breath following mild exercise, and fullness in the upper abdomen caused by an enlarged spleen. Because the enlarged spleen crowds the stomach, people with the disease may feel full after eating small amounts. Abnormal bleeding and bruising, swollen lymph nodes, tenderness in the sternum (breastbone), pallid skin, low fever, and enlargement of the liver are other possible symptoms.

In one of three cases, chronic myeloid leukemia is discovered before symptoms appear, usually through blood tests performed during routine physical examinations. Diagnosis is confirmed through a series of additional blood tests, and a biopsy of bone marrow and bone. Imaging studies, such as X rays, ultrasound scans, CT (computed tomography) scans, and MRI (magnetic resonance imaging), may be used to see whether the leukemia is affecting the spleen, lymph nodes, and liver.

Treatment of chronic myeloid leukemia aims to suppress the bone marrow with CHEMOTHERAPY. The spleen may be removed to relieve symptoms, but this surgery does not extend survival.

Bone marrow transplant (see BONE MARROW TRANSPLANT, ALLOGENEIC) from a donor is used for some people with the disease, particularly those who have not yet entered the blast crisis and are younger than 40. This treatment cures the disease in about half the people who receive it.

Leukemia, hairy cell

A rare cancer of the blood-forming tissues, particularly the bone marrow. The number of all types of blood cells falls, while abnormal cells (known as hairy cells because of their unusual appearance under the microscope) proliferate in the blood and bone marrow. Symptoms include fatigue, weakness, easy bleeding and bruising, recurrent infections, excessive sweating, swollen lymph nodes, and an enlarged spleen. The disease progresses slowly and is treated with CHEMOTHERAPY plus antibiotics to stop infections and transfusions of platelets to stop bleeding episodes. In many cases, the spleen is removed to resolve symptoms. Although the disease is not curable, most people with hairy cell leukemia live 10 years or longer after diagnosis.

Leukocyte

A blood cell that helps fight infection; also called a white blood cell. Any blood cell that contains a nucleus is a leukocyte. Leukocytes are capable of moving independently, as when they travel through blood vessel walls to a wound site to protect the body against foreign substances. Leukocytes are able to engulf foreign particles, such as bacteria, and this process causes an increase in the number of leukocytes in the blood during infection. Laboratory testing to determine whether infectious disease is present is based on the number of leukocytes in the blood.

In the healthy body, there are five types of leukocytes: neutrophils, lymphocytes, basophils, eosinophils, and monocytes. Monocytes defend against infection by engulfing foreign substances of all sorts, while lymphocytes react to specific infectious agents. The neutrophils, basophils, and eosinophils are also involved in the immune response. Lymphocytes are either B cells, which produce antibodies, or T cells, which attack virus-infected or foreign cells.

Leukoencephalopathy, progressive multifocal

Also known as PML, an aggressive infection of brain cells caused by the JC virus (JCV). In PML, JCV infects and destroys the cells that produce myelin, the substance that forms the sheath that normally surrounds and protects nerve cells. This disease develops most frequently in people who have compromised immune systems as a result of HIV (human immunodeficiency virus) infection or long-term chemotherapy for cancer. The occurrence of PML in the presence of HIV constitutes a diagnosis of AIDS (acquired immunodeficiency syndrome).

The symptoms of PML include extreme weakness; hemianopia, or blindness in half of the normal visual field; mental impairment; lack of coordination; paralysis on one side of the body; and language difficulties. Diagnosis is usually made by a neurologist with the aid of tests such as MRI (magnetic resonance imaging) and CT (computed tomography) scanning.

There is no known cure for PML, and the period between the onset of symptoms and death can be a matter of months. However, in some cases anti-HIV drugs, such as zidovudine (also known as AZT), have proven helpful.

Leukopenia

An abnormally low number of white blood cells circulating in the blood; commonly known as a low white blood cell count. Leukopenia is diagnosed by taking a sample of blood and counting the number of white blood cells per microliter (a millionth [1/1,000,000] of a liter). The normal white blood cell count is 4,000 to 10,000 per microliter of blood. Leukopenia usually occurs when white blood cells are used up at a rapid rate and production of new cells falls behind. This happens most commonly in response to chemotherapy; cancers affecting the bone marrow; enlargement of the spleen; infection; autoimmune diseases; and nutritional deficiencies.

Treatment is aimed at the underlying disease, for example, using antibiotics to combat a bacterial infection. If the leukopenia is severe, the growth factors G-CSF (granulocyte colony–stimulating factor) and GM-CSF (granulocyte-macrophage colony–stimulating factor), which stimulate white blood cell production, are given as medications.

Leukoplakia

Raised white patches on the inside of the cheek, tongue, or lips. In the mouth, leukoplakia may be due to irritation from poorly fitted dentures, chronic cheek biting, or tobacco. In its early stages, leukoplakia usually causes no symptoms and is diagnosed during the course of a routine physical or dental examination. Because it is a potentially cancerous condition, leukoplakia must be closely monitored by a physician; a biopsy may be necessary. Treatment consists of eliminating all tobacco products and other irritants.

Leukorrhea

A vaginal discharge consisting of mucus and pus cells. The discharge may be white or yellowish. Leukorrhea sometimes occurs at or just before each menstrual period.

Levothyroxine

A thyroid hormone. Levothyroxine, a naturally occurring hormone produced by the thyroid gland, is associated with metabolism and energy. Levothyroxine medication is used to replace a thyroid hormone deficiency and to treat goiter, or enlarged thyroid gland.

LH

Luteinizing hormone; also known as luteotropin in females and interstitial cell–stimulating hormone in males. LH is produced by the pituitary gland. Together with estrogen, LH in women stimulates the follicles in the ovaries to release a developed egg. LH also prepares the uterus to support a fertilized egg. Also in women, LH promotes the formation of the tissue in the ovary that secretes another female sex hormone, progesterone, and prepares the mammary glands for milk secretion.

In men, LH stimulates the interstitial cells in the testicles to produce and release large amounts of testosterone, the major male sex hormone.

Testosterone influences a man's body shape, voice, body hair, sex drive, and ability to achieve an erection.

LH-RH

Luteinizing hormone–releasing hormone. LH-RH is released in response to estrogen, progesterone, and testosterone; regulates the hormone levels; and triggers sexual and reproductive functions. LH-RH stimulates the release of LH (luteinizing hormone), the pituitary hormone that triggers a woman's ovaries to produce estrogen, which stimulates female sex characteristics and the growth of the uterine lining in preparation for pregnancy. Progesterone maintains pregnancy, in part by inhibiting FSH (follicle-stimulating hormone) and LH release. Testosterone in males stimulates male sex characteristics and promotes sperm production in the testicles.

Lice, head

Small parasites that feed on blood from the scalp. Head lice are tiny gray insects (about the size of sesame seeds) that cause an intensely itchy scalp, are extremely contagious, and affect primarily schoolchildren.

Head lice are treated by applying over-the-counter or prescription shampoos or lotions to the scalp and hair. It is also important to remove nits, the whitish eggs of lice. Nits can be seen firmly attached to hair shafts and must be removed with a fine-tooth comb or with the fingernails. To prevent lice from reattaching to the hair of the scalp, clothes and bedding must be washed in very hot water. Items that cannot be easily washed (such as stuffed animals) should be sealed in plastic bags for 3 weeks.

Upholstered furniture and carpets should be vacuumed.

Licensure, medical

The granting of a license allowing a person to practice medicine. Licensure is granted by a state agency, frequently a state board of medicine in the state where a person wishes to practice medicine. To obtain a medical license, a person must have a diploma from an accredited medical college, pass an examination that reflects knowledge of his or her branch of medicine, and be of good moral character.

Lichen planus

A benign (not cancerous) skin condition consisting of shiny flat papules (small superficial bumps on the skin) that vary from pink to red to violet. The itchy bumps of lichen planus usually develop on the arms and legs but may occur anywhere on the body. Diagnosis is made through physical examination, medical history, and sometimes a skin biopsy. Treatment of the rash is with topical and, in severe cases, oral corticosteroids. Retinoids (forms of vitamin A) and phototherapy (treatment with light) have also been used.

Lichen sclerosus

A skin disorder of the vulva, or external female genitalia. The skin surface of the vulva becomes thin, wrinkled, and papery and red or purple in appearance. The affected area can include the skin at the top of the thighs, the inner buttocks, under the arms, beneath the breasts, on the neck, on the back, and on the arms. The chief symptom is intense itching. Lichen sclerosus may develop into cancer, and a biopsy of affected skin is recommended for precise diagnosis. Treatment focuses on management of the itching, usually with creams containing corticosteroids. Ointments containing testosterone are also used.

Lichen simplex

A localized area of skin thickening caused by rubbing and scratching; a form of DERMATITIS. The skin patches are thick, dry, and leathery and may be darker or redder than the surrounding skin. The areas most commonly affected are easily reached, such as the nape of the neck and the outer part of the lower legs.

Diagnosis of lichen simplex is based on the appearance of the skin and a medical history. Doctors may perform a skin biopsy to confirm the diagnosis. Sometimes lichen simplex is the result of chronic irritation. It may start with an insect bite or rough clothing that irritates the skin, which leads to an urge to rub or scratch the area. Antihistamines to reduce itching and sedatives to reduce stress are sometimes prescribed. Depending on the severity, other treatments may include soothing lotions and topical corticosteroids. In severe cases, corticosteroids are injected into lesions.

Life support

A system involving equipment and procedures that provides all or some of the bodily functions necessary to maintain life. Life support may involve providing oxygen, nutrients, and water and eliminating carbon dioxide and other body wastes. The most commonly used form of life support is a ventilator, which is designed to breathe for a person with respiratory failure.

Ligament

A strap of tissue that connects bones at joints. Ligaments may allow some movement, as in the joints between the vertebrae, or may fix the joint so firmly that the bone will break before the ligament will detach. See JOINT.

Ligament injuries, knee

Stretching or tearing injuries, sometimes referred to as sprains, involving one of the knees' ligaments. The knee includes two cruciate ligaments, the anterior and the posterior, which attach internally within the joint in a crisscross pattern. The medial collateral and lateral ligaments also help stabilize the joints.

An injury to the cruciate ligament often produces a "popping" sound with swelling, but may not be painful. The leg may buckle or "give out" when weight is put on it. Diagnosis is made by physical examination and several maneuvers of the leg by the doctor to test the knee's capacity to maintain its proper position when pressure is applied. MRI (magnetic resonance imaging) can detect a complete tear in the ligament; a partial tear can be detected by arthroscopy. See ARTHROSCOPIC SURGERY.

Exercises to strengthen surrounding muscles and a protective knee brace may be prescribed for a partial tear of a cruciate ligament. Surgery is sometimes recommended when the ligament is completely torn, especially in the case of an active athlete or exerciser. Reconstruction is generally accomplished using a combination of open surgery and arthroscopic surgery.

With injuries to the medial collateral ligament, there is often pain and swelling. Diagnosis involves a physical examination in which pressure is applied to the side of the knee to gauge the looseness of the joint and the amount of pain. Ice may be recommended to ease pain and swelling. Exercise may be prescribed, and a sleeve-type brace or non-weight-bearing crutches are used during this time. If both ligaments are torn, surgical repair is usually necessary.

Ligation

Tying up or binding of a blood vessel or duct to prevent bleeding of another structure. Ligature is the threadlike material used in ligation to tie off the blood vessel or duct.

Light therapy

The use of natural or artificial light to treat various ailments such as depression or sleep disorders by affecting chemicals in the brain and hypothalamus. Light therapy is used to treat people with seasonal affective disorder (SAD) and workers who have shift-related sleep disorders.

Light treatment

See PHOTOTHERAPY.

Lightning injuries

Injuries caused by lightning from thunderstorms. Lightning strikes about 1,800 people per year in the United States. It is the cause of more deaths—anywhere from 100 to 450 each year—than any other weather hazard. Injuries can include severe burns, nervous system damage, broken bones, the cessation of heartbeat, and loss of hearing or eyesight. People holding onto metal objects, such as golf clubs or baseball bats, are at highest risk. Lightning injuries can be prevented by simple, common sense measures. If no shelter is available, a person should remove metal objects, crouch down in a ball position, and stay at least 15 feet away from other people. A person should not seek a tall tree to stand under during a lightning storm.

Limp

A characteristic, unsteady gait that favors one leg over the other because of pain or problems with the muscles or bones of the hips, legs, or feet. Limping may be related to pain or problems in the lower back, a simple injury or bruise, a strain or fracture, ill-fitting shoes, a plantar wart on the sole of the foot, a splinter in the foot, or an inflamed joint. See also JUVENILE RHEUMATOID ARTHRITIS.

Lip cancer

Cancer that usually occurs on the lower lip. Lip cancer is associated with long-term sun exposure and using tobacco and alcohol. A biopsy is required to make the diagnosis.

Squamous cell carcinoma of the lip begins as actinic cheilitis (a sun-induced inflammation) or leukoplakia (raised white patches). The most common symptom is an enlarging growth that at first is not painful. Over time, it becomes an infected open sore. There may also be numbness of the lower lip. Lip cancer may grow rapidly and invade other tissues. Treatment is with surgical excision (cutting).

Lipid-lowering agents

See CHOLESTEROL-LOWERING DRUGS.

Lipids

A broad category of substances in the body that includes fats and fatlike compounds such as sterols (including CHOLESTEROL). Although not all lipids are fats, the two terms are often used interchangeably.

Lipoma

A benign tumor that develops from fatty tissue. Most lipomas occur on the thigh, trunk, or shoulder, although they can develop in any fatty tissues. They commonly appear as slow-growing soft swellings and usually require no treatment. See also LIPOSARCOMA.

Lipoprotein

A substance that is made of varying amounts of cholesterol, triglycerides, lipids, and protein. Since fats are not soluble in water, lipoproteins carry fats through the blood.

Liposarcoma

A cancerous tumor that develops from fatty tissue. Liposarcomas are usually found in the thigh or the back of the abdominal cavity and tend to be large and to recur. Some liposarcoma cells may travel to the lungs or to the interior surface of the abdomen. Treatment of liposarcoma varies. Some tumors can be easily removed surgically, while others require more extensive surgery and aggressive chemotherapy, with or without radiation therapy. See also LIPOMA.

Liposuction

A surgery that uses a suction device to permanently remove unwanted deposits of fat tissue and reshape specific body parts. Liposuction can be performed on the abdomen and waist, hips, buttocks, back, chest, neck, chin, and cheeks. The procedure works best on healthy individuals with normal body weight, firm skin, and pockets of excess fat.

The improved body contour is usually apparent in 2 to 6 weeks, after most of the swelling has subsided.

Lisp

The defective pronunciation of the sibilant letters s and z. See SPEECH DISORDERS.

Listeriosis

A serious bacterial infection that is common in livestock and infects humans when food contaminated with the bacterium *Listeria monocytogenes* is ingested. The bacterium that causes listeriosis is found in the intestines of several different animals, including nonhuman mammals, birds, arachnids, and crustaceans, as well as in soil and water.

An infected person has fever, muscle aches, and sometimes nausea and diarrhea. The infection can spread to the nervous system, possibly producing headache, stiff neck, confusion, loss of balance, and seizures. When infections occur in women who are pregnant, symptoms may be mild and flulike; however, the consequences of an infection during pregnancy can be serious, leading to premature delivery, infection of the newborn, or even spontaneous abortion and stillbirth.

Severe forms of the infection are rare but may produce bacteremia with high fever, meningitis, inflammation of the eyes, lymph node enlargement, and skin inflammation caused by direct contact with infected animal tissues. Diagnosis depends on a physical examination, clinical history of symptoms, and blood tests.

The infection is treated with antibi-

otics. When antibiotics are given promptly to a woman who is pregnant, infection of the fetus or newborn can be prevented.

Lithotomy position

The position in which women lie on their backs with their legs or feet raised in stirrups, commonly used for gynecological examinations. The lithotomy position is also used for childbirth.

Lithotripsy

A procedure in which kidney stones are broken up into smaller pieces so they can be removed or flushed out in the urine. There are several ways of performing lithotripsy.

Extracorporeal shock wave lithotripsy (ESWL), the most common approach to treating kidney stones, uses shock waves, generated outside the body, to break up the stones. The shock waves travel through the skin and other tissues to break the kidney stones into tiny sand-like particles that are then excreted in urine.

Percutaneous nephrolithotripsy, which is used when the stone is large, is performed by passing a narrow tubelike instrument through a small incision in the back to remove the stone. If the stone is very large, a small ultrasonic or electrohydraulic energy probe may be used to fragment the stone; the small pieces are then removed.

Laser lithotripsy uses a laser to break up stones that have traveled to a ureter. The small fragments can then be flushed out in the urine. Ureteroscopy uses a tiny fiberoptic telescope passed up a ureter from the bladder to view the kidney stone, fragment the stone, or remove it.

Liver

An organ that performs complex functions relating to the processing, filtering, and regulating of chemicals in the blood. The liver—the largest internal organ in the body—lies in the upper right side of the abdomen, just under the diaphragm, over the intestine on the right side and the stomach on the left.

Important functions of the liver include eliminating toxins, promoting absorption of fats, manufacturing proteins, and storing and releasing of energy. It also filters and processes waste products. The liver manufactures numerous chemical proteins that contribute to the body's defenses against infection. Clotting factors, also called coagulation factors, are produced in the liver to help prevent blood loss in case of injury.

The liver regulates the level of amino acids in the blood, of cholesterol (a fatlike substance), and of blood sugar (glucose). Further, the liver metabolizes toxic substances, including alcohol and other drugs, from the blood. After chemically detoxifying them, the liver cells secrete them into bile, which is then sent to the digestive system to be removed from the body. SEE BILIARY SYSTEM; BLOOD.

Liver abscess

A pus-filled sac in the liver that may be caused by an amebic infection, a bacterial infection, or trauma. Symptoms include night sweats, fever, chills, nausea, vomiting, loss of appetite, weight loss, and abdominal pain. Diagnosis is made through blood tests, X rays, and ultrasound scanning. Depending on the underlying cause of an abscess, anti-amebic drugs such as metronidazole or antibiotics are prescribed. Treatment for a liver abscess may include draining it by needle aspiration (removal of fluid by suction), catheter drainage, or open surgical drainage.

Liver biopsy

A diagnostic procedure in which a needle is used to remove a small piece of the liver for testing. The tissue is examined under a microscope for abnormalities or to assess the damage to the liver. This procedure may be performed to diagnose cirrhosis, hepatitis, liver cancer, or other diseases.

Liver cancer

Liver cancer is categorized as either primary or secondary. Primary liver cancer, which originates in the liver, is relatively rare in the United States. It is usually associated with a history of hepatitis B, hepatitis C, or some other chronic liver disease. Secondary liver cancer, the more common type, is metastatic, meaning that it has spread to the liver from other parts of the body (most commonly from cancer of the breast, lung, or intestinal tract). The symptoms of liver

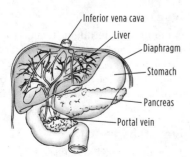

Inferior vena cava
Liver
Diaphragm
Stomach
Pancreas
Portal vein

Anatomy of the liver

The liver is a large, spongy organ of the digestive system lying over the stomach on the upper right side.

cancer include appetite loss, weight loss, fatigue, weakness, and abdominal discomfort.

Diagnosis of liver cancer is made by physical examination and tests, such as a complete blood cell (CBC) count, liver function tests, imaging studies, and a liver biopsy. Because cancer is usually advanced once it has spread to the liver, the outlook is often poor, and liver failure often results. However, if the cancer is localized in a small area, a surgeon may perform a partial removal of the liver.

Liver disease, alcoholic

Progressive liver damage due to excessive alcohol consumption. Alcoholic liver disease progresses through three stages of rising severity: a fatty liver (in which fat accumulates inside liver cells), alcoholic hepatitis (inflammation of the liver due to excessive alcohol use), and finally cirrhosis (a severe liver disease in which healthy cells are destroyed and replaced by scar tissue). Eventually, liver cancer and liver failure may result. Nonalcoholic steatohepatitis (NASH) has symptoms similar to those of alcoholic liver disease, but is not due to alcohol.

People who have a fatty liver often experience no symptoms. However, the liver may be tender and enlarged, and results of liver function tests are often abnormal. If alcohol use ceases, the problem is reversible.

If, despite increasing signs of damage, a person continues to consume alcohol, alcoholic hepatitis can develop. As with a fatty liver, there may be no early symptoms other than elevated liver function test results. Later symptoms may include losses of appetite and weight, weakness, fatigue,

nausea, vomiting, and pain around the liver. Severe alcoholic hepatitis is a life-threatening condition characterized by fever, bleeding in the gastrointestinal tract, ascites (accumulation of fluid in the abdomen), and eventually liver failure. See also CIRRHOSIS.

Liver failure

A condition in which a damaged liver can no longer meet the many demands placed upon it. When a major portion of the liver is destroyed and the liver fails to function properly, the final treatment option is a liver transplant. See CIRRHOSIS; LIVER.

Liver function tests

Blood tests that assess the general health of the liver or biliary system. Abnormal results denote the possibility of liver damage or inflammation. Liver function tests, in combination with a physical examination and a medical history, are used to diagnose and plan treatment for a variety of liver diseases, including hepatitis (inflammation of the liver), cirrhosis (a severe liver disease), and alcoholic liver disease.

Liver scan

A noninvasive technique that uses radioactive compounds to record and display an image of the liver. Liver scans are useful in the diagnosis of problems such as abscesses and tumors.

Liver transplant

Surgery in which a damaged liver is replaced with a healthy liver from a donor. The procedure is performed in cases of liver failure, a condition in which the liver can no longer perform important functions, such as eliminating toxins, promoting absorption of fats, manufacturing proteins, and storing and releasing energy.

The transplant operation takes place in a hospital under general anesthesia. After a liver transplant, powerful immunosuppressive drugs are administered to prevent rejection of the new organ by the patient's immune system. Although early immunosuppressive medications had many dangerous side effects, newer ones such as tacrolimus and cyclosporine, are much safer.

Liver, cirrhosis of the

See CIRRHOSIS.

Living will

A document that a person completes while still mentally competent, which directs his or her physician to withhold or withdraw life-sustaining treatment that would prolong life without the chance for meaningful recovery. A living will, a type of advance directive, normally becomes effective when a person is no longer capable of expressing his or her wishes and has become incapacitated or irreversibly unconscious or is in a persistent vegetative state (see ADVANCE DIRECTIVES).

Lobectomy, liver

Surgical removal of one lobe or part of the liver. The liver is the one internal organ that can regenerate; it grows back to its normal size within 6 to 8 weeks after surgery.

A liver lobectomy is performed to remove a tumor, to remove a portion of a liver that has been so severely damaged that it cannot be saved, or to remove a portion of the liver from a donor who has agreed to donate his or her organ to another person. See LIVER TRANSPLANT.

Lobectomy, lung

Surgical removal of one lobe of a lung. The right lung is divided into three distinct sections, or lobes; the smaller left lung has two lobes. A lung lobectomy involves the removal of one of these lobes, leaving the person with more lung tissue intact after surgery than would be the case with complete removal of the lung.

A lung lobectomy is performed to treat a malignant tumor or to treat a lung abscess, which is a severe, localized infection of the lung that can develop from inhaling contaminated material.

Lobotomy, prefrontal

A procedure, now considered obsolete, to cut the nerves connecting the frontal lobe to the rest of the brain. The procedure gained popularity in the mid-1930s and was hailed as a major step forward in treating patients with severe mental disease, such as schizophrenia. The surgery had severe side effects, leaving patients with harmful personality changes. The development of effective medication for mental illness has made prefrontal lobotomy a treatment of last resort.

Local anesthesia

See ANESTHESIA, LOCAL.

Lochia

The vaginal discharge that normally occurs after delivery of a baby. The lochia consists of mucus, blood, and tissue from the lining of the uterus.

Usually, the lochia is bright red and as heavy or heavier at first than a menstrual period. The discharge tapers off and stops within 3 to 6 weeks after delivery. A sudden increase in the flow of lochia or the return of the bright red color can be signs that a woman is overexerting herself. A foul-smelling discharge or chills and fever may be signs of infection. A woman should contact her doctor immediately about any of these symptoms.

Lockjaw

See TETANUS.

Long QT syndrome

A rare, inherited, sometimes fatal disorder of the heart's electrical system. Under great emotional or physical stress, this abnormality may weaken the ability of the heart to maintain a normal rhythm and pump effectively. The result can be reduced blood flow to the brain, which may cause sudden fainting. People with this disorder may also develop a very fast heartbeat, which can accelerate to 350 beats per minute (ventricular fibrillation). This quickly tires the heart and, if untreated, causes it to stop pumping and death results.

Individuals with long QT syndrome must take care not to overexert or to engage in hard, strenuous exercise. Beta blockers, a family of medications that slow heartbeat and decrease the number of nerve impulses affecting the heart, help protect against ventricular fibrillation under stress. If medication alone is insufficient, a pacemaker or an implantable cardioverter defibrillator—devices that monitor the heartbeat and correct it if it becomes abnormal—can be put in place surgically. Emergency equipment should be kept on hand to prevent oxygen deprivation in the event of fainting or ventricular fibrillation.

Long-term care facility

A number of types of facilities designed for people who require custodial care for a longer period than is possible in a hospital. Long-term care is generally provided to people who have a chronic, progressive illness or disability. Many long-term care residents are older adults. There are several types of care facilities, including:

- *NURSING HOME* A facility that offers care for older people or those with chronic diseases for a longer period than is possible in a hospital.

- *SKILLED CARE (OR NURSING) FACILITY* An institution that provides physician coverage; 24-hour nursing services; and complete assistance with daily living, including feeding and hygiene. Long-term skilled care may also be administered in rehabilitation hospitals.

- *INTERMEDIATE CARE FACILITY* A residential facility for people who may need some health services; minimal nursing care; and limited help with eating, dressing, or getting around.

- *ASSISTED LIVING* Nonmedical housing with private apartment-style living and 24-hour services provided to individuals who cannot maintain their own households without assistance but do not require constant medical attention.

- *BOARD-AND-CARE HOMES* Group homes that provide rooms, meals, and limited assistance with daily activities such as bathing, grooming, dressing, and bathroom use. Board-and-care homes are an alternative for older people who do not require constant medical attention.

- *CONTINUING CARE RETIREMENT COMMUNITIES* These organizations, often called CCRCs, provide a range of services and housing options on one campus. These include independent living, assisted living, and skilled nursing care. Older people may move from one component of a CCRC to another.
- *HOSPICE* A facility or service that provides care for terminally ill people.

Loose bodies

A joint injury in which pieces of bone or cartilage break off into unattached fragments. Loose bodies usually cause pain, restricted range of motion, and increased damage to the joint. The fragments must be removed, usually by arthroscopic surgery, to restore the joint's normal function and movement.

Lou Gehrig disease

Amyotrophic lateral sclerosis, or ALS, the most common form of MOTOR NEURON DISEASE. Lou Gehrig disease is characterized by progressive loss of muscle function.

Lumbar

Having to do with the lower back. The lumbar region of the human body is situated between the thorax, or chest, and the pelvis. This area includes the lower back and the loins, or the back and side of the body between the lowest rib and the pelvis.

The five lumbar vertebrae in the spinal column are those located be-

tween the thoracic or chest vertebrae and the sacral vertebrae (endpoint of the vertebral column) and are sometimes referred to as L1 through L5.

Lumbar puncture

Also known as a spinal tap, a procedure that involves inserting a needle into the spinal canal to remove a sample of cerebrospinal fluid (CSF). A lumbar puncture is most commonly performed to diagnose problems such as a subarachnoid hemorrhage (see HEMORRHAGE, SUBARACHNOID), encephalitis, meningitis, multiple sclerosis, Guillain-Barré syndrome, Reye syndrome, polio, and tumors or inflammation of the brain or spinal cord. Less commonly, it is done to administer drugs, such as antibiotics or anesthetics, or to remove spinal fluid in order to decrease spinal fluid pressure.

Lumbosacral spasm

A tightening of the muscles that surround the lower part of the spine. Lumbosacral spasm can be prolonged or intermittent and is a common cause of back pain. It may result in temporary scoliosis, an S-shaped curvature of the spine. Treatment for back pain due to lumbosacral spasm depends on the cause, duration, and severity of discomfort.

Lumpectomy

The removal of a lump in a woman's breast and some of the tissue around it to evaluate for or treat breast cancer. In cases of breast cancer, a lumpectomy is usually followed by radiation therapy to the remaining part of the breast to reduce the chance of the cancer coming back. Most doctors also remove some of the lymph nodes under the arm. Many doctors now perform a lumpectomy for small tumors instead of a mastectomy in women with breast cancer; a lumpectomy is less deforming than and as effective as a mastectomy in treating early breast cancer.

Lung

The major organ of the respiratory system, in which oxygen from the air enters the bloodstream and is exchanged for the waste product carbon dioxide. The two lungs lie in the chest cavity, protected by the ribs. The upper end of each lung lies just above the collarbone, and the bottom ends rest on the diaphragm (the sheet of muscle that separates the chest cavity from the abdomen).

Air enters and leaves the lungs through the trachea (windpipe). The trachea branches into two large bronchial tubes that lead directly into the lungs. Within each lung, the bronchial tube divides into three air-

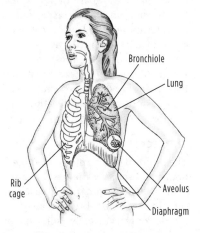

Anatomy of the lung
The lungs lie in the chest, protected by the rib cage. The fundamental process of respiration occurs in the bronchioles, the smallest airways in lung tissue.

ways called main stem branches; each branch leads into one of three lobes (upper, lower, and middle) of the lung.

In medical terms, the mechanical process of breathing—inhaling oxygen and exhaling carbon dioxide—is called ventilation. Respiration refers to the total process of bringing oxygen into the body, transporting it to the bloodstream in the lung tissue and exchanging it for the waste products of metabolism, absorbing oxygen into blood cells, and expelling the waste product carbon dioxide. The lungs are the principal organs involved in these processes. See also RESPIRATORY SYSTEM.

Lung cancer

Cancer that originates in the lung. Lung cancer accounts for only about 15 percent of all new cancers in the United States, but is responsible for 25 percent of all cancer deaths, because it is frequently incurable. Early detection is difficult because symptoms often do not appear until the disease is advanced. Warning signs may include a persistent cough, coughing up blood, shortness of breath, hoarseness, persistent pain in the chest or upper back, and a persistent chest infection, such as pneumonia or bronchitis.

Tests used in the diagnosis of lung cancer include the following types of imaging tests: chest X ray; CT (computed tomography) scanning and MRI (magnetic resonance imaging); BRONCHOSCOPY; and mediastinoscopy. A needle biopsy of a lung lesion, in which a very thin needle is inserted through the chest wall, may also be used.

Most lung cancers are caused by smoking. Even people who do not smoke are at risk of developing lung cancer if they are exposed to second-hand or environmental tobacco smoke (the smoke left in the air by smokers). Exposure to radon and asbestos may also cause lung cancer.

The two main types of lung cancer have different characteristics, requiring different treatment approaches:

- Small cell lung cancer cells multiply quickly to form large tumors, which spread to the lymph nodes and other organs, such as the bone marrow, brain, liver, and adrenal glands. Small cell lung cancer is usually caused by smoking. This type of cancer usually responds to chemotherapy and radiation therapy, although the response may last for only a limited amount of time. When small cell lung cancer is limited to the chest, it can be cured with radiation therapy and chemotherapy.

- The three types of non-small cell lung cancer are named for the types of cells in which they develop: squamous cell carcinoma; adenocarcinoma; and large cell carcinoma. Surgery, chemotherapy, and radiation therapy are all used to treat all types of non-small cell lung cancers. Early-stage non-small cell lung cancers can be cured with surgery alone.

Overall, 13 percent of people with lung cancer survive more than 5 years after diagnosis. See also LOBECTOMY, LUNG.

Lung disease, chronic obstructive

See CHRONIC OBSTRUCTIVE PULMONARY DISEASE.

Lung imaging

Diagnostic techniques for viewing the lung tissue. Several procedures allow a doctor to examine the lungs, including chest X rays, CT scanning (computed tomography scanning), MRI (magnetic resonance imaging), ultrasound scanning, nuclear scanning using radioactive contrast materials, and angiography.

Lung surfactant

See SURFACTANT.

Lung transplantation

A complicated, high-risk surgical procedure in which a healthy lung or lungs replace damaged or diseased lungs. Lung transplantation is performed only as a lifesaving measure on people who have not responded to other treatment options, will not survive without the transplant, and have a high probability of a positive outcome from the transplant. Most people who successfully receive a transplanted lung or lungs can recover to live relatively normal lives, but long-term outcomes are not yet known. Single lung transplantation is more common than bilateral lung transplantation. Finding appropriate donor lungs is difficult because the organs must match exactly the recipient's body size, blood type, and tissue.

Lung tumors

See LUNG CANCER.

Lung, collapsed

A physical event that occurs when air or gas collects in the chest cavity, exerting pressure on the lung and causing it to collapse. Collapsed lung is also referred to as PNEUMOTHORAX.

Lupus erythematosus, discoid

A form of lupus that most commonly causes red, round plaques (patches of thick raised skin) on the face, scalp, or ears. Discoid lupus erythematosus (DLE) is an inflammatory autoimmune disease that is less severe than systemic lupus erythematosus. It occurs when an unknown trigger causes the immune system to attack parts of the body as if they were foreign substances. DLE is suspected by its appearance and diagnosed through a biopsy of the rash. Treatment of the skin rash is with corticosteroid creams or oral medications. Because sun sensitivity can be a problem, sunscreen, sunglasses, and protective clothing should be worn.

Lupus erythematosus, systemic

An autoimmune disorder that can cause arthritis and also affects several tissues and internal organs. Systemic lupus erythematosus, which is commonly called SLE or lupus, causes the body's antibodies to damage cells and tissues in the body, which may include the joints, skin, kidneys, heart, lungs, pancreas, blood vessels, and brain.

Affected individuals may have a wide variety of symptoms that range from mild to severe. The most commonly experienced of these are extreme fatigue, painful or swollen joints due to arthritis, unexplained fevers, anorexia, anemia, skin rashes, and kidney problems. Skin rashes are common among those with SLE, and most have sun sensitivity. Like other rheumatic diseases, lupus can cause aches, pain, and stiffness in the joints, muscles, and bones. It is also characterized by intermittent episodes of symptoms, called flares, and periods of wellness, called remission.

Diagnosis is based on a medical history, a physical examination, and laboratory test results. There is presently no known cure for lupus, but symptoms can be managed with medication. Treatment is aimed at preventing flares, treatment of flares when they occur, and minimizing the risk of complications. Mainstays of treatment for lupus are nonsteroidal anti-inflammatory drugs (NSAIDs), antimalarial medications, corticosteroid medications, immunosuppressive medications, or intravenous gamma globulin.

Luteinizing hormone

See LH.

Luteinizing hormone-releasing hormone

See LH-RH.

Lyme disease

A bacterial infection that is transmitted to humans by the bite of infected deer ticks and infected western black-legged ticks. Lyme disease is an inflammatory disorder that causes a rash, which may be followed by symptoms that appear weeks or months after the initial infection. The infection can affect the skin, joints, heart, and nervous system, with symptoms that persist for months or even years without treatment.

There are three different stages of illness, with possible overlapping and apparent recovery between each stage.

The first stage occurs in as few as 3 days or as many as 28 days after exposure, may last for months, and begins with general flulike symptoms that may include fatigue, headache, fever, chills, a stiff neck, aching muscles, joint pain, backache, sore throat, swollen glands, nausea, vomiting, and dizziness.

During this first stage, most infected people develop an expanding, circular skin lesion surrounding the reddened site of the tick bite. Periodic rashes may also appear.

During stage two of Lyme disease, the nervous system and heart can become affected. Symptoms include extremely severe headaches, neck pain, sleep disturbances, poor concentration and memory, emotional instability, irritability, double vision, numbness and weakness in the extremities or the face, eye pain, and ear pain. Within several weeks of infection, a small percentage of infected people develop an unusually strong, rapid, or irregular heartbeat; this symptom is generally temporary.

Stage three of Lyme disease involves arthritic complications, experienced as joint pain. The joint pain usually occurs in the larger joints, such as the knees and hips and may last for a few days, recur a few weeks later, or become chronic. Other ongoing symptoms may include chronic fatigue or psychological problems.

Initial diagnosis may be made by a doctor's identification of the characteristic skin lesion and a clinical history that includes a reported tick bite or fleabite and residence in or travel to an area that has ticks. Blood tests for the bacteria that cause Lyme disease may be negative early in the course of the illness, but later antibodies to the bacteria may be found in the blood. When the joints have become involved, tests may be performed on the synovial fluid and membrane, along with X rays of the joint. Treatment outcome is improved by the early use of antibiotics. If cardiac, joint, or neurological disease has developed, treatment with intravenous ceftriaxone or penicillin may be needed.

To relieve inflammatory and painful symptoms, nonsteroidal anti-inflammatory drugs (NSAIDs), including aspirin, may be recommended to infected persons older than 18 years. (Aspirin should never be given to children under 18 because of the risk of developing Reye syndrome, a potentially fatal disease.) A temporary pacemaker may be required if there are significant cardiac symptoms. Swollen knee joints may be aspirated to remove excess fluid.

Lymph node

A small, hollow structure found along a lymph vessel, generally occurring in clusters in some parts of the body. Lymph nodes contain concentrations of lymphocytes, white blood cells that attack invading organisms such as bacteria and viruses. Lymphocytes travel in and out of the lymph nodes via lymph vessels to circulate freely throughout the bloodstream, searching for harmful organisms and repairing damaged cells. Inside the lymph nodes, the white blood cells trap and kill microorganisms. See LYMPHATIC SYSTEM; IMMUNE SYSTEM.

Lymphadenitis

An inflammation of one or more lymph nodes that may be caused by infection with bacteria, viruses, fungi, or other microorganisms that produce disease. Lymphadenitis occurs when these microorganisms are trapped in the lymph nodes, and white blood cells congregate to attack them. Pus, abscesses, and inflammation can occur as a result. The infection produces swollen, red areas of skin that are sometimes painful to the touch.

Lymphadenitis may be diagnosed by blood tests and a culture or biopsy of the person's lymph nodes. The treatment varies according to the microorganism that has caused the infection. Bacteria are a common cause and can be controlled with antibiotic therapy.

Lymphadenopathy

Abnormal enlargement of the lymph nodes. Lymphadenopathy most commonly occurs in the lymph nodes located in one area of the body, but it may also occur simultaneously in several unconnected areas. Widespread lymphadenopathy is usually a result of a generalized infection in the body, an autoimmune disease, or a malignancy (cancer).

A complete medical history and a physical examination are the initial basis for diagnosing the cause of lymphadenopathy. Usually this will produce a readily identifiable source of the problem such as an upper respiratory tract infection, pharyngitis, periodontal disease, conjunctivitis, lymphadenitis, tinea, infected insect bites, a recent immunization, or some form of dermatitis. When no cause can be found, a surgical biopsy or fine-needle aspiration of the affected node may be recommended to confirm a diagnosis. Treatment of lymphadenopathy depends on the cause of the condition.

Lymphangioma

A benign (not cancerous) tumor in the skin composed of dilated lymph vessels. Lymphangiomas primarily occur on the arms and chest. They are usually removed by excision (cutting away the tumor) for cosmetic reasons.

Lymphangitis

An inflammation of the channels of the lymph system that are located below the skin. Lymphangitis is commonly caused by *Streptococcus* bacteria that have entered the lymphatic channels through openings in the skin such as cuts or wounds.

Symptoms of lymphangitis include red, irregular, warm, and tender streaks that appear on an arm or leg near the infected skin lesion. The streaks appear to travel from the lesion toward the lymph nodes closest to the extremity involved, generally those in the armpits or the groin. The lymph nodes become enlarged and tender (see GLANDS, SWOLLEN).

Symptoms may include fever, chills with tremor, rapid heartbeat, and headache. In some instances, these symptoms can precede signs of local infection.

Diagnosis of lymphangitis is based on symptoms and signs. It may be possible to determine the infectious organism if cells can be cultured for laboratory evaluation. It is important to treat lymphangitis promptly with antibiotics.

Lymphatic system

A drainage system of vessels, glands, and ducts that channels a body fluid called lymph from tissues all over the body back into the bloodstream. The lymphatic system is a major part of the body's immune system, which fights infection and cancer.

The lymphatic system is composed of a network of vessels running throughout the body, interspersed with small organs or glands called lymph nodes (see LYMPH NODE). Each lymph node includes its own artery and vein connecting it to the circulatory system. Lymph nodes tend to be clustered throughout the body—for example, in the armpits and groin. When a particular part of the body is infected, the lymph vessels carry white blood cells and the harmful microorganisms to the lymph nodes closest to the site of the infection to be destroyed. The lymph nodes may become inflamed themselves as they fight off the invading organisms.

Lymphatic vessels also help absorb fats in the intestine. See DIGESTIVE SYSTEM; INTESTINE.

Lymphocytes

A type of white blood cell that is the basic functional unit of the body's immune system, which fights disease-causing microorganisms that invade the body.

There are about 1 trillion lymphocytes in the human body, all of which look similar under the microscope. They are differentiated by the distinctive molecules or markers they carry on their cell surface. These markers determine whether a lymphocyte is a B cell or a T cell, and within the two classes of cells, the markers determine specific behaviors of the cells.

The two types of lymphocyte work in different ways to destroy microorganisms: B cells manufacture antibodies, and T cells release toxic chemicals. These lymphocytes are "smart cells": as part of the immune system, they recognize a specific invader and develop a specialized attack.

After an infection has been successfully fought off, both T cells and B cells have the capacity to reserve some of their number to remain in the body as memory cells. These memory cells can quickly recognize the same invading organism if it enters the body again and multiply immediately to destroy it. This built-in protection against disease is called immunity. See LYMPHATIC SYSTEM.

Lymphogranuloma venereum

One of the sexually transmitted diseases (STDs); caused by specific types of the bacterium *Chlamydia trachomatis*. Lymphogranuloma venereum (LGV) occurs when these strains of bacteria invade and reproduce in the lymph nodes. This STD occurs mostly in tropical and subtropical areas; it is rare in the United States.

The first sign of infection is a small blister that forms in the genital area, possibly on the cervix or the vagina in women. It is followed by enlarged, tender lymph nodes, or swollen glands (see GLANDS, SWOLLEN), on one side of the groin. This swelling develops into a large, tender mass within the tissues below the skin that produces inflammation of the skin's surface. A number of sores may develop on the skin's surface and produce a discharge.

Antibiotic medications, including doxycycline, erythromycin, and tetracycline, taken for about 3 weeks can rapidly treat the early stages of LGV. Surgery may be required to treat abscesses. All sexual contacts of an infected person need to be informed of the disease.

Lymphoma

A group of more than 24 types of cancers that develop in the lymphatic system, primarily in the lymph nodes and spleen. Different types of lymphoma behave differently. Some grow slowly, while others grow very quickly and can cause serious illness in a short time if they go untreated. Lymphomas are classified by their appearance when examined under a microscope, and they are generally divided into two categories. If characteristic Reed-Sternberg cells are present, the lymphoma is Hodgkin disease; all other lymphomas are considered non-Hodgkin lymphoma (see LYMPHOMA, NON-HODGKIN).

Lymphomas normally produce two types of symptoms: those related to the enlarged lymph nodes and generalized symptoms that affect the entire body. The first sign of lymphoma is usually an enlarged lymph node in the neck, the armpit, or the groin.

Generalized symptoms include feeling unwell, sweating heavily during the night, and unintentionally losing weight and having lapses in energy and appetite.

Diagnosis begins with a biopsy of an affected lymph node. The lymph node is removed and sent for microscopic examination to classify the type of lymphoma. If a lymphoma exists, further tests can detect whether it has spread beyond the lymph nodes. Depending on the type of lymphoma and the extent of the disease, it may be treated with radiation, chemotherapy, immunotherapy, or bone marrow transplantation.

Lymphoma, non-Hodgkin

The cancers that develop in lymphatic tissue that are not Hodgkin disease. Non-Hodgkin lymphoma accounts for about 5 percent of all cases of cancer in the United States. Symptoms usually include painless swelling of the lymph nodes in the neck, groin, or underarm; unexplained fever; night sweats; constant fatigue; unexplained weight loss; itchy skin; and reddened patches on the skin. Diagnosis requires several tests, including a biopsy of an affected lymph node, blood tests, X rays, CT (computed tomography) scanning, and MRI (magnetic resonance imaging) scanning.

Treatment depends on the type of lymphoma and the extent of the disease. Non-Hodgkin lymphomas are categorized as low-, intermediate-, or high-grade, and their treatment varies accordingly.

- *LOW-GRADE LYMPHOMA* is slow-growing and widespread. They are almost always incurable. Treatment of low-grade lymphomas usually involves chemotherapy or radiation therapy when the person is experiencing symptoms. Bone marrow transplantation (see BONE MARROW TRANSPLANT, ALLOGENEIC; BONE MARROW TRANSPLANT, AUTOLOGOUS) is sometimes performed. A new therapy (immunotherapy) using antibodies that attack the cancerous cells has been shown to shrink lymphomas. Stage I (localized) low-grade lymphoma sometimes can be cured with radiation therapy alone.

- *INTERMEDIATE- AND HIGH-GRADE LYMPHOMAS*, also known as aggressive lymphomas, progress more rapidly than low-grade lymphomas and can be cured with chemotherapy in about half of all cases. Intensive courses of several drugs are often necessary, and radiation therapy may be used.

Lynch syndrome

See COLON CANCER.

Lysis of adhesions

A surgical procedure performed under general anesthesia to cut away adhesions, which are composed of scar tissue formed after earlier surgery. Those adhesions are most common in the abdomen. Because fibrous scar tissue is inelastic, adhesions in the abdomen can cause pain when they are stretched. In addition, adhesions involving the intestine can block or obstruct the digestive system, a condition that can be fatal if left untreated.

Macrocephaly

A congenital condition in which the head and brain are abnormally large in comparison with the rest of the body. Macrocephaly is associated with enlarged ventricles (hydrocephalus) or increased fluid and failure to develop parts of the brain (hydranencephaly).

Macrolides

A class of antibiotics produced naturally by *Streptomyces*, a type of aerobic bacteria. The macrolides have a wide spectrum of activity and are used to treat infections in people who are allergic to penicillin. Among the infections treated with macrolides are *Streptococcus* infections, legionnaires disease, and chlamydial infections. Macrolides are also used to improve digestive activity in people with diabetes and to control severe cases of acne.

Macular degeneration

A progressive disease of the eyes that affects the central portion of the retina (the macula) and causes a gradual loss of vision. In macular degeneration, the insulating layer between the retina and the underlying network of blood vessels (choroid) breaks down. Abnormal blood vessels may develop, which can rupture or leak blood and cause scar tissue to form; this, in turn, causes the macula to degenerate. Central vision fades as a result of this process, but vision to the sides (peripheral vision) remains unaffected. The disease may affect one or both eyes.

People with the disease may become visually impaired but do not become totally blind since their peripheral vision remains intact. However, as the disease progresses, they may lose the ability to drive and to read.

There are two basic types of macular degeneration: dry (or atrophic) degeneration, in which the degeneration usually proceeds slowly and vision loss is gradual, and wet degeneration, in which new blood vessels develop from the choroid, which can leak fluid under the retina, creating a large blind spot and rapid loss of central vision. Nine of 10 cases are the dry type. The signs of macular degeneration are blurry or fuzzy vision, a dark or empty area in the center of the visual field, and the wavy appearance of straight lines (for example, sentences on a printed page or telephone poles along a road). A diagnostic device called an Amsler grid, which consists of dark lines forming a square grid around a dot in the center, is used to diagnose and monitor the disease. Blurring of the grid or distortion of its lines into wavy, fuzzy, or missing areas can indicate macular degeneration.

There is no proven treatment for dry macular degeneration. Rather, the person is taught how to adapt to the loss of central vision with low-vision aids, such as magnifiers and reading lamps.

Some cases of wet macular degeneration can be treated with laser surgery, although this treatment cannot be used if leaks occur in the very center of the macula.

Mad cow disease

Also known as bovine spongiform encephalopathy (BSE); a chronic, degenerative disorder that affects the central nervous system of cattle. Since 1996, concerns have arisen that there is a link between a disease in humans called new variant Creutzfeldt-Jakob disease and mad cow disease. Both are fatal brain diseases with unusually long incubation periods, and both are caused by unconventional transmissible agents.

Magnet therapy

The use of magnetic devices placed on or near the body, thought by some to relieve pain and speed healing. Magnet therapy is used to treat arthritis (especially osteoarthritis), insomnia, carpal tunnel syndrome, and headaches and is popular among professional athletes.

Magnetic resonance imaging

See MRI.

Malabsorption syndrome

Impaired absorption of nutrients in the small intestine due to a number of diseases and conditions, each of which can damage the structure of the small intestine or diminish the presence of the enzymes that aid digestion. Pale, greasy, foul-smelling stools are a common symptom of malabsorption. Additional symptoms include abdominal bloating, flatulence, and diarrhea. Signs of vitamin and mineral deficiencies due to malabsorption are a sore tongue, numbness and tingling sensations in the arms and legs, muscle cramps, and bone pain.

Conditions that commonly cause malabsorption include celiac disease, Crohn disease, lactose intolerance, lactase deficiency, and damage to the pancreas.

Malabsorption is diagnosed by a complete physical examination and tests, such as stool analysis, blood tests, a gastrointestinal (GI) series, and gastroscopy. Once malabsorption has been diagnosed, treatment depends on its underlying cause. For example, the only effective treatment for celiac disease is avoiding all foods that contain gluten.

Malaria

A protozoal disease caused by a microscopic, single-celled parasite that is transmitted from person to person by a female *Anopheles* mosquito. Malaria is caused by infection with one of four different types of parasitic protozoa called plasmodia. Female Anopheles mosquitoes carry an infectious form of this parasite in their saliva. The parasite is transmitted to a person who has been bitten by an infected mosquito, and the parasite enters the person's bloodstream.

Symptoms of malaria tend to occur from 1 week to 1 month after a person has been bitten by a mosquito. In the less severe forms of malaria, symptoms may include headache, fatigue, nausea, vomiting, and diarrhea lasting for 24 hours, followed by high fever, trembling, and chills lasting for 12 to 24 hours. Sudden chills may alternate with episodes of fever, marked by rapid breathing and an absence of perspiration. When the fever breaks, there is profuse perspiration. This syndrome is repeated each time the parasite is released again from the liver into the bloodstream, usually every 2 or 3 days.

Malaria is diagnosed by blood tests that can detect the plasmodia parasite. In the presence of severe symptoms, malaria may be treated immediately with antiprotozoal medications without waiting for blood test results. Chloroquine is a standard treatment for malaria.

Male sex hormones

See ANDROGEN.

Malformation

Congenital defect resulting from abnormal prenatal development. Malformation can occur in a single organ or a larger area of the body and usually refers to a structural defect, such as a cleft lip. Malformation stems from abnormal differentiation of cells and tissues during early embryo development.

Malignant

In medicine, the term used to describe a condition that becomes progressively worse over time and may result in death. In reference to a tumor, malignant signifies a cancerous growth or one that is likely to penetrate the tissues in the organ in which it originates. Malignant tumors tend to sink roots into the tissues around them, as well as to grow and spread. Malignant tumors invade surrounding tissues; nonmalignant cancers seldom spread to other parts of the body. See METASTASIS.

Malignant melanoma

See MELANOMA, MALIGNANT.

Mallet finger

See BASEBALL FINGER.

Malnutrition

A nutritional disorder that results from an imbalanced, inadequate, or excessive diet. Malnutrition may also be due to an underlying medical condition that interferes with the ability to obtain nutrients from foods.

Malpractice

In medicine, a single act or ongoing conduct of a medical professional that does not meet established standards of care and that results in verifiable harm or damage to the person receiving treatment. Medical malpractice may involve an error or omission as a result of negligence, intentional wrongdoing, or ignorance.

Malpresentation

A position of the fetus immediately before childbirth that is not ideal and may cause problems during delivery. The part of the baby that is situated at the opening of the mother's pelvic cavity is called the presenting part and is normally the head, facing the mother's back.

The most common malpresentations are breech presentation and occipital posterior presentation, in which the baby's head is down but facing toward the mother's front. Usually, the fetus rotates naturally to the correct position during delivery. Malpresentation can usually be diagnosed well in advance by pelvic examination, ultrasound, or X ray. Once a doctor has confirmed malpresentation, the mother will be monitored closely to see if the fetus spontaneously turns to the normal presentation. If it does not, careful management during labor is essential.

MALToma

Lymphomas that arise particularly in the gastrointestinal tract, but also in other organs. MALToma is a type of lymphoma that has only recently been recognized. (MALT stands for mucosa-associated lymphoid tissue.) It is associated with a particular bacterium and sometimes responds to treatment with antibiotics. MALTomas can also affect lymph nodes, where they tend to be localized and easily removed.

Mammogram

An X ray of a woman's breasts. The resulting breast X rays, or mammograms, can help a doctor to diagnose breast cancer. Doctors recommend a mammogram for women younger than age 40 years for specific reasons (helping to evaluate an abnormality) or if there is a strong family history of breast cancer. Women ages 40 to 50 years should have a mammogram done every 1 to 2 years. Women older than 50 years should have a mammogram annually.

Mandible

The bone of the lower jaw.

Mandibulofacial dysostosis

A birth defect (see BIRTH DEFECTS) characterized by a group of deformities affecting the size and shape of the ears, eyelids, cheekbones, and jaw. Also called Treacher Collins syndrome. Physical features of mandibulofacial dysostosis may include down-slanting eyes; notches in the lower eyelids; a prominent nose; a broad mouth; a small chin with a steeply angled lower jaw; underdeveloped, malformed, or prominent ears; and growth of hair extending in front of the ears. Hearing loss often accompanies the syndrome, and the person may also have problems breathing and eating. Less frequently, physical features include cleft lip or cleft palate, heart defects, and crossed eyes.

Early diagnosis and treatment of hearing loss can prevent possible developmental and educational disabilities. Reconstructive facial surgery can improve the appearance of the face and close a cleft palate. It is recommended that a craniofacial center (medical facility devoted to disorders of the skull and face) be consulted if possible.

Mania

A mood state characterized by a persistently euphoric mood, frequently accompanied by decreased need for sleep, high physical energy, overspending, increased sexual activity, rapid speech, loss of self-control and judgment, unrealistic beliefs in one's abilities, racing thoughts, and disturbed appetite lasting for at least 1 week. Mania is a sign of BIPOLAR DISORDER. An underlying serious medical condition should be considered if mania occurs in an older person.

Manic-depressive illness

A mental disease characterized by extreme mood swings from high to low. See BIPOLAR DISORDER.

Mantoux test

See TUBERCULIN SKIN TEST.

MAOIs

See MONOAMINE OXIDASE INHIBITORS.

March fracture

A break or fracture of a bone, most commonly in the metatarsal bones of the feet or in the lower leg, that occurs as a result of prolonged or repeated marching, running, or other stress. It produces pain in the ball of the foot or in the leg and is made worse by activity. A doctor may diagnose a March fracture on the basis of an X ray, bone scan, and MRI scanning, in combination with a physical examination and clinical history. Treatments include reducing physical activity, braces, crutches, or a short-leg walking cast.

Marfan syndrome

An inherited disorder of the connective tissue primarily affecting the eyes and the skeletal, cardiovascular, and central nervous systems.

People with Marfan syndrome usually have tall, lanky frames with long arms and slender, tapering spidery fingers (arachnodactyly). They tend to be nearsighted and have lenses of the eye that are slightly off-center. Cardiovascular abnormalities, curvature of the spine (scoliosis); flat feet; vision problems; thin, narrow face; and sunken chest are also associated with the syndrome.

Marfan syndrome cannot be cured. Visual defects can often be corrected. Children with Marfan syndrome should be watched carefully throughout adolescence for signs of developing scoliosis. During medical examinations, chest X rays and echocardiograms are usually performed. Most people may need to take medication to lower the heart rate, blood pressure, or both, which reduces the risk of serious problems with the aorta. In cases involving major problems with the aorta or aortic valve, surgery may be required.

Marital counseling

See COUPLES THERAPY.

Masculinization

The normal process by which a male acquires sex-specific attributes during sexual maturation as a result of the response of the body to the male hormones called androgen hormones. Androgen hormones, including testosterone, are produced in the testicles in response to stimulation by the pituitary hormone LH (luteinizing hormone).

Massage

A technique that may be used in physical therapy or by a massage therapist involving a kneading with the hands of certain soft tissues of the body, especially the muscles, ligaments, and tendons. The purpose of massage is to promote relaxation of the body part being massaged and to relieve overall physical tension in the person receiving the massage.

Massage therapy

Holistic medical therapy that uses hands-on massage to promote healing. Massage therapy is used to improve blood circulation; to relax tense muscles and help stimulate weak ones; to stimulate secretions, such as lymph; to stimulate the nervous system; and to help release toxic metabolic by-products from body tissues.

There are several types and categories of massage used by massage therapists: traditional European massage, which includes Swedish massage and is the most commonly used method in the United States; contemporary Western massage, which focuses on creating deep relaxation; deep tissue massage, which is used to release chronic patterns of tension; and trigger point massage, which applies concentrated finger pressure directly to individual muscles.

Mast cell

A tissue cell that is part of the immune system and originates as a stem cell. Mast cells contain large amounts of histamine and other chemicals that trigger many of the symptoms of allergies.

Mastectomy

Surgical removal of all or part of the breast, usually as a treatment for breast cancer. The principal goal of surgery for breast cancer is to re-

move the primary tumor from the breast. Depending on the size and location of the primary tumor, any of four basic types of surgery will be selected: lumpectomy, partial mastectomy, subcutaneous mastectomy, and modified radical mastectomy. The selection of the procedure depends on the person's condition and preference.

In a lumpectomy, only the tumor and a small amount of surrounding tissue are removed. The procedure leaves a barely noticeable scar and a small depression in the breast. The surgery usually is followed by radiation therapy and often by chemotherapy, to reduce the risk of recurrence.

In a partial mastectomy, a segment of breast tissue containing the primary tumor is removed, including the overlying skin, a portion of the tissue surrounding the tumor, and some of the underlying tissue. Some lymph glands in the armpit will also be removed, and radiation therapy will usually follow to reduce recurrence.

Subcutaneous mastectomy is used to prevent breast cancer in women at high risk for developing the disease. All the inner tissue of the breast is removed, leaving the nipple and as much skin as possible intact. The lymph glands in the armpit are examined and may be removed for biopsy. A silicone implant is inserted, to recreate the appearance of the original breast.

In a modified radical mastectomy, the entire breast and all lymph glands under the arm are removed in a single block of tissue, if possible. The chest muscles are almost always left in place. Healing leaves a long scar across the chest, but the breast can usually be reconstructed later.

Radical mastectomy, in which the breast, lymph nodes in the armpit, and chest muscles are all removed, is almost never performed, because it is no more effective than a modified radical mastectomy.

Mastitis

An inflammation of the breast due to a bacterial infection; usually, but not always, found in breast-feeding mothers. The infection is diagnosed by a physical examination. Characteristic physical signs of mastitis include a swollen, hard, red area of the breast that is intensely painful, accompanied by fever. Mastitis responds successfully to antibiotic therapy.

Mastopexy

See BREAST LIFT.

Masturbation

Touching the genitals and other sexually responsive areas of one's own body for pleasure, stimulation, and release of sexual tension.

Measles

A highly contagious, viral, respiratory infection that produces a characteristic rash. Measles, which is also called rubeola, usually spreads from person to person through contact with airborne respiratory droplets that occur when an infected person coughs or sneezes or via physical contact with items and surfaces that have been contaminated by the virus.

The symptoms of measles generally begin 10 to 14 days after exposure to the virus. In children, measles usually causes only mild symptoms, but otitis media, inflammation of the middle ear, is a common complication. Initial symptoms may include a runny nose, nasal congestion, fever, and cough.

Within 2 to 4 days, tiny lesions called Koplik spots develop on the inside of the cheeks near the back molars. At the same time or soon thereafter, the typical measles rash appears as very red eruptions that start on the forehead near the hairline and behind the ears, then spread over the trunk and to the extremities, including the palms of the hands and the soles of the feet. The rash is not painful and does not itch.

Treatment of people who are otherwise healthy includes taking acetaminophen to reduce fever and relieve discomfort, bed rest, and the use of a cool-mist humidifier to alleviate cough and nasal congestion. Aspirin should not be given to children with measles because of the associated risk of Reye syndrome.

The antiviral medication ribavirin is used to treat some people with weakened immune systems. Antibiotic therapy may be required to treat bacterial complications such as middle ear infections in children.

There is an effective measles vaccine, which is generally given to children as part of the measles-mumps-rubella, or MMR, injection (see VACCINATION). Women who are planning a pregnancy and who have never been immunized should be immunized before becoming pregnant.

Meckel diverticulum

A congenital malformation in which a pouch of tissue forms near the lower end of the small intestine. Often, a Meckel diverticulum causes no symptoms and requires no treatment. About one third of cases contain the same type of tissue that lines the stomach. In those cases, the gastric tissue may secrete acid and ulcerate, leading to bleeding. The pouch can also become infected or obstructed and cause bleeding, abdominal pain, vomiting, and fever.

Diagnosis of a Meckel diverticulum is made by physical examination and tests such as radionuclide scans. Severe symptoms often prompt an abdominal operation called an exploratory laparotomy (see LAPAROTOMY, EXPLORATORY). If a Meckel diverticulum is discovered during a laparotomy, surgeons remove it.

Meconium

A newborn's first stool, consisting of a combination of swallowed amniotic fluid and mucus from the baby's gastrointestinal tract. Sometimes, meconium is released into the amniotic fluid before birth, which is usually considered a sign of fetal distress.

Medial

The center, or middle, of the body. The opposite of medial is lateral.

Mediastinoscopy

An endoscopy of the chest in which the area between the lungs and above the heart is visually examined using a lighted instrument inserted through a small incision. A mediastinoscopy is performed in the hospital under general anesthesia and is used to diagnose diseases such as lung cancer and tuberculosis.

Mediastinum

The central body cavity between the lungs, occupying the area between the breastbone and the spine, down to the diaphragm. Within the mediastinum are the heart and the major vessels leading in and out of it, the trachea, the esophagus, thymus gland, lymph nodes and vessels, and the vagus and phrenic nerves.

Medicaid

A federal- and state-funded health insurance program for low-income people of all ages. Medicaid money funds state programs that provide health services to people who qualify for welfare in their state.

Medical records

A detailed accounting of a person's health status over time. Medical records include information about vital signs, illnesses, injuries, test results, diagnoses, and treatments. Other pertinent information such as allergies to medications is also included. Medical records are confidential documents protected by federal law.

Medicare

A federal health insurance program for people over 65. Every American over age 65 is eligible for Medicare, regardless of income or assets. To receive Medicare, older adults file an enrollment application with the local Social Security office as they near age 65. Medicare covers much of the cost of inpatient hospital care, skilled nursing facility care, some forms of home health care, and hospice care. However, strict conditions must be met. Recently Medicare added a new program, Part D, that provides drug coverage for enrollees.

Individuals are advised to check on what is and what is not covered. Doctors are called participating providers when they agree to accept Medicare's payment rates (assignment) for medical services.

Medication

See DRUG.

Meditation

A mind-body technique that uses controlled breathing and quiet contemplation to induce a state of mental and physical tranquility. Meditation is used by conventional and alternative medical practitioners as a way to lower blood pressure, to help people with asthma breathe, to combat chronic chest pain, and generally to relax. Meditation has been used effectively to treat hypertension, anxiety, headaches, irritable bowel syndrome, and insomnia.

Mediterranean diet

The term refers to the type of food typically consumed by Europeans who reside near the Mediterranean Sea. Its principal components are plentiful vegetables and fruits, seafood, dried peas and beans, and olive oil. Very little red meat and few fatty dairy products are consumed. See also FATS AND OILS.

Medulla oblongata

The lower portion of the brain stem just above the spinal cord. The medulla oblongata contains nerve centers that control breathing, heart rate, and blood pressure. See BRAIN.

Medulloblastoma

A rapidly growing, cancerous brain tumor, most often seen in children, that usually develops in the back of the brain. Symptoms associated with it include headaches, apathy, and unexplained vomiting, soon followed by difficulty in walking as the tumor grows larger.

Treatment starts with surgery to remove as much of the cancer as can be safely removed. After the surgery, tests are performed to see how many cancer cells remain; these include MRI (magnetic resonance imaging), bone scans, and analysis of cerebral spinal fluid. Radiation therapy and chemotherapy may be given.

Megacolon

A distended colon. Symptoms of megacolon include severe constipation. Diagnosis is made by X rays or a lower gastrointestinal (GI) series (also known as a barium enema). In severe cases, surgery is required.

Meiosis

A type of cell division that takes place during germ cell (egg or sperm cell) formation and produces four daughter cells, each with half the number of chromosomes of the original cell. In meiosis, which occurs during the formation of gametes (mature male or female germ cells) in humans, the 46 chromosomes in the germ cell divide to make two new cells, each with 23 chromosomes that pair with corresponding chromosomes to exchange bits of genetic material. In women, X chromosomes inherited from both parents form a pair, while in men, one X chromosome inherited from the mother pairs with one Y chromosome inherited from the father. Once the genetic exchange is complete, meiosis continues. When the chromosomes of a cell duplicate in a single division to produce two new daughter cells each with the same number of chromosomes as the parent cell, the process is called mitosis.

Melanoma, eye

See EYE TUMORS.

Melanoma, malignant

A skin cancer that begins in the melanocytes, the cells that produce melanin. Melanomas are usually dark brown or black and can resemble dark freckles or moles. Typically, they are unevenly colored, irregular-shaped tumors that bleed easily.

Often, the first sign of malignant melanoma is a change in the size, shape, color, or feel of an existing mole. It can become larger or irregular in shape where one-half does not match the other. The edges can become ragged, blurred, or irregular, and the pigment can spread into surrounding skin. The color of a mole can become uneven, incorporating shades of black, brown, tan, white, gray, red, pink, or blue.

Melanomas are usually larger than healthy moles, exceeding 1/4 inch in width. Malignant melanomas may also appear as new moles. Such new moles are usually black, abnormal in appearance, and noticeably unattractive.

Treatment includes surgery to remove the entire melanoma and some surrounding skin to prevent recurrence. In its early stages, melanoma is usually curable by surgery. How-

ever, as a melanoma becomes more advanced, it becomes more difficult to treat and can be deadly. Chemotherapy, immunotherapy with interleukin 2 (IL-2), or interferon may be used in some cases of advanced disease.

Preventing malignant melanoma generally requires screening for abnormal moles and avoiding the direct rays of the sun. Using a sunscreen with a minimum SPF of 15 is essential (see SUNSCREENS).

Melatonin

A hormone responsible for regulating the body's biological clock. Melatonin is produced in larger quantities at night than in the day by the pineal gland at the base of the brain. Because people produce less melatonin as they age, this relative deficiency may contribute to the sleep problems that many older people experience. Melatonin supplements may help people sleep better.

Melena

Partly digested blood in the stool (see also FECES, BLOOD IN THE). Melena is considered a medical emergency because it indicates internal bleeding, which may be a symptom of peptic ulcer disease or other disorders of the stomach, intestines, or esophagus.

Membrane

A thin layer of tissue that covers a body surface, lines a cavity, divides a space or organ, lubricates joining parts, or anchors a body structure. There are two principal types of membranes. Mucous membranes are mucus-secreting tissue such as those that line the nose and mouth; they lubricate the cavity and protect against infection. Connective membranes cover bone or hold body parts in position (for example, the synovial membrane lines the cavities of the joints).

Memory, loss of

Forgetfulness that can result from brain damage or severe emotional trauma; amnesia. Pathological loss of memory can be caused by DEMENTIA, ALZHEIMER'S DISEASE, alcoholism, head injury, seizures, stroke, brain surgery, ECT (electroconvulsive therapy), the use of barbiturates or other tranquilizers, and other physical events or conditions. Depending on the cause, loss of memory can occur gradually or all at once, and it may be permanent or temporary.

A certain amount of forgetfulness is normal as people age. Normal aging is also associated with difficulty in learning new material.

Menarche

The onset of menstruation, or a woman's first menstrual period.

Meniere disease

A disorder of the ear caused by an increase of fluid in the part of the inner ear called the labyrinth, which controls a person's sense of balance. The cause of Meniere disease is unknown.

Meniere disease occurs as discrete episodes, or attacks of vertigo, which may last a few hours or an entire day. The episodes may be preceded by a feeling of fullness in the ears. During attacks of the disorder, symptoms may include dizziness, nausea and vomiting, distorted hearing or hearing loss, ringing in the ears (see TIN-

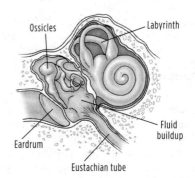

Pressure from fluid buildup
Meniere disease involves an excessive buildup of fluid in the labyrinth, a system of passageways in the inner ear that regulates balance.

NITUS), and the feeling of pressure in one ear. The frequency and severity of attacks vary widely.

A person experiencing symptoms of Meniere disease should see an ear, nose, and throat specialist (otolaryngologist). Tests may include a caloric test (a balance test of the labyrinth), as well as MRI (magnetic resonance imaging), to help determine whether a person has this disorder. The physician may prescribe medication to control nausea and vomiting, a diuretic to prevent excess fluid from accumulating in the labyrinth, and medications placed in the middle ear to control dizzy spells. Surgery may be recommended.

Meninges

The three, thin membranes that cover the brain and spinal cord. The innermost layer of tissue is called the pia mater, which lies against the surface of the brain and spinal cord. The middle layer, the arachnoid mater, is separated from the pia mater by the subarachnoid space, which is filled with cerebrospinal fluid. The dura mater is the tough outer layer that lines the inside of the skull and loosely encloses the spinal cord.

Meningioma

A benign tumor arising from the membranes, or meninges, that surround the brain and spinal cord. Meningiomas are rare tumors that can occur at any age. Depending on size and location, meningiomas may cause symptoms such as headache, vomiting, impaired mental function, speech loss, and visual disturbances. However, many meningiomas do not cause any symptoms. If the tumor penetrates the overlying bone, thickening and bulging of the skull may occur. Depending on the size and location of the meningioma, surgical removal may be required. When this is not possible, tumors are treated with radiation therapy. Asymptomatic meningiomas may not require treatment.

Meningitis

Inflammation of the membranes or meninges that surround the brain and spinal cord. Viral meningitis is a relatively mild disease; bacterial meningitis is life-threatening and requires immediate treatment. Meningitis is usually caused by infections that originate elsewhere in the body and travel in the bloodstream to the brain or spinal cord.

The symptoms of bacterial meningitis, which are most commonly caused by *Streptococcus, Staphylococcus, Haemophilus influenzae* (*H. influenzae*), and *Meningococcus* bacteria, often come on suddenly and include fever, severe headache, nausea, vomiting, stiff neck, and sensitivity

to light. There can also be changes in behavior, such as confusion and sleepiness. These are important symptoms that indicate a need for emergency treatment. In infants, there may be irritability, lethargy, poor feeding, and fever. In viral meningitis, symptoms can range from mild to severe, but often resemble influenza.

Meningitis is diagnosed by lumbar puncture and examination of cerebrospinal fluid. Other useful tests include blood tests, X rays, and CT (computed tomography) scanning. Early diagnosis and treatment of bacterial meningitis are imperative to prevent neurological damage or death. Antibiotics are administered intravenously to control the infection. Corticosteroids may be used to reduce brain inflammation, and anticonvulsants, to prevent or treat seizures.

With early diagnosis and treatment, most people recover from bacterial meningitis, although some develop complications such as deafness. Since the introduction of *H. influenzae* immunization, and the development of a vaccine against *Pneumococcal* bacteria, the incidence of this type of meningitis has decreased dramatically in the United States.

Meningocele

A birth defect in which the membranes of the brain or spinal cord protrude through abnormal gaps in the skull or spinal column. See also NEURAL TUBE DEFECT.

Meningomyelocele

A severe form of spina bifida, a neural tube defect. Meningomyelocele occurs when the bones of the spine do not form completely, leaving the spinal canal incompletely closed. The protrusion of the spinal cord affects neurological function below the site of the defect. Most defects occur in the lowest areas of the back (lower lumbar or sacral areas), because in normal development they are the last parts of the spine to close. Symptoms of muscle weakness, paralysis, loss of sensation, and impaired bladder and bowel control are caused by damage to the spinal cord. Symptoms also include the presence of a sac protruding from the spinal cord on the back of a newborn baby. The exposed spinal cord is susceptible to infection, especially meningitis.

Surgical repair of the defect is usually recommended and is generally successful. Before surgery, the newborn must be handled with care to reduce damage to the exposed spinal cord. Antibiotics may be used to treat or to prevent infections. Physical therapy may be useful to reduce muscle weakness, but neurological damage is usually permanent and irreversible.

Some success has been reported in treating meningomyelocele with experimental fetal surgery (performed during pregnancy within the uterus). The meningomyelocele is closed, and the pregnancy continues.

The root cause of meningomyelocele is not known. One possible cause is folic acid deficiency. Maternal use of valproic acid, a medication used to treat seizures and migraine headaches, increases the risk.

Meniscal tears

A break or rupture in the crescent-shaped pad of cartilage, called the meniscus, located in the knee where the ends of the thighbone and lower leg bone meet to form the knee joint. An impact injury or a rapid twisting motion from a squatting position are the usual causes of meniscal tears. A slight swelling typically occurs within several hours of the injury. There may be episodic, recurrent swelling, an inability to fully extend the knee ("locking"), and an instability of the knee causing it to give way.

Meniscal tears are diagnosed by physical examination, specifically by a swelling of the knee joint, a limited ability to fully extend the leg, and localized tenderness to the touch. Treatment may be easily remembered by the acronym RICE—rest, ice, compression, and elevation. Physical therapy may be recommended. Crutches may be used if there is swelling and pain with movement. Arthroscopic surgery may be considered.

Meniscectomy

The surgical removal of a portion of one of the two pads of cartilage, called the menisci, which are located in the knee joint. The procedure is usually performed as arthroscopic surgery under local or general anesthesia on an outpatient basis. Meniscectomy becomes necessary as a treatment for tears in the meniscus. Injuries requiring meniscectomy are usually diagnosed with MRI (magnetic resonance imaging).

Meniscus

A disk of loosely attached cartilage that helps protect the joint by absorbing shock and registering pressure against the joint. The knee joints contain menisci.

Menopause

The process during which a woman stops menstruating; literally, a woman's final menstrual period. Menopause generally occurs between ages 40 and 55; the average age is 51. Menopause is considered premature when it occurs before age 40.

The process is lengthy and gradual, beginning during perimenopause, when the ovaries' production of estrogen and other hormones slows down. Perimenopause can last for several years. Menopause is over at the point in time when a woman has not had a menstrual period for a minimum of 6 months. The most important hormonal change during menopause is a profound drop (by about 75 percent) in the production of estrogen. Changes in estrogen levels are responsible for the common physical complaints associated with menopause, such as hot flashes (the most common symptom), vaginal dryness, night sweats, and urinary problems. During menopause women may experience sudden mood changes or depression. Many women feel nervous, irritable, or very tired beginning in perimenopause, either because of lack of sleep or the change in their hormone levels.

Some women going through menopause may consider hormone replacement therapy (HRT), which alleviates menopausal symptoms and may reduce the risk of osteoporosis, but HRT use increases the risk of heart disease and breast cancer. See also HORMONE THERAPY.

Menorrhagia

See MENSTRUATION, DISORDERS OF.

Menstruation

The monthly discharge of blood and other secretions from a woman's uterus. Menstruation heralds the beginning of the reproductive years in a woman's life. Most women have their first period (menarche) around age 12. Menstruation usually stops around age 50 (menopause). The length of the menstrual cycle for most women is 28 days. A woman's menstrual cycle is the time from the first day of one period to the first day of the next. Normal cycles can vary from 21 to 35 days. The number of days a woman menstruates also may vary. Most women have periods lasting from 3 to 7 days, with an average of about 5 days. Most women have monthly periods; but others have irregular periods. Many different factors can change a woman's menstrual cycle, including weight gain or loss, an illness, stress, excessive exercise, pregnancy, or menopausal and adolescent transitions. See MENSTRUATION, DISORDERS OF.

Typically each month, the lining of the uterus thickens in response to the hormones estrogen and progesterone. During a 28-day menstrual cycle, ovulation (the release of an egg by an ovary into a fallopian tube) occurs about halfway through the cycle, on about day 14. Only at this point can pregnancy occur. As the egg moves into one of the fallopian tubes, a man's sperm can fertilize it. A fertilized egg will usually move into the uterus and attach to the uterine lining, where it begins developing into a fetus. An unfertilized egg will move into the uterus and eventually be absorbed or disintegrate. Estrogen and progesterone levels will then decrease, and the lining of the uterus will be shed during menstruation.

Menstruation, disorders of

Problems related to menstruation. A doctor can help identify the causes and suggest treatment options. Disorders can include disruptions in the cycle itself, differences in the discharge, or other problems.

HEAVY BLEEDING Menstrual bleeding is abnormal if it lasts for more than a week or if it is different from a woman's usual menstrual pattern. Heavy bleeding can have many causes, including hormone imbalance, cancer of the uterus (see UTERUS, CANCER OF), miscarriage, infection of the uterus, or blood clotting problems. Heavy bleeding can result in deficient iron, causing anemia. A woman who experiences heavy bleeding should contact her doctor.

IRREGULAR MENSTRUATION A woman may experience a change in her regular pattern of menstruation for a number of reasons, especially when she first begins having periods and when she nears menopause. Irregular cycles can also occur because of illness, weight gain or loss, stress, heavy exercise, or other reasons. Since pregnancy can halt menstruation, a woman should see her doctor if she misses a period.

AMENORRHEA Amenorrhea is the absence of a woman's menstrual periods. Primary amenorrhea is a condition in which a girl has not yet started menstruating by age 16. Secondary amenorrhea is the temporary or permanent absence of menstrual periods in a woman who has previously menstruated regularly; its most frequent cause is pregnancy. A woman should see a doctor if she misses her period.

PREMENSTRUAL SYNDROME (PMS) Some women experience this specific type of physical and mental distress as the menstrual period approaches. Common PMS symptoms include swollen and tender breasts, bloating (retention of water), headache, depression, mood swings, and irritability. The exact cause of PMS is unknown; however, most doctors believe it is related to hormonal changes in a woman's body throughout her menstrual cycle. Most treatments are geared toward relieving the symptoms of PMS. The best response to treatment occurs with a class of drugs called serotonin reuptake inhibitors, or SRIs.

DYSMENORRHEA Severely painful menstruation is called dysmenorrhea. Most often, it is treated with analgesics (painkillers) such as ibuprofen. Sometimes, severe menstrual pain may be caused by a tumor, infection, or endometriosis, a condition in which tissue that lines the uterus also grows outside its usual location, such as outside the uterus. When a specific cause for the pain is diagnosed, treatment for the underlying problem may be needed.

Mental illness

Any of a number of disorders that disturb a person's thoughts, emotions, and behavior. Some mental illnesses cause relatively mild distress, while others result in severe impairment and may require hospitalization. Treatment depends on the nature of the illness and the severity of the symptoms.

Mental retardation

A disorder characterized by below-average intellectual function accompanied by deficits in behavior that occurs before age 18 years. The cause of retardation in most children is not known. However, some of the most common causes include genetic disorders such as Down syndrome and fragile X syndrome and environmental factors (such as maternal alcohol abuse during pregnancy). Other causes include brain damage from head injury or infection, such as bacterial meningitis.

Parents are often the first to notice that an infant is not developing on schedule. He or she may lag in developmental milestones such as rolling over, sitting, crawling, smiling, or walking. This is usually known as developmental delay and is a sign of possible mental retardation.

If mental retardation is suspected, an assessment of intellectual function and age-appropriate adaptive behavior must be made by a qualified professional. Indications of a problem are low scores (below 70) on a standard intelligence quotient (IQ) test. There is no cure for mental retardation. Treatment focuses on helping each individual reach his or her own maximum potential.

Mental status examinations

Careful examination by a physician, usually a psychiatrist or neurologist, to determine how well and how normally a person's mind is functioning. The physician checks the person's appearance and behavior, rapport, mood and emotional state, speech, thinking, content of thoughts, cognitive functions, and judgment.

Mercury

A metallic element that is liquid at room temperature. Mercury was used widely in medications and as disinfectants for many years, but its use has been greatly reduced because of concerns about toxic effects.

Mercury poisoning occurs when metallic mercury is absorbed through the skin or its vapor taken in through the lungs. Acute poisoning causes vomiting, bloody diarrhea, and severe abdominal cramps in addition to the inability to produce urine. Chronic poisoning causes loose teeth, loss of appetite, sores in the mouth, tremors, anemia, and irritability. If someone is suspected of having consumed or absorbed metallic mercury, a poison center should be contacted immediately.

Mesentery

A supporting membrane that attaches various internal organs to the abdominal wall. The term is most frequently used to refer to the part of the peritoneum that enfolds most of the small intestine and attaches it to the rear wall of the abdominal cavity. The mesentery contains the arteries, veins, nerves, and lymphatic

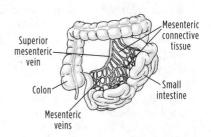

Superior mesenteric vein

Mesenteric connective tissue

Colon

Small intestine

Mesenteric veins

Supporting and connecting
The mesentery is a heavily veined tissue that supports the organs in the abdomen and connects them to the abdominal wall.

vessels that supply the large and small intestines.

Mesothelioma

A rare cancerous tumor of the membranes that line the abdominal and chest cavities and cover the lungs. Mesothelioma is strongly associated with long-term exposure to asbestos. Symptoms of mesothelioma of the lung can include shortness of breath, vague chest pain that may radiate to the shoulders or upper abdomen, loss of appetite and weight, fatigue, hoarseness, and general weakness. Symptoms of mesothelioma in the abdominal cavity can include nausea, vomiting, bowel and urinary obstruction, swelling of the legs and feet, and fever. Symptoms of pleural mesothelioma (in the chest cavity lining) may include pain in the lower back or chest or shortness of breath.

Diagnosis of mesothelioma involves chest X rays and CT (computed tomography) scans. Biopsy may be needed. Surgery is the most common treatment of mesothelioma, although radiation therapy is frequently used, too.

Mesothelium

A type of epithelium (surface cell layer) that lines the body cavities of the peritoneum (the membrane lining the abdominal cavity), the pleura (the membranes that cover the lungs), and the pericardium (the membrane surrounding the heart). Malignant tumors of this lining are often related to asbestos exposure.

Metabolism

The entire range of biochemical processes by which living things transform substances into energy.

Metabolism is commonly used to refer to the breakdown of food and its transformation into energy, but it incorporates all chemical and physical changes that take place within the body and enable it to grow and function.

Metabolism incorporates two component processes: catabolism and anabolism. Catabolism refers to the breakdown of nutrients or other organic constituents of the body by which energy is liberated and used for other physical processes. Anabolism refers to the building of complex substances from simple ones. The body uses these complex substances to make up tissues and organs.

Metabolism, inborn errors of

A group of inherited disorders of metabolism, many of which are associated with mental retardation. Inborn errors of metabolism usually involve deficiencies of enzymes needed to carry out an important chemical reaction. In most cases, affected infants appear normal at birth, but over time their development slows and symptoms emerge. These may include behavioral disorders, mental retardation, and muscular abnormalities. Inborn errors of metabolism vary in their symptoms and severity.

Some progress has been made in the treatment of some metabolic disorders, whether by providing supplements to counteract the inborn deficiency or by regulating the diet to minimize the effect of the metabolic or enzyme deficiency.

Metaplasia

Cells that appear abnormal under a microscope yet do not show signs of malignancy. Metaplasia is an acquired condition, in which normal tissue is transformed into what may or may not be premalignant tissue. For example, squamous metaplasia of the cervix refers to a change in the cells on the surface of the cervix that is part of a normal repair process.

Metastasis

The spread of disease, usually cancer, from one part of the body to another; a growth of cancer cells far from the original cancer site. When cancer spreads, it is still named after the part of the body where it first developed. If prostate cancer has spread to the lungs, for example, it is still considered prostate cancer. Metastasis involves the spread of cancer cells through the bloodstream or the lymphatic system. Surgeons removing cancerous tumors usually try to remove nearby lymph nodes as well. Metastases are responsible for many cancer deaths. Early treatment of cancer helps prevent metastasis.

Methadone maintenance

Treatment of a person with heroin addiction to reduce withdrawal symptoms and a craving for the drug. Methadone is a long-acting synthetic narcotic painkiller.

Methanol

Wood alcohol; also called methyl alcohol. Methanol is used as a solvent or fuel and is a clear, colorless, flammable liquid with a characteristic odor. Consumption of even a very small amount of methanol can produce permanent blindness, and 100 milliliters (about 1/2 cup) is likely to be fatal for an adult.

The symptoms of poisoning from methanol include weakness, leg cramps, seizures, breathing difficulties, blurred vision, bluish lips and fingernails, nausea, headache, dizziness, and coma. Permanent blindness can occur after methanol ingestion. If a person is suspected of having consumed methanol, a poison center should be called immediately.

Metrorrhagia

Bleeding from the uterus that occurs between menstrual periods. Causes may include polyps or cancer of the endometrium (see ENDOMETRIAL CANCER), cervicitis, and cancer of the cervix (see CERVIX, CANCER OF). Spotty bleeding sometimes occurs during ovulation. Women who take estrogen therapy may experience metrorrhagia from the medication. See MENSTRUATION, DISORDERS OF.

Microalbuminuria

A condition in which small amounts of the blood protein albumin leak into the urine. Microalbuminuria occurs during the early stages of kidney failure in people with diabetes. The first stage of microalbuminuria and kidney disease in people with diabetes is characterized by an elevated rate of filtration in the kidneys, with the glomeruli (filtering units of the kidneys) showing damage.

At first, microalbuminuria may occur only periodically. However, as the rate of albumin leakage into the urine increases, the condition becomes more constant. People who have type 1 or type 2 diabetes mellitus can remain in the early stages of kidney failure with microalbuminuria for a long time without further kidney damage. Maintaining normal blood pressure and controlling the blood sugar level help prevent rapid progression of the condition.

Microangiopathy

A disease of the very small blood vessels.

Microbe

Any living organism so small it can be viewed only under a microscope. Often, the word is used to describe disease-causing organisms, such as viruses, bacteria, protozoa, and fungi. The words microbe and microorganism have the same meaning. Also, the study of microbes is called microbiology.

Microcephaly

In a newborn, an abnormally small head. Microcephaly is associated with fetal alcohol syndrome, the rare disorder phenylketonuria, Down syndrome, rubella, malnutrition, and exposure to radiation. Once the cause is established, the doctor will help the family determine the appropriate care necessary to help the child develop, because many children born with microcephaly may be developmentally delayed.

Microorganism

See MICROBE.

Microsurgery

Any delicate procedure in which a surgeon views the operation site through a special surgical microscope to operate on small structures within the body. Microsurgical techniques are used on the ear, brain, larynx, and reproductive system, in reconstruction of facial features, and in reattaching severed limbs.

The advantage of microsurgery is that it allows the surgeon accurate and precise access to very small structures.

Middle-ear effusion, persistent

See OTITIS MEDIA.

Midwife

A person trained to assist women in childbirth. Midwives typically provide care and education to women during the prenatal period (see PRENATAL CARE), through labor and delivery, and after the birth of the baby. They promote a noninterventional process of childbirth. While minimizing drug use, they use other approaches to labor pain management such as relaxation methods and breathing techniques. Midwives often handle home deliveries and assist in birthing centers, where they work with a physician.

Migraine

A common form of primary headache. Migraines that are preceded by an aura are known as classic migraines. Other forms of migraine include complicated migraine (with focal neurological symptoms), basilar migraine (with vertigo and occasional loss of consciousness), and ophthalmic migraine (with eye pain and vision loss).

Migraine pain is typically associated with alternate constricting and relaxing of blood vessels in the brain. However, in recent years researchers have also focused attention on alterations in nerve pathways and imbalances in brain chemistry.

There are many possible triggers of migraine pain. Triggers themselves do not cause pain; instead, they activate already existing brain chemical imbalances. Triggers may include hormonal fluctuations caused by birth control pill use, hormone replacement therapy, and premenstrual syndrome. In women who have migraines, more than half occur right before, during, or directly after their period. Migraines diminish in many women following menopause.

Other triggers include physical or mental stress, changes in sleep patterns, allergic reactions, smoking or exposure to secondhand smoke, bright lights, loud noises, alcohol, caffeine, and missed meals. Diet is also widely implicated in migraine.

Migraine headaches are characterized by throbbing pain that most commonly begins on one side of the head. It can start on either side, beginning as a dull ache that gradually worsens into disabling pain, or it can begin abruptly with severe pain from the onset. Migraine attacks occur on a sporadic basis and can last from several hours to several days. Severe pain may be accompanied by other symptoms, such as nausea, vomiting, dizziness, chills, or loss of appetite.

In some cases, migraine pain is preceded by fatigue, depression, or an aura. An aura may consist of dreamlike perceptions or visual disturbances.

Diagnosis of a migraine is based on the nature of the pain, its frequency and duration, location, severity, and accompanying symptoms. In rare cases, a migraine is a warning sign of a potentially serious problem. Diagnostic tests such as CT (computed tomography) scanning, MRI (magnetic resonance imaging), electroencephalogram (EEG), and blood studies may be performed to rule out serious underlying causes of symptoms, such as a ruptured aneurysm, brain tumor, stroke, or meningitis. Doctors recommend immediate medical evaluation for those who experience migraines accompanied by a loss in consciousness; sudden, violent head pain; head pain that worsens over time and is accompanied by symptoms such as nausea, vomiting, fever, and a stiff neck; and head pain that is associated with abnormal neurological functions (including changes in speech, vision, balance, or movement).

Doctors treat migraines with two categories of medications: abortive (to relieve pain and other symptoms) and prophylactic (to prevent migraines from developing). Abortive medications include triptans, vasoconstrictors, lidocaine nasal drops, muscle relaxants, narcotic analgesics, and aspirin and other nonsteroidal anti-inflammatory drugs (NSAIDs). Prophylactic medications include tricyclic antidepressants, serotonin antagonists, cardiovascular drugs (beta blockers and calcium channel blockers), and antiseizure drugs (such as valproic acid).

The mainstay of home care is rest in a dark, quiet room. Many people benefit from regular sleep, exercise, a healthy diet, and avoidance of smoking, alcohol, and caffeine.

Milia

Small, firm, superficial, benign (not cancerous), white bumps typically found on the cheeks and forehead. They are a common condition in newborns that generally disappear without treatment after several weeks. In adults, they may be removed by a dermatologist.

Mind-body medicine

A way of approaching health and illness that emphasizes the intricate relations among mind, body, and spirit and their mutual effects. Many conventional and alternative mind-body interventions exist:

PSYCHOTHERAPY Therapy is the treatment of a person's emotional and psychological health with medication, behavioral modification or reeducation, and ongoing discussion of the person's concerns.

SUPPORT GROUPS Groups such as Alcoholics Anonymous or groups for people who have the same disease help members form bonds with each other and promote sharing of information and experiences.

MEDITATION A self-directed practice for relaxing the body and calming the mind, meditation helps reduce pain, anxiety, and high blood pressure and provides useful techniques for coping with stress.

HYPNOSIS The induction of trance states and the power of suggestion can help a person manage pain, reduce bleeding in people with hemophilia, and lessen the severity of hay fever and asthma attacks, among other common ailments.

YOGA Yoga is a way of life that seeks enlightenment and incorporates dietary practice, physical exercise, and ethical concerns. Yoga is used to reduce anxiety levels, lower blood pressure, reduce cholesterol levels, and help people stop smoking.

Mineral supplements

Dietary supplements containing essential minerals, usually in combination with vitamins. Together, minerals and vitamins are called "micronutrients," substances required in tiny amounts to promote essential biochemical reactions in the cells. The lack of a particular micronutrient for a prolonged period causes a deficiency disease or condition, which can generally be reversed by supplying the lacking micronutrients.

Minerals

Inorganic nutrients that are important for good health.

The human body needs minerals to help regulate cell function and provide structure for cells. Major minerals include calcium, phosphorus, and magnesium. Lesser amounts of other minerals are needed, such as chromium, copper, fluoride, iodine, iron, manganese, molybdenum, selenium, zinc, potassium, and sodium.

Minilaparotomy

A procedure used in tubal ligation, a sterilization method for women. The doctor makes a small incision near the pubic bone and pulls the fallopian tubes (see FALLOPIAN TUBE) through the opening, ties them off with bands or surgical clips, and stitches the incision closed. This procedure is common in other countries but is rarely used in the United States, where laparoscopy is preferred.

Minipills

Birth control pills that contain only progestin. See CONTRACEPTION, HORMONAL METHODS.

Miscarriage

Spontaneous abortion; loss of a pregnancy before the fetus is developed enough to survive outside the uterus, or before approximately 20 weeks of gestation. Fifteen to 20 percent of all pregnancies result in miscarriage. It is more common in women older than 35 years of age and in pregnancies with more than one fetus. A miscarriage often resembles an especially heavy menstrual period.

A pregnant woman who is bleeding should contact a doctor to find out if she is having a miscarriage. Typically, an ultrasound will be conducted; symptoms will be monitored to control bleeding and pain and to confirm that the cervix remains closed. The woman will probably be advised to rest and to avoid intercourse. When bleeding and pain are accompanied by the rupture of the amniotic sac surrounding the fetus and the opening of the cervix, a miscarriage is certain and the process is described as an inevitable miscarriage.

In an incomplete miscarriage (also called an incomplete abortion), a miscarriage occurs, but some of the fetal tissue remains in the uterus. In the condition called a missed miscarriage, or missed abortion, the uterus fails to expel the fetus after it has died. In both incomplete and missed miscarriages, symptoms of pregnancy may begin to disappear. In both situations, a procedure may be performed to remove the contents of the uterus. Most often, when a pregnancy has ended early, a D and C (dilation and curettage) procedure is performed.

Miscarriages can be caused by chromosome abnormalities, anatomical problems in the mother or trauma to the abdomen. The risk for miscarriage is higher in women who smoke or have certain illnesses or conditions, including diabetes; lupus (a disorder of the connective tissue); a hormone imbalance; high blood pressure; and certain infections, such as German measles (rubella), herpes simplex (a sexually transmitted viral infection), and chlamydia (a sexually transmitted bacterial infection).

A woman has a 70 to 80 percent chance of carrying a pregnancy to term after a miscarriage, unless there is a problem with autoimmune antibodies, chromosomal abnormalities, or a weak cervix.

Mitochondrial diseases

Disorders caused by mutations affecting the mitochondria (components of cells that oxidize food for them) in the cells of the body. When genetic mutations affect the mitochondria, disruption in energy supply can be devastating. The most vulnerable cells are those requiring the most energy, such as those in the brain, heart, and skeletal muscles. Most mitochondrial diseases are inherited.

The chief problems associated with mitochondrial diseases are low energy, the production of free radicals (highly charged molecules that can damage DNA and cell membranes by oxidizing them), and a buildup of lactic acid. Because mitochondria are present in cells of all types, mitochondrial diseases can affect many organ systems. For example, in the cardiac system, mitochondrial diseases can cause arrhythmias and heart failure.

There is no simple diagnostic test or procedure for mitochondrial diseases. Blood and urine tests, ECG (electrocardiogram, EKG) or audiogram (hearing test), and ophthalmologic examination may be helpful, as may MRI (magnetic resonance imaging) of the brain, electroencephalogram (EEG), and muscle biopsy.

Mitochondrial diseases cannot be

cured but are managed by treating specific symptoms, both to alleviate them and to slow the progression of the disease. There are few treatments for the underlying diseases.

Mitral insufficiency

Failure of the mitral valve of the heart to close tightly, causing it to leak (regurgitate), decreasing the flow of blood into the body. To compensate, the ventricle pumps harder, and over time it enlarges to compensate. Eventually, the ventricle begins to fail, and lung congestion can result from the pooling of blood in the left atrium. A type of rapid heartbeat known as atrial fibrillation can also develop, and a blood clot may form in the atrium, travel through the bloodstream, and lodge in a blood vessel (see EMBOLISM).

Early in the course of the disease there may be no symptoms, but as the leakage continues, symptoms may include breathlessness (especially during mild exercise or at night), fatigue, and edema (the accumulation of fluid) in the ankles.

Mitral insufficiency can be caused by any condition that weakens or damages the mitral valve, including heart attack, endocarditis (inflammation of the lining of the heart that often involves the heart valves), or rheumatic fever. In some cases, babies are born with mitral insufficiency.

The symptoms of mitral valve insufficiency can be lessened with medications. Diuretics are used to drain excess fluid from the lungs and lower extremities, cardiotonics can strengthen the heartbeat, anticoagulants can prevent blood clots, antibiotics can prevent infection, and angiotensin-converting enzyme (ACE) inhibitors can reduce the workload of the heart and prevent failure. Surgery to repair or replace the valve is also an option. See HEART VALVE SURGERY.

Mitral stenosis

Narrowing of the heart's mitral valve, which connects the atrium (upper chamber) and the ventricle (lower chamber) on the left side of the heart. Since the narrowed valve restricts blood flow, blood pools in the atrium and backs up into the lungs. As the atrium stretches over time, a type of rapid heartbeat known as atrial fibrillation is likely to develop. A blood clot may form in the pooled blood in the atrium and then travel through the bloodstream and lodge in a blood vessel (see EMBOLISM), causing serious damage, particularly to the brain or lungs.

Mild forms of mitral stenosis produce no symptoms, but over time breathlessness with little or no exercise, constant fatigue, frequent bronchitis, chest pain, and palpitations (uncomfortably rapid heartbeat) may occur.

The severity of symptoms of mitral valve stenosis can be reduced with medications such as diuretics or digoxin. Surgery may be needed (see HEART VALVE SURGERY).

Mitral valve prolapse (MVP)

An abnormal bulging backward of the mitral valve when the heart contracts. MVP is the most common heart valve problem, affecting approximately 1 person in 20. It is most likely to occur in women between the ages of 20 and 40 who are thin and have mild forms of back or chest deformities. MVP can also be a sign of Marfan syndrome.

MVP is generally not serious and causes no symptoms; however, it must be monitored to detect those few people in whom complications occur. In a small percentage of cases, MVP causes the mitral valve to regurgitate (leak) excessively. It can also lead to rapid heartbeat, chest pain, fatigue, anxiety and panic attacks, shortness of breath, syncope (fainting), and, rarely, heart failure or sudden death.

If symptoms develop, medications such as beta blockers or antiarrhythmics may be used. In severe cases, surgery is called for. See HEART VALVE SURGERY.

Mittelschmerz

Acute abdominal pain around the time of ovulation.

Mohs surgery

A type of surgery used in the treatment of skin cancer; also known as microscopically controlled surgery.

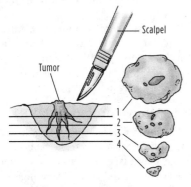

Revealing boundaries of a tumor
Mohs surgery enables the surgeon to see the full extent of a tumor as it grows under the skin. Tint indicates extent of tumor.

In Mohs surgery, which is performed on an outpatient basis using a local anesthetic, a cancerous tumor is removed one thin layer at a time until only healthy tissue remains.

Mold

A parasitic fungus that exists in multicellular colonies; the deposit or growth produced by molds. Molds and their spores are the cause of allergies for many people. Molds thrive in damp locations.

Mole

A colored spot on the skin derived from cells that contain melanin, the pigment that gives skin its color; also known as a nevus. When a mole changes color or shape, it may indicate malignant melanoma (see MELANOMA, MALIGNANT), a serious form of skin cancer.

All abnormal moles should be closely monitored through regular self-examination and periodic appointments with a dermatologist.

Molluscum contagiosum

A viral infection of the skin that produces multiple, firm eruptions that range in color from pearly pink to white and have a central, sunken opening that oozes a white, waxy substance.

The virus is transmitted both by close physical contact and indirectly via contact with contaminated towels or water in a swimming pool. The outbreak can occur almost anywhere on the body, especially in children. Treatment involves removal of the soft central tissue of the eruptions; the surrounding elevations of skin may be removed by freezing or by electrical or chemical burning.

Moniliasis

A fungal infection caused by *Candida* microorganisms, most frequently by *Candida albicans*. Moniliasis rarely causes lesions in the liver, spleen, kidneys, bone, skin, but more commonly is seen in the tissues of the mouth (where it is referred to as oral thrush) or the vagina (when it it called a vaginal yeast infection). Moniliasis is not a contagious infection. *Candida* fungi exist normally not only in the mouth and vagina, but also in the gastrointestinal tract, where their growth is controlled by the presence of normally occurring bacteria. Uncontrolled overgrowth of the fungus may be caused by factors that reduce natural resistance, including illness, stress, and certain medications.

Symptoms of oral thrush include painful, raised sores in the mouth, usually on the tongue or inner cheeks, that have a creamy white appearance. It is diagnosed by evaluation of these characteristic signs; microscopic examination of the tissue from a sore in the mouth can confirm a diagnosis of moniliasis. Antifungal medications including nystatin, clotrimazole, and miconazole, used for 7 to 14 days, can successfully treat the infection. Improved oral hygiene techniques can aid in healing. In adults the presence of thrush suggests as immune deficiency disease such as HIV infection or cancer, so further testing may be required.

The symptoms of moniliasis in the vagina are local itching; irritation; swelling; a thick, white, odorous discharge; discomfort during vaginal intercourse; and frequent urination with stinging or burning. The infection is diagnosed by physical examination and may be confirmed by a culture of cells taken from the vaginal wall. Moniliasis is generally treated successfully with over-the-counter antifungal topical medications (creams or suppositories) for a period of about 7 days.

Monoamine oxidase inhibitors

Antidepressant drugs. Monoamine oxidase inhibitors, also called MAOIs, relieve depression by blocking the action of a chemical substance in the nervous system called monoamine oxidase. There are currently only three MAOIs available orally for prescription in the United States: isocarboxazid, phenelzine, and tranylcypromine.

Monoclonal antibody

See ANTIBODY, MONOCLONAL.

Mononucleosis, infectious

An acute viral disease characterized by fever, sore throat, and swollen glands. Infectious mononucleosis is usually caused by the Epstein-Barr virus (EBV), but may also be caused by the cytomegalovirus (CMV). Both viruses are members of the herpes family. Infectious mononucleosis can be transmitted in saliva, via airborne infectious droplets, or via blood transfusion. Because of the transmission via saliva, mononucleosis is sometimes called "the kissing disease."

The infection occurs in people of all ages, but frequently affects young people between the ages of 15 and 25 years. Symptoms are generally mild in young children, but in older teens and young adults, more severe and prolonged symptoms tend to occur, usually within 4 to 6 weeks of exposure. Typically, the first symptoms to appear include fever, headaches, night sweats, muscle aches, and severe fatigue that requires up to 16 hours of sleep a night. After several days, further symptoms may include sore throat and swollen tonsils, lack of appetite and weight loss, aching joints, abdominal pain, chills, swollen glands in the neck and armpits, and a red rash that generally appears on the chest.

Most symptoms tend to lessen in severity within 10 days but may persist for up to 4 weeks. Fatigue, in particular, may be prolonged. A person who has infectious mononucleosis that enlarges the spleen should be careful to avoid strenuous contact sports for at least 4 weeks after the illness begins, to prevent the risk of a ruptured spleen.

A clinical history, physical examination, and blood tests will confirm diagnosis of mononucleosis. An antiviral medication to treat infectious mononucleosis is not available. Treatment is limited to relieving symptoms with corticosteroid or antibiotic medications.

Bed rest and increased fluid intake are recommended, as is use of ibuprofen or acetaminophen for body aches and fever. Children younger than 18 years should not take aspirin because of the associated risk of Reye syndrome.

Monosodium glutamate

See MSG.

Monounsaturated fats

A type of unsaturated fat that can lower levels of harmful LDL (low-density lipoprotein) cholesterol without also decreasing levels of HDL (high-density lipoprotein cholesterol).

Olive and canola oils are good sources of monounsaturated fats. Avocados and nuts are also sources. See FATS AND OILS.

Morbidity

Loss of physical and psychological health and well-being, whether temporary or permanent. Often morbidity is stated as a rate determined by dividing the total number of people in a group into the number of people who suffer illness or injury. For example, if a sample population of 1,000 people lives in a given city and 50 of them develop influenza (flu), the morbidity rate is 0.05.

Morning sickness

A common set of symptoms, including nausea, vomiting, and food and smell aversions, that affect many pregnant women during the first trimester, usually in the mornings, although they can occur at any time of day. For some women, morning sickness lasts throughout the pregnancy. Morning sickness becomes a serious problem if a woman is unable to keep food or fluids down and begins to lose weight or become dehydrated (see HYPEREMESIS GRAVIDARUM), in which case hospitalization or hydration and medication may be needed.

Morning-after pill

A series of hormonal pills that a woman can take to prevent pregnancy for up to 72 hours after having had unprotected sex or having been the victim of sexual assault. Hormones in the pills inhibit the development of a fertilized egg in the uterus. Taking a morning-after pill does not guarantee that a woman will not become pregnant but significantly reduces the risk. See CONTRACEPTION, EMERGENCY POSTCOITAL.

Mortality rate

A statistic that measures the frequency at which death occurs in a population within a given time.

Morton neuroma

A benign, swollen enlargement of the sheath of nerve that runs across the bottom of the foot and out to the toes. Morton neuroma typically develops in the ball of the foot in the space between the third and fourth toes. The principal symptom is a burning pain in the ball of the foot, often occurring during weight-bearing activities such as walking or using stairs. The pain may also be experienced as an aching, shooting, or tingling pain in the toes. The condition is diagnosed by physical examination or X rays.

Nonsteroidal anti-inflammatory drugs (NSAIDs) such as aspirin or ibuprofen may be recommended. Icing the foot several times a day; wearing wider, low-heeled, and soft-soled shoes; and using a metatarsal pad may help relieve pressure on the nerve and diminish the pain. Orthotics (specially designed shoe inserts) may be recommended, or a cortisone injection may be considered. In some cases, outpatient surgery may be necessary.

Mosaicism

An anomaly of chromosome division resulting in two or more types of cells containing different numbers of chromosomes; also, the occurrence of two or more genetically distinct cell lines in a single organism. Mosaicism may occur normally, as in the case of certain sex-linked genetic traits, or pathologically, as a result of gene mutation.

Motion sickness

A disorder brought on by certain kinds of motion such as being on a boat or ship during rough seas, traveling on an airplane when there is air turbulence, or riding in a car on curving or steep, hilly roads. Mild motion sickness produces a slight upset stomach. When motion sickness is severe, there may be nausea, vomiting, dizziness, sweating, loss of balance, loss of coordination, and physical and mental exhaustion. The cause of motion sickness is excessive stimulation of the vestibular system in the labyrinth (part of the inner ear that controls balance). Overstimulation of the system produces an abnormal perception of the body's movement and position in relation to the environment, creating a sensation of disorientation that produces the symptoms. Medications containing meclizine, cyclizine, scopolamine, diphendydramine, or dimenhydrinate can often be effective for preventing motion sickness when taken before or during travel, but drowsiness is a frequent side effect. The scopolamine skin patch should not be used by children.

Motor neuron disease

A group of rare, progressive disorders in which the nerves that control muscle activity degenerate within the brain and spinal cord. This results in muscle wasting (atrophy) and weakness. The cause of motor neuron disease is unknown.

Amyotrophic lateral sclerosis, or

ALS, is the most common form of motor neuron disease. Other motor neuron diseases include progressive muscular atrophy and progressive bulbar palsy. In younger people, forms include infantile progressive spinal muscular atrophy (Werdnig-Hoffmann paralysis) and chronic spinal muscular atrophy. For symptoms of motor neuron disease, see ALS. Diagnosis of motor neuron disease is made through neuromuscular examination that indicates muscle weakness. Weakness often begins in a single limb or in the shoulders or hips. Examination may also reveal tremors, spasms, fasciculation, and atrophy. There may be abnormal reflexes and a clumsy gait (walk). Tests to confirm diagnosis and rule out other causes include electromyogram (EMG; measurement of muscle electrical activity), blood tests, CT (computed tomography) scanning, and MRI (magnetic resonance imaging).

As there is no cure, the goal of treatment is to control symptoms. Medication may be prescribed to manage spasticity and the ability to swallow. Helpful measures include physical therapy, rehabilitation, and orthopedic appliances (such as a wheelchair). To prevent choking, a tube may eventually be placed into the stomach for feeding. Because mental functioning remains intact, emotional support is vital for the person who is coping with a motor neuron disease.

Mouth cancer

See ORAL CANCER.

Mouth ulcer

A break in the mucous membrane lining the mouth. Traumatic ulcers are those that occur due to injury (such as contact with a jagged tooth or denture). A canker sore generally develops when a person is fatigued, under stress, or ill. A cold sore in or around the mouth is a type of herpes infection. If a sore does not heal within 10 days, it is important to see the doctor. Rarely, a mouth ulcer is a symptom of a more serious underlying condition such as a tumor.

Mouth-to-mouth resuscitation

A technique used to restore oxygen to the lungs of someone who has stopped breathing. Mouth-to-mouth resuscitation is the quickest way to get oxygen into a person's lungs.

The person assisting should begin by tilting the person's head back and lifting the chin, both to open the airway and to move the tongue away from the back of the throat. The person's nose is pinched shut with the rescuer's fingers while a tight seal is made around the person's mouth by the rescuer's mouth. The rescuer will breathe slowly and gently into the person until the chest rises. A breath should be given approximately every 5 seconds, with pauses in between to let the air flow out. If the person remains unresponsive, not breathing or moving, then chest compressions should be started. Rescue breathing should continue until the person begins to breathe on his or her own or until the rescuer is too tired to continue.

Movement disorder

Disorders of the nervous system, muscles, joints, and bones that may impair movement. There are many different types of movement disorders: apraxia is a loss or impairment of the ability to perform purposeful movements; tremor is involuntary, rhythmic muscle movement caused by alternate contraction and relaxation of the muscles. In many cases, problems with movement are a symptom of an underlying medical problem, such as Parkinson disease, multiple sclerosis, head injury, or emotional disorders.

MRI

Magnetic resonance imaging; a diagnostic imaging technique that uses powerful magnetic fields and radio-frequency waves to produce computer-enhanced, cross-sectional images of internal organs and structures. MRI allows physicians to visualize interior body parts with great clarity and without exposure to the radiation involved in the use of X rays. An MRI is generally used to obtain two-dimensional views of an internal organ or structure, particularly of soft tissues (for example, muscles) that do not show up well on regular X rays. The technique is particularly helpful for visualizing internal areas of the nervous system, including the brain and spinal cord. It may also be used to evaluate injuries to the bones and joints. MRI is often used to monitor response to chemotherapy, radiation therapy, or other treatments for cancer and other diseases.

MRI takes between 15 and 60 minutes, depending on the area being examined. A contrast medium may be injected. During the MRI, the person must lie as still as possible on a narrow table that slides into a tubelike chamber. People with claustrophobia may need a sedative to be enclosed in this tubelike chamber for the test.

Newer open MRIs are less claustrophobic.

MRI is considered a safe procedure. The only known risks are for people who have cardiac pacemakers, aneurysm clips in the brain, or specific types of metal implants in the body. The radio-frequency waves of the magnet can cause a pacemaker to malfunction or an aneurysm clip to shift. It is generally safe to undergo an MRI if a person has orthopedic metal implants or surgical clips in the body, but it is important that the radiologist be notified.

MS

See MULTIPLE SCLEROSIS.

MSG

Monosodium glutamate; a food additive that has been reported to cause adverse reactions in susceptible people. Reactions to MSG include headache, nausea, diarrhea, sweating, chest tightness, and a burning sensation at the back of the neck.

Mucocele

A swollen sac or cavity filled with mucus secreted from cells in its inner lining. Also known as mucus cysts, mucoceles consist of clear fluid trapped beneath a thin layer of mucous membrane. They usually appear on the inner surface of the lips. Although mucoceles are harmless and usually painless, they can be bothersome. Treatment may involve surgery.

Mucous membrane

A thin, soft tissue (found throughout the body) that lines a body cavity, passageway, or structure. A mucous membrane secretes mucus, a thick fluid that lubricates the tissue.

Mucus

A thick, viscous fluid produced by mucous glands. Mucus is secreted by glandular cells located within the moist mucous membranes that line many of the body's organs, cavities, and structures, where it functions as a protective barrier, a lubricant, and a carrier of enzymes. Mucus is secreted within the nasal sinuses, the respiratory tract, the gastrointestinal tract, and other structures.

Multi-infarct dementia

See VASCULAR DEMENTIA.

Multiple births

A pregnancy in which a woman is carrying more than one fetus. It occurs when two or more eggs are released simultaneously from the ovaries and are fertilized or when a single fertilized egg divides into two eggs early in development. A pregnancy with two or more fetuses is considered a higher risk pregnancy because multiple fetuses have greater nutritional needs than a single baby and place extra strain on the mother's body.

The risks of certain disorders, including high blood pressure, hydramnios, and postpartum hemorrhage, are higher in multiple-baby pregnancy. Preterm labor is common in multiple births; about half of all multiple births are premature. Premature births are those that occur before the 37th week of pregnancy (full term is considered to be around 40 weeks for one fetus, shorter for multiple births) because the fetuses grow too large for the uterus and trigger uterine contractions.

While twins may sometimes be delivered by vaginal delivery, triplets and quadruplets are usually delivered by cesarean section. Multiple-birth babies are more likely to be of lower than average birth weight.

Multiple chemical sensitivity (MCS)

A syndrome in which a person reports multiple symptoms that he or she believes are due to low-level chemical exposure and that interfere with daily life and work. People with this condition often report symptoms after they have been exposed to an environmental chemical, such as a pesticide or chemical used in a building remodeling. The exposure level is typically low enough that it should not cause symptoms, but after a suspected exposure, the person may have multiple symptoms in response to previously tolerated low-level exposures. Symptoms include fatigue, difficulty concentrating, a depressed mood, memory loss, weakness, taste disturbance, dizziness, headaches, and heat intolerance. In severe cases, people with MCS will alter their behavior to avoid what they presumed brought on their symptoms.

The condition may cause or be associated with psychiatric conditions such as depression and anxiety. Treatment of MCS focuses on helping the person control and manage symptoms, treating any psychiatric illness, and encouraging the person to remain active.

Multiple myeloma

A cancer of the plasma cells. Normal plasma cells are found in the bone marrow and are the part of the body's immune system that produces antibodies. Abnormal plasma cells cause several problems. They compromise the body's ability to fight infections. By multiplying excessively, they reduce the ability of the bone marrow to function properly. Myeloma cells attack and weaken surrounding bone, causing pain and fractures, resulting in elevated calcium levels. The disease can also interfere with kidney function and cause renal failure.

The growth of the plasma cells can produce tumors, usually in the bone marrow and often in more than one site. Called multiple myeloma, the condition commonly produces back pain, which can be mild or severe. Other symptoms include anemia, abnormal bleeding, infections, and poor kidney function.

Multiple myeloma is usually treated with chemotherapy, which can often control the disease for several years but does not cure it. Individuals can be treated with medications that help to prevent bone fractures. Bone marrow transplantation is done on younger patients and can allow them to survive for many years. Radiation therapy is used to reduce bone pain associated with the disease. About a quarter of the people who have been diagnosed with this cancer survive for at least 5 years.

Multiple personality disorder

Another name for a rare dissociative identity disorder, an emotional condition in which a person has two or more distinct identities that surface regularly, control the person's actions, and know little about the other identities; the identities are in conflict with one another. Multiple personality is considered a dissociative disorder because the individual becomes detached, or dissociated, from reality.

When a person is under the control of one of his or her personalities, he or she cannot remember events that happened when another personality was in control. The change from one personality to another is often triggered by stress, and it usually occurs in a matter of seconds. The number of personalities varies from two to more than 100, with fewer than ten being most common.

Multiple personality disorder usually emerges in early life, at approximately age 5 or 6, and is more common in females than males. Physical or sexual abuse is commonly associated with the disorder. The diagnosis remains scientifically controversial. Treatment consists of psychotherapy to help break down the barriers between the different personalities and allow the person to create a single, unified identity.

Multiple sclerosis

Also known as MS, a chronic, often disabling disease of the central nervous system. The symptoms of MS range from mild (such as numbness in the limbs) to severe (including paralysis and loss of vision). The disease is twice as common in women as in men.

Multiple sclerosis is an autoimmune disease (a disease caused by the reaction of a person's immune system against his or her own tissues).

In normal nervous tissue, a fatty substance called myelin protects and coats nerve fibers. In MS, the myelin becomes swollen and inflamed. Eventually, damaged myelin is detached from fibers and is destroyed (demyelination), resulting in the symptoms of MS.

The initial signs of MS are often abnormal sensations, such as pins and needles, and difficulty walking. Some people experience more serious pain and loss of vision as a result of optic neuritis (inflammation of the optic nerve). Less common initial symptoms include tremor, lack of coordination, slurred speech, the sudden onset of paralysis, and a decline in cognitive function (the ability to think, reason, and remember).

As MS progresses, the primary symptoms, which are the result of demyelination, include weakness, numbness, tremor, paralysis, pain, loss of vision, loss of balance, and bowel and bladder dysfunction. The secondary symptoms of MS occur as complications of the primary symptoms. For example, inactivity can lead to decreased bone density, poor posture and trunk control, and weakness from disuse. Paralysis can result in pressure sores.

The tertiary (third-level) symptoms of MS include the social and vocational consequences of the primary and secondary symptoms. Depression is a common problem. Tertiary symptoms are managed by psychologists, social workers, physical and occupational therapists, and public health agencies.

Diagnosis is based on symptoms, medical history, and neurological examination. Tests such as lumbar puncture, evoked responses, and MRI (magnetic resonance imaging) may be performed to confirm the diagnosis. The progression of MS is variable and does not always result in complete disability. Flare-ups (attacks) are often self-limited in the early stages of MS. Some people with MS may have very few attacks and experience few problems. Although there is no cure, medications such as corticosteroids are available to help control symptoms and to slow the progression of the disease. Interferon beta and glatiramer acetate are given to decrease the frequency of flare-ups and ultimately decrease disability.

Mumps

A contagious viral infection that produces swelling in one or both of the two salivary glands located above the angle of the jaw in front of each ear and in the salivary gland located under the tongue.

The virus that causes mumps is spread from person to person via infectious respiratory secretions or saliva. Once it has entered the body, the virus spreads into the bloodstream and may migrate to many different glands, including the testes in a man, the ovaries in a woman, and in both sexes, the pancreas and the brain.

Mumps is very rare in the United States as a result of the effective vaccine against it, generally given to young children as part of the MMR (measles-mumps-rubella) vaccination. However, outbreaks can occur, highlighting the importance of continued vaccination.

The symptoms of mumps tend to be vague but can include fever, headache, sore throat, muscle aches, poor appetite, and fatigue. Most people who have symptoms develop the characteristic painful swelling in one or more salivary glands, often producing tender fullness between the earlobe and the angle of the jaw. Chewing and swallowing can make eating uncomfortable. These symptoms may last for 10 days.

Some postpubertal males develop symptoms of inflammation and infection of the testes, including localized swelling, tenderness, and pain. If a woman's ovaries are involved, she may have pain in the lower abdomen.

Mumps is diagnosed by taking a clinical history to determine possible exposure and by performing a physical examination. The diagnosis can be confirmed by blood tests for antibodies; samples of urine, saliva, or spinal fluid may be tested to detect the virus itself.

There is no antiviral medication to cure mumps. Treatment is based on easing symptoms: acetaminophen for fever and body aches and warm or cold compresses for swollen glands.

Most healthy people who contract mumps recover completely. There is a small risk of sterility in males when both testicles are affected, but this is rare.

Munchausen syndrome

The intentional feigning or production of physical or psychological symptoms out of a deep-seated need to assume the sick role; a mental disorder also known as factitious disorder and pathomimicry. A person with Munchausen syndrome may make up the complaint and support it with lies or inflict injuries on his or her own body, such as injecting material under the skin to produce abscesses. The motivation behind Munchausen syndrome is an unconscious need to be cared for as a sick person. The disorder may result in unneeded medical tests and exploratory surgeries.

In a related disorder known as Munchausen syndrome by proxy, an individual produces or feigns physical or emotional symptoms in another person under his or her care. Usually the victim is a young child, and the person producing the symptoms may be the child's parent or caretaker, most often the mother.

Murmur

See HEART MURMUR.

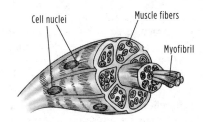

Skeletal muscle
There are three kinds of muscle tissue: skeletal, cardiac, and smooth. Skeletal muscles are thick and thin muscle fibers that permit a person to move when his or her brain tells them to.

Muscle

A fibrous structure in the body composed of cells that can contract or relax to generate movement. Different types of muscles can cause movement of the skeletal framework of the body (skeletal muscle), movement of the tissues of body organs (smooth muscle), or the specialized pumping action of the heart (cardiac muscle). The skeletal muscles, attached to bone, make up slightly less than half of the total body weight of an average person.

Muscle relaxants

Drugs used to relieve pain caused by sprains, spasms, or injuries to skeletal muscles. Skeletal muscle relaxants work by relaxing muscles to relieve stiffness, pain, and spasm. Most muscle relaxants work by acting on the central nervous system. Muscle relaxants include carisoprodol, chlorzoxazone, and methocarbamol. Muscle relaxants can impair a person's ability to drive.

Muscle spasm

Persistent involuntary tightening of one or more muscles, usually causing pain from excessive rigidity. Muscle spasm may be caused by a strain, injury, fracture of a related bone, or chronic overuse of a muscle. It may also be due to a muscle's protective action in the prevention of movement of a body part that is stressed. Pain-relieving and antispasm medications may be prescribed; physical therapy may be helpful.

Muscular dystrophy

A group of genetic diseases characterized by progressive muscle weakness and loss of muscle tissue, particularly of the muscles used to control movement. There are nine major forms of muscular dystrophy (MD). The type called Duchenne MD is the most common and most devastating and usually affects children, while the myotonic form most often occurs in adults.

The chief symptoms are related to progressive muscle weakness that gets worse over time. Depending on the type of MD, frequent falls, delayed development of motor skills, difficulty walking, drooping eyelids, drooling, and difficulty using specific muscle groups may be symptoms. Other symptoms may include skeletal deformities, muscle deformities, clawfoot, clawhand, and hypotonia, or decreased muscle tone. Muscle tightness is common and involves shortened muscle fibers around the joints, inhibiting joint mobility. Loss of muscle mass, or wasting, is also common. Some types of MD are associated with mental retardation.

The primary method by which MD is diagnosed is muscle biopsy. Other diagnostic aids include electromyography (EMG), a test used to determine whether muscle weakness is caused by destruction of muscle tissue or by damage to nerves, and a blood test to determine the level of serum creatine kinase (CK) an enzyme found in muscle cells. Because MD is inherited, there is usually a family history of the disorder.

There is no known cure for MD. Treatment is aimed at controlling symptoms to improve the person's quality of life. Physical therapy is used to prevent shortening of the muscles and to maintain muscle strength.

Muscular system

The more than 600 muscles that are attached to and supported by the bones of the skeleton. These muscles shorten or lengthen to move the bones to which they are attached. These movements are voluntary, or under conscious control. Together, the muscles and bones form the moving framework of the body referred to as the musculoskeletal system.

Musculoskeletal system

The muscles, bones, and joints that form the moving structural frame of the body. See JOINT; MUSCULAR SYSTEM; and SKELETAL SYSTEM.

Mutagen

An agent that can cause a change in a gene. Mutagens can alter the genetic makeup of cells by changing the structure of their DNA; these changes can increase the rate of mutation. Examples of mutagens include several kinds of radiation, X rays, ultraviolet light, many chemicals, and some viruses.

Mutation

A permanent structural change in the genetic material of a cell that can be passed on to subsequent generations.

Mutations usually appear in single genes and result from changes in the DNA (deoxyribonucleic acid). Most mutations either have no effect or are harmful, causing cancers, birth defects, and hereditary diseases. Some mutations, however, can improve the survival chances of an organism.

A mutation can originate from a fault in the copying of a cell's DNA during cell division. Mutations can also occur from direct damage to the DNA by a MUTAGEN.

Myalgia

Muscle pain, often due to an overuse stress injury, that is generally caused by using the muscles in a new or unusual activity for a prolonged period of time. Myalgia is also common in people with a fever or viral infection.

Myasthenia gravis

Also known as MG, a chronic neuromuscular disease that affects the voluntary muscles of the body. Myasthenia gravis is an autoimmune disease (a disease caused by the reaction of a person's immune system against his or her own tissues). Myasthenia gravis can affect anyone, but is most common in young adult women and older men. In this disease, the voluntary muscles become weak and tire easily. Chronic weakness improves with rest and worsens with activity. Certain muscles are involved more often than others. These include the muscles that control eye movement, chewing, coughing, swallowing, and facial expression. Muscles that control the arms and legs may also be affected. Shortness of breath occurs when the breathing muscles become weakened.

Diagnosis is based on symptoms and medical history. The doctor may also order tests such as an electromyogram (EMG), which is a special test to evaluate muscle strength; nerve conduction studies; and blood tests for abnormal antibodies.

There is no known cure for myasthenia gravis. However, long-term remission is possible. Treatments include anticholinesterase medications and plasmapheresis (a blood-cleansing technique). If symptoms are severe, prednisone, a corticosteroid, may be prescribed. In some cases, surgical removal of the thymus is recommended.

Mycoplasma

A group of very small bacteria. Three types of Mycoplasma cause disease in humans. *Mycoplasma pneumoniae* is responsible for a mild type of bronchitis and pneumonia that is particularly common in adolescents and young adults. *Mycoplasma hominis* causes kidney disease, pelvic inflammatory disease, vaginal infections, and postpartum fever (after childbirth). *Ureaplasma urealyticum* infects the lower urinary tract, producing inflammation and a burning sensation upon urination. Mycoplasma infections are usually treated with antibiotics.

Mycosis

A system-wide fungal infection or disease. In people who are otherwise in good health, mycosis tends to be chronic, usually with mild symptoms, but sometimes produces fever, chills, night sweats, loss of appetite and weight, malaise, and psychological depression. When the fungus causing mycosis is inhaled into the lungs and spreads from there it can affect various organs of the body. The liver, spleen, and bone marrow may be involved; when the brain becomes involved, chronic meningitis develops.

Blood tests can detect mycosis by isolating antibodies to the specific fungus involved. The causative fungus can be detected in samples of sputum, urine, blood, bone marrow, or infected tissues. Mycosis can be treated with systemic antifungal medications.

Myectomy

The surgical removal of all or a part of a muscle.

Myelin

The fatty substance covering and protecting nerves. The sheath of myelin formed around the nerves speeds the transmission of electrical impulses along the nerve cells and acts as an electrical insulator.

Myelitis

Inflammation of the spinal cord. Myelitis is often the result of a viral disease, such as polio, measles, or herpes. Transverse myelitis is a type of myelitis in which there is demyelination (loss of the fatty tissue around the nerves) of the spinal cord. It may be caused by viral infection, spinal cord injury, an immune reaction, insufficient blood flow through the blood vessels in the spinal cord, or as a complication of diseases (for example, multiple sclerosis, smallpox, or chickenpox). Symptoms may include low back pain, spinal cord dysfunction, muscle spasms, discomfort, headache, loss of appetite, and numbness or tingling in the legs. Although there is no specific treatment for transverse myelitis, recovery usually

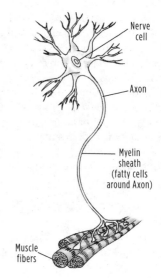

Insulating sheath
Myelin assists the function of a nerve cell by protecting and insulating the axon that carries the cell's electrical impulse. The so-called myelin sheath is composed of fatty cells surrounding the axon at intervals along its length.

begins within 2 to 12 weeks after its onset and may continue for up to 2 years. However, most people are left with considerable disability. Depending on the cause, the disabilities include motor, sensory, and sphincter (bowel) deficits.

Myelocele

A developmental defect of the central nervous system in which a portion of the spinal cord protrudes through a congenital cleft in the vertebral column. See SPINA BIFIDA.

Myelodysplastic syndrome

A group of related, progressive disorders of the bone marrow characterized by low populations of abnormally developed blood cells. Since myelodysplastic syndrome precedes the development of acute leukemia in approximately one case in four, it is sometimes called preleukemia. The current understanding of this disease is that all blood cells (white, red, and platelets) develop from a single line of precursor cells, and this single line is abnormal. At about the time the abnormal cells are ready to enter the bloodstream, they self-destruct. Thus, the bone marrow is packed tight with abnormally developing blood cells, but the number of cells in the blood is unusually low. The cells that do appear in the bloodstream typically do not perform their functions as well as normal cells.

Exposure to radiation and benzene are known to increase the risk of developing myelodysplastic syndrome. In many cases, however, there is no clear-cut cause.

All forms of myelodysplastic syndrome produce severe anemia (low number of red blood cells), pallid skin, fatigue, and breathlessness after mild exertion. Leukopenia (low white blood cell count) increases susceptibility to infection, which often causes fever. The population of platelets, which have key roles in clotting the blood, is also low, leading to nosebleeds, unusually heavy bleeding after injury or surgery, or petechiae (small hemorrhages under the skin), and possibly an enlarged spleen.

A significant number of cases are discovered before symptoms develop, usually as a result of routine blood tests during a medical examination. The diagnosis is confirmed by a bone marrow biopsy or bone biopsy.

In younger people, myelodysplastic syndrome is treated in the same way as acute leukemia. See LEUKEMIA, ACUTE MYELOGENOUS, for details.

Myelography

X-ray examination of the spinal cord. Doctors perform myelography when more commonly used tests such as MRI (magnetic resonance imaging) and CT (computed tomography) scanning do not provide enough information to make a diagnosis of problems such as herniated disks.

Myeloma, multiple

See MULTIPLE MYELOMA.

Myelomeningocele

The most severe form of spina bifida. In this developmental defect of the central nervous system, a portion of the spinal cord itself protrudes through the back. Tissues and nerves may be covered by skin or exposed. It can be associated with a defect called Chiari malformation type II, in which the base of the brain pushes down through the foramen magnum (the opening in the skull for the spinal cord).

Surgery is performed in the first 48 hours of life to drain spinal fluid and protect children against hydrocephalus, an accumulation of fluid in the brain. If hydrocephalus occurs, it is controlled by shunting (the implantation of a shunt or drain to relieve fluid buildup and prevent complications, such as brain damage, seizures, and blindness). Infants can survive myelomeningocele, but usually with serious problems.

Myelopathy

Symptoms of spinal cord impairment from spinal cord disease. Types of myelopathy include syphilitic myelopathy and cervical spondylotic myelopathy.

Syphilitic myelopathy

This is a rare form of neurosyphilis, which is a progressive, destructive, life-threatening infection of the brain and spinal cord that occurs in some cases of untreated syphilis. Syphilitic myelopathy causes a progressive degeneration of the spinal cord and peripheral nerve tissue. There is increasing weakness of the arms and legs that may lead to paralysis.

Diagnosis of neurosyphilis is made with blood tests, a cerebrospinal fluid VDRL test, lumbar puncture, CT (computed tomography) scanning or MRI (magnetic resonance imaging), and a cerebral angiogram. Treatment is with antibiotics such as penicillin.

Cervical spondylotic myelopathy

Compression of the spinal cord in the neck affects primarily older adults. Symptoms develop slowly and may include stiffness, numbness, pain, and weakness. Cervical spondylotic myelopathy causes problems with walking. Diagnosis is made through physical examination and tests such as MRI. Treatment of mild cases is with neck braces or traction; more serious cases may require surgery.

Myelopathy can also be caused by multiple sclerosis, transverse myelitis, spinal cord ischemia (loss of blood flow), or a tumor. When patients have symptoms of myelopathy, tests including MRI of the spinal cord, myelogram, and lumbar puncture should be performed.

Myeloproliferative disorders

A group of related and highly similar diseases that involve abnormally high production of certain kinds of blood cells because of malfunction of the bone marrow. The myeloproliferative diseases differ from one another in the primary type of blood cell affected. Normal bone marrow contains cells, known as hematopoietic cells or stem cells, that have the ability to reproduce themselves into what is known as a clone. Each clone can produce different cell lines that develop into red blood cells, one of several kinds of white blood cells, and platelets (cells that have key roles in blood clotting). In normal bone marrow, a number of clones are active in producing normal blood cells in normal proportions. In the myeloproliferative disorders, an abnormal clone takes over from the others, producing blood cells of one type that are essentially normal yet far too abundant, while the number of other blood cell types may be too low.

All myeloproliferative disorders are diagnosed by means of blood tests to count the numbers of different types of blood cells and examination under a microscope of a small sample (biopsy) of bone and bone marrow.

Polycythemia vera

The distinguishing characteristic of polycythemia vera is an abnormally high number of red blood cells. In most cases, the numbers of granulocytes, which are a type of white blood cell, and platelets, which have key roles in blood clotting, are also too high. The added mass of blood cells causes the blood to be thicker and stickier than normal and increases the blood volume. In a sense, a person with polycythemia vera has too much blood. Symptoms include headache, ringing in the ears, vertigo, blurred vision, hypertension (high blood pressure), nosebleeds, abnormally heavy menstrual periods in women, pain in the upper digestive system, gout, difficulty concentrating, inflamed veins because of blood clots (thrombophlebitis, which principally affects the legs), numbness or tingling in the hands or feet, and enlargement of the spleen and liver. Polycythemia vera usually develops slowly and insidiously.

The primary treatment for polycythemia vera is periodic removal (phlebotomy) of a limited amount of blood to reduce the volume of the blood and lower the red blood cell count. Drugs that suppress the bone marrow and slow blood cell production, such as hydroxyurea and interferons, are often used, too.

In many cases, these treatments are sufficient, and the person lives a normal life. In some people, however, the disease becomes more severe, entering what is known as the spent phase, when the bone marrow becomes heavily scarred and blood cell production falters and fails. If this occurs, a bone marrow transplant (see BONE MARROW TRANSPLANT, ALLOGENEIC) is a possible treatment.

Chronic myeloid leukemia

A myeloproliferative disease characterized by an abnormal increase in white blood cells. This disease is also known as chronic myelocytic leukemia, chronic myelogenous leukemia, and chronic granulocytic leukemia. Chronic myeloid leukemia (see LEUKEMIA, CHRONIC MYELOID) is a progressive disease that is most common among the middle-aged.

Essential thrombocytosis

An excessively high number of platelets is the identifying characteristic of this myeloproliferative disease. These platelets tend to clump together in the blood. The result is both unusual bleeding, such as from the nose, gums, and digestive tract, and blood clots that can block blood vessels, causing blood clots in the legs, heart attack, or stroke. Other symptoms include visual disturbances, fatigue, heavy menstrual periods in women, enlargement of the liver and the spleen, numbness or tingling, skin itching, and ringing in the ears.

Medication is the primary treatment. Aspirin is used to lower the risk of clotting, while hydroxyurea and interferons suppress the bone marrow and reduce the number of platelets. Unless essential thrombocytosis progresses to acute leukemia, prospects for long-term survival are good with consistent monitoring.

Myelofibrosis with myeloid metaplasia

In this myeloproliferative disorder, the normal bone marrow is replaced by scar tissue, and blood cell formation occurs outside the marrow in the spleen and liver; the spleen is usually enlarged. Myelofibrosis with myeloid metaplasia occurs primarily in middle-aged and older adults and rarely in children. The only cure for myelofibrosis with myeloid metaplasia is a bone marrow transplant (see BONE MARROW TRANSPLANT, ALLOGENIC).

Myocardial infarction

The medical term for heart attack.

Myocarditis

Inflammation of the myocardium (the heart muscle). Myocarditis is uncommon and usually causes few or no symptoms, with recovery in several weeks. In a small percentage of cases, symptoms are severe enough to require hospitalization and treatment for heart failure and other complications, such as cardiac arrhythmia (irregular heart rhythm), cardiomyopathy (impaired heart muscle function), pulmonary embolism (a blood clot that can lodge in the lungs), or stroke. The disease is most common among middle-aged men, but can affect both sexes at any age.

Myoclonus

A spasm of a muscle or group of muscles. In epilepsy (a brain disorder in which clusters of nerve cells in the brain sometimes signal abnormally), myoclonic seizures cause twitches or jerks of the arms, legs, or upper body. In most people, seizures are controlled with antiepileptic drugs such as carbamazepine, valproate, and phenytoin.

Myoglobin

A protein found in muscle cells containing iron. Myoglobin takes oxygen from the blood and releases it to muscles during strenuous exercise, where it generates energy by burning the blood sugar (glucose). Normally myoglobin is continually released in small amounts into the bloodstream. However if muscle tissue is damaged as in a heart attack, larger amounts of myoglobin are released and blood levels rise rapidly. Myoglobin is one of the first tests done to determine if a person with chest pain is having a heart attack, because it may be one of the first blood tests to become abnormal.

Damage or injury to skeletal muscle also causes myoglobin to be released into the blood usually in even larger amounts than seen in a heart attack. In a crush injury, for example, myoglobin released in large amounts because of extensive muscle damage can cause kidney damage.

Myomectomy

A surgical procedure for removing uterine fibroids (also called myomas). In this procedure, only the fibroids are removed, leaving the remaining uterus intact. Women who have had myomectomies are more likely to require delivery by cesarean section if they become pregnant. Fibroids recur in about 20 percent of women who have undergone myomectomy. See also FIBROID, UTERINE.

Myopathy

Any primary disease or disorder of the muscle tissue, including fibromyalgia, muscular dystrophy, and myositis.

Myopia

See NEARSIGHTEDNESS.

Myositis

Inflammation of muscle.

Myositis ossificans

Abnormal bone formation in a muscle usually located near the elbow joint. It usually occurs from muscle damage or as a complication of a fracture. It can also be a common complication of thigh muscle injuries from contact sports. Treatment may include taking nonsteroidal anti-inflammatory drugs (NSAIDs), such as aspirin or ibuprofen, with a gradual return to range-of-motion exercises. Surgery is usually not considered unless conservative therapy fails to improve symptoms within 6 months.

Myotonia

A disorder of abnormally prolonged contractions of a muscle or group of muscles. Myotonia is a symptom of disorders such as myotonic muscular dystrophy.

Myringitis, bullous

A bacterial or viral inflammation of the eardrum that produces small water or blood blisters on the eardrum and sudden, severe pain in the ear. There may be a yellowish or bloody discharge if the blisters rupture. Bullous myringitis is sometimes mistaken for a ruptured eardrum (see EARDRUM, PERFORATED). Bullous myringitis is generally treated with oral antibiotic medication or ear drops containing one of the corticosteroids and antibiotics. The goal of treatment is to prevent infection of the blisters as they break open. Although bullous myringitis can be extremely painful, it is not considered serious, and the eardrum usually heals within a week or two with proper treatment.

Myringoplasty

A surgical procedure to reconstruct a perforation in the eardrum's membrane when there is no middle ear infection or disease of the ear bones. The procedure seals the middle ear and usually improves hearing. The surgery is performed under local anesthesia through the ear canal.

Myringotomy

A surgical procedure involving an incision into the eardrum to promote drainage of fluid from the middle ear to improve hearing and relieve pain. Myringotomy is generally performed on children who have an accumulation of fluid in the middle ear, called middle ear effusion, which causes pain and impairs hearing. The fluid buildup in the middle ear is often caused by otitis media (inflammation of the middle ear). It may also be caused by a common cold (see COLD, COMMON), allergies, or a respiratory tract infection. The buildup of pus and mucus puts pressure on the eardrum, causing pain, swelling, and redness. Because the eardrum does not vibrate properly, hearing is impaired. In some cases, the eardrum may rupture as a result of the pressure against it (see EARDRUM, PERFORATED).

If myringotomy alone is performed, the incision made in the eardrum is likely to heal and close before the infection is gone and the fluid has drained. To prevent this, the surgeon usually inserts a tube, called a ventilation tube, into the middle ear.

Myxedema

A condition characterized by dry, puffy skin and swelling around the lips and nose. It is a feature of the most severe type of HYPOTHYROIDISM (a slowing of metabolism due to decreased activity of the thyroid gland). Other symptoms include intolerance of the cold, hair loss, decreased energy, hoarseness, muscle aches, constipation, weight gain, and memory loss. Left untreated, myxedema can lead to coma and death. Myxedema is diagnosed with thyroid function blood tests. Synthetic thyroid hormones are used to treat myxedema.

Myxoma

A noncancerous tumor occurring in soft tissue, such as muscles and ligaments. Myxoma is a jelly-like tumor that usually develops under the skin. The uncommon tumors may also appear in the jaw bones or within muscles. Myxomas can grow very large.

Narcolepsy

A disabling neurological sleep disorder characterized by overwhelming daytime drowsiness and sudden collapses into sleep. (See also SLEEP DISORDERS.) Narcolepsy is related to REM (rapid eye movement) sleep, the dreaming state of sleep.

Symptoms generally develop after age 15. Narcolepsy has four classic symptoms: excessive daytime sleepiness, cataplexy (sudden loss of voluntary muscle control, ranging from slurred speech to total physical collapse), sleep paralysis (a temporary inability to move or speak while sleeping or upon waking up), and hallucinations.

Although early diagnosis and treatment are important, narcolepsy is often misdiagnosed. Diagnosis is made according to medical history and with tests such as an overnight polysomnogram (PSG, which records
various physiological functions while a person sleeps) and the multiple sleep latency test (MSLT, to test how quickly and deeply people fall asleep).

Other possible tests include an electroencephalogram (EEG).

There is no cure for narcolepsy. However, symptoms can be controlled through medications and lifestyle changes. The goal of treatment is to keep a person alert during the day and to minimize occurrences of cataplexy. Amphetamines and other stimulants have traditionally been used to treat excessive daytime sleepiness. Today the new nonamphetamine drug modafinil is available to promote wakefulness.

Narcotics

Analgesics (painkillers); sleep-inducing drugs. Narcotics act on the central nervous system to relieve pain. No matter what the reason for their use, any narcotics used for a long time can potentially cause physical and psychological dependence. Physical dependence can cause symptoms of withdrawal when the narcotic is stopped.

Narcotics are prescribed in the United States to relieve pain, help anesthesia work more effectively, treat severe diarrhea, relieve coughs, treat pulmonary edema, and suppress heroin dependence.

The most widely used illegal narcotic is the opioid heroin: 90 percent of all street drug narcotic abuse involves heroin. Other opiates that are abused include morphine, codeine, and methadone. Long-term effects include the loss of resistance to disease and infection, inflammation of veins, bronchial congestion, hepatitis, blood infection, and skin abscesses.

Nasal polyps

Small saclike growths on the mucous membrane lining the inside of the nostrils. Nasal polyps protrude into the nasal cavity, appearing singly or in clusters, and are pearly gray. The polyps originate near the sinuses at the top of the nose and grow into the open areas of the nasal cavity. They are not true polyps because the growth is not new or abnormal tissue, but rather swollen tissue inside the nose. One-sided nasal polyps tend to be nonmalignant, while bilateral (two-sided) polyps may be malignant.

The symptoms of nasal polyps include difficulty breathing, an impaired sense of smell and taste, headache, and a runny nose. The nasal passages tend to feel blocked and never seem to clear completely. Large polyps can obstruct the airways. Nasal polyps can cause recurrent sinus infections. While antihistamines and decongestants may help prevent nasal polyps by keeping the nasal passages dry and clear, these medications will not relieve the symptoms when nasal polyps are already established.

Polyps are a consequence of chronic inflammation of the nasal lining, possibly from asthma, hay fever, nasal allergies, chronic sinus infections or, sometimes, CYSTIC FIBROSIS. Polyps will usually respond to a corticosteroid drug. When nasal polyps do not respond to medication, surgery becomes an option.

NASH

See NONALCOHOLIC STEATOHEPATITIS.

Nasogastric tube

A thin, flexible, plastic tube that is passed through the nose down into the stomach. Its purpose is to provide a pathway for nourishment or to drain away secretions. Doctors may insert a nasogastric tube in cases such as a gastrectomy, surgical removal of all or part of the stomach; intestinal perforation, a hole or erosion most often caused by a peptic ulcer; or pyloric stenosis, partial or complete blockage of the outlet from the stomach to the duodenum.

Nasopharynx

The area connecting the nasal passages with the part of the pharynx (throat) that lies above the soft palate in the back of the mouth. The nasopharynx is part of the respiratory tract through which air passes into the lungs. When a person swallows, the soft palate moves back against the top of the throat to seal off the nasopharynx so that food does not enter it.

Nasopharynx, cancer of

A disease in which malignant cells are found in the tissues of the nasopharynx. It occurs most commonly among people who are heavy cigarette smokers. Cancer of the nasopharynx usually occurs after the age of 50 and is more common in men than in women. One known risk factor for this cancer is infection by the Epstein-Barr virus (a herpesvirus that causes mononucleosis).

There may be no symptoms, or early symptoms might be similar to the symptoms of infections of the respiratory tract. If these symptoms linger for 2 weeks or more, a physician should be consulted. Symptoms that may appear as the cancer progresses include difficulty with breathing or speaking, frequent headaches, a lump in the nose or neck, pain or ringing in the ear, recurrent blood in the saliva or nasal secretions, and impaired hearing.

Cancer of the nasopharynx is most effectively treated when diagnosed and treated in its early stages. Possible treatments for cancer of the nasopharynx include radiation therapy; surgery; chemotherapy; and participation in a clinical trial, possibly using biological therapy or IMMUNOTHERAPY.

National Institute of Occupational Safety and Health (NIOSH)

The federal agency responsible for conducting research and making recommendations about the prevention of work-related disease and injury. NIOSH is part of the Centers for Disease Control and Prevention (CDC).

National Institutes of Health (NIH)

One of the eight health agencies of the Public Health Service, which is part of the US Department of Health and Human Services. Founded in 1887, the NIH is the focal point for medical research in the United States. The NIH's goal is to acquire new knowledge to help prevent, detect, diagnose, and treat disease and disability.

Natural childbirth

Methods of vaginal delivery that emphasize pain management using relaxation and other techniques rather than pain-relieving drugs. Pain management techniques may include massage, changing of body positions, meditation, taking a warm shower, or breathing techniques. Part of natural childbirth includes eliminating fear and tension through preparation. It usually involves a partner or coach, usually the father, who provides emotional support and helps the mother use the various relaxation techniques in labor. Typically, a few months before the baby is born, the mother and partner attend childbirth classes where both learn what to expect during childbirth, as well as techniques for breathing and relaxation intended to make labor more comfortable.

Natural family planning

Prevention of pregnancy by abstaining from sexual intercourse when conception is likely to take place. Most women ovulate and are most fertile in the middle of the menstrual cycle. Complicating matters, the first half of the menstrual cycle is more variable than the second half, making it difficult to predict exactly when a woman will ovulate. Using the rhythm method successfully requires a couple's absolute ability to identify the fertile time and follow the rules of the method. However, about 25 percent of those using the rhythm method have an unintended pregnancy within a year.

In natural family planning, there are three methods commonly used to find out when a woman is ovulating. In one method, the woman takes her temperature every morning before getting out of bed and records it on a chart. A second method involves the woman's monitoring of the changes in her vaginal secretions. The third method involves a combination of taking the woman's temperature every day and checking for signs of ovulation, including breast tenderness, abdominal cramps, vaginal spotting, and changes in the firmness of the cervix. See CONTRACEPTION, OTHER METHODS.

Nausea

For symptom chart, see NAUSEA OR VOMITING, page xxv.

A sensation of having an upset stomach or needing to vomit. Nausea can be a symptom of a wide variety of conditions ranging from the morning sickness of pregnancy to a stomach virus or indigestion.

Navel

The scar on the abdomen that marks the site where the umbilical cord connecting mother to fetus during pregnancy was attached to the fetus. The medical word for the navel is the umbilicus.

Nearsightedness

A focusing (refractive) error of the eyes that makes it difficult to see distant objects clearly; also known as myopia. In most cases of nearsightedness, the eyeball is overly long from front to back. As a result, the distance

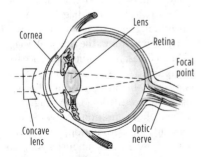

Correcting Nearsightedness

Eyeglasses or contact lenses refocus light rays so that the focal point falls on the retina.

is too great for the lens to focus incoming light rays on the retina (the thin, light-sensitive layer of nerve tissue at the back of the eye that relays visual information to the brain). Nearsightedness can also result from too much focusing power in the lens and cornea (the clear covering on the exposed surface of the eye). In both types of nearsightedness, distant objects are blurry while close ones are clear.

Nearsightedness is most frequently treated with glasses or contact lenses that correct the focusing error. People who do not wish to wear glasses or contact lenses may choose refractive surgery, which permanently alters the shape of the eye to correct faulty vision.

Neck

The narrow structure of the body that connects the trunk to the head. The neck is a complex structure of muscles, organs, blood vessels, and nerves surrounding the upper spine. Seven bones called the cervical vertebrae form the core of the neck and support the head. The cervical vertebrae fit together like a stack of rings, allowing them to rotate the head and move it back and forth. The spinal cord passes through the cervical vertebrae and into the trunk. A number of nerves, such as those connecting with the arm, branch off the spine in the neck.

Neck dissection, radical

A surgical procedure to remove lymph nodes, which are small glands that act as a filter and as a barrier to infection (see LYMPH NODE) and that may be involved in cancer of the head and neck. There are about 300 lymph nodes located in the head and neck. Cancers in the head and neck may spread to the lymph nodes in the neck and need to be removed.

Neck injuries

Injuries to the neck or cervical spinal cord. Symptoms of a neck injury include stiff neck, a head held in an unusual position, weakness, difficulty walking, paralysis of legs or arms, neck pain, loss of bladder or bowel control, or numbness or tingling in an arm or leg. Neck injuries can be extremely serious and can lead to loss of sensation and function in the parts of the body below the site of the injury. When someone has a cervical spinal injury, any additional movement can cause further damage to the spine. The purpose of first aid for any neck injury is to prevent further harm to the person while emergency medical care is sought. The person should be kept absolutely immobile. Headgear, such as a helmet, should not be removed. The person should be kept warm to help prevent shock. Breathing should be checked and arti-

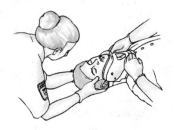

Placing a collar
A person who may have a neck injury should not be moved until trained help arrives, if possible. The medical team may apply a plastic collar to help prevent further injury from neck movement.

ficial respiration or cardiopulmonary resuscitation (CPR) administered if necessary. Any external bleeding should be stopped by applying pressure.

Necrosis

The death or decay of tissue in a part of the body, such as a bone. Necrosis occurs when not enough blood is supplied to tissue. See also GANGRENE.

Necrotizing enterocolitis

A life-threatening intestinal disease in infants. Necrotizing enterocolitis can cause the death of intestinal tissue and can lead to scarring, narrowing, or rupture of the bowel. The disease is most common in low-birthweight and premature infants. Its symptoms include intolerance to baby formula, a distended abdomen, and gas in the muscular layers of the intestinal wall. Some infants experience vomiting, diarrhea, blood in the stool, lethargy, and fluctuations in temperature. Severe enterocolitis can create a hole in the intestine. When that happens, an infant may develop peritonitis (a painful inflammation of the lining of the abdominal cavity), go into shock, and possibly die.

The typical infant diagnosed with necrotizing enterocolitis is a newborn who is still in the hospital. Diagnosis is based on the presence of symptoms. X rays, ultrasound scanning, and blood and stool tests are used in confirming the diagnosis. When the condition is suspected, feeding by mouth is stopped, and fluids are given intravenously. A small tube is inserted into the infant's nose, extending down into the stomach, to relieve trapped gas and to allow the bowel to rest.

Necrotizing fasciitis

A severe, life-threatening infection caused by bacteria that attack the soft tissue beneath the top layers of skin, including the fibrous tissue that covers the muscles. Necrotizing fasciitis is usually caused by group A *Streptococcus* and other bacteria that enter the body via an infection or minor cut or lesion on the surface of the skin.

The bacteria causing this infection are sometimes referred to as "flesh-eating bacteria" because they attack the body's soft tissue, moving very rapidly under the top layers of skin and killing the soft tissue they infect. Small blood vessels in this tissue may be blocked, and the loss of blood supply to the dead tissue causes gangrene of the skin.

Underlying tissues affected by the infection are usually severely painful, and the skin's surface is red, hot, and swollen. As it progresses, the skin becomes discolored, gangrene progresses, and the person can develop a high fever and low blood pressure.

In its early stages, the dead tissue, including outer layers of skin, underlying soft tissue, and fat, can be surgically removed. Cultures of pus from underlying tissue can determine the specific type of antibiotic required to treat the causative bacteria.

Limb amputation is sometimes essential to prevent death, which is not uncommon with advanced stages of the condition. Insufficient removal of infected tissue can allow the infection to continue spreading. Repeated surgeries within 1 to 2 days may be necessary to make sure the bacteria and affected tissue have been removed.

The decay of tissue with severe infection may progress to systemic shock, which causes respiratory failure, heart failure, low blood pressure, and kidney failure. Necrotizing fasciitis is one of the fastest spreading infections known. Prompt medical evaluation and treatment are essential to preventing death.

Needle biopsy

Insertion of a special needle into a lump, cyst, or other area of concern in order to remove a specimen of tissue for microscopic evaluation. A needle biopsy is performed to determine whether or not a growth is cancerous or to find the cause of infection or inflammation.

Needle localization

A procedure used to locate the place where a biopsy specimen will be taken from the breast. Using mammography (see MAMMOGRAM), the radiologist finds the precise area from which the biopsy sample will be taken and marks the skin directly above it. A thin, hollow needle containing a wire about the size of a strand of hair is inserted into the spot and then removed, leaving the wire in the breast. The function of the wire is to show the surgeon performing the biopsy where the "suspicious" tissue is, because it cannot be seen with the naked eye.

Neonatal intensive care

Hospital care that focuses on the problems of the distressed newborn. Neonatal intensive care units, or NICUs, are designed to meet the unique needs of immature and ill newborns. These include special fluid requirements, oxygen management (see OXYGEN, SUPPLEMENTAL), temperature control, and drug dosages. Located primarily in major medical centers, NICUs are staffed by teams of neonatologists and nurses who are specially trained in the care of newborns.

Neonatology

The branch of pediatric medicine that focuses on the care of neonates, babies from birth to 4 weeks of age, and treatment of their disorders. Areas of interest include treatment of prematurely born infants, infants who have experienced birth trauma or are ill or underweight, and the early detection and treatment of congenital (present from birth) disorders such as spina bifida. A neonatologist is a physician who specializes in the care of neonates.

Neoplasia

An abnormal growth or tumor. Neoplasia is the result of a malfunction in the process of cell reproduction in which too many cells are created. The overgrowth of new cells may form a tumor, a type of neoplasm. Neoplasms can be benign or malignant, although the term is commonly used to mean a malignant or cancerous tumor.

Nephrectomy

Surgical removal of a kidney. Nephrectomy is generally undertaken only if the person's other kidney is functioning normally. It is indicated when there is irreversible damage to a kidney. Cancer is the most common reason to perform a nephrectomy, but damage may be a result of traumatic injury to a kidney; chronic infection, obstruction, or pain caused by a large kidney stone; and kidney failure. Nephrectomy is also performed to obtain a kidney for a kidney transplant.

Nephritis

Inflammation of one or both kidneys. Nephritis is among the most common of kidney diseases and occurs more frequently in childhood and adolescence than in middle age. It may result from an infection, particularly streptococcal infections, or an abnormal immune response. Disorders such as lupus erythematosus are associated with nephritis.

A urinalysis will reveal elevated levels of the protein albumin, indicating the condition albuminuria. Red and white blood cells and hyaline or granular casts are also present in the urine of people with nephritis.

There are two forms of nephritis: acute and chronic. People who have the acute form, especially children, usually recover. Symptoms include fatigue, appetite loss, facial swelling, pain in the abdomen or side, and a reduced quantity of dark urine. Acute kidney inflammation can progress to chronic nephritis, which can gradually destroy the kidney. In chronic nephritis there may be few symptoms early in the course of the disease. However, when kidney function is severely impaired by chronic nephritis, high blood pressure may develop, which can damage the heart or the kidneys and possibly result in death from kidney or heart failure.

Nephrocalcinosis

A kidney disorder that is characterized by deposits of calcium oxalate or calcium phosphate in the tubules of the kidneys and the areas between the tubules. Nephrocalcinosis may result in kidney stones and reduced kidney function. Nephrocalcinosis may be caused by an excess excretion of calcium by the kidneys, acidosis of the tubules of the kidneys, a rare congenital condition called sponge kidney, an elevated calcium level in the blood, necrosis of the kidneys, or tuberculosis.

Nephrology

The branch of medical study and practice that specializes in the function, diseases, and disorders of the kidneys. A nephrologist is a physician who specializes in the study and treatment of kidney disorders.

Nephron

Tiny structures of the kidneys that filter blood to remove waste products, regulate fluid and electrolyte content of the blood, and form urine. Nephrons are the working units of the kidneys. Each kidney is made up of approximately 1 million nephrons. The nephrons are composed of glomeruli (the filtering units of the kidneys), renal tubules, and their abundant supply of blood vessels.

Nephropathy, analgesic

Disease of the kidneys associated with excessive use of over-the-counter painkillers, or analgesics. Nonprescription analgesics—including aspirin, acetaminophen, ibuprofen, and naproxen—do not cause kidney damage in most people when the recommended dosage is taken. For people who have risk factors such as advanced age, systemic lupus erythematosus, or chronic kidney conditions, and for those who have recently binged on alcohol, analgesic nephropathy can result in acute kidney failure.

Nephropathy, diabetic

Kidney disease caused by an elevated level of blood glucose, the primary characteristic of diabetes mellitus. Diabetic nephropathy eventually affects a significant proportion of people with type 1 or type 2 diabetes mellitus. If the damage is significant, it impairs the ability of the kidneys to remove waste products from the body.

Diabetic nephropathy may take many years to develop. It is the leading cause of end-stage renal disease (see KIDNEY FAILURE) in the United States. People who have diabetes can slow the pace of kidney damage by keeping their blood sugar level as close to normal as possible, maintaining a normal blood pressure, not smoking, and avoiding medications that might harm the kidneys.

Nephropathy, IgA

A chronic, progressive kidney disorder that can lead to end-stage renal disease (see KIDNEY FAILURE) and is caused by abnormal deposits of various proteins and products of inflammation inside the glomeruli. Glomeruli normally filter waste products and excess water out of the blood. The deposits associated with IgA nephropathy interfere with this filtering process, causing blood and protein to accumulate in the urine. Early symptoms include swelling of the hands and feet.

Treatment is based on slowing the progression of the underlying disorder and preventing complications such as high blood pressure, which contributes to more damage to the glomeruli. Recommended dietary restrictions for people who have nephropathy may include limiting protein and lowering cholesterol levels.

Nephrosis

A condition produced by abnormalities in the glomerular membrane, the membranous part of the glomeruli (the filtering units of the kidneys). Nephrosis allows large amounts of protein in the blood to escape into the urine. It can occur in people of all ages but tends to be more common in children. Excessive protein loss can cause water and sodium to accumulate in the body, resulting in edema (swelling) around the ankles, feet, and eyes and in the abdomen. While nephrosis cannot always be cured, some forms of it can be suppressed by the use of corticosteroid hormones such as prednisone.

Nephrostomy

Surgical formation of an opening that allows the introduction of a small tube into a kidney to drain urine to the surface of the abdomen. Nephrostomy allows urine to bypass a ureter (one of the two narrow tubes connecting a kidney and the bladder). The procedure may be performed after surgery on the ureter to remove urine from the body and to allow the ureter to heal.

Nephrotic syndrome

A combination of signs and symptoms caused by disorders that result in injury to the glomeruli (the filtering units of the kidneys). Damage to these structures results in abnormal excretion of protein in the urine.

Nephrotic syndrome may be the result of diabetes mellitus, an infection, exposure to certain medications, a cancerous tumor, and autoimmune or hereditary disorders. Nephrotic syndrome is diagnosed by blood and urine tests. The findings include abnormally high levels of protein in the urine, a decreased level of protein in the blood, and, in many cases, a high blood cholesterol level. Fat globules may be observed in the urine. Clinically, the loss of protein may cause fluid retention, resulting in edema (swelling) around the ankles and, in severe cases, ascites (accumulation of fluid in the abdominal cavity) and pulmonary edema.

Nerve

A cable of fibers that carries electrochemical impulses to and from the brain or spinal cord to a specific point in the body. The nervous system is a network of nerves passing throughout the body.

At a cellular level, a single nerve is composed of thousands of nerve fibers; each fiber is the tail (axon) of an individual nerve cell called a neuron. Each nerve fiber is insulated by a covering called the myelin sheath. The fibers are bundled together in groups called fascicles; a fascicle contains the types of nerve fibers—sensory, motor, and autonomic (involuntary)—needed to serve a particular site in the body.

Nerve block

A method of making an area of the body numb and pain-free by injecting anesthetic medication around the nerves that control sensation in the area. A nerve block is performed when it is not possible to inject an anesthetic agent directly into the area being treated because of an inflammation or the risk of infection. Or, if the area that needs to be anesthetized is very large, anesthesia of the legs and lower part of the body can be achieved by blocking the lower spinal nerves with spinal or epidural anesthesia (see ANESTHESIA, SPINAL; ANESTHESIA, EPIDURAL) or a caudal block.

Nerve entrapment

The compression of a nerve. Nerve entrapment causes symptoms such as numbness, tingling, and pain in the area supplied by the nerve. See PINCHED NERVE; CARPAL TUNNEL SYNDROME.

Nerve injuries

Crush or cut injuries to nerves that damage some or all of their conducting fibers. Tingling is a symptom of damage or irritation to a nerve or nerves. Numbness suggests that the affected nerve may be severed or dead. A brief tingling sensation, as when a person's hand or foot "falls asleep," is not a cause for concern. However, numbness or persistent tingling may indicate a significant nerve injury and require medical attention.

In crush injuries, individual fibers within a peripheral nerve are damaged, but the nerve trunk remains intact. This means that new fibers can regenerate along the path left by degenerated fibers. Surgery to reconnect the nerve may be needed. However, when a nerve is completely severed, the fibers cannot regenerate, and there is no recovery of function.

Nervous system

The vast body system that gathers information, stores it, and controls the body's responses to it. The nervous system gathers data about both the external environment and the body's own internal state, analyzes the data, and initiates and directs the body's responses, ranging from automatic adjustment of body functions to complex motor movements and emotional or intellectual activity.

The basic unit of the nervous system is the NEURON, or nerve cell, that detects sensory information and conveys it in the form of an electrochemical impulse. Anatomically, the overall nervous system includes both the central nervous system (CNS), made up of the brain and spinal cord, and the peripheral nervous system, composed of all the nerves that branch out from the central nervous system and carry information between the brain and spinal cord and the rest of the body. Within the CNS, the brain is the body's computer and control center, constantly receiving sensory information, analyzing it, and deciding on reaction.

Neural tube defect

A birth defect that is the result of the failure of the spinal cord or brain to develop normally in an embryo. In a normal embryo, the neural tube eventually develops into the spinal cord and brain. When neural tube defects occur, the degree of deformity and disability depends on the level of neural involvement. Neural tube defects range from anencephaly (a fatal birth defect in which an infant's brain and skull fail to develop) to spina bifida (a crippling but not fatal defect in which the backbones, or vertebrae, do not form a complete ring to protect the spinal cord). Adequate folate levels in the first month after conception are important in the prevention of neural tube defects.

Neuralgia

Pain caused by irritation of or damage to a nerve. The pain of neuralgia occurs in brief bouts and may be severe, intense, burning, and stabbing. There are a number of different types of neuralgia: trigeminal neuralgia (which causes severe pain on one side of the face); glossopharyngeal neuralgia (an intense pain that is felt in the throat, ear, and back of the tongue), and occipital neuralgia (in which there is pain, tingling, or numbness at the base of the skull). Treatment depends on diagnosis of the underlying disorder. Medications such as anticonvulsants, antidepressants, and topical painkillers may be helpful.

Neuroblastoma

A cancerous tumor of the adrenal glands or sympathetic nervous system. Neuroblastoma, the fourth most common cancer in children, occurs most frequently in children younger than 5 years. Although the adrenal gland is the most common site, tumors may develop in the sympathetic nerve tissue located in the abdomen, pelvis, neck, or chest. Symptoms depend on the location of the tumor, but may include pain, paralysis, anemia, fever, and high blood pressure. Diagnosis of neuroblastoma is made through tests such as CT (computed tomography) scanning, MRI (magnetic resonance imaging), and biopsy. Treatment options include surgical removal of the tumor, radiation therapy, chemotherapy, and bone marrow transplantation.

Neurofibromatosis

Genetic disorders characterized by changes in skin pigment, tumors growing on the nerves, and dysplasias (abnormal tissue development). Neurofibromatosis (NF) exists in two forms, NF1 and NF2. The disease can be severely disabling, be mildly disfiguring, or not cause any symptoms. NF is found in every racial and ethnic group and affects males and females equally.

A common early sign of NF1, also known as von Recklinghausen disease, is the presence at birth of six or more tan spots on the skin, called café au lait (coffee with milk) spots. During adolescence, benign tumors begin to grow under the skin or deeper. Called neurofibromas, these tumors also grow on nerves and are made up of cells that normally surround the nerves. Neurofibromas can vary in size and may or may not be painful. Tumors growing on the optic nerves can affect vision. Most people with NF1 have mild symptoms and live a normal life. Scoliosis, or curvature of the spine, is common in NF. Children with NF1 may have learning disabilities, speech problems, and seizures; and they may have psychological problems related to their illness and deformities. Occasionally benign tumors may become malignant; regular examination by a physician is critical.

NF2 is associated with benign tumors that grow on the eighth cranial nerve (auditory nerve), one of 12 pairs of nerves serving the brain. The tumors, called schwannomas because they arise from Schwann cells, often put pressure on the auditory nerves, causing hearing loss, which is frequently the first symptom of the disease. Other symptoms include ringing in the ears, dizziness, or balance problems. Tumors may also develop in the brain or on the spinal cord, causing numbness, seizures, or headaches.

There is no cure for NF. Treatment is directed at alleviating symptoms. Painful or disfiguring tumors on the skin can be removed surgically. Tumors on the optic or auditory nerves that are causing symptoms can sometimes be removed or treated with chemotherapy or radiation. Scoliosis can be treated with surgery or by wearing a brace. The only treatments available for the tumors of NF2 are surgery and radiation therapy.

Neurology

The branch of medical science that deals with the diagnosis, treatment, and management of disorders of the brain and nervous system. Examples of neurological disorders include ALS (amyotrophic lateral sclerosis), Alzheimer's disease, brain tumors, epilepsy, headache, multiple sclerosis, Parkinson disease, spinal cord injuries, stroke, and tremor. A neurologist is a physician with specialized training in the diagnosis, treatment, and management of disorders of the brain and nervous system.

Neuroma

A noncancerous tumor composed of nerve cells and fibers. A neuroma may affect any nerve in the body. Symptoms may include pain, numbness, and tingling in parts of the body supplied by the nerve. If the symptoms are troubling, the neuroma is surgically removed. See also ACOUSTIC NEUROMA.

Neuron

A nerve cell; the basic conducting cell of every structure in the nervous system. Neurons receive, interpret, and transmit information in the form of electrochemical impulses.

There are three types of neurons: motor neurons, sensory neurons, and interneurons. A motor neuron connects to a muscle or organ to convey instructions from the central nervous system (brain or spinal cord). A sensory neuron carries information about sensations such as heat, light, touch, or sound waves to the central nervous system. An interneuron connects cells within the structures and pathways of the central nervous system.

Neuropathic joint

Damage to the nerves of a joint, which may eventually lead to joint damage that interferes with normal mobility. The nerve damage may produce sensations of tingling, numbness, burning, or pain in the joint. Because of loss of sensation, there is no signal to warn the body that activities might be damaging the joint. As a result, a neuropathic joint is easily damaged, and bony destruction can rapidly occur. Inherited disorders, nutritional deficiencies, alcoholism, syphilis, and diabetes mellitus may be associated with nerve damage.

Neuropathy

Disease, inflammation, or damage to any of the peripheral nerves that carry messages between the brain and spinal cord and the rest of the body. The peripheral nervous system includes all nerves not in the brain or spinal cord. Neuropathy typically involves damage or injury to nerve cell axons (the conducting fibers that make up nerves) or the myelin sheaths that protect them. Neuropathy is not a specific disease, but a condition associated with many disorders, including vitamin and dietary deficiencies, diabetes, and HIV (human immunodeficiency virus) infection.

Common symptoms of neuropathy include numbness, tingling, pain (neuralgia), abnormal or burning sensations, muscle weakness, and atrophy. There are different types of neuropathy. Treatment depends on the underlying disease, but often includes pain medication, physical therapy, occupational therapy, and orthopedic surgery.

Neurosurgery

Surgical treatment of the brain, spinal cord, or other parts of the nervous system. Conditions managed by neurosurgery include tumors of the brain, spinal cord, or meninges (the membranes that surround and protect the brain and spinal cord); an aneurysm (a weak point or bulge in an artery); brain abscess; hemorrhage; birth defects; or otherwise unmanageable pain. A neurosurgeon is a physician who specializes in operating on the brain and nervous system.

Neurosyphilis

A progressive, destructive, life-threatening infection of the brain and spinal cord that occurs in some cases of untreated syphilis. Neurosyphilis is a complication that develops many years after a primary syphilitic infection.

Diagnosis of neurosyphilis is made through blood tests, lumbar puncture to analyze spinal fluid, CT (computed tomography) scanning or MRI (magnetic resonance imaging), and occasionally a cerebral angiogram. Treatment is with a long course of antibiotics, such as penicillin.

Neurotransmitter

A nerve-signaling chemical in the brain. There are more than 50 different neurotransmitters. Their function is to carry nerve impulses across synapses (small gaps) between nerve cells (neurons). Neurotransmitters can either stimulate or inhibit electrical impulses. Examples of neurotransmitters include acetylcholine, dopamine, norepinephrine, and serotonin.

Nevus

See MOLE.

NGU

See URETHRITIS, NONGONOCOCCAL.

Niacin

Also known as nicotinic acid or vitamin B3, a water-soluble vitamin of the B complex. (See VITAMIN B.) Niacin improves blood circulation by dilating arteries and is important for the skin, gastrointestinal tract, nervous system, and sex hormones. It is also a key element in the metabolism of nutrients such as carbohydrates and fats that create energy. Dietary sources of niacin include meats, poultry, fish, eggs, nuts, peanut butter, brewer's yeast, and wheat germ.

A deficiency of niacin can lead to symptoms such as weakness, fatigue, insomnia, irritability, depression, nausea, headaches, skin rashes, and tender gums.

In amounts available only by prescription, niacin lowers the levels of total and LDL (low-density lipoprotein) cholesterol and triglycerides.

Nicotine gum

Smoking cessation chewing gum. Nicotine gum is available without a prescription to help people quit smoking. As a person chews the gum, nicotine is released and passes into the bloodstream through the lining of the mouth, reducing the withdrawal effects of not smoking.

Nicotine patch

A drug in patch form that helps people stop smoking. The nicotine in a nicotine patch passes through the skin into the bloodstream, taking the place of nicotine obtained by smoking in order to gradually reduce the physical withdrawal effects of not smoking. Nicotine patches are available with and without a prescription.

Nicotinic acid

See NIACIN.

Night sweats

Hot flashes that occur at night. Most women experience hot flashes, or sudden, brief increases in body temperature for about 1 to 2 years during menopause, as the body begins to produce less estrogen. In addition to an increase in the temperature of the skin, hot flashes cause a slight increase in the heart rate, which can lead to heart palpitations and dizziness. See MENOPAUSE.

Among the other causes of night sweats are tuberculosis, AIDS (acquired immunodeficiency syndrome), drug withdrawal, lymphomas, and bacterial and parasitic infections.

Nit

The egg of a small insect, usually a louse (see LICE, HEAD).

Nitrites

Food additives used to protect processed foods against bacterial growth and to preserve color and flavor. Nitrites are chemical salts of nitrous acid that are converted by the body into compounds called nitrosamines. Foods that contain nitrites include bacon, ham, and pickles. Because laboratory animals have developed tumors after consuming large amounts of nitrites, there has long been concern that nitrites may cause cancer in humans.

Nitrogen

A colorless, gaseous element found in the air. Nitrogen forms about four fifths of the Earth's atmosphere. Nitrogen is a constituent of protein and nucleic acids and is therefore present in all living cells. Nitrogen is responsible for a serious condition (the bends, compressed air illness, or decompression sickness).

Nitrosamines

Chemical compounds that may have a role in cancer cell formation. Nitrosamines are formed in the stomach and intestines through reactions of nitrites and proteins. Nitrites are produced from nitrates that are naturally present in vegetables or added as preservatives to meat, poultry, and fish. Antioxidants, which interfere with the formation of nitrosamines, can prevent this conversion from taking place and may offer protection against some cancers.

Nocturia

The need to urinate during the night. Nocturia is common in older people and pregnant women. The condition may also be a symptom of other diseases, such as an enlarged prostate, infection of the bladder, kidney failure, uncontrolled diabetes, or congestive heart failure.

Nocturnal emission

Involuntary ejaculation of semen (the sperm-containing fluid expelled from a man during sexual climax) during sleep. Nocturnal emissions are normal in adolescent boys and men who do not have sex.

Nodule, cold

A growth on the thyroid gland that does not absorb radioactive iodine during a diagnostic imaging procedure called radioactive iodine uptake because it is composed of nonfunctioning thyroid tissue. Nonfunctional nodules containing a gelatinous substance or consisting of cancer cells do not absorb radioactive iodine and are not detected on the thyroid scan.

Nodule, hot

A growth on the thyroid gland that absorbs radioactive iodine during a diagnostic imaging procedure called radioactive iodine uptake. A hot nodule absorbs radioactive iodine because it is composed of functioning thyroid tissue, which attracts and holds iodine. This generally indicates that the tissue is not cancerous.

Nonalcoholic steatohepatitis

An inflammation of the liver that resembles alcoholic liver disease, but is not caused by alcohol. It may occur in a person with fatty liver, cirrhosis, and other forms of hepatitis. Nonalcoholic steatohepatitis (NASH) may be the most common liver disorder in the United States.

Nongonococcal urethritis

See URETHRITIS, NONGONOCOCCAL.

Noninvasive

A term describing a medical procedure that does not involve penetration of the skin or entry into the body through one of the natural openings.

Nonnucleoside reverse transcriptase inhibitors (NNRTIs)

Anti-AIDS (acquired immunodeficiency syndrome) drugs. NNRTIs are a class of drugs being used in combination with nucleoside analogue drugs, such as zidovudine (AZT), ddI (didanosine), and others. NNRTIs work by blocking the ability of HIV (human immunodeficiency virus) to infect new cells; this is accomplished by preventing viruses from replicating.

Nonprescription drugs

Drugs that are available without a doctor's prescription; also called over-the-counter (OTC) drugs. OTC drugs tend to be medications that relieve minor symptoms at doses that are effective and safe.

Nonsteroidal anti-inflammatory drugs

Drugs used to relieve symptoms associated with arthritis and other painful conditions. Nonsteroidal anti-inflammatory drugs, or NSAIDs, are used to relieve inflammation, swelling, stiffness, and joint pain. They are also used to treat attacks of gout; bursitis; tendinitis; sprains, strains, or other injuries; and menstrual cramps. In addition to their pain-relieving properties, some NSAIDs, including aspirin and ibuprofen, have fever-reducing properties. Aspirin should not be given to children under 18 because of the risk of contracting Reye syndrome, a potentially fatal disease.

Nonstress test

In pregnancy, external monitoring of a fetus, using ultrasound (see

ULTRASOUND, SCANNING). A non-stress test is painless, requires no drugs or anesthesia, can be performed in the doctor's office or in a hospital labor room, and takes between 20 and 40 minutes. The non-stress test shows whether the fetus is reactive, meaning that its heart speeds up in response to a uterine contraction or its own movements, or nonreactive, meaning the heart rate neither varies nor speeds up with a contraction or movement. About 20 percent of nonreactive babies are actually in danger. See also PRENATAL TESTING.

Norepinephrine

One of the two principal hormones synthesized by the adrenal medulla (the inner layer of the adrenal glands). Norepinephrine and epinephrine regulate heart rate and blood pressure. They stimulate the sympathetic nervous system, the part of the autonomic nervous system that predominates at times of stress. The two hormones are largely responsible for the fight-or-flight response and help the body resist stress.

Nose

The facial structure that is the main organ of smell and the primary opening into the respiratory system. The supporting bones of the nose, the nasal bones, protrude from the skull. The nose is not actually a part of the skull, but is made up of a number of cartilages that attach to the nasal bones.

One of the principal functions of the nose is to cleanse inhaled air. The air brought into the nose also stimulates the sense of smell.

Nose reshaping

A surgical procedure, also known as rhinoplasty, to change the shape and contour of the nose.

A nose reshaping is often done in the office of a physician or an outpatient surgery center as ambulatory surgery, with the patient returning home the same day. Complicated procedures may require a 1- or 2-night hospital stay. The surgery usually takes 1 to 2 hours, with complex reshapings requiring more time. Anesthesia can be by either a local, combined with conscious sedation, or a general anesthetic.

For the first day after surgery, the face feels puffy and the nose is sore and achy. There may also be a dull headache. Stitches and splints are removed after 1 week. If dissolvable sutures have been used, they will disappear in the same period.

Nosebleed

A flow of blood from the nose, a frequent occurrence in children between ages 2 and 10. Also called epistaxis, a nosebleed is commonly due to dryness caused by low humidity in the home, nose picking, inflammation of the nasal lining from a cold or allergies, a foreign object in the nose, blowing the nose too hard, or falling on or hitting the nose. Rarely, abnormal growths or a problem with blood clotting causes nosebleeds. Minor nosebleeds can be treated at home. A person with a nosebleed should sit straight up and tip his or her head forward, so blood will not flow down the throat. The individual should not lie down or tilt his or her head back. The sides of the nose should be pinched together for 5 to 10 minutes, while the person breathes through the mouth. Afterwards, an ice pack can be applied to the nose.

If bleeding continues despite these measures, a doctor should be consulted. A child or adult who has very frequent nosebleeds or whose nosebleed was caused by an injury or is accompanied by dizziness should see a physician.

Nosocomial infections

Infections that are acquired by people while they are hospitalized. To be categorized as nosocomial, the infection must not be present and the causative organisms must not be incubating at the time a person is admitted to the hospital. The primary element in controlling nosocomial infections is preventing transmission as early as possible.

NSAIDs

See NONSTEROIDAL ANTI-INFLAMMATORY DRUGS.

Nuclear medicine

The branch of diagnostic and therapeutic RADIOLOGY that involves the use of very small amounts of radioactively tagged compounds, called radionuclides or radioisotopes, to create images of parts of the body and visualize biochemical processes within the body. These compounds can be injected, ingested, or inhaled. Nuclear medicine enables physicians to obtain information about organ function, blood flow, and other physiologic activity.

Nucleus

The center portion of a living cell that contains DNA (deoxyribonucleic acid) and RNA (ribonucleic acid). The nucleus of a cell controls its metabolism, growth, and reproduction. The nucleus is separated from the surrounding cytoplasm by a double membrane called a nuclear envelope.

Numbness

Partial or total loss of sensation in part of the body that is caused by interference with the passage of impulses along sensory nerves. Numbness suggests that the affected nerve is damaged. It is a more serious condition than tingling or a pins and needles sensation, which suggest that a nerve is compressed but not damaged. Possible causes of numbness include nerve injury; lack of blood supply; diabetes mellitus, type 1 and type 2; thyroid problems; vitamin B12 (cyanocobalamin) deficiency; carpal tunnel syndrome; transient ischemic attack; stroke; and multiple sclerosis.

Nurse

A person trained in nursing care. Nurses work in hospitals, nursing facilities, clinics, birth centers, physicians' offices, schools, workplaces, and home-care settings. Registered nurses (RNs) are licensed by the states to care for the sick and promote health. Licensed practical nurses (LPNs) provide basic care under the supervision of RNs and doctors. Nurses' aides assist nurses in the provision of care.

Nurse anesthetist

A nurse trained and qualified to administer anesthetic agents. Nurse anesthetists, designated by CRNA (certified registered nurse anesthetist), have completed 2 to 3 years of training in anesthesia at the master's degree level. They must pass a national examination to become a CRNA.

Nurse practitioner

Also known as an NP, an advanced practice nurse specially trained for a role in primary care. Types of nurse practitioners include family nurse practitioners, pediatric nurse practitioners, school nurse practitioners, adult nurse practitioners, women's health care nurse practitioners, and geriatric nurse practitioners.

Nursemaid elbow

Also known as pulled elbow, a painful injury in which nearby soft tissue slips into the elbow joint and is trapped there. Nursemaid elbow is most common among children under age 4. The injury can occur when a small child is lifted, yanked, or swung by the hand or wrist or falls on his or her outstretched arm. A suspected nursemaid elbow injury should promptly be supported by a sling and examined by a doctor. X rays may be taken to rule out a fracture. If there is no fracture, the doctor will carefully manipulate the elbow joint to release the trapped tissue.

Nurse-midwife

An advanced practice nurse specializing in women's health care needs, including prenatal care, labor and delivery, and postpartum care. Nurse-midwives work in health maintenance organizations, private practices, public health clinics, and birth centers.

Nursing facility

Formerly known as a nursing home, a facility that offers a combination of housing, personal services, and health care to older or disabled people who are unable to care for themselves independently. Today a wide spectrum of nursing facilities is designed to fit different levels of needs. See LONG-TERM CARE FACILITY.

Nursing home

See LONG-TERM CARE FACILITY.

Nutrient

A chemical substance in food that is essential to health maintenance, normal body function, growth, and reproduction. Vitamins, minerals, carbohydrates, fats, proteins, and water all are essential nutrients.

Nutrition

The study of the food people eat and its digestion and assimilation for growth, tissue repair, and physical activity. Areas of focus include diet, dietary deficiencies, and establishing minimum daily requirements for necessary nutrients (see DIETARY REFERENCE INTAKES).

Nutritional supplements

Products intended to supplement the body's nutritional requirements. Nutritional supplements include vitamins, minerals, herbal products, and dietary aids. They are sold without prescription and are sometimes advertised as providing miraculous benefits, such as curing disease or stopping the aging process. There is considerable debate as to whether people need to take nutritional supplements, and they are not without risk—especially in high doses.

Nystagmus

Involuntary, rapid, and repetitive movement of the eyes. Nystagmus usually involves both eyes, and it often increases when the person looks in a particular direction. The movement can be side to side (horizontal nystagmus), up and down (vertical), or circular (rotary). The condition may be present at birth or acquired later in life. Some forms of nystagmus accompany poor vision, as is found in albinos, people with extreme nearsightedness or farsightedness, or people who have scarred retinas (the light-sensitive tissue in the back of the eye) or optic nerves.

In some cases, treating the cause of the nystagmus resolves the condition; often, however, it is permanent. Reduced vision can be improved with glasses that decrease eye movement and with low-vision aids. Or surgery can be performed on the eye muscles to position the eyes for best vision.

Obesity

A body weight 20 percent or more above an individual's ideal weight or a BODY MASS INDEX (BMI) of 30 or higher. Obesity is a serious medical problem linked with high blood pressure (see HYPERTENSION), elevated cholesterol levels, heart disease, cardiovascular disease, type 2 diabetes, stroke, and some cancers. Weight-related cancers include colon and prostate cancer in men and breast,

uterine, and endometrial cancer in women. Obesity is also linked to back pain, sleep apnea (a potentially life-threatening condition in which a person stops breathing for short periods during sleep), gallstones, osteoarthritis, heartburn, gout, and varicose veins. See WEIGHT LOSS.

Obesity-hypoventilation syndrome

Also known as pickwickian syndrome; a group of symptoms that may accompany extreme obesity. Obesity-hypoventilation syndrome is characterized by shortness of breath, a flushed face, nighttime sleep disturbances such as SLEEP APNEA SYNDROME, and an irresistible urge to take short naps during the day. Because massive obesity interferes with breathing, people with this condition may also experience chronic HYPOXIA or decreased blood oxygen concentration. Obesity-hypoventilation syndrome can lead to serious complications such as pulmonary hypertension (see HYPERTENSION, PULMONARY), or COR PULMONALE (right-sided heart failure).

Obsessive-compulsive disorder

A mental disorder characterized by mild to severe persistent, intrusive thoughts, images, or impulses (obsessions) that a person tries to compensate for with repetitive actions (compulsions) he or she feels driven to perform. Obsessions are not usually related to real-life problems. The most common obsessions concern contamination (for example, from handling money or shaking hands); recurring doubts (for example, about having locked a door or turned off a stove); a need for objects to be ordered or arranged in a particular way; violent or shocking impulses (for example, hurting someone); and unusual sexual images.

In most cases, obsessive-compulsive disorder (OCD) begins gradually and develops slowly. Symptoms tend to worsen at times of stress and can improve markedly when the stress is removed. A pattern of flare-up and remission is common. In some cases, the obsessions or compulsions become the major focus of the person's life and result in major disability.

A number of medications have proven effective for treating OCD, including antidepressants, anti-anxiety medications, and mild tranquilizers. Behavior therapies can also be effective.

Obstetrics

The medical specialty involved in the care of pregnant women. Obstetrics includes care given during the period in which a woman is trying to conceive; during pregnancy, labor and childbirth; and just after a baby is born. Family physicians, certified nurse-midwives, and obstetricians are all trained in obstetrics. An obstetrician is a doctor who specializes in caring for women during pregnancy, labor, and childbirth. Most obstetricians are also gynecologists, doctors who specialize in treating the female reproductive system.

Obstructive airways disease

A pathological process that involves narrowing of the bronchial airways. Obstructive airways disease may affect the windpipe (trachea), as well as its smaller branches (the bronchi), which are connected to the lungs and supply air to them.

The most common obstructive airways diseases are ASTHMA, chronic BRONCHITIS, and EMPHYSEMA. Asthma is characterized by reversible spasms in the airways and a person may have periods with no symptoms. Chronic bronchitis and emphysema are closely associated with smoking and are less likely than asthma to be reversible.

Occult

A term meaning hidden or obscure. For example, a FECAL-OCCULT BLOOD TEST detects the presence of blood in the feces that is not visible to the naked eye.

Occult blood test, fecal

See FECAL-OCCULT BLOOD TEST.

Occupational lung disease

Lung disorders caused by repeated exposure to hazardous agents in the workplace that are inhaled into the lungs. These diseases include asbestosis, coal worker's pneumoconiosis, silicosis, byssinosis, hypersensitivity pneumonitis, and occupational asthma. See DUST DISEASES.

People can experience the symptoms of these diseases in different ways, but the most common symptoms—regardless of the agents that caused them—are cough, shortness of breath, chest pain, and chest tightness. These symptoms resemble those of other disorders, so it is important to inform a doctor of possible occupational exposures when giving a medical history.

The first line of treatment is to reduce the person's exposure by removing him or her from the work environment that is causing the illness or, in some cases, to ensure that proper protective equipment is used.

Occupational medicine

The branch of medicine that is concerned with the effects of a person's job on his or her health. Occupational medicine emphasizes the prevention of work-related disease and injury and the promotion of general health in workers. It encompasses problems ranging from lung disease in miners to carpal tunnel syndrome in computer users.

Occupational therapy

Treatment to help people with a temporary or permanent physical or mental impairment restore, maintain, or improve their ability to perform daily tasks in their living and working environments.

OCT

See OXYTOCIN CHALLENGE TEST.

Oligohydramnios

An abnormally small amount of AM-NIOTIC FLUID (the fluid that surrounds the fetus in the uterus during pregnancy). Mild oligohydramnios is usually not a serious problem but severe oligohydramnios often signals the presence of an abnormality. Oligohydramnios in early pregnancy may result in a miscarriage; late in pregnancy, it can cause birth defects or the death of the fetus. If oligohydramnios is suspected, the doctor will want to diagnose the underlying problem and treat it. If the pregnancy

is advanced beyond the 37th week, the doctor may induce labor.

Oligomenorrhea

Irregular and infrequent menstrual periods that are more than 45 days apart. Reduced bleeding and lack of ovulation may occur. See MENSTRUA-TION, DISORDERS OF.

Omentum

A double fold of the membrane lining the abdominal cavity. The greater omentum attaches to the stomach and hangs down over structures close to it, including the duodenum and colon. The lesser omentum covers the liver and parts of the stomach and small intestine. These folds store fat and may also prevent the spread of infection between abdominal organs. See PERITONEUM.

Oncogenes

Genes that contribute to the transformation of normal cells into cancerous cells. Normal cell growth can go wrong when a gene that stimulates cell growth becomes hyperactive and turns into an oncogene. As a rule, a single oncogene is not sufficient to change normal cells into cancer cells: many mutations in many different genes are usually required.

Oncology

The medical specialty concerned with the diagnosis, treatment, and study of cancer. A doctor who is trained in oncology is called an oncologist.

Oncology, surgical

The treatment of cancer with surgery. Surgical procedures are commonly used to treat cancer by removing it. Surgery to remove cancerous tissue, whether for biopsy or therapy, is generally performed by surgical oncologists.

Oocyte

A human egg; also called a female gametocyte or ovocyte. An oocyte carries the female half of the chromosomes that, when united with the complementary chromosomes from a sperm, form a zygote.

Oophorectomy

Surgical removal of one or both ovaries (see OVARY). Oophorectomy is usually performed as part of a HYSTERECTOMY, although it is sometimes performed alone. The procedure is used to treat cancer of the ovary, large ovarian cysts or tumors, and some cases of ENDOMETRIOSIS. When a woman has a very small benign tumor or cyst on an ovary, it can sometimes be removed while leaving the ovary intact in a procedure called a partial oophorectomy.

Open-heart surgery

A procedure in which the heart is operated on after it is exposed through a surgical incision in the chest wall. During the surgery, a heart-lung machine takes over the work of the heart and lungs, circulating and oxygenating the blood. The most common open-heart procedure is BYPASS SURGERY. Other types include procedures to replace heart valves (see HEART VALVE SURGERY) and HEART TRANSPLANTS.

Ophthalmology

The branch of medical science that studies the structure, function, and diseases of the eye. A physician who specializes in ophthalmology is an ophthalmologist.

Ophthalmoplegia

Paralysis of the eye muscles. There are three types of ophthalmoplegia: internuclear (affecting the structures in the central nervous system that coordinate eye movements), external, and internal. Internuclear ophthalmoplegia, a type of motor disturbance of the eye, results from damage to the area of the brain that coordinates eye movement and can be caused by multiple sclerosis, ischemic vascular disease, or brain stem tumor. External ophthalmoplegia involves dysfunction of the extraocular muscles (which control the movement of the eye). Internal ophthalmoplegia involves disorders associated with dysfunction of the pupillary muscles (which control constriction of the pupils).

Ophthalmoscope

A handheld device with a magnifier and a strong, focused light that is used to examine the interior of the eye. The light shines through the pupil to the back of the eye to view the retina (the thin layer of nerve tissue that detects light and relays visual information to the brain), the retinal blood vessels, and the optic disc (the point where the optic nerve joins the retina).

Opioids

See NARCOTICS.

Opportunistic infections

Infections that occur in people with a weakened immune system. These infections can be caused by viruses, bacteria, parasites, or fungi. A weakened or suppressed immune system may be caused by a number of factors, including long-term treatment with corticosteroids or antibiotics and anticancer treatments such as chemotherapy. Diseases such as LEUKEMIA, SICKLE CELL DISEASE, and DIABETES can weaken a person's immune system, making him or her more susceptible to infection. Infection with human immunodeficiency virus, or HIV, the virus that causes AIDS, severely weakens the immune system and leads to a high risk of opportunistic infections such as PNEUMOCYSTIS PNEUMONIA. Common opportunistic infections include herpes infections and CYTOMEGALOVIRUS (or CMV).

Optic neuritis

Inflammation of the optic nerve. If the inflammation affects the nerve where it connects with the back of the eye, it is called papillitis and the sole symptom is usually gradual or sudden blurred vision or blindness of the affected eye. If the inflammation affects the optic nerve outside the eye, it is called retrobulbar neuritis and causes pain as the eye is moved and often leads to blurred vision or blindness. Optic neuritis can be caused by a viral infection, autoimmune disease, or multiple sclerosis. In most cases, optic neuritis disappears on its own within 2 to 8 weeks. Corticosteroid medications may be prescribed to hasten healing. In rare cases, surgery may be performed to relieve pressure on the nerve.

Optometrist

A professional trained to diagnose and correct focusing errors of the eyes. Optometrists graduate from a school of optometry and hold a doctor of optometry (OD) degree. The scope of optometry practice is regulated by state law. In all states, optometrists examine eyes and prescribe glasses or contact lenses to correct focusing problems. In some states, optometrists can also prescribe medication to treat certain eye diseases. Optometrists do not perform surgery.

Oral cancer

Cancer in any part of the mouth or oral cavity, including the lips, tongue, floor of the mouth, lining of the cheeks, tonsils, and gums. Also known as mouth cancer, oral cancers are common and can be detected during examination of the mouth by a doctor or dentist. The most frequent cause of oral cancer is tobacco use, including chewing tobacco and smoking cigarettes, pipes, or cigars.

Early signs of oral cancer may be red, slightly raised areas with poorly defined borders; a lump that can be felt with the tongue; or a sore inside the mouth that does not heal. A symptom of lip cancer may be a growth that forms a dry crust that bleeds when removed. Cancer of the gum may cause a toothache, loose teeth, or a sore on the gum that does not heal. Tongue cancer may cause mild irritation, pain during eating or drinking, and difficulty speaking or swallowing. Cancer of the tonsils may cause a persistent sore throat and an earache.

Because the symptoms of oral cancer can occur in many other disorders, a physical examination is essential for a diagnosis. A diagnostic workup of suspected oral cancer may include X rays, CT (computed tomography) scanning, MRI (magnetic resonance imaging), and biopsy. Treatment usually involves surgery and radiation therapy, sometimes in combination with chemotherapy. Laser therapy is sometimes used.

Oral contraceptives

See CONTRACEPTION, HORMONAL METHODS.

Oral sex

Sexual stimulation of the genitals by a sex partner's mouth and tongue. Cunnilingus is oral stimulation of the female genitals; fellatio is oral stimulation of the penis. Certain SEXUALLY TRANSMITTED DISEASES (such as chlamydia, herpes simplex, genital warts, syphilis, gonorrhea, and HIV) can be transmitted through oral sex.

Oral surgery

A branch of dentistry that involves the diagnosis and surgical treatment of disorders of the teeth, mouth, and jaws. The removal of teeth is an important part of the practice of oral surgery. An oral and maxillofacial surgeon is a dental surgeon who specializes in diagnosing and surgically treating problems related to the jaw and related facial structures, including the teeth.

Orbital fracture

A break in any of the seven bones that form the eye socket (orbit). Orbital fractures commonly result from blunt trauma, such as a blow from a fist or impact against a dashboard in an automobile collision. The rim of the orbit breaks only with significant force, while the bones deeper within the orbit are thinner and break more easily.

Symptoms of an orbital fracture include blood accumulating in the socket and pressing against the eye and optic nerve; impairment of the muscles that control the eyeball, causing double vision or difficulty moving the eye; numbness in the upper teeth; protrusion of the eyeball from the socket; or collapse of the eye within the socket.

Minor orbital fractures that cause only temporary symptoms are allowed to heal on their own. Severe fractures require surgical repair. See BLOW-OUT FRACTURE.

Orchiectomy

Surgical removal of one or both testicles. A testicle may be removed because of cancer in the testicle (see TESTICLE, CANCER OF THE), dead testicular tissue (see TESTICLE, TORSION OF THE), or an undescended testicle (see TESTICLE, UNDESCENDED). Removal of one testicle usually does not affect sexual activity or fertility. Both testicles are sometimes removed as treatment for advanced prostate cancer.

Orchiopexy

An operation performed to bring an undescended testicle down into the scrotum or to restore blood flow to a testicle that has twisted around its blood vessels. In a fetus, the testicles develop in the abdomen and descend into the scrotum shortly before birth or, in some cases, during the first year of life (see TESTICLE, UNDESCENDED). If this does not occur, orchiopexy is usually performed before age 2. Also, a normal testicle can become twisted and cut off its own blood supply (see TESTICLE, TORSION OF THE); orchiopexy is performed to prevent this condition.

Organ

A body part composed of more than one tissue that performs a specific function or functions. The specific function of an organ, such as the heart, lungs, and liver, is essential to the functioning of the whole body. In animals, organs are usually made up of several tissues, one of which generally predominates and determines the chief function of the organ.

Organ donation

The agreement to take healthy organs or tissues from one person to replace damaged organs or tissues in another person. In most cases, the organ is taken from someone who has recently died, but there are procedures for transplanting portions of the liver, lung, and pancreas from a living donor as well. People who want to donate their organs upon death can sign a donor card (available with driver's licenses in some states) and carry it with them; they should also tell family members of their wishes.

Organs and tissues that can be donated include the kidneys, heart, liver, lungs, pancreas, intestine, corneas, skin, bone, middle ear, bone marrow, connective tissues, and blood vessels.

Organism

Any living thing.

Orgasm

The climax stage of sexual response that follows the arousal and plateau stages in both men and women. It lasts for a few seconds and consists of rhythmic muscular contractions and pleasurable sensations.

Orgasm, lack of

A persistent absence of the climax phase during sexual activity despite adequate sexual stimulation. Lack of orgasm is also known as anorgasmia, and it can affect both men and women. The condition may be lifelong or it may arise only in certain situations. Causes can be physical or psychological. Physical causes include diseases such as diabetes and multiple sclerosis, cancer in the pelvic region, tumors of the spinal cord, surgery to the genitals, and drugs (alcohol or sedatives).

Treatment of anorgasmia depends on cause. If the cause is physical, treatment of the underlying condition or a change in medication may alleviate the problem. Psychological causes are best addressed in COUPLES THERAPY or SEX THERAPY.

Orphan drugs

Drugs used to treat rare diseases. Orphan drugs are defined by the Food and Drug Administration (FDA) as those used to treat diseases or conditions affecting fewer than 200,000 people in the United States. Because so few people need them, the drugs are unlikely to prove profitable for manufacturers, and it is sometimes difficult to find sponsors for them.

Orthodontics

The branch of dentistry that involves the diagnosis, prevention, and treatment of irregular positions of the teeth and abnormal relationships between the upper and lower jaws in children and adults. The practice of orthodontics involves straightening the teeth and treating problems related to the growth and development of the jaw. A dentist who specializes in orthodontics is called an orthodontist. See also BRACES, DENTAL.

Orthopedics

The medical specialty that studies, diagnoses, and treats disorders of the musculoskeletal system, including the bones, joints, muscles, ligaments, tendons, and nerves. An orthopedist is a physician who is trained in this medical specialty. See also JOINT REPLACEMENT; SPORTS MEDICINE.

Orthopnea

Difficulty breathing that occurs while lying down. People with orthopnea wake up at night feeling short of breath, and they find they can sleep restfully only when sitting upright or with several pillows under their head. Orthopnea is often a sign of heart failure, but it can be caused by other heart and lung problems or by anxiety.

Orthotics

Special devices that are used or worn to control, correct, or compensate for irregularities or injuries of the bones, muscles, or joints. They may be purchased commercially or custom-made for an individual.

Osgood-Schlatter disease

Inflammation in the upper part of the shin bone that connects to the tendons around the kneecap. It is most common in active adolescents. Symptoms include pain, swelling, and tenderness in the shin, just below the knee. There may also be pain above the knee. Pain worsens during activity, especially running, bicycling, and stair climbing.

With rest and limited activity, the pain, swelling, and tenderness gradually subside. Ibuprofen (not aspirin) can also help control pain and swelling. Applying an ice pack after activity reduces the pain and inflammation. Other treatments include a temporary brace (see BRACE, ORTHOPEDIC) to support the knee and special exercises to strengthen the surrounding muscles. Children generally outgrow the problem by late adolescence.

Ossification

The process by which bone is formed from cartilage or fibrous tissue. The human skeleton is gradually transformed from cartilage to hard bone during infancy and childhood by ossification. As cartilage becomes bone, it is said to ossify.

Osteitis

Inflammation or infection of the bone.

Osteitis deformans

See PAGET DISEASE.

Osteoarthritis

A condition caused by wear and tear on the joints accompanied by an erosion of their lubricated sliding surface, called the articular cartilage. As the cartilage flakes and cracks, the joint loses the cushioning that allows it to move smoothly. Cracking or popping of the joint often occurs. The bone of the joint becomes flattened, thickened, eroded, and distorted. Extra bone tissue develops at the joint margins. Osteoarthritis is present to some degree in most adults older than 40. The weight-bearing larger joints, including those of the hips, knees, and lower spine, are commonly affected, as are the small joints of the fingers.

Osteoarthritis may or may not cause pain. Often, the condition is discovered during a physical examination that includes X rays. Limited and minor pain of osteoarthritis may occur at intervals of a few months or a year and can be treated by resting the joint, applying heat, and taking acetaminophen or a nonsteroidal anti-inflammatory medication (NSAID) such as aspirin, ibuprofen, or naproxen.

People with osteoarthritis who are overweight can reduce the extra stress on affected joints by losing weight. Strengthening the muscles surrounding affected joints can also help relieve symptoms. Physical therapy, including exercise and massage, may be recommended.

Severe and persistent pain may be treated with prescription painkillers. Corticosteroid drugs can be injected into a painful joint to relieve discomfort, but this carries the risk of damaging the joint cartilage if performed too frequently. Injectable joint fluid supplements are also available. If more conservative treatment has not been effective, joint replacement surgery may be an option. See also JOINT REPLACEMENT, HIP; JOINT REPLACEMENT, KNEE.

Osteochondritis dissecans

A condition that develops from stress fractures of the underlying cartilage of a joint, often the knee, elbow, or ankle. See OSTEOCHONDROSIS.

Osteochondrosis

A chronic condition, also called osteochondritis, in children involving inflammation and deformity of growing bone. It is caused by an inadequate blood supply to the developing bone, which causes the bone to progressively deteriorate over a period of 2 to 3 years. Generally, only one bone is affected. Symptoms may include pain in the affected area and restriction of movement. X rays are often used to make the diagnosis.

Treatment generally emphasizes containment of the hip with a reduction of pressure on the affected joint. A CALIPER SPLINT or other special brace may need to be worn for as long as 2 years while the bone heals naturally. Surgery is sometimes recommended. There is a more optimistic prognosis for children who develop osteochondrosis before the age of 6.

Osteogenic sarcoma

See OSTEOSARCOMA.

Osteoid osteoma

A benign bone-forming tumor, which may occur anywhere but usually occurs in the legs, particularly the thighbone (femur). It occurs most often between ages 5 and 25, affecting more boys than girls. Symptoms include a dull aching pain that becomes progressively more severe over time. The pain can be felt when the body is at rest and is aggravated by activity, though movement itself does not necessarily cause the pain. The tumor can produce inflammation in surrounding soft tissues, creating the sensation of swelling or a lump in the area. Nonsteroidal anti-inflammatory drugs (NSAIDs) such as ibuprofen, can help relieve the pain. If the pain is severe and interferes with everyday activities, the tumor may be treated with radiofrequency ablation or be surgically removed.

Osteoma

A benign bone tumor that may be found in any bone in the body and that usually produces a painless swelling.

Osteomyelitis

Inflammation of the bone marrow and adjacent bone. Also a medical term for all the infectious diseases of the bone, including the bone marrow. Osteomyelitis may be localized or widespread and may include the cartilage and the periosteum (a fibrous membrane that covers the surface of bones, except at the joints). Bone infections may be caused by microorganisms, most commonly bacteria from a staphylococcal infection, that reach bone tissue via the bloodstream, a fracture, an injury, or a sinus infection or dental abscess.

Symptoms include fever, pain, and redness and swelling of the affected area. X rays are not useful early in the course of this infection, but a bone scan or MRI can be useful in making the diagnosis. Antibiotics are prescribed for several weeks to treat osteomyelitis and prevent its spread through large areas of bone. Surgery may be needed to drain the pus or to stabilize the bone in cases of significant bone destruction.

Osteopathic medicine

A branch of medicine that focuses on the interactive relationships among the many body systems and the shifting balance among them as it relates to a person's health. In all 50 states, osteopaths receive the same medical license that physicians do.

Osteopenia

Thinning of the bones or low levels of bone calcium. A woman is diagnosed with osteopenia by a bone density test (see DUAL-ENERGY X-RAY ABSORPTIOMETRY, DEXA). Treatment includes increasing calcium and vitamin D intake and performing regular weight-bearing and resistance exercises to prevent it from progressing to OSTEOPOROSIS.

Osteophyte

An outgrowth of bone tissue that forms at the edge of a joint that has been affected by osteoarthritis. It is commonly known as a SPUR.

Osteoporosis

A bone disease, usually diagnosed in postmenopausal women, characterized by a decrease in bone density and bone tissue that is thin, brittle, porous, and more vulnerable to fracture.

Osteoporosis often causes no symptoms and goes undiagnosed until an affected bone breaks. Fractures most often occur in the spine, hip, and wrist bones. When a spinal fracture occurs, the primary symptom is a severe backache. A stooped, round-shouldered posture can result from the gradual compression of several weakened vertebrae in the spine. As a result, normal height may become diminished.

Causes and contributing factors

Not all of the causes of osteoporosis are known, but aging is thought to be a major factor. The loss of estrogen at menopause is one known risk factor for women because estrogen has a vital role in incorporating calcium into the bone structure. Other risk factors include a small body frame, alcohol abuse, cigarette smoking, a family history of osteoporosis, inadequate intake of calcium and protein, and, in younger women, excessive exercise that causes a woman to stop having menstrual periods.

Certain medical conditions may make a person more susceptible to developing osteoporosis. These conditions include the use of corticosteroid medications and hormonal disorders such as hyperthyroidism, hyperparathyroidism, and Cushing disease.

Diagnosis and treatment

Osteoporosis is diagnosed with a bone density test. DUAL ENERGY X-RAY ABSORPTIOMETRY (DEXA), the most commonly used test, is painless and is considered the most sensitive and accurate. DEXA measures the bones' mineral content, which indicates their strength and density. People whose test results indicate that they have reduced bone density should be evaluated by their physician for testing and treatment.

There are two major classes of prescription drugs to treat osteoporosis: antiresorptives (which can slow, and sometimes stop, the loss of bone minerals) and bone-building drugs (which help to rebuild bone). Commonly used antiresorptive drugs include bisphosphonates (which inhibit bone resorption) and estrogen analogs (which act like the female hormone estrogen to maintain bone density without estrogen's possible side effects). Other antiresorptives include calcitonin (which comes in a nasal spray or injection). HORMONE REPLACEMENT THERAPY (HRT) is an option for some women with osteoporosis. Parathyroid hormone is the only bone-forming medication currently approved for treating osteoporosis.

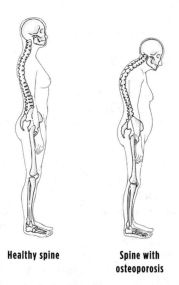

Healthy spine **Spine with osteoporosis**

Compression fractures in spine

The bone-thinning effects of osteoporosis can cause a compression fracture, a type of fracture in which the front portion of the vertebra collapses. The result of compression fractures is a weakened and often abnormally curved spine—a condition commonly called dowager's hump.

Osteosarcoma

A cancerous tumor in the bone. Found primarily in adolescents, osteosarcomas may be painful and weaken the bone, making it vulnerable to fracture under slight pressure. Cancerous bone tumors tend to spread rapidly to other parts of the body, especially to the lungs. If a lump develops on a bone, a doctor should be consulted. Treatment involves chemotherapy to shrink the tumor and surgery to remove it. Additional chemotherapy is often given for several months after surgery.

Osteotomy

A surgical procedure in which a bone is cut to shorten, lengthen, or change its alignment. The procedure is often used to help improve the stability of a joint or correct deformities caused by osteoarthritis.

Ostomy

A surgical procedure that creates an opening, or STOMA, in a body tissue. This opening may be in the wall of the abdomen to allow the discharge of wastes, or it may be in the windpipe to allow air to enter and leave the lungs without going through the nose or mouth (tracheostomy). An ostomy is usually performed when a person has lost normal function of the bladder, bowel, or upper airway because of cancer or another disease, a birth defect, or an injury.

In some ostomies of the urinary tract, a pouch is created inside the body, and accumulated urine is drained off by inserting a tube (catheter) through the stoma. In a colostomy (which connects the colon to the abdominal wall), the person wears a pouch that seals in place over the stoma to collect feces; the pouch is emptied periodically. In a TRA-CHEOSTOMY, a permanent opening is created between the windpipe and the skin through a special tube.

Otitis externa

See SWIMMER'S EAR.

Otitis externa, malignant

Inflammation of the external ear canal due to a bacterial infection that produces tenderness and severe pain in the ear, as well as constant fluid discharge from the ear. Usually there is no fever. Malignant otitis externa does not mean the condition is cancerous; the term "malignant" refers to the infection's tendency to spread into surrounding tissue and bone. The diagnosis is usually confirmed by a bone scan. People who have symptoms should see an ear specialist for treatment. Large doses of antibiotics may be prescribed for as long as 3 months. In rare cases, surgery may be necessary. Left untreated, malignant otitis externa may result in damage to the facial nerves and other cranial nerves. It may also lead to a brain abscess. In severe cases, it may be fatal.

Otitis media

Inflammation of the middle ear resulting from infection, affecting one or both ears. Otitis media is most common in young children but may also affect older children and adults.

Causes and symptoms

When the eustachian tube (which connects the middle ear cavity to the back of the nose and throat) becomes inflamed and swollen as the result of a common cold (see COLD, COMMON), allergies, or a respiratory tract infection, the passageway between the ear and the nose can become blocked. Secretions can accumulate behind the eardrum and become infected, increasing pressure in the middle ear and causing an earache, as well as swelling and redness of the eardrum. The pressure may become sufficiently severe to rupture the eardrum and allow the fluid to drain out of the ear.

In some cases, the fluid remains in the middle ear, trapped by the blocked eustachian tube. This condition is called chronic middle ear fluid, or otitis media with effusion. The accumulated fluid can remain in the middle ear for weeks, months, or even years, causing recurring ear infections and difficulty hearing.

Symptoms of otitis media may include earache, problems with hearing, feelings of fullness or pressure in the ear, a discharge from the ear, dizziness and loss of balance, loss of appetite, nausea, vomiting, and fever. Because ear infections can damage the hearing structures within the ear, a physician should be consulted.

Diagnosis and treatment

A physician will examine the ears using an OTOSCOPE (lighted viewing instrument inserted into the ear) to look for redness, swelling, and the presence of fluid behind the eardrum. Hearing tests and measurements of air pressure in the middle ear may be performed.

If otitis media is diagnosed, medication may be prescribed. If the condition is caused by a bacterial infection, the doctor will prescribe an antibiotic. If, after treatment, fluid remains in the middle ear, most doctors wait to see if the fluid clears up on its own. When fluid remains in the middle ear for 3 months or longer or when hearing loss develops that could interfere with a child's speech development, a

doctor may recommend MYRINGOTOMY. If chronic infections of the adenoids or tonsils are involved, the doctor may recommend removing them at the time the ventilation tube is inserted. See also ADHESIVE OTITIS MEDIA, CHRONIC.

Otolaryngology

The science, academic study, and medical practice of the field of diseases and disorders of the ears, nose, and throat and other structures of the head and neck. An otolaryngologist is a physician who specializes in this field of medicine. Otolaryngologists are also called ENT (ear, nose, and throat) physicians.

Otosclerosis

A disorder of the middle ear that causes progressive hearing loss, generally affecting both ears. The disorder results from changes in the composition of the stapes (the sound-conducting bone in the inner ear). These changes cause the stapes, a normally movable bone in the middle ear, to become cemented to the surrounding bone and to stop vibrating; the vibrations conduct sound waves that are essential to hearing. Otosclerosis usually develops during the teen or early adult years.

The disorder is generally diagnosed with hearing tests, including AUDIOMETRY, that evaluate the hearing loss. The disease is most effectively treated by a surgical procedure called a STAPEDECTOMY (replacement of the stapes with an artificial bone), which usually restores normal functioning to the middle and inner ear. One ear is operated on at a time.

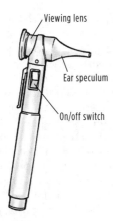

Viewing lens

Ear speculum

On/off switch

Otoscope

An otoscope has a speculum that can be inserted into the ear canal. The device is equipped with a light and a magnifying lens.

Otoscope

A lighted instrument inserted into the external ear canal to allow a physician to examine the ear and observe changes in the external ear canal and eardrum. The use of a pneumatic otoscope is considered the best method for early detection of middle ear fluid, especially in children.

Ototoxicity

Damage to tissues of the inner ear caused by medications or chemicals, resulting in disturbances in hearing and balance. Affected tissues can include the COCHLEA, the cochlea's hair cells (sensory cells that transform sound waves into nerve impulses), and the vestibulocochlear nerve that sends balance and hearing information from the inner ear to the brain. Ototoxicity may be caused by a class of antibiotics called aminoglycosides; certain anticancer drugs; certain diuretics; aspirin and aspirin-containing compounds; certain quinines including tonic water; and environmental chemicals including arsenic, lead, and carbon monoxide. The effects can be temporary or permanent.

The symptoms of ototoxicity may range from mild to severe and from intermittent ringing in the ears to hearing loss in both ears. Hearing loss is often first experienced in the higher frequencies and can progress to difficulty comprehending speech. Usually, job exposure to hazardous chemicals can cause hearing loss after about 2 to 3 years.

Treatment usually focuses on reducing the effects of the damage. Hearing aids or a COCHLEAR IMPLANT may benefit people who have profound hearing loss in both ears. PHYSICAL THERAPY can aid people experiencing balance problems.

Outpatient treatment

Medical care in a hospital that does not include an overnight stay. Outpatient treatment may also be provided at a clinic or doctor's office.

Ovarian cysts

Small, fluid-filled sacs that form on the ovaries, most commonly in women during their childbearing years. They result from changes in hormone levels related to the menstrual cycle, as well as the production and release of eggs from the ovaries (ovulation). The cysts can range in size from that of a pea to that of a grapefruit. Symptoms can include severe abdominal pain, irregular or delayed periods, a dull ache in the lower abdomen, or pain during sexual intercourse.

If a cyst is small and causing no symptoms, the doctor may monitor it for a few weeks, because most cysts go away by themselves over one or two menstrual cycles. Large or painful cysts can be treated with hormones or surgery. The surgical procedure used to remove ovarian cysts is called an OOPHORECTOMY.

Ovary

One of the pair of the female sex glands that contain eggs (female reproductive cells) and produce the female sex hormones estrogen and progesterone. Each ovary is about the size and shape of a walnut. The ovaries are situated in the pelvis, one on either side of the uterus and connected to the uterus by the fallopian tubes. See REPRODUCTIVE SYSTEM, FEMALE.

Ovary, cancer of the

Cancer that begins in the ovaries. Ovarian cancer is the sixth most common cancer in women. Because it is difficult to detect at an early stage, ovarian cancer is more likely to spread from the ovary and be fatal than is cancer of the cervix or endometrium (the lining of the uterus). Early stages of ovarian cancer usually have no symptoms. A tumor may first be detected when a doctor feels an enlarged ovary as part of a routine pelvic examination. At later stages, a woman may have vague intestinal problems, a feeling of fullness in her abdomen, or abdominal or pelvic pain or discomfort.

If ovarian cancer is suspected, a doctor may order an ultrasound or CT scan or take a blood sample to measure the level of the protein CA-125, which is elevated in the blood of most women with ovarian cancer. However, no test is completely reliable for detecting ovarian cancer and a doctor may need to use a laparoscope, a surgical device inserted through a small abdominal incision that allows viewing of the internal organs. A laparotomy, a procedure that requires a larger abdominal incision, may be performed to diagnose and find out if the cancer has spread to other organs or tissues.

For most women with ovarian cancer, surgery is performed to remove the uterus (HYSTERECTOMY) and the fallopian tubes and ovaries (SALPINGO-OOPHORECTOMY). If the cancer is confined to one ovary, the doctor may remove only that ovary, particularly if the woman is young and wants to have children. At times, some lymph nodes and parts of the intestine may be removed. Surgery is usually followed by chemotherapy and, in rare cases, radiation therapy.

Overdose, medication

Excessive consumption of prescription or nonprescription medications, either by accident or deliberately. An overdose can involve seemingly harmless drugs sold over the counter—such as aspirin, acetaminophen, iron, vitamins, antihistamines, and sleep aids—which in large enough doses can be fatal. Children and older people are at particular risk for medication overdose, but any person who fails to read a drug label and follow a doctor's instructions may be at risk.

An overdose may also occur if a child takes a drug of any kind, including iron supplements, thinking it is candy. Any medication overdose requires a call to a POISON CENTER or a trip to the nearest hospital emergency department.

Over-the-counter (OTC) drugs

See NONPRESCRIPTION DRUGS.

Overweight

Body weight that is 10 to 20 percent higher than the average for a certain height and that represents an increased percentage of body fat. Being 20 percent or more overweight is considered obesity. A person who has a BODY MASS INDEX (BMI) of 25 to 29.9 is considered overweight; a BMI over 30 is considered obesity. BMI correlates weight with body fat percentage. Exceptions may be athletes, whose extra weight is more likely to be due to excess muscle than fat.

Ovulation

The process by which a mature egg is released from an ovary into the fallopian tube, through which it travels to the uterus. Ovulation takes place during a woman's reproductive years at around day 15 of the 28-day menstrual cycle. If fertilized by a sperm, the egg may be implanted in the wall of the uterus and produce a pregnancy. See MENSTRUATION.

Ovulation stimulants

Drugs used to cause more frequent ovulation; fertility drugs. Ovulation stimulants are prescribed when a woman has difficulty conceiving because she ovulates irregularly or not at all. The drugs do not improve fertility in women who ovulate regularly. Ovulation stimulants may be used to control the time of ovulation in a woman undergoing artificial insemination or other assisted reproductive technology.

Ovulation, lack of

Anovulation; the inability of the ovaries (see OVARY) to produce mature eggs or to release mature eggs on a regular basis. Among the most common causes of infertility in women, anovulation usually results from hormone imbalances, which may be caused by excessive weight loss, obesity, stress, or strenuous exercise. It also frequently occurs in women with POLYCYSTIC OVARIAN SYNDROME (a condition in which cysts develop in the ovaries). The most common cause of anovulation is excessive weight loss, which can result from the eating disorder anorexia bulimia or from excessive exercise. In many cases, treating the underlying cause and restoring the woman's weight to normal is enough to restore fertility.

Ovum

The female reproductive cell—also known as an egg—found in the ovaries. Typically, after puberty, a woman's body releases one ovum during each menstrual cycle; this

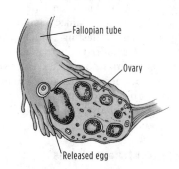

Fallopian tube

Ovary

Released egg

Female reproductive cell
The ovum, released each month from a female ovary, has the potential to be fertilized by a sperm (male reproductive cell) and develop into a fetus.

process is called OVULATION. See RE-
PRODUCTIVE SYSTEM, FEMALE.

Oximetry

A painless diagnostic test that measures the amount of oxygen in a person's blood. The test does not require
a blood sample. Instead, a small device is placed on the finger, toe, or
ear lobe. The device contains a sen-
sor that is connected to a machine
that displays the oxygen saturation
and pulse rate of the person being
tested.

Oxygen, supplemental

Oxygen administered as a form of
therapy when the oxygen level in the
blood is significantly decreased. Supplemental oxygen may be helpful for
people who have lung diseases that
reduce lung function. It is most commonly prescribed to people who have
emphysema, chronic obstructive pulmonary disease (COPD), sarcoidosis,
interstitial pulmonary fibrosis, and
occupational lung diseases.

There are several approaches to dis-
pensing oxygen in the home—in
large steel or aluminum tanks or in
smaller, portable tanks. Liquid oxygen is longer lasting and can be
stored in smaller tanks that are con-
veniently transported. Oxygen con-
centrators are devices that produce
oxygen by concentrating the oxygen
that is present in the air and eliminating other gases.

Oxygen free radicals

Unstable molecules formed as by-
products of the body's normal chemical processes. In excess, oxygen free
radicals can damage cell membranes,
disrupt the immune system, and contribute to the development of diseases such as cancer, cataracts, and
heart disease. The supply of oxygen
free radicals in the body can be increased by factors such as smoking,
stress, exposure to radiation, inflammation, and air pollution. Antioxidant vitamins such as vitamins A, C,
and E are scavengers of oxygen free
radicals. To include antioxidants in
their diet, people are advised to include plenty of fruit, vegetables, and
whole grains.

Oxytocin

A hormone released by the pituitary
gland in the brain to stimulate contractions of the uterus during labor
and production and release of milk
during breast-feeding.

Oxytocin challenge test

External fetal monitoring performed
on pregnant women to assess the
health of the fetus using the hormone oxytocin to stimulate uterine
contractions. The pregnant woman
is given an intravenous solution of
oxytocin and the doctor observes the
reaction of the fetus to the stress of
the contractions to help determine
how well the fetus will handle the
stress of labor. Labor contractions
tend to reduce the available supply
of oxygen by compressing the placenta. A normal response to the oxytocin challenge test (OCT) suggests
that the fetus is healthy, is receiving
enough oxygen, and will be able to
withstand the stress of labor. If the
fetus is experiencing difficulties, the
doctor may decide to deliver the
baby early.

Pacemaker

An electronic device that causes the heart to beat by releasing small electrical discharges. A temporary external pacemaker can be used to regulate an abnormally slow heartbeat for a short time. It is connected to the heart by wires threaded through a narrow tube inserted into a vein in the neck, chest, or groin. An internal, permanent pacemaker is implanted in the chest wall. Pacemakers are often used to correct bradycardia (an abnormally slow heartbeat) by electrically stimulating the heart to maintain a sufficient, predetermined heart rate. In some cases, pacemakers are used to correct tachycardia (an abnormally fast heartbeat). Pacemakers can increase the heartbeat automatically during increased physical activity.

Paget disease

An irregular thickening and softening of the bones of unknown cause. It is most common in adults older than 50. The bones most often affected by Paget disease are the hip bones, shin bones, thighbone, skull, spine, and collarbone. The disease makes these bones enlarged, deformed, and easily fractured. Bone pain is the most common symptom. The chronic aching sensation tends to worsen at night. The affected areas may feel warm and tender. When Paget disease affects the skull bones, it may cause deafness. Increased blood flow through the diseased bones may strain the heart, which can cause heart failure. Rarely, a bone tumor may develop.

Paget disease is diagnosed by physical examination, X rays, and various blood tests. There is no cure, but symptoms may be treated by pain-relieving medication such as aspirin or ibuprofen. Injections of the hormone calcitonin may be given to relieve severe pain. Some oral medications may also be effective.

Paget disease of the vulva

A form of skin cancer in the area of the vulva. Symptoms include recurrent severe itching and soreness. Red velvety lesions with clearly defined borders or white patches may appear on the vulva, anus, vagina, or the area between the anus and vagina. It is diagnosed by biopsy, and surgical removal is usually required.

Pain management, acute

Methods for controlling pain that has a limited duration (usually no more than 1 month), resulting from an injury, surgery, or illness. In most cases, acute pain resolves when the affected tissues heal. Cancer pain is generally classified as acute even though it may be long-lasting.

Medications

In most cases, acute pain responds well to medication. Three classes of medications are available, depending on the type and severity of the pain.

OPIOIDS Derived from the poppy plant, these are the most powerful anti-pain medications. They include codeine and morphine, as well as closely related synthetic compounds, such as oxycodone, hydromorphone, and hydrocodone. When used correctly, they are highly effective at controlling even severe pain. Opioids block the transmission of pain signals through the spinal cord and the perception of pain in the brain. They also may provide a sense of diminished anxiety. When used for pain control under medical supervision, opioids rarely cause addiction.

The drawback to opioids is their side effects. They depress the respiratory system, may cause nausea and itching, and often result in constipation and an inability to urinate. Adjusting doses and taking other measures, such as increasing the amount of fiber in the diet, can alleviate or counter the side effects.

NONOPIOIDS This group of medications includes aspirin and other nonsteroidal anti-inflammatory drugs (NSAIDs) such as ibuprofen and naproxen and newer drugs called Cox-2 inhibitors. NSAIDs can reduce inflammation and pain from sprains, strains, or other injuries; menstrual cramps; gout attacks; tendonitis; and other painful conditions. Some NSAIDs (such as aspirin, ibuprofen, and naproxen) can reduce fever. Acetaminophen is a pain reliever and fever reducer but not an NSAID because it does not relieve inflammation. Side effects of NSAIDs include irritation to the stomach lining, sometimes leading to severe bleeding. In large doses, these drugs may be toxic to the liver and kidneys. Cox-2 inhibitors appear to increase the risk of heart attack or stroke and should only be taken after discussing the benefits and risks with the doctor who prescribes them.

COMBINATION DRUGS These medications mix a non-narcotic pain reliever with an opioid such as co-deine. They are generally effective against relatively mild to moderate pain and are particularly useful for patients during their initial recovery at home after surgery.

Anesthesia

For moderate to severe pain of limited duration, local or regional anesthesia (see ANESTHESIA, LOCAL; ANESTHESIA, REGIONAL) can often provide excellent relief. After surgery, many surgeons inject local anesthetic agents into the area surrounding the incision to block the sensation of pain as the surgical anesthesia wears off. This also controls discomfort during the first few hours after surgery, when pain is likely to be the worst. For pain in the legs and lower portion of the body, a single dose of long-acting medication can be injected along with the anesthetic medication in spinal or epidural anesthesia (see also ANESTHESIA, SPINAL; ANESTHESIA, EPIDURAL).

Pain management, chronic

Methods for controlling pain that continues after an injured tissue has healed. Chronic pain often begins as acute pain (see pain management, acute). It can be caused by diseases such as shingles, osteoarthritis, diabetes, or cancer; traumatic injury, such as from an automobile collision or a gunshot wound; or from surgery, such as the phantom limb pain following amputation. Every case of chronic pain is unique, so a treatment plan must be developed by a physician and a team of specialists.

Medications

Opioid medications, such as codeine and morphine, are highly effective at stopping acute pain, but carry the risk of chemical dependency over the long term. Acetaminophen and nonsteroidal anti-inflammatory drugs (NSAIDs) do little to relieve severe or chronic pain. Some antidepressants help with chronic pain, even in people who are not depressed. Amitriptyline, trazodone, and imipramine can be combined with analgesic medications such as NSAIDs, but unwanted side effects may include drowsiness, constipation, and dry mouth. Anticonvulsants, developed originally to treat epilepsy, are effective in controlling chronic nerve pain, such as TRIGEMINAL NEURALGIA.

Other medications are used for specific kinds of pain. CORTICOSTEROIDS work well against pain caused by inflammation and swelling, such as in osteoarthritis. Long-term use of corticosteroids, however, can cause serious problems, such as bone thinning (see OSTEOPOROSIS), cataracts, and high blood pressure. Capsaicin is a cream that works well against shingles pain in the skin, osteoarthritis, and neuropathy caused by diabetes.

Other approaches

In some cases, local anesthetics can be injected around nerves or into joints to reduce swelling, irritation, spasms in the muscles, or abnormal nerve transmissions that cause pain. The anesthetic medication can be mixed with corticosteroids to amplify its benefits. However, local anesthetics last for a limited time and may provide only temporary relief.

Transcutaneous electrical nerve stimulation (TENS) involves the use of a small battery-operated device that blocks the transmission of pain impulses by stimulating nerve fibers through the skin with low-level elec-

trical energy; it can sometimes provide significant pain relief. Risks are minimal but the electrodes can irritate the skin, and the electrical current may cause local discomfort.

ACUPUNCTURE and ACUPRESSURE are recommended by some physicians who treat chronic pain, but their effectiveness is not uniform for all pain conditions. Physical therapy techniques, can help to alleviate pain in the muscles and joints.

Since stress makes pain worse, relaxation techniques, such as meditation and yoga, can help lessen pain. BIOFEEDBACK is useful for teaching a person how to be aware of, and learn to control, unconscious responses to pain.

Palate

The roof of the mouth. The palate separates the oral cavity from the nasal cavity (see NOSE). The front portion of the palate is hard and bony (hard palate); the back portion is soft and fleshy (soft palate).

Palliative care

Any procedure or medication intended to ease pain and otherwise improve quality of life but that does not cure disease. For example, a physician may perform palliative surgery on a person with advanced cancer in order to ease pain and treat other symptoms, even when it is not possible to cure the cancer.

Palpate

To examine by means of touch to evaluate the health of an organ or body part.

Palpitations

The sensation of a strong, fast, or irregular heartbeat. Palpitations can be unpleasant, but they usually last for only a few seconds. They may occur alone or with other symptoms, such as sweating, chest pain, dizziness, shortness of breath, nausea, and light-headedness.

Palpitations may be related to an underlying heart condition. Possible causes include hypertension (high blood pressure), cardiac arrhythmia (irregular heartbeat), mitral valve prolapse, hyperthyroidism (an overactive thyroid gland), anemia (a shortage of red blood cells), and coronary artery disease. They can also be brought on by stress, anxiety, panic attack, stimulants such as caffeine and nicotine, excessive alcohol, and some medications.

Treatment may include measures to alleviate or eliminate symptoms, such as deep breathing, relaxation exercises, splashing cold water on the face, or drinking cold water. If a substance or medication is causing the problem, it can be reduced or eliminated. Palpitations caused by heart disease, anxiety, or stress often improve as that condition is treated. Medications to prevent or control palpitations are available.

Palsy

PARALYSIS in any part of the body that is sometimes accompanied by involuntary tremors.

Pancreas

A long, tapered gland located in the abdomen behind the stomach and beneath the liver. The pancreas has important roles in digestion and regulation of blood sugar. It contains both exocrine tissue and endocrine tissue. The exocrine tissues, which comprise most of the pancreas, secrete digestive enzymes into a network of ducts that lead to the main pancreatic duct. This main duct joins the common bile duct and enters the duodenum (the first part of the small intestine). In the small intestine, these digestive enzymes help break down proteins, fats, and carbohydrates.

The endocrine tissues in the pancreas secrete the hormones INSULIN, glucagon, and somatostatin into the blood to regulate the blood sugar (glucose) level. See BILIARY SYSTEM.

Pancreas, cancer of the

Cancer originating in the PANCREAS. Pancreatic cancer is the fourth most common cause of cancer death in the United States. Depending on which part of the pancreas is affected, symptoms may include abdominal pain, loss of appetite, weight loss, nausea, vomiting, and JAUNDICE (a yellowing of the skin and the whites of the eyes). Pain usually centers in the upper abdomen and may penetrate to the back. However, when cancer occurs in the head of the pancreas, there may be no pain. Other symptoms usually are not apparent until the cancer has advanced to an incurable stage.

Diagnosis of pancreatic cancer is made by blood tests and imaging procedures, such as CT (computed tomography) scanning and endoscopy. Early detection and pancreatectomy (surgical removal of all or part of the pancreas) provide the best chance of a cure. Pancreatectomy is generally used only in the early stages of the disease. Chemotherapy and radiation may be recommended before or after surgery.

Pancreas transplant

Replacing a diseased, nonfunctioning pancreas with a healthy pancreas from a donor. The pancreas, located in the upper abdomen near the stomach, produces insulin to regulate sugar levels in the blood. In people with type 1 diabetes, the insulin-producing cells of the pancreas no longer function. Most recipients of pancreas transplants are people with type 1 diabetes who have kidney disease requiring a kidney transplant or who have severe, frequent hypoglycemia (low blood sugar) that is disabling. For other people with type 1 diabetes and for people with type 2 diabetes, pancreas transplants are experimental because of the serious side effects of the immune-suppressing medications that must be taken for life to prevent organ rejection.

Pancreatectomy

Surgical removal of all or part of the PANCREAS. A pancreatectomy is the most effective treatment for pancreatic cancer. It is also performed in some cases of chronic pancreatitis (long-term inflammation of the pancreas) and following traumatic injury to the pancreas.

Pancreatitis

Inflammation of the PANCREAS. Pancreatitis may be sudden and acute or chronic and long-lasting. Most cases are associated with alcohol abuse or gallstones (hardened masses of cholesterol or bilirubin that develop in the gallbladder). Acute pancreatitis usually comes on rapidly and can result in life-threatening disease. Intense pain develops in the upper abdomen and can penetrate to the back. Other symptoms include nausea, vomiting, fever, and abdominal distension. Internal bleeding may cause bruises to appear on the abdomen.

Recurrent attacks of acute pancreatitis can lead to chronic inflammation of the pancreas, damaging it and eventually making it unable to produce enzymes and hormones. An impaired pancreas can cause insulin deficiency, diabetes, and malabsorption (reduced absorption of nutrients through the small intestine).

The doctor may prescribe insulin if the blood glucose level is elevated. Complete abstinence from alcohol is vital to recovery from both forms of pancreatitis.

Cases of acute pancreatitis usually require hospitalization. Treatment may include pain relievers, drugs to control pancreatic juices, and possibly antibiotics. Surgery is sometimes necessary if there are complications such as bleeding, infection, or cysts. If gallstones are the underlying cause, they are usually removed. Severe cases of pancreatitis are life-threatening.

In chronic pancreatitis, the doctor may also prescribe pain relievers, along with digestive enzyme medication and insulin as needed. Eating a special low-fat diet is also essential. In severe cases, a PANCREATECTOMY (surgical removal of all or part of the pancreas) can provide pain relief.

Pandemic

A disease that affects greater numbers of people than usual across a major geographical area, such as a region, a country, a continent, or the whole world. An example is the AIDS (acquired immunodeficiency syndrome) pandemic in Africa, which affects a large portion of the population. See EPIDEMIC.

Panic attack

A sudden, unexpected, overwhelming, and terrifying episode of anxiety in which the person feels as if he or she is out of control and threatened with imminent harm. Physical symptoms can include a sensation of shortness of breath, dizziness or faintness, rapid pounding heartbeat, trembling, sweating, shakiness, chills, choking, nausea, heartburn, numbness or tingling in the hands or feet, chest pain or discomfort, flushed or clammy skin, paralysis of the face, and agitation. The symptoms come on rapidly, usually peak within seconds or minutes, and subside. Usually the whole episode peaks within 10 minutes and is over within 30 minutes. Panic attacks may recur. They can be a symptom of any of the ANXIETY DISORDERS, depression, and a number of physical conditions, including impaired breathing and heart disease.

Panic disorder

A mental illness causing repeated, frequent, unexpected episodes of extreme anxiety called PANIC ATTACKS and resulting in severe anxiety about further attacks. There are three key components of panic disorder: the presence of panic attacks, the unexpectedness of the panic attacks, and fear and anxiety over further panic attacks for at least 1 month following an attack. Physical symptoms of panic attacks can include chest pain, shortness of breath, heart palpitations, dizziness or faintness, sweating, nausea, flushed or clammy skin, and agitation. The symptoms come

on rapidly, usually peak within seconds or minutes, and subside, usually within minutes.

Untreated panic disorder can make it difficult for the individual to function in job, social, or family roles. Approximately one of five people with panic disorder attempts suicide.

Panic disorder is highly treatable. The usual approach combines medication and psychotherapy. Medications effective against panic disorder include antidepressants and antianxiety drugs.

Pantothenic acid

See VITAMIN B.

Pap smear

A screening test for cancer of the CERVIX usually performed during a woman's annual health examination. To perform a Pap smear, a doctor inserts a speculum into a woman's vagina and, using a tiny brush or cotton swab, removes cells from the surface of the cervix. The sample is sent to a laboratory where the cells are examined microscopically for abnormalities, such as atypical cells, precancerous cells, and cancerous cells. Many laboratories also test for certain strains of the human papillomavirus (HPV), which increases a woman's risk of cervical cancer.

A negative (normal) result from a Pap smear test means a woman's cervix is probably healthy. An abnormal result does not necessarily mean a woman has cancer because a Pap smear can detect precancerous cell changes that have not yet become cancerous. If a woman has a mildly abnormal Pap smear, the doctor may recommend retesting in 3 months to see if the abnormalities persist. See also CERVICAL DYSPLASIA; CERVIX, CANCER OF.

Papilledema

Swelling of the region where the optic nerve joins the retina (the thin, light-sensitive area in the back of the eye). Papilledema is caused by increased intracranial pressure, and both eyes are usually involved. Papilledema can result from a brain tumor, bleeding into the brain tissue, or pseudotumor cerebri. Malignant hypertension, a medical emergency, may also cause disc swelling.

Papilloma

A small, soft, flesh-colored growth that protrudes from the skin. See also SKIN TAG.

Paracentesis

Also known as an abdominal tap; a procedure in which fluid is removed from the abdominal cavity with a needle inserted through the abdominal wall. The abdominal cavity normally contains little fluid but excess fluid can be present in people with conditions such as chronic liver disease or neoplasms (abnormal growths) in the abdomen. Paracentesis is performed to remove a sample of fluid to determine why it is present or to help relieve symptoms when a large accumulation of fluid causes discomfort or affects a person's breathing.

Parainfluenza virus

Any one of three related viruses that cause a variety of respiratory infections ranging in severity from the common cold to CROUP to a type of pneumonia. Parainfluenza viruses tend to cause illness predominantly in young children. By adulthood, most people have established immunity to the viruses and have no symptoms or only mild infections. Different types of the virus cause different forms of disease. The most common infection in children is the common cold. See COLD, COMMON.

Bed rest and treating symptoms with acetaminophen and cough medications are generally recommended. (Aspirin should not be given to children younger than 18 years because of the risk of REYE SYNDROME.)

Paralysis

The complete or partial loss of the power of motion or sensation. Paralysis occurs when there is a loss of nerve impulses to a muscle, resulting in an inability to move that muscle. Sudden paralysis is usually the result of STROKE or trauma (such as a broken neck or back). Spinal cord injuries commonly result from car or motorcycle injuries, falls, sporting injuries, or gunshot wounds. Paralysis from spinal cord injuries can be irreversible.

Paralysis can be temporary or permanent, localized or widespread, or sudden or spreading. PARAPLEGIA is paralysis that affects the lower extremities and most often occurs after injury to the lower spinal cord. Quadriplegia affects both the upper and lower extremities; it occurs as a result of damage to the upper spinal cord. Hemiplegia (paralysis of one side of the body) is usually caused by brain damage, often as the result of a stroke. Palsy is partial paralysis in any part of the body that is sometimes accompanied by involuntary tremors. Other symptoms that can accompany paralysis include numbness, tingling, pain, and problems with speech, vision, or balance.

Treatment of paralysis is based on its underlying cause. A long-term rehabilitation program involves physical therapy and occupational therapy. Treatment with other specialists—such as speech therapists, respiratory therapists, social workers, or psychiatrists—may also be required.

Paramedic

A medical professional trained to perform emergency medical procedures. Paramedics are the most highly trained of all emergency medical technicians. See EMERGENCY MEDICAL TECHNICIAN.

Paraneoplastic syndrome

Symptoms related to a tumor that are not due to direct invasion by the tumor, but usually from substances secreted by the cancer cells of the tumor. These substances usually produce symptoms in organs unrelated to the site of the tumor. Paraneoplastic syndromes can play a role in the diagnosis of cancer, because their appearance can be the first sign of disease, making it possible for the cancer to be detected early.

Paranoia

Extreme, pervasive, and unwarranted distrust of other people's actions and motivations and an exaggerated sense of self-importance. Paranoia occurs in many mental disorders but is rare as an isolated mental disorder. The cause of paranoia is unknown. Treatment is usually behavior therapy to try to reduce the person's sensitivity to criticism and improve his or her social skills.

Paraplegia

PARALYSIS of the legs, often as a result of a spinal cord injury. In addition to paralysis, other symptoms frequently include numbness, tingling, pain, and problems with speech, vision, or balance. There may be a loss of bladder and bowel control, as well as sexual dysfunction.

Paraplegia is diagnosed by a physical examination and tests such as blood studies, CT (computed tomography) scanning, MRI, electromyogram (EMG), myelography, and X ray. The immediate goals of treatment are to stabilize the injured spine, restore proper alignment, and decompress any affected neurological structures. Long-term treatment is a rehabilitation program involving physical and occupational therapy.

Parasite

An organism that obtains nourishment by living in or on other organisms, called hosts, producing disease in human or animal hosts. Parasites that cause infections in humans are most common in areas of the world where water safety standards are poor, such as developing countries. In the United States, some kinds of parasites have been found in well water, rivers, lakes, and streams. The most common symptoms caused by parasitic infection include diarrhea, weight loss, loss of appetite, abdominal cramps, and mild fever.

Parasympathetic nervous system

A division of the autonomic nervous system (part of the nervous system that controls unconscious body functions) that is dominant in the body's normal, resting state (that is, in the absence of stress). Parasympathetic nerve activity includes narrowing the air passages in the lungs, constricting the pupils, decreasing the heart rate, lowering blood pressure, maintaining normal digestive activity, and enabling the bladder to empty. See NERVOUS SYSTEM.

Parathyroid glands

Four small glands located behind the thyroid gland that are important in regulating the levels of calcium in the blood. The parathyroids are part of the ENDOCRINE SYSTEM because they release parathyroid hormone directly into the bloodstream.

Parathyroid hormone

A hormone produced by the parathyroid glands that helps control the level of calcium in the blood; also known as PTH. Parathyroid hormone increases calcium in the blood when levels are too low by releasing calcium from the bones and decreasing calcium excretion from the kidneys. When blood calcium levels are elevated, the parathyroid gland is signaled to stop producing parathyroid hormone to reduce and normalize the amount of calcium in the blood. Parathyroid hormone also stimulates the kidney's production of vitamin D, which helps increase intestinal absorption of calcium.

Parathyroid tumor

A growth on the parathyroid glands that usually results in excessive production of PARATHYROID HORMONE. Excess levels of parathyroid hormone produce elevated calcium in the blood

and urine, which can lead to kidney damage and the formation of calcium-containing kidney stones. When the kidneys excrete large amounts of calcium, extreme thirst and frequent urination are often symptoms. Increased stomach acid secretion may cause heartburn or acid reflux.

Parathyroid tumors that secrete excess parathyroid hormone and cause problems are generally surgically removed. If the tumor causes no problems, surgery may not be necessary. In this case, monitoring the blood calcium level, screening for kidney stones, and evaluating bone density must be done periodically.

Parathyroidectomy

Surgical removal of parathyroid gland tissue for the treatment of HYPERPARATHYROIDISM. In hyperparathyroidism, the parathyroid glands, for unknown reasons, become enlarged and produce excessive amounts of PARATHYROID HORMONE. To determine which of the glands are involved, DIAGNOSTIC IMAGING, including an ultrasound scan, an isotope scan, and possibly an angiogram, may be performed. Parathyroidectomy usually cures the disorder. See HYPERPARATHYROIDISM.

Parenteral nutrition

The administration of a nutritional solution through a catheter into the blood stream. Total parenteral nutrition (TPN), also called hyperalimentation, is used in prolonged coma, severe malabsorption, burns, and other conditions in which feeding by mouth is not possible or does not provide adequate nutrition. Problems that may require parenteral nutrition in children include intestinal obstruction, structural abnormalities of the digestive tract, and severe chronic diarrhea.

The solutions that are used contain glucose, amino acids, lipids, vitamins, minerals, and other substances needed by severely ill people.

Paresthesia

An abnormal sensation of numbness, tingling, prickling, or pins and needles on the skin. Paresthesias are usually experienced in the extremities and can be an indication of nerve damage or poor circulation.

Parkinson disease

A chronic degenerative disease characterized by tremors, rigidity, postural instability, and slowness of movement. Parkinson disease is the most common form of parkinsonism (the term for a group of disorders with these symptoms). Parkinson disease occurs when nerve cells (neurons) in parts of the brain stem (particularly the substantia nigra) die or degenerate. These neurons normally produce dopamine, an important neurotransmitter that transmits signals about movement within the brain. In Parkinson disease, the loss of dopamine causes the corpus striatum part of the brain to fire out of control. This leaves affected people unable to direct or control their movements in a normal manner.

The early symptoms of Parkinson disease are subtle and gradual. People may notice fatigue, malaise, irritability, or a slight shakiness. As the disease progresses, shaking and tremor begin to interfere with daily activities. Tremors may be worse with rest and improve with movement. Bradykinesia, or the slowing of automatic move-

ment, may prevent a person from performing routine activities, such as washing and dressing. Postural instability can lead to suddenly freezing in place and to falling.

Parkinson disease can be difficult to diagnose in its early stages, before symptoms become prominent. There is no cure for Parkinson disease but medication can usually improve the symptoms and may slow the progression of the disease. Doctors frequently prescribe levodopa (which the brain uses to make dopamine) combined with carbidopa (which prevents the body from metabolizing the levodopa before it can reach the brain). Because this treatment can become less effective over time, drugs called dopamine agonists may also be prescribed to help control the symptoms. Drugs that reduce tremors, such as benztropine (which is an ANTICHOLINERGIC AGENT), may also be prescribed.

If symptoms become severe and do not respond to treatment, surgery to implant a brain "pacemaker" may be recommended. For the pacemaker, wires are implanted in the brain to stimulate a specific area with a mild electric current to help control the tremors. Surgery is sometimes done to destroy the small area of brain tissue that is causing the symptoms.

Parkinsonism

A term referring to a group of disorders characterized by four primary symptoms: tremor, rigidity, postural instability, and slowness of movement (see also PARKINSON DISEASE). Parkinsonism also is the term usually used to describe the symptoms of Parkinson disease that are not caused by the degeneration of dopamine-producing cells in the brain; people with parkinsonism produce enough dopamine but do not seem to process it correctly. Strokes in the basal ganglia may damage nerve cells that use dopamine, resulting in parkinsonian symptoms, or parkinsonism.

Paroxysm

An acute attack or intensification of the symptoms of a disease; also a sudden seizure or spasm.

Parvovirus

See FIFTH DISEASE.

Passive smoking

Nonsmokers' exposure to smoke emitted by burning cigarettes or cigars and exhaled by cigarette or cigar smokers. Passive smoking, also referred to as secondhand smoke, puts people who do not smoke but live or work in the same indoor environment as smokers at risk of developing lung cancer, heart disease, stroke, bronchitis, and pneumonia. Children exposed to passive smoking have an increased prevalence of fluid in the middle ear, which is a symptom of chronic middle ear disease. They are also susceptible to irritation of the upper respiratory tract and may have significantly reduced lung function. Passive smoking may cause asthma in children who do not already have it.

Passive-aggressive personality disorder

See PERSONALITY DISORDERS.

Patch test

A test used to detect hypersensitivity to a substance that comes in contact with the skin. The patch test consists of applying a substance suspected to be the cause of a CONTACT DERMATI-TIS to an unaffected area of skin. The substances causing the allergies are identified if the skin reacts to them.

Patellar tendinitis

Inflammation of the tendon that connects the kneecap to the shinbone. The cause of patellar tendinitis is overuse, usually during athletic activity, which produces microscopic tears in the tiny fibers of the tissue. These tears can stretch the patellar tendon and cause painful inflammation. Symptoms include pain when running or jogging and localized tenderness when pressure is applied to the point just below the kneecap where the patellar tendon connects the kneecap to the shinbone.

Initial discomfort is generally treated by resting the area, applying ice, and elevating the knee. Patellar tendinitis usually heals on its own within 3 weeks.

Paternity testing

Testing of blood or DNA to identify the biological father of a child. Most often, blood samples are taken from an infant soon after birth, the possible father, and sometimes the mother. These samples are then analyzed for compatibility. For DNA testing on blood or a swab of cells from inside the cheek, the DNA of the child and potential father are analyzed to see if they match.

Pathogen

An agent that causes disease, usually referring to a microorganism such as a virus, bacterium, or fungus.

Pathology

The branch of medicine concerned with diagnosis of disease, its effects on bodily functions, and causes of death. Pathology can involve laboratory examination of bodily fluids (clinical pathology), cell samples (cytopathology), and tissues (anatomical pathology). Pathology can involve the study of DNA (genetic material) to detect inherited genetic abnormalities, establish the paternity of a child, or identify criminal suspects. A pathologist is a doctor who specializes in pathology.

Pathophysiology

The study of changes in body function caused by disease. Pathophysiology is concerned with changes in how organs function, rather than with disease-related changes in body structures.

Patient-controlled analgesia

See ANALGESIA, PATIENT-CONTROLLED.

Peak flow meter

A device that measures airflow, called peak expiratory flow rate, which is one measure of lung function. The person being tested blows quickly and forcefully into the device, and a reading indicates how open the airways are. Peak flow meters are used primarily to determine the severity of ASTHMA and may be used as a diagnostic tool to detect an asthmatic condition before other symptoms appear. See REACTIVE AIRWAY DISEASE.

Pediatrics

The medical specialty that concerns children's physical and emotional development, the diagnosis and treatment of diseases and disorders in children, and their growth and development from birth usually to age 18. A physician who specializes in pediatrics is called a pediatrician.

Pediculosis

An infestation with lice, which are ectoparasites that live on the human body. Pediculosis may affect the head, the body, or the pubic area (see CRAB LICE). It is transmitted person to person by close physical contact or by contact with infested surfaces, including clothing, towels, bed linens, combs, and hats. Head lice (see LICE, HEAD) infestation is common among school children. Overcrowded environments promote transmission.

Pedophilia

A chronic mental disorder in which an older teen or adult is sexually attracted exclusively or in part to prepubescent children. Pedophilia is more common in males than females. Risk factors include having been sexually abused as a child, having other mental disorders, and substance abuse. Because pedophilic behaviors are illegal, an affected person is dealt with by both the criminal justice system and health-care professionals.

Treatment focuses on stopping the behavior and achieving long-term control of the person's behavior in the community. Common treatment methods are cognitive-behavioral therapy and group therapy to help the person develop strategies to resist acting on the pedophilic impulses. When appropriate, medications such as androgen-lowering agents, which reduce the body's production of the male hormones, are prescribed to suppress the person's sex drive. Successful management of the condition usually requires continuing collaboration between the criminal justice and health-care systems.

Pelvic examination

An examination of a woman's reproductive system. Periodic pelvic examinations are recommended for all women beginning at age 18 or when they become sexually active. The examination includes both the external and internal parts of the reproductive system. The doctor performs a PAP SMEAR and may test for various sexually transmitted diseases, depending on a woman's risk factors.

Pelvic floor exercises

See KEGEL EXERCISES.

Pelvic inflammatory disease (PID)

An infection in women that has spread to the internal reproductive organs, usually as a result of an untreated SEXUALLY TRANSMITTED DISEASE (STD), most commonly GONORRHEA and CHLAMYDIA. Even if these infections do not produce any symptoms, the bacteria that cause them can travel to the uterus, fallopian tubes, and ovaries, resulting in PID. Scarring of tissues inside the fallopian tubes can damage the tubes or block them completely, resulting in infertility. Pelvic inflammatory disease is currently the most common preventable cause of infertility in women in the United States.

PID may produce no symptoms at all, minor symptoms, or severe symptoms. When symptoms occur, they may include mild aching in the lower abdomen, pain during intercourse, painful urination, discomfort during menstruation, irregular menstrual periods, breakthrough bleeding, and an abnormal vaginal discharge with a foul odor. There may also be fever or chills, nausea, vomiting, and weight loss. The diagnosis of PID and the extent of the disease may be first determined during a pelvic examination, which usually reveals tender or swollen reproductive organs.

Milder cases of PID are usually treated with oral antibiotic therapy for 14 days. Over-the-counter or prescription pain medication and hot baths or heating pads placed on the abdomen or lower back may be used to relieve discomfort. Sexual partners should be informed of possible infection and need treatment whether they have symptoms or not. Abstinence from sexual activity or the use of condoms is recommended until the infection is cleared in both partners. Scarring or the rupture of an abscess may require surgery.

Pelvic pain

For symptom chart, see ABDOMINAL PAIN, page viii.

Pain in the pelvic region in women that may indicate illness. Pelvic pain can be acute, chronic, intermittent, or constant. Diagnosis will depend on the timing, severity, and location of the pain, along with other symptoms. Sudden and severe pain in the pelvis accompanied by nausea, vomiting, faintness, and rapid pulse is considered a medical emergency.

Diagnosing the cause of pelvic pain is based on the woman's medical history and a physical examination, followed by laboratory tests that may include tests of the blood and urine, a pregnancy test, Pap smear, and an ultrasound. If the pain is thought to involve the reproductive system but initial tests are not conclusive, exploratory surgery or LAPAROSCOPY may be necessary. When a diagnosis, such as an ectopic pregnancy or endometriosis, is made surgically, treatment can be performed at the same time.

Women who have chronic discomfort can be helped to adapt to their symptoms with counseling; the discomfort may also be reduced by taking nonsteroidal anti-inflammatory drugs (such as aspirin or ibuprofen), antidepressants, or oral contraceptives, depending on the cause of the pain. Relaxation techniques can also be helpful.

Pelvis

The ringlike framework of bones in the lower trunk that supports the upper body and protects abdominal organs such as the bladder, rectum, and, in women, the uterus.

Pemphigus vulgaris

A blistering disease caused by an autoimmune reaction toward proteins in the skin. Typically, men or women between 40 and 60 years old are affected. Painful and itchy blisters and sores may cover a significant portion of the body. Blisters may first appear in the mouth. Diagnosis is made through biopsy and blood tests. Treatment is with oral corticosteroids and drugs that suppress the immune system. Pemphigus vulgaris can lead to a life-threatening skin infection and is fatal if untreated.

Penicillins

A class of ANTIBIOTICS, used to treat some bacterial infections. They work by killing bacteria or preventing their growth. There are many different kinds of penicillin, all of which share a common chemical makeup.

Penile implant

Surgical insertion of semiflexible plastic rods or an inflatable prosthesis in the penis. A penile implant provides erections in men who have difficulty obtaining or maintaining erections (see ERECTILE DYSFUNCTION). The semiflexible plastic rods provide a permanent semierection; the inflatable implant can be inflated temporarily for sexual activity. The surgery is performed under general or spinal anesthesia.

Penile warts

See CONDYLOMA ACUMINATUM; GENITAL WARTS.

Penis

The male sex organ through which urine and semen pass. The penis consists of three cylinders of spongy tissue that can engorge with blood and become erect during an erection. Through the center of the penis runs the urethra, the tube that carries urine out of the body. The urethral opening is at the tip of the penis. The end of the penis is covered with a flap of skin called the foreskin, which is sometimes surgically removed (see CIRCUMCISION, MALE). During sexual arousal, semen (a thick liquid containing sperm), passes into the urethra; during ejaculation, muscles at the base of the penis contract and propel the semen out of the penis. Although both semen and urine pass through the urethra, they cannot pass through it simultaneously because an internal valve shuts during ejaculation to allow only semen to pass into the urethra. See REPRODUCTIVE SYSTEM, MALE.

Penis, cancer of

A very rare cancer that affects mainly uncircumcised men older than 50. The most common form of the cancer begins as a persistent, painless, raised sore on the foreskin or the head (glans) of the penis. As the cancer invades, symptoms include pain, bleeding, discharge from the tumor, discomfort on urination, and enlarged lymph nodes in the groin.

A tumor confined to the foreskin can be removed with circumcision (see CIRCUMCISION, MALE). More extensive tumors require removal of part or all of the penis; lymph nodes in the groin are removed if the cancer has spread or, sometimes, to check for possible spread of cancer. Radiation of the groin and pelvis may be recommended after surgery. Anticancer drugs (chemotherapy) may be prescribed if the cancer has spread to other parts of the body.

Peptic ulcer disease

A disease in which one or more raw areas develop in the membranes lining the esophagus, stomach, and duodenum. The affected areas are damaged by strong acids and digestive enzymes secreted by stomach glands. The two main types of peptic ulcer disease are DUODENAL ULCERS and GASTRIC ULCERS. Duodenal ulcers occur primarily on the duodenal bulb, which is the first part of the duodenum, the part of the small intestine into which the stomach empties. Gastric ulcers can occur anywhere in the stomach.

Although the symptoms of duodenal and gastric ulcers differ slightly, the disease processes are largely the same. Upper abdominal pain is the most common symptom of both. Burning, gnawing pain typically occurs after meals. Other possible symptoms, such as nausea, vomiting, and loss of appetite and weight, are more characteristic of gastric ulcers than duodenal ulcers. Infection with the bacterium *Helicobacter pylori* is responsible for most cases of peptic ulcer disease. Other factors that play a role are the long-term use of nonsteroidal anti-inflammatory drugs (NSAIDs), such as aspirin and ibuprofen, and smoking.

Diagnosis is usually made through a careful medical history of symptoms and a variety of tests. Because ulcer pain and nausea tend to follow a pattern, the doctor will want to know when symptoms occur and how they are relieved. Pain and nausea are typically eased by food, milk, antacids, or vomiting.

Over-the-counter or prescription antacids often can provide relief. However, prolonged use of antacids can disrupt body chemistry. Therefore, many doctors prefer to prescribe drugs that reduce acid secretion: histamine blockers, anticholinergic agents, and proton pump inhibitors. Although these drugs relieve symptoms, treating the underlying *H. Pylori* infection can cure the ulcer. A regimen called triple therapy (using three medications at once) can eradicate most of the bacteria. The regimen usually includes two antibiotics, and the third medication is usually a PROTON PUMP INHIBITOR.

When peptic ulcer disease fails to respond to treatment or if complications develop, surgery may become necessary, but only rarely.

Percutaneous umbilical cord blood sampling

A prenatal diagnostic test to detect genetic abnormalities and infection in the fetus. Percutaneous umbilical cord blood sampling (PUBS) is used after the 17th week of pregnancy and only when other diagnostic procedures have not provided a definitive result. Because it is a very complicated and difficult procedure, PUBS is performed exclusively by physicians who are specially trained in maternal-fetal medicine. Guided by ultrasound, the doctor uses a sterile needle to take blood from the fetus's umbilical cord. PUBS is associated with more complications, such as injury to the umbilical cord, than other prenatal tests such as AMNIOCENTESIS or CHORIONIC VILLUS SAMPLING.

Perforation

An abnormal hole in an organ or tissue caused by disease or injury. A perforation usually produces sudden and severe pain, inflammation, and possible shock. Although perforation can occur anywhere, it is most common in the stomach, duodenum, sigmoid colon (the final part of the colon that connects with the rectum), or the appendix. In the case of intestinal perforation, which is life-threatening, doctors treat the shock, administer antibiotics, and insert a tube to remove gas and fluid. Surgery is usually required to repair a perforation. The surgeon usually removes the affected area of the intestine, reattaches the remaining parts of the intestine, and performs a temporary COLOSTOMY (a surgically created opening or stoma in the abdominal wall for stool to pass through into a bag).

Pericarditis

Inflammation of the pericardium, the thin, fluid-filled sac that surrounds the heart. When the pericardium becomes inflamed, it may cause pain as the heart moves against it. In addition, excess fluid can accumulate inside the pericardium and restrict the ability of the heart to beat. If fluid buildup prevents the heart from pumping sufficient blood to the body, an emergency situation known as tamponade results and the person requires immediate treatment. Pericarditis may be either acute (temporary) or chronic (persistent and recurring).

Symptoms include a characteristic sharp pain that begins behind the sternum (breastbone) and sometimes spreads to the neck and left shoulder. The pain often worsens if the person takes a deep breath or lies down. Sitting up and leaning forward can reduce the severity of the pain. Occa-

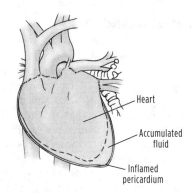

Pressure on the heart

The fluid-filled pericardium is a thin, flexible cushion encasing the heart. In a person with pericarditis, excess fluid can build up and cause pain or restrict the muscular expanding movements of the heart. Some types of pericarditis cause the sac to stiffen, enclosing the heart in a rigid, constrictive container.

sionally the pain is dull and persistent rather than sharp and piercing. Other symptoms can include shortness of breath, swollen abdomen, low fever, coughing, weakness, and pain when swallowing.

Treatment of pericarditis depends on the cause. Antibiotics are used for bacterial infections, and aspirin or ibuprofen is used to alleviate pain and reduce inflammation. Strenuous activity should be avoided during treatment. If fluid accumulation inside the pericardium prevents the heart from pumping sufficient blood to the body, the fluid needs to be drained by inserting a needle into the pericardium; sometimes a catheter (a thin tube) is implanted to continue the drainage.

Pericardium

The sac that encloses the heart and the origin of the large blood vessels leading into and out of the heart. The pericardium has a thick, protective outer bag (called the fibrous pericardium) that keeps the constantly moving heart in position. Within that is an inner sac of membrane (the serous pericardium) that has two layers. The outer layer is separated from the inner layer by a cushion of lubricating fluid. The thin, inner layer secretes this fluid and is a smooth lining that allows the heart to move without friction as it beats.

Perimenopause

A transition period leading to MENO-PAUSE, the cessation of menstruation. Symptoms of perimenopause usually begin in a woman's 40s, about 3 to 5 years before her final menstrual period. The initial symptom is commonly irregular menstrual cycles.

Other symptoms include hot flashes, night sweats, insomnia, mood swings, and vaginal dryness, most of them the result of reduced levels of the hormone ESTROGEN. Oral contraceptives are sometimes prescribed to regulate the menstrual cycle during this time. Many of the symptoms of perimenopause are associated with a variety of pelvic disorders. For this reason, any significant changes in the menstrual cycle should be reported to a doctor. See also MENSTRUATION, DISORDERS OF.

Perinatal

Referring to the period beginning with the 20th week of pregnancy and ending after the first 28 days following delivery.

Perineum

Internally, the floor of the pelvic area. Externally, the perineum is the area of skin and underlying muscle between the genitals and the anus. In women, the perineum stretches during childbirth.

Period, menstrual

See MENSTRUATION.

Periodontal disease

Gum disease characterized by inflammation and infection of the gums, ligaments, bone, and other tissues that surround and support the teeth. Gingivitis and periodontitis are the two primary forms of periodontal disease, which is also called pyorrhea. Gingivitis results from the buildup of plaque (see PLAQUE, DENTAL) and calculus (see CALCULUS, DENTAL) on the teeth. This buildup can cause the gums to pull away from the teeth and lead to the formation of pockets, called periodontal pockets, between the gums and the teeth. The accumulation of plaque and calculus on the teeth that causes periodontal disease is the result of poor oral hygiene in general and, specifically, inadequate or infrequent brushing and use of dental floss to clean the teeth.

Periodontitis

See PERIODONTAL DISEASE.

Periosteum

A sheath of connective tissue that covers all bone surfaces except the ends. Its rich supply of blood vessels delivers oxygen and nutrients to bone cells, it contains nerve pathways, and it has cells that can develop into bone.

Periostitis

Inflammation of the PERIOSTEUM. The causes of periostitis include infection, injury to the area, or an abnormal growth in the tissue. It is diagnosed by X rays and bone scanning. Symptoms include bone pain, localized tenderness and warmth, and swelling of the soft tissue. Periostitis is generally treated by medication to relieve the pain and inflammation. When necessary, medication is prescribed to fight any associated infection.

Peripheral vascular disease

Any disorder of the blood vessels that lie outside the heart. Peripheral vascular disease can affect arteries (which carry oxygen-rich blood from the heart to the body) or veins (which carry oxygen-poor blood from the extremities to the heart).

Peripheral vascular disease is most commonly caused by ATHEROSCLEROSIS. Blood clots (see EMBOLISM; THROMBUS), vasculitis (inflammation of the blood vessels), a tear between the inner and outer layers of the artery (aortic dissection), thrombophlebitis, varicose veins, or chronic venous insufficiency are less common types of vascular disease. Risk factors include smoking, eating a high-fat diet, uncontrolled hypertension (high blood pressure), uncontrolled diabetes, and obesity.

When a person is diagnosed with peripheral vascular disease, the first recommendation the doctor will make is to stop smoking if the person smokes. If the person has high blood pressure or high cholesterol, the doctor will prescribe antihypertensives or cholesterol-lowering medications. He or she may also prescribe platelet inhibitors to reduce the risk of heart attack. Medications may also be prescribed to help reduce some symptoms in the legs and improve the person's ability to walk. People with diabetes need to strictly control their blood glucose level. If these measures are not effective in reducing symptoms, a doctor may recommend ANGIOPLASTY or inserting a STENT in the affected blood vessel in the leg to help improve circulation. In some cases, BYPASS SURGERY around the leg artery is necessary.

Peristalsis

Wavelike, rhythmic, muscle contractions that carry food through the digestive tract. Peristalsis occurs from the moment food enters the mouth until waste matter is expelled from the rectum.

Peritoneal dialysis

A procedure that takes over the functions of the kidneys to remove waste products and maintain the body's water and chemical balance. Peritoneal dialysis uses the lining of the abdomen, called the peritoneal membrane, and a cleansing solution, called dialysate, to filter the blood through a catheter to remove excess water, waste products, and chemicals from the body.

There are two main types of peritoneal dialysis: continuous ambulatory peritoneal dialysis (CAPD) and continuous cycling peritoneal dialysis (CCPD). CAPD is the most common type and involves the passage of dialysate from a plastic bag into the catheter where it enters the abdomen. The solution is drained from the abdomen after 4 to 6 hours; the draining process takes 30 to 40 minutes. The process is repeated three to four times every day. Because there is no machinery involved, a person can perform CAPD when it is most convenient. CAPD can be done at home in a variety of locations without help. CCPD is similar to CAPD except that a machine is connected to the catheter to fill and drain the dialysate from the abdomen automatically. CCPD is generally done at night while a person is sleeping and lasts between 10 and 12 hours every night.

Peritoneum

The two-layered membrane that lines the interior of the abdominal cavity. It brings blood vessels, lymph vessels, and nerves to the organs. It supports the abdominal organs, anchors some of them to the abdominal wall, and completely surrounds some of them. It secretes a lubricating fluid so that organs can slide against each other, and it may help protect against infection. In some areas of the abdomen, the peritoneum forms multilayered membranes called the omentum and the mesentery.

Peritonitis

Inflammation of the PERITONEUM. Peritonitis usually occurs when bacteria contaminate the abdominal cavity. The resulting inflammation may be acute or chronic.

Acute peritonitis generally occurs as a secondary infection, most commonly caused by a perforation of structures in the gastrointestinal (GI) tract. This may be due to trauma to the abdomen, foreign bodies in the GI tract, severe intestinal obstruction, peptic ulcer disease, appendicitis, diverticulosis, pancreatitis, pelvic inflammatory disease (PID), ectopic pregnancy, or severe vascular conditions such as a blood clot (embolism).

Chronic peritonitis is caused by repeated infections or illnesses such as PID, certain postoperative infections, and chronic infections that affect the abdominal area. One cause of chronic peritonitis is TUBERCULOSIS. Fungal peritonitis usually occurs in people who had surgery or a bowel perforation and were treated with antibiotics, or people who have weakened immune systems.

Symptoms of peritonitis vary in severity depending on the extent of the infection. Abdominal pain may be experienced suddenly over the entire abdominal region or in a localized area. There may be vomiting and high fever.

X rays of the abdomen are taken to detect signs of perforation in the gastrointestinal tract. In some cases, fluid from the peritoneal cavity may be drawn out (aspirated) with a fine needle, cultured, and examined under a microscope.

Peritonitis is generally treated with antibiotics, the use of a nasogastric tube (which is passed through the nose, into the esophagus, and into the stomach to remove fluids), treatment of any respiratory symptoms, and replacement of fluids and electrolytes. Surgery may be necessary to repair a perforation or to drain any pus.

Peritonsillar abscess

An acute infection that produces a collection of pus between the tonsils and the muscle at the back of the mouth. Peritonsillar abscess occurs most commonly in young adults and is usually caused by a *Streptococcus* infection (see STREPTOCOCCAL INFECTIONS), but may be due to other types of bacteria. Symptoms include severe pain when swallowing, fever, and lockjaw (painful spasm of the jaw muscle that makes it difficult or impossible to open the mouth). The soft palate becomes reddened and swollen, and the uvula (the appendage of the soft palate) is enlarged and repositioned to one side.

Treatment consists of antibiotic therapy, usually oral penicillin, taken for 15 days. Drainage of pus from the peritonsillar area may become necessary and is performed by surgical incision or aspiration. If abscesses recur, removal of the tonsils (tonsillectomy) may be required.

Pernicious anemia

See ANEMIA, PERNICIOUS.

Personality disorders

A group of mental illnesses that is characterized by persistent, inflexible, and dysfunctional patterns of thought, action, emotion, and attitude that cause significant distress in social roles, job performance, family relationships, and other key areas of day-to-day living. Individuals with a personality disorder differ markedly from the norm in the ways they think, feel, relate to others, and control emotional impulses.

Types

ANTISOCIAL People with this personality disorder have a complete disregard for the rights of others.

AVOIDANT Social discomfort, fear of criticism, and timidity are the principal features of the disorder.

BORDERLINE The key features of this personality disorder are unstable personal relationships, shifting self-image, and impulsive behavior.

DEPENDENT People with this personality disorder have such an excessive need for others to take care of them that they submit and cling out of a pervasive fear of abandonment.

HISTRIONIC Extreme yet superficial emotions are the key feature of histrionic personality disorder.

NARCISSISTIC This personality disorder is characterized by self-centeredness, grandiosity, a need for admiration, and a lack of empathy.

OBSESSIVE-COMPULSIVE The principal characteristic of this personality disorder is preoccupation with orderliness, perfectionism, and control of others, even when it undercuts efficiency, flexibility, and openness.

PARANOID A person with this mental illness exhibits extreme, pervasive, and unwarranted distrust of other people's actions and motivations.

PASSIVE-AGGRESSIVE People with this personality disorder resent responsibility and express their resentment through forgetfulness, inefficiency, complaining, blaming others, procrastination, and other behaviors rather than expressing how they feel.

SCHIZOID The key feature of this personality disorder is detachment from social relationships and restricted emotions in social settings.

SCHIZOTYPAL Characterized by discomfort with, and reduced capacity for, close relationships, this personality disorder also involves eccentric or superstitious ways of thinking and behaving.

Causes, course, and treatment

The precise causes of personality disorders remain unclear. They usually begin during adolescence and peak in early adulthood. In some cases, symptoms become less pronounced in middle age. Treatment varies with the disorder. Counseling can help some individuals understand their personality patterns and learn how to change them in positive ways. Some individuals with personality disorders may have other mental illnesses, such as depression or anxiety, which can be treated with medication. Mood-stabilizing drugs such as lithium, carbamazepine, or antidepressants may be used when severe symptoms such as anxiety or depression develop.

Perthes disease

See OSTEOCHONDROSIS.

Pertussis

A serious bacterial infection of the lining of the breathing passages, particularly in the windpipe area. Pertussis, also called whooping cough, is caused by *Bordetella pertussis* bacteria and is extremely contagious. Symptoms of the infection include prolonged, violent coughing spasms followed by a long inhaling of breath with a characteristic high-pitched, crowing, or whooping sound. Pertussis can be fatal, but in the United States, widespread vaccination has made it rare.

A history of symptoms and physical examination leads to a diagnosis, which may be confirmed by detecting the bacteria in cultures or smears of secretions from the nose and upper throat. Treatment is based on antibiotic therapy, which may also be prescribed to other members of an infected person's household to prevent the spread of infection. Infants younger than 3 months who have pertussis are hospitalized; infants between 3 and 6 months may also need to be hospitalized.

Respiratory complications can be severe in infants and may include suffocation (asphyxiation). Seizures can also occur in infants. Middle ear inflammation, called OTITIS MEDIA, may occur. A potentially fatal form of pneumonia is a complication in an infected person of any age.

Pervasive developmental disorders

See DEVELOPMENTAL DISORDERS, PERVASIVE.

Pessary

A prosthesis placed in the vagina to tighten and support the pelvic floor. The purpose is usually to hold a prolapsed (dropped) uterus in place. Pessaries are used less often now that surgery for uterine prolapse is an effective treatment.

PET scanning

Positron emission tomography scanning; an imaging technique that combines NUCLEAR MEDICINE and chemical analysis to enable physicians to observe the function of certain organs of the body. After the person has an injection of a radioactive compound, cross-sectional images are taken by a special camera to demonstrate how an organ or tissue is metabolizing the injected substance. This can be useful for identifying and staging some cancers and diseases that cannot be detected by CT SCANNING or an MRI.

Petechiae

Pinpoint, round, red spots in the skin caused by bleeding in the skin; a single spot is a petechia. Petechiae can be a sign of various blood diseases, such as leukemia, immune thrombocytopenic purpura, and myeloproliferative disorders.

Petit mal

An older term for an ABSENCE SEIZURE. See also SEIZURE.

Peyronie disease

Severe curvature of the erect penis. (A minor bend is normal and not a sign of disease.) In severe cases, the penis can form a slight hook or corkscrew shape that makes sexual intercourse impossible. The condition is caused by a scar or plaque that forms in the spongy tissue that fills with blood when the penis becomes erect. Because the plaque fails to stretch as the surrounding tissue expands during erection, the penis bends or curves.

In approximately half of the cases, Peyronie disease clears up on its own, usually within a year. If the condition persists, medication can be prescribed for pain. In severe cases, surgery may be needed.

pH

A measure of the degree to which a solution is either an ACID or an alkali. The pH measures the hydrogen ion (H+) concentration in a substance: the more acidic a substance is, the greater the concentration of hydrogen ions and the lower the pH. A pH of 7 is neutral; a pH of less than 7 indicates acidity; and a pH of more than 7 indicates alkalinity. The pH measurement is used in medicine to measure the body's ACID-BASE BALANCE.

Phagocyte

A white blood cell that attacks foreign substances such as microorganisms that have entered the body. Phagocytes are able to engulf and digest antigens (see ANTIGEN), and some may also be able to transfer antigens to other white blood cells called T LYMPHOCYTES, or T cells. This is an essential component of the body's immune response. Phagocytes trigger the inflammatory response and produce and distribute a wide variety of powerful chemicals, including enzymes, complement proteins, and regulatory factors. They also carry receptors that enable them to be activated to attack specific microorganisms and tumor cells.

Pharmacology

The study and science of drugs; the characteristics of a drug that make it medically effective. Pharmacology includes the study of the discovery, chemistry, effects, uses, and manufacture of drugs.

Pharyngitis

See SORE THROAT.

Pharynx

The passageway that connects the nose and mouth with the trachea (leading to the lungs) and the esophagus (leading to the stomach). The pharynx, also called the throat, is lined with a mucous membrane. The pharynx has three sections: the nasopharynx, the oropharynx, and the laryngopharynx. The nasopharynx leads from the soft palate at the back of the mouth to the nasal cavity and is a passage for air only. The oropharynx lies behind the nasopharynx and behind the base of the tongue; both air and food pass through it. The laryngopharynx is the lowest portion that connects with the esophagus and is a passage for food only.

Phenylketonuria

See PKU.

Pheochromocytoma

A tumor of the adrenal gland that causes the release of excessive amounts of the adrenal hormones EPINEPHRINE and NOREPINEPHRINE. The tumors occur with equal frequency in men and women. Only about 10 percent of them are cancerous.

Symptoms may be sporadic and can increase in severity and duration over time, although some pheochromocytomas do not cause symptoms. Headache and excessive perspiration are the most common symptoms.

Pheochromocytomas may be difficult to diagnose because their symptoms mimic the symptoms of other conditions, including high blood pressure, anxiety disorders, and heart disease. Diagnosis depends on the results of tests that detect excessive amounts of adrenal hormones or of breakdown products in blood or urine.

The majority of these tumors can be removed through surgery. Medication to control blood pressure may be necessary, too.

Pheromone

A substance secreted by the bodies of animals, including humans, which identifies them to members of the same species. Pheromones are often detected by smell. Specific instinctive behaviors, such as mating and aggression, are involved in the response to pheromones.

Phimosis

An abnormal condition in which the foreskin is too tight to be pulled back over the head (glans) of the penis. The condition can occur in adolescents and adults who fail to clean under the foreskin, which causes an infection called BALANITIS with swelling, tenderness, and discharge. The foreskin bulges during urination, and the urine stream is narrow and slow. In extreme cases, urination is blocked; the backup of urine can cause kidney damage, called HYDRONEPHROSIS. If there is an infection, phimosis can be treated with antibiotics and corrected permanently by removing the foreskin surgically. See CIRCUMCISION, MALE.

Phlebitis

See THROMBOPHLEBITIS.

Phlebotomy

The removal of blood from a vein. A phlebotomy may be performed to obtain a sample of blood for analysis, to remove blood for donation (see BLOOD DONATION), or to treat blood disorders such as HEMOCHROMATOSIS.

Phobia

A persistent, irrational, exaggerated, and involuntary fear of a specific object, place, activity, or situation. Examples of specific phobias are fear of heights (ACROPHOBIA), open spaces (AGORAPHOBIA), snakes, closed spaces (CLAUSTROPHOBIA), and water. Social phobias include fears of meeting new people and of being embarrassed, humiliated, or ridiculed in front of others. Contact with the focus of the fear can prompt a PANIC ATTACK.

Phobias that severely restrict or interfere with a person's life require treatment. Since a phobia is an extreme anxiety reaction, medications that control anxiety can help alleviate the symptoms of phobia. Antidepressants are useful in some cases as well. Often, behavior therapy is combined with cognitive therapy, which teaches the person to recognize and change the mistaken beliefs that lead to the fear. Relaxation training can help individuals with a phobia.

Phosphorus

An essential mineral present in every cell of the body. Phosphorus is found mainly in bones and teeth and has a role in the breakdown of carbohydrates and fats, the synthesis of protein, muscle contraction, kidney function, nerve conduction, and heartbeat regulation. Dietary phosphorus is found in protein, principally in meat and dairy products. If a person's diet is adequate in calcium and protein, it is likely to be adequate in phosphorus.

Photocoagulation

A surgical technique that uses a laser to condense protein in the eye. Photocoagulation is used to reattach a detached retina (the thin layer of light-sensitive tissue at the back of the eye; see RETINAL DETACHMENT), seal or destroy abnormal blood vessels in the retina (see MACULAR DEGENERATION), or destroy eye tumors.

Photophobia

Abnormal sensitivity to, and intolerance of, light. Photophobia can be a symptom of a variety of diseases and conditions, such as excessive wear of contact lenses, eye injury or infection, inflammation, migraine headache, meningitis (inflammation of the brain covering), and reaction to certain medications. Photophobia should be evaluated by a medical professional if it is unexplained, persistent, or accompanied by blurry vision or red eyes.

Photorefractive keratectomy

A laser-surgery operation on the clear surface (cornea) of the eye to correct nearsightedness, farsightedness, or astigmatism; also known as PRK. The procedure has largely been replaced by LASIK.

Photosensitivity

Heightened sensitivity to the sun. Photosensitivity may occur as a result of disease, medications, or chemical components of the skin. Conditions that lead to photosensitivity include systemic lupus erythematosus, xeroderma pigmentosum, and a number of metabolic disorders. Photosensitizing medications include quinolone antibiotics, sulfonamides, tetracyclines, thiazide diuretics, tretinoin, tricyclic antidepressants, and some medications used to treat cancer, diabetes, and high blood pressure.

Diagnosis is made according to the appearance of the skin and a medical history. Goals of treatment are to identify and treat any underlying disorder and eliminate exposure to possible photosensitizing chemicals or medications. It can be helpful to avoid exposure to the sun between the hours of 10 AM and 4 PM (when rays are at their most intense), use a broad-spectrum sunblock, and wear protective clothing.

Phototherapy

The treatment of disorders with the use of light, primarily ultraviolet A (UVA) and ultraviolet B (UVB) light. Phototherapy is used to treat skin problems such as DERMATITIS, PSORIASIS, and VITILIGO, and to treat jaundice in newborns. Although phototherapy is often effective, long-term treatment is associated with an increased risk of skin cancer and premature skin aging.

In photochemotherapy, phototherapy is used in combination with topical or systemic medications. In some cases, photochemotherapy may involve the drug puva (psoralen plus UVA). Psoralen is a photosensitizing agent that maximizes the effect of ultraviolet light on the skin.

Jaundice in newborns is usually due to elevated levels of bilirubin (a by-product of the breakdown of red blood cells). This is a potentially serious condition because high bilirubin levels are associated with problems such as mental retardation, cerebral palsy, delayed or abnormal motor development, deafness, problems with perception, and behavioral disorders.

Physiatry

See PHYSICAL MEDICINE AND REHABILITATION.

Physical examination

See EXAMINATION, PHYSICAL.

Physical medicine and rehabilitation

Also known as physiatry, the field of medicine that focuses on restoring function in people with various musculoskeletal and neurological disorders. Physiatrists—physicians who specialize in the field of physical medicine and rehabilitation—treat acute and chronic pain resulting from a wide range of problems, from back pain to carpal tunnel syndrome to quadriplegia.

Physical therapy

Specialized treatment for a person who has a disability, disease, or injury with the goal of restoring and maintaining function or preventing malfunction or deformity. A doctor may prescribe physical therapy to a person who has an orthopedic, neurological, vascular, or respiratory condition resulting from congenital disorders, an inherited dysfunction, or a disability caused by trauma or disease.

Physical therapy involves diagnostic testing as well as treatment. The diagnostic tests may include muscle testing, electrical testing, perceptual and sensory testing, and measurements of the joints' range of motion. Functional activity tests evaluate a person's ability to carry out the everyday tasks required for self-care. Treatments may include heat treatments using water, melted paraffin, or ultrasound devices that generate heat internally and the application of electric current to generate heat in body tissues.

Therapeutic exercise is a cornerstone of physical therapy and is used to increase strength and endurance, improve the coordination and functional movement that allow a person to engage in the activities of everyday life, and increase and maintain range of motion in joints.

Physician

A person licensed to practice medicine; a doctor of medicine. Physicians must successfully complete a rigorous course of instruction and training, including 4 years of graduate medical education. After graduating from medical school, all states require that a physician complete at least one year of postgraduate training in order to become eligible for licensure. Doctors who specialize in various fields (such as pediatrics, family medicine, or dermatology) receive additional postdoctoral residency training.

Physiology

The branch of biology dealing with the functions and vital processes of the human body.

Phytochemicals

A broad group of chemicals found in plants that are thought to provide considerable health benefits. There are hundreds of phytochemicals, such as flavonoids, isoflavones, indoles and other phenols, and protease inhibitors. Scientists are investigating the role these chemicals may have in the prevention and control of cancer, heart disease, and other diseases.

Pica

An eating disorder in which a person has an abnormal craving to consume substances that are inorganic, such as chalk, clay, paint chips, plaster, dirt, or coal. Pica is most common in children younger than age 6 and the exact cause is unknown. Counseling can often help change the behavior. Although most children outgrow pica, it can continue into adulthood.

Pick disease

A type of irreversible dementia in older people characterized by frontal lobe degeneration in the brain and the presence of distinctive Pick cells in brain tissue. Symptoms include impaired speech, inability to name objects, loss of insight, apathy, impulsiveness, dietary changes, and lack of inhibitions. As in ALZHEIMER'S DISEASE, over time people who have Pick disease grow unable to perform the usual activities of daily living and eventually become incapacitated.

PID

See PELVIC INFLAMMATORY DISEASE.

Pigeon toes

See INTOEING.

Pigmentation

Coloration of the skin, hair, and eyes with the pigment melanin. Pigmentation can be affected by many factors, including heredity, hormones, injury, and exposure to heat or radiation. Skin conditions characterized by altered pigmentation include freckles, melasma, pityriasis alba, suntans, tinea versicolor, and vitiligo. In most cases, the skin changes are cosmetic and do not affect general health. Treatments for severe pigment disorders include bleaching creams, topical corticosteroids, and PHOTOTHERAPY (treatment with light).

Pill, birth control

See CONTRACEPTION, HORMONAL METHODS.

Pilonidal sinus

A hairy bump in the cleft of the buttocks in tissue near the tailbone; also known as a pilonidal cyst. A pilonidal sinus can become infected and form a painful abscess (pus-filled sac). Treatment is with antibiotics and, as necessary, either surgical incision and drainage or surgical excision (cutting out the cyst).

Pinched nerve

The compression or "trapping" of a nerve, causing numbness, tingling, weakness, and pain in the area supplied by the nerve. The primary treatment for improving the symptoms is to relieve the pressure on the nerve. Physical therapy, injections of corticosteroids, and medication to reduce the inflammation and pain may be used. In some cases, surgery may be necessary. See NERVE ENTRAPMENT.

Pineal gland

A small, hormone-producing organ located near the base of the brain. The pineal gland secretes MELATONIN, which has a role in daily biological cycles that are involved in sleep and mood. The secretion of the hormone varies during a 24-hour period and is heaviest at night. The gland also signals the onset of men-

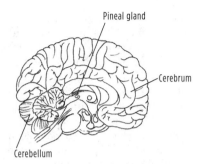

Hormonal clock
The tiny pineal gland, which secretes hormones that are involved in daily cyclical behavior, is located at the base of the brain.

struation in girls and is involved in the menstrual cycle.

Pinkeye

See CONJUNCTIVITIS.

Pinna

The portion of the ear that projects from the head; the external ear.

Pins and needles sensation

See PARESTHESIA.

Pinworm infestation

An infection caused by the parasitic roundworm *Enterobius vermicularis*, which lays its eggs in the human intestines. Pinworm infestation is common in temperate zones and usually affects children between the ages of 2 and 12. The infection is transmitted by the transfer of the eggs, which may be present on the hands or under the fingernails of an infected person or on clothing, bath towels, or bed linens.

Pinworm infestation frequently does not cause any symptoms, or there may be itching in the anal region, usually at night when the female roundworms migrate to that area. Other symptoms may include loss of appetite, irritability, and abdominal pain.

Pinworm infestation is diagnosed by microscopic identification of eggs collected in the perianal area. Medications, including mebendazole or albendazole, are generally used to treat pinworm infestations, but they cannot be taken by a woman during pregnancy. Another medication, pyrantel pamoate (or pyrantel emboate), may be recommended for pregnant women who have a pinworm infestation.

Pituitary gland

A small, two-lobed gland at the base of the brain that secretes hormones that stimulate other glands throughout the body to produce hormones; a major part of the ENDOCRINE SYSTEM. Because the nervous system and the endocrine system work together so closely, they are sometimes referred to collectively as the neuroendocrine system.

Pituitary tumors

Abnormal growths that arise in the pituitary gland located at the base of the brain. Most pituitary tumors are not malignant. However, they can enlarge and damage nearby tissue. Symptoms of a pituitary tumor include headache, seizures, personality changes, visual disturbances, drooping eyelids, weakness, lethargy, irritability, and cold intolerance. Some pituitary tumors secrete an excess of hormones leading to gigantism or acromegaly (from excess of growth hormone), HYPERTHYROIDISM, or CUSHING SYNDROME.

A pituitary tumor is diagnosed through physical examination and tests, such as CT (computed tomography) scanning of the skull, MRI (magnetic resonance imaging), angiogram, spinal tap, and endocrine function tests. Surgical removal is indicated if the tumor is large and pressing on the optic nerves or if it causes serious hormone imbalances.

Pityriasis alba

A common asymptomatic disorder characterized by round or oval, white, scaly patches on the skin. Patches most commonly occur on the cheeks but may also occur elsewhere on the face or on the upper arms, thighs, and neck. The patches may disappear and then return. Pityriasis alba occurs most often in young children and usually resolves by early adulthood.

Pityriasis rosea

A benign (noncancerous) skin rash that usually begins with a single oval patch and then spreads. The original patch, which may be rosy pink, salmon, or tan, commonly appears on the trunk. Within a week or two after the emergence of the first patch, smaller, similar plaques (patches of thick, raised skin) appear more generally over the trunk. Pityriasis rosea is most common in children and young adults and affects both sexes equally. It usually disappears on its own without treatment and leaves no permanent marks. Treatment with ultraviolet B light, antihistamines, and hydrocortisone cream may be prescribed to relieve itching.

PKU

Phenylketonuria; a rare genetic disorder characterized by the inability of the body to use the essential amino acid phenylalanine because of the absence or deficiency of an enzyme, phenylalanine hydroxylase. This deficiency leads to very high phenylalanine levels in the blood and tissues. Because excessive phenylalanine is toxic to the central nervous system, PKU results in mental retardation and neurological problems if not treated within the first few weeks of life. When treatment is begun shortly after birth and maintained consistently, children with the disease can expect normal development and a normal life span. Because treatment of PKU is so effective and its consequences so severe, newborn screening for PKU with a blood test is routine, even though the disorder is very rare.

Infants with PKU appear normal at birth, although they may have fairer skin and hair than other family members. Untreated PKU may be associated with early symptoms of vomiting, irritability, a rash, and urine with an earthy odor, although most infants have no symptoms until brain damage has occurred. Later symptoms include seizures and mental retardation.

The goal of treatment of PKU is to maintain a normal blood level of phenylalanine. This requires a very special diet, one that eliminates high protein foods, since all protein contains phenylalanine.

It is important for women with PKU who are of childbearing age to seek nutritional guidance before they become pregnant. Eating a special diet before and during pregnancy that lowers their phenylalanine level can help ensure a healthy pregnancy and baby.

Placebo

A substance used in medical research that resembles a drug but has no medical action; also called a sugar pill or dummy pill. Researchers can determine whether an experimental drug is effective by comparing the response to the drug with the response to the placebo. The experimental drug must produce better results than the placebo to be considered effective.

Placenta

The organ that links the blood supplies of the mother and fetus during pregnancy. The placenta is connected to the fetus by the UMBILICAL CORD. Although the blood of the fetus and the blood of the mother do not actually mix, the placenta supplies the developing fetus with oxygen and nutrients from the mother's bloodstream.

Placenta previa

In pregnancy, a placenta that has grown abnormally low in the uterus, partly or completely covering the cervix. The condition is unusual, occurring in only one of every 200 pregnancies, and its cause is unknown. Depending on how much of the cervix is covered by the placenta, it may cause problems toward the end of the pregnancy. Symptoms do not always occur, but if the placenta begins to separate from the uterus, the woman may experience sporadic, painless bleeding from the vagina, usually late in the pregnancy.

Treatment usually includes bed rest to prevent excessive bleeding. In severe cases, a cesarean section will be needed.

Placenta, retained

A placenta that is not expelled by the uterus after birth. To remove the placenta, the doctor usually administers an anesthetic to the mother, reaches inside the uterus, and removes the placenta. The mother is then given a drug to encourage the uterus to contract to prevent excessive bleeding.

Plantar wart

A hard, rough-surfaced area on the sole of the foot that is caused by a virus. See WART.

Plaque

A fatty deposit inside an artery wall. As the plaque builds, it may develop a thick covering of calcium, which causes the characteristic hardening of the artery in ATHEROSCLEROSIS. The growing plaque can narrow the opening in the artery and restrict blood flow, sometimes causing blood to pool behind the restriction and ballooning the artery into an ANEURYSM.

Plaque, dental

A sticky deposit of bacteria, saliva, and food debris that forms on the teeth, particularly in the spaces between the teeth and gums. When plaque accumulates and hardens on the teeth, it forms calculus (see CALCULUS, DENTAL).

Plasma

The liquid portion of the blood. A straw-colored fluid, plasma represents a little over half of the body's total volume of blood. Mostly water, plasma serves as the medium that transports the blood cells. It also contains proteins, hormones, acids, salts, nutrients, oxygen, carbon dioxide, and cellular waste products.

Plasmapheresis

A process for separating out specific blood components from the plasma, the liquid portion of blood. Plasmapheresis is used to treat certain blood diseases and autoimmune diseases.

Plasminogen activator

Any of a group of substances able to convert plasminogen into plasmin. Plasminogen is a substance normally present in blood; plasmin is an enzyme that digests the blood-clotting protein fibrin. Tissue plasminogen activator (tPA) is a medication used to dissolve blood clots immediately after a heart attack or stroke. Because TPA acts directly on clots, it rarely causes systemic bleeding.

Plastic surgery

Any operation that repairs, restores, or improves parts of the body; the surgical specialty that includes both COSMETIC SURGERY and RECONSTRUCTIVE SURGERY. A plastic surgeon is a physician who specializes in plastic surgery.

Platelets

Blood cells that help repair injured blood vessels. Also known as thrombocytes, platelets stop the loss of blood by plugging holes in blood vessels, the first step in the formation of a clot. Like most blood cells, they form in the bone marrow and then migrate into the blood.

Pleura

The double-walled membrane that covers the surface of the lungs and lines the wall of the chest cavity. The space between the two layers is filled with a lubricating fluid that helps the lungs move easily as they expand and contract.

Pleural effusion

An abnormal collection of fluid in the pleural space, the space between the two membrane layers (pleural membranes) that cover the lungs and line the chest cavity. When fluids accumulate in the pleural space, lung volume is reduced. Congestive heart failure, cirrhosis, and pneumonia are among the most common causes of fluid collection in the pleural space. Some cancers, such as those of the lung or breast, can spread to the pleural membrane and cause pleural effusion. The fluid buildup can also result from injury.

Chest pain and breathing difficulties are the most common signs of pleural effusion. However, the condition may be asymptomatic and discovered by chance during a physical examination or diagnostic testing. Chest X rays are considered the most accurate method for confirming the presence of pleural effusion. Some of the fluid is usually removed and examined to find the cause or to remove a fluid buildup.

If the cause of the effusion is a bacterial infection, antibiotic therapy is given. As the infection clears, the condition resolves spontaneously. If there is pus in the pleural effusion, it is drained through a chest tube. Alternatively, a surgical procedure to open the chest, either thoracoscopy or THORACOTOMY may be used.

Pleurisy

Inflammation of the two thin, transparent membranes, called the pleura or pleural membranes, that cover the lungs and line the chest wall. Pleurisy most commonly occurs when a virus or bacterium infects the membranes. The primary causes of pleurisy are pneumonia, tissue death produced by a pulmonary embolism, cancer, tuberculosis, rheumatoid arthritis, and systemic lupus erythematosus.

Sudden chest pain is the most common symptom of pleurisy. This may be experienced as discomfort or as severe, stabbing pain that occurs continually or only when a person breathes deeply or coughs. Pain may be localized at the site of inflammation or felt as pain in the abdomen or neck and shoulder area. A person may have labored breathing.

Treatment of pleurisy is based on the cause. Antibiotics are prescribed to treat a bacterial infection. No treatment is required for a viral infection. If an autoimmune disease is the cause, treatment of the disease will usually help resolve the pleurisy.

Plexus

A tightly organized network of veins, lymphatic vessels, or nerves.

PMS

See PREMENSTRUAL SYNDROME.

Pneumoconiosis

Inflammatory lung diseases caused by the long-term inhalation of naturally occurring or synthetic mineral dusts, such as coal or silica dust. There may be no symptoms, or there may be coughing and shortness of breath. If the disease becomes severe and progressive, it can cause massive pulmonary fibrosis (scarring of the lungs), a severe cough, and disabling shortness of breath.

A clinical history, especially a history of exposure to dust, and a chest X ray that reveals the characteristic spots on the lungs, are the principal elements for a diagnosis of pneumoconiosis. There is no cure for this disease. Medications that keep airways open and free of secretions, such as those used to treat chronic obstructive pulmonary disease (COPD), may offer help with breathing. Some people with advanced disease are treated with oral corticosteroids.

Pneumocystis pneumonia

An OPPORTUNISTIC INFECTION caused by a one-celled organism believed to be a fungus called *Pneumocystis jiroveci*. The fungus rarely causes infection in healthy people. But in people who have weakened immune systems, the organism can invade the lungs and multiply. As a result, the tiny air sacs in the lungs called alveoli (which enable the exchange of oxygen and carbon dioxide between the bloodstream and the lungs) can become thickened and enlarged and their function impaired. The infection occurs almost exlusively in people whose immune system is suppressed, such as people with AIDS.

Symptoms include difficult and labored breathing, dry cough, and fever. A chest X ray generally reveals involvement of both lungs. Diagnosis can be confirmed by identification of the infection-causing fungus in respiratory secretions. The infection can be life-threatening and is treated with antimicrobial medications.

Pneumonectomy

The surgical removal of a lung, performed as a treatment for LUNG CANCER or when a lung has irreparable damage from severe trauma. Because pneumonectomy reduces breathing capacity by half, surgeons often attempt to perform more localized surgeries, such as LOBECTOMY (removal of a lobe of the lung), de-pending on the location and extent of the cancer.

Recovery from pneumonectomy tends to be slow, and tolerance for exercise tends to remain significantly limited by shortness of breath for up to 6 months or longer. Survival rates following pneumonectomy depend on the underlying condition and are generally good. Temporary postoperative complications may include a prolonged need for a ventilator; heart problems, such as cardiac arrhythmia and myocardial infarction; pneumonia; infection of the surgical site; PULMONARY EMBOLISM; and problems with the severed airway.

Pneumonia

For symptom chart, see CHEST PAIN, page xiv.

A serious infection of the lungs that causes inflammation of the lung tissue. Pneumonia causes the air sacs in the lungs to fill with pus and other fluid, obstructing the flow of oxygen into the bloodstream. The depletion of oxygen in the blood interferes with normal functioning of the body's cells. If this occurs in combination with the infection's spread throughout the body, pneumonia can cause death. The use of antibiotics has greatly reduced the life-threatening potential of pneumonia. Even so, pneumonia is still the leading cause of death from infectious disease in the United States.

Pneumonia may be caused by one of a number of different organisms; the most common are bacteria, viruses, and mycoplasma (a group of microorganisms similar to bacteria). Other causes include various chemicals and other infectious agents, such as the fungus that causes PNEUMO-CYSTIS PNEUMONIA. Pneumonia may also be caused by inhaling food, liquid, gases, foreign bodies, or dust. Tuberculosis pneumonia is extremely serious and requires immediate medical treatment.

Symptoms

Symptoms of bacterial pneumonia may come on suddenly or gradually. They include a fever as high as 105°F, profuse perspiration, chills, severe chest pain, and coughing that produces mucus that is green or rust-colored. Other symptoms may include an increase in pulse rate and breathing, and bluish discoloration of the lips and nail beds.

The symptoms of viral pneumonia are similar to those of the flu, including fever, dry cough, headache, muscle pain, and weakness. Although viral pneumonia is often milder than bacterial pneumonia, the symptoms generally escalate within 12 to 36 hours, progressing to difficulty breathing, a more severe cough with mucus, and possible bluish discoloration of the lips. In severe cases, viral pneumonia can be fatal.

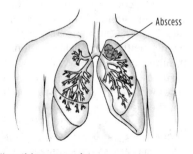

Necrotizing pneumonia

Necrotizing pneumonia, the death of lung tissue caused by bacterial pneumonia, occurs when an inflammation of the bronchial tubes and lungs forms pus-filled abscesses in the lungs.

The principal symptom of mycoplasma pneumonia is violent, sporadic coughing that produces a small amount of pale mucus. Fever and chills may be the first symptoms, and there may be nausea or vomiting, but rarely. Recovery may be prolonged with feelings of extreme weakness.

Diagnosis and treatment

When there is a suspicion of pneumonia, a physical examination by the doctor includes listening to the person's chest with a stethoscope to detect distorted breathing sounds. Bronchial and other forms of pneumonia are detected by chest X rays. A sample of sputum may be tested to try to identify the pathogen causing the infection. Blood tests and measurement of the oxygen level in the blood may be needed.

Early treatment with antibiotics generally cures bacterial infection and speeds recovery from mycoplasmal pneumonia. Antiviral medications may be used to treat certain kinds of viral pneumonia, but for most forms of viral pneumonia there is no specific treatment available.

Pneumonitis

Inflammation of the lungs generally caused by hypersensitivity to repeated or prolonged inhalation of natural or chemical agents. In its acute form, the symptoms resemble those of a flulike illness with a cough. It may also take the form of recurrent pneumonia or chronic shortness of breath, a productive cough, and weight loss. These symptoms may appear within 4 to 12 hours following exposure to the causative irritant. Pneumonitis can improve or resolve completely within a few days when exposure to the irritant is stopped. When exposure is continued, the inflammation may progress to PULMONARY FIBROSIS. See also DUST DISEASES; OCCUPATIONAL LUNG DISEASE.

Pneumothorax

The presence of air in the space between the pleural membranes, the two membranes that cover the lungs and line the chest cavity. Pneumothorax occurs when air leaks into the space from inside a lung. The air can increase pressure on the lung, resulting in a collapsed lung.

A small pneumothorax may cause only mild discomfort. Initial symptoms are usually a sudden sharp chest pain, shortness of breath, and sometimes a nonproductive, hacking cough. Pain can also occur in the shoulder and abdomen on the affected side. Severe pneumothorax can be life-threatening, causing intense shortness of breath and shock.

Pneumothorax may be suspected if breath sounds heard through the stethoscope are diminished. Blood tests may reveal a lack of adequate oxygen supply in the blood. A chest X ray can reveal a collapsed lung and the presence of air outside structural outlines. If a pneumothorax is small, the air is generally reabsorbed within a few days and no treatment is needed. If the air space is larger, there is a risk of complications, including PLEURAL EFFUSION (a collection of fluid in the pleural space); the condition is generally treated by placement of a chest tube to aspirate the air and to expand the collapsed lung.

Podiatry

The branch of medicine concerned with the care of the feet, especially foot disorders. A podiatrist is a health care provider who specializes in this branch of medicine.

Poison center

A facility staffed by health professionals trained in the prevention and treatment of poisoning. Most communities have a poison center; the phone number is usually listed on the inside cover of the local phone book. In the event of a poisoning or suspected poisoning, a telephone call to the poison center will elicit instructions from a trained health professional (usually a nurse or pharmacist) on how to handle the emergency at home.

Poison ivy

A type of CONTACT DERMATITIS caused by skin exposure to an oily substance in the sap from the poison ivy plant. Poison ivy is characterized by red, intensely itchy patches of skin that soon begin to swell and blister. A rash can also develop if a person touches clothing, shoes, or a pet that has been exposed to poison ivy.

After exposure to poison ivy, immediate action can prevent a rash from developing. Doctors recommend rinsing the exposed skin thoroughly with cold water within 5 minutes of contact. Washing with soap is not necessary and may spread the oil. Contaminated clothing should be laundered.

Poison ivy develops within 12 to 48 hours after exposure to the plant; the rash peaks after 5 days and generally disappears within 14 to 20 days without treatment. Itching and discomfort can be relieved by applying cool compresses, soothing lotions (such as calamine lotion), and prescription topical corticosteroids; taking oatmeal baths; and taking oral antihistamines. Severe cases are treated with oral corticosteroids.

Poisoning, carbon monoxide

Poisoning from the inhalation of carbon monoxide (CO). Carbon monoxide is a tasteless, odorless, colorless gas produced by the incomplete burning of carbon-based fuel. Carbon monoxide can take the place of oxygen in the blood. The symptoms of carbon monoxide poisoning include headache, fainting, confusion, unconsciousness, chest pain, breathing difficulties, bluish color of lips and fingernails, pale skin, nausea and vomiting, low blood pressure, abnormal heartbeat, hyperactivity, seizures, coma, and shock. When the concentration of carbon monoxide is very high, muscle paralysis, seizures, coma, and death can occur.

If carbon monoxide poisoning is suspected, the person should be moved out into the fresh air immediately and the suspected area ventilated. Emergency medical assistance should be sought, and the local POISON CENTER should be called. ARTIFICIAL RESPIRATION may be required. Electronic carbon monoxide detectors installed in the home can alert residents when an excessive amount of carbon monoxide is present.

Poisoning, chemical

Ingestion, inhalation, or absorption of toxic chemicals. The signs of poisoning from swallowed chemicals include burns around the lips and mouth, excessive salivation, and difficulty swallowing. When cleaning or petroleum products have been swallowed, the breath could have an odor resembling the offending chemical. Signs of chemical poisoning by inhalation include choking, coughing, and headache. Signs of chemical absorption poisoning through the skin include itching and burning at the site of absorption. In all cases of chemical poisoning it is essential to follow the instructions of a POISON CENTER professional and to seek emergency medical assistance.

Polio

An acute infection caused by an enterovirus called poliovirus that can affect the nervous system and the skeletal muscles. Polio, which is a shortened term for poliomyelitis, has become a rare disease since polio immunization has become widespread in developed countries. It is highly contagious, spreading through direct contact with an infected person or infected respiratory secretions or feces.

In some polio infections, there may be no symptoms or mild symptoms that last for 72 hours or less and include mild fever, headache, sore throat, abdominal pain, and vomiting. Nonparalytic polio causes symptoms that persist for 1 to 2 weeks and may include moderate fever, headache, stiff neck, vomiting, diarrhea, fatigue, muscle tenderness and spasm, and pain or stiffness in the torso, neck, back, and extremities. Paralytic polio causes fever 2 to 7 days before other symptoms appear, such as headache, stiff neck and back, general sensitivity to touch, difficult urination, constipation, difficulty swallowing and breathing, drooling, and muscle contractions or spasms, especially in the calf, neck, or back.

A diagnosis of polio is made by a physical examination and confirmed by cultures of throat secretions, stool, or cerebrospinal fluid that reveal the presence of the poliovirus. The symptoms are treated based on their severity. In severe cases when paralysis affects the muscles involved in breathing and swallowing, emergency breathing assistance in a hospital may be a lifesaving measure. When muscle function or strength are lost or impaired, treatment may include physical therapy, the use of braces or corrective shoes, and orthopedic surgery.

Lifelong immunity to polio depends on the type of poliovirus a person has contracted. POSTPOLIO SYNDROME is a condition that can affect people many years or even decades after their initial infection.

Pollen

An airborne, fertilizing agent that carries a plant's male genetic material to a female plant. Pollen can be inhaled, producing the symptoms of allergies such as hay fever and asthma in susceptible people. The pollens that are most powerful at producing allergic symptoms are those of the grass family, ragweeds, and birch and oak trees.

Polychondritis, relapsing

An inflammatory, autoimmune disorder that affects the cartilage and other connective tissues of the joints, as well as the ears, nose, larynx, trachea, eye, heart valves, kidney, and blood vessels. When the disorder affects the joints, the symptoms include pain and arthritis in large and small joints on both sides of the body. It is diagnosed by clinical history and laboratory tests. Mild cases are generally treated with nonsteroidal anti-inflammatory drugs (NSAIDs), such as aspirin and ibuprofen, to relieve pain and inflammation. More severe cases may be treated with a corticosteroid drug such as prednisone and the most severe cases with immunosuppressive agents such as cyclophosphamide.

Polycystic kidney disease

An inherited disorder in which the kidneys are enlarged and contain clusters of fluid-filled cysts (see KIDNEY CYST). Polycystic kidney disease may produce only a few small cysts or many cysts. Over time, the cysts tend to destroy kidney tissue, eventually leading to KIDNEY FAILURE.

There may be no symptoms early in the disease. For this reason, polycystic kidney disease may go undiagnosed in many people. One of the first signs is likely to be high blood pressure, which can result when enlarging cysts compress blood vessels or when the cysts produce hormones that increase blood pressure. Other symptoms may include blood in the urine (called HEMATURIA) or feelings of heaviness or pain in the back, sides, or abdomen.

Indications that a person may have polycystic kidney disease include a family history of the disease, certain signs and symptoms, and the discovery of cysts in the kidneys. Imaging tests that may be used for diagnosis include ultrasound scanning, CT SCANNING, and MRI.

There is no known treatment or cure for polycystic kidney disease. LAPAROSCOPIC SURGERY may be recommended for people who have severe pain from cysts larger than 5 centimeters in diameter. Laparoscopic surgery offers relief from pain but does not preserve kidney function. A low-protein diet that eliminates red meat and limits salt and alcohol is generally recommended.

Polycystic ovarian syndrome

A condition in which the ovaries become enlarged and contain multiple cysts. Polycystic ovarian syndrome (PCOS) is linked to an inherited resistance to the effects of the hormone insulin, which regulates the blood sugar glucose. Insulin resistance causes the pancreas to produce more and more insulin, which, in turn, stimulates the ovaries to produce an excessive amount of testosterone and other male hormones.

PCOS typically appears around the time of puberty. Women with PCOS tend to be overweight and to carry fat around their abdomen. Because women with PCOS rarely or never ovulate, their menstrual periods are irregular, often separated by several months. When they have periods, they are often very heavy. Other symptoms include excess hair on the face and body and acne. The cysts are usually painless, and the diagnosis is often made during an evaluation of infertility.

Treatment depends on whether the woman wishes to become pregnant. Fertility drugs may be prescribed to stimulate ovulation in a woman who wants to become pregnant. For women who do not want to become pregnant, either progesterone or birth control pills may be prescribed to regulate the menstrual cycle and reduce the woman's risk of developing uterine cancer.

Polycythemia

An increase in the number of red blood cells circulating in the bloodstream; also known as erythrocytosis (from erythrocyte, the medical term for red blood cell). The added mass of blood cells causes the blood to be thicker than normal and increases blood volume. A person with polycythemia is at increased risk of blood clots that can lead to heart attack, stroke, or thrombophlebitis (inflammation of the veins).

Polycythemia occurs most often in people who live at high altitudes or who have respiratory diseases such as chronic obstructive pulmonary disease, which reduce oxygen levels in the blood. Smoking is also a common cause. Polycythemia can also arise as a result of a disease that increases production of red blood cells, such as kidney disease and tumors of the brain, liver, ovary, uterus, prostate, thymus, or adrenal glands. Polycythemia can also occur when a person loses a significant portion of plasma (the liquid portion of the blood), increasing the relative proportion of red blood cells in the bloodstream. See also MYELOPROLIFERATIVE DISORDERS.

Polyhydramnios

In pregnancy, an excess amount of amniotic fluid, which can increase either gradually or suddenly. Maternal symptoms of polyhydramnios include a larger than expected abdominal size, abdominal discomfort, breathlessness, nausea, or swelling of the legs. It is diagnosed by physical examination and ultrasound. Tests may be done to check for fetal abnormalities. In most cases, the fetus is normal and no treatment is required. Sometimes, excess fluid is removed to relieve symptoms, using a procedure similar to AMNIOCENTESIS.

Polymyalgia rheumatica

An inflammatory disorder that causes aching and stiffness around the upper arms, neck, and thighs and is the most common hematologic disorder among people over age 50. The cause is unknown. Typically, the pain is most severe in the morning but may continue throughout the day and disturb sleep at night.

There is no known cure for polymyalgia rheumatica (PMR), which generally improves on its own within a year or two. Treatment of the symptoms, however, can provide relief. Diagnosis is made by a history of the symptoms and a blood test to measure the degree of inflammation. If symptoms are mild, nonsteroidal antiinflammatory drugs (NSAIDs) may be recommended. In more severe cases, the doctor might prescribe a corticosteroid such as prednisone.

Polyp

A mass of tissue that develops on the inside wall of a hollow organ. Polyps are usually benign and are commonly found in the nose or sinuses, the ear, the stomach, and the colon. Some types of polyps in the colon can become cancerous and are usually removed (polypectomy).

Polyposis, familial

An inherited condition in which numerous POLYPS form in the large intestine (colon). In familial polyposis, the polyps begin as precancerous adenomas, usually during puberty, but often become cancerous by age 40. Harmless cysts may appear on the skin of the scalp, face, arms, or legs. Bony growths in the jaw or on the skull sometimes appear. Other symptoms include blood or mucus in the stool, diarrhea, and occasional abdominal cramps, with or without weight loss. But by the time these symptoms develop, cancer may already be present, so it is particularly important that people with a family history of familial polyposis be examined for the condition early in childhood or adolescence.

A genetic test can identify the disease-causing gene in people with a family history of polyposis. Each child of a person with familial polyposis has a 50 percent risk of inheriting the defective gene and developing the disease. Familial polyposis is diagnosed by direct examination of the colon with SIGMOIDOSCOPY or COLONOSCOPY. There is no cure for familial polyposis. Surgical removal of the colon, or COLECTOMY, is standard treatment and is the only way to prevent the development of more adenomas in the colon.

Polyuria

The passing of an abnormally large volume of urine. Polyuria is associated with a number of diseases or disorders including KIDNEY FAILURE and SICKLE CELL ANEMIA. It is also a sign of excess glucose in the blood in people with diabetes mellitus (see DIABETES MELLITUS, TYPE 1; DIABETES MELLITUS, TYPE 2). Polyuria requires medical attention if it persists over several days and does not have an apparent cause such as an increased intake of fluids or taking certain medications that stimulate thirst or urination.

Pore

A small opening, particularly in the skin.

Port-wine stain

A type of vascular BIRTHMARK or blood vessel malformation. Port-wine stains can be pink, red, or purple and of any size, and they occur most often on the face, neck, arms, and legs. They tend to increase in size as a child grows and do not disappear on their own. It is essential for a doctor to diagnose this type of birthmark and monitor its growth, especially if it is on the forehead, eyelids, or sides of the face. Large port-wine stains at these sites are associated with an increased risk of glaucoma or seizures. A port-wine stain may also form a pyogenic granuloma (a small, inflamed bump on the skin that bleeds easily), which usually must be surgically removed. Many port-wine stains can be removed with LASER SURGERY, which destroys the blood vessels.

Positron emission tomography scanning

See PET SCANNING.

Postmaturity

A condition in which pregnancy lasts longer than 42 weeks. Although risks to the health of mother and baby increase after 42 weeks of pregnancy, 95 percent of postmature babies are born healthy and without incident.

Postmortem examination

See AUTOPSY.

Postpartum cardiomyopathy

Heart failure after pregnancy caused by a disorder of the heart muscle. The cause is unknown. The condition occurs mostly in women over age 30 who have had several pregnancies or in women who have had PREECLAMPSIA, ECLAMPSIA, or a multiple pregnancy. Postpartum cardiomyopathy usually occurs in the first month after childbirth, but it can occur as much as 5 months later. Symptoms include moderate respiratory distress and left-sided chest pain.

Treatment includes standard care for PULMONARY EDEMA (fluid in the lungs) and digitalis drugs, which make the heart work more efficiently. The doctor may also prescribe anticoagulant (blood-thinning) drugs.

Postpartum depression

Severe depression after childbirth that does not resolve within a few weeks. Signs of this form of depression may include feelings of guilt, anxiety, or hopelessness that do not go away; inability to sleep or sleeping too much; anxiety or panic attacks; lack of interest in the baby or other family members; fear of harming the baby; suicidal thoughts; changes in appetite; or extreme fatigue.

Support from family, friends, and a woman's partner is vital and may help her cope with the stresses contributing to the depression. If the depression persists or interferes with her ability to function, a woman should seek help from a doctor.

Postpartum hemorrhage

Excessive loss of blood from the uterus or vagina after delivery. Postpartum hemorrhage often occurs when the muscles of the uterus do not contract enough to cause it to shrink and compress the blood vessels inside. It can also occur if bits of the placenta remain inside the uterus and prevent it from tightening up sufficiently. Cervical or vaginal tissue is sometimes torn during delivery, which can also lead to bleeding. Treatment includes medications that help the uterus contract. Any fragments of placenta are removed, and any tears are stitched closed.

Postpolio syndrome

Also known as PPS, a condition that affects some people who have previously had POLIO. PPS occurs 20 to 30 years after the original disease and causes slow, progressive weakening of the muscles. Other symptoms include fatigue, decrease in muscle size, involuntary twitching of muscles, muscle and joint pain, respiratory and sleep problems, trouble swallowing, and cold intolerance. There is no cure for PPS. Treatment focuses on relieving the symptoms

Posttraumatic stress disorder

An ANXIETY DISORDER that involves the re-experiencing of a traumatic event evoking intense fear, helplessness, and horror through hallucinations, flashbacks, or nightmares. Commonly abbreviated PTSD, it can arise after accidents involving death, natural disasters, a fire, war, physical abuse, assault, rape, or torture. PTSD usually develops within 3 months of the trauma, but can begin years later. Antianxiety and antidepressant medications are often used to treat PTSD. Hypnosis may also be used. Psychotherapy that helps the person express grief over the traumatic event is also helpful, as is participation in a support group with people who have been through similar experiences.

Postural drainage

A form of RESPIRATORY THERAPY in which special positioning of the body allows mucus to drain from the lungs. Postural drainage is used to provide relief to people who produce excessive mucus as a result of conditions including cystic fibrosis, bronchiectasis, and lung abscess.

Postural hypotension

See HYPOTENSION.

Potassium

A mineral involved in electrical and cellular functions in the body. Potassium is an ELECTROLYTE involved in the regulation of water and ACID-BASE BALANCE. Potassium also helps in protein synthesis, carbohydrate metabolism, building of muscle, and normal growth processes. The most common problems associated with potassium deficiency are hypertension, cardiac arrhythmias, and fatigue. Potassium supplements should be taken only by prescription and can be life-threatening.

Prader-Willi syndrome

A genetic disorder that causes incomplete sexual development, short stature, cognitive disabilities, and an insatiable appetite that leads to obesity. Characteristics of PWS may include infantile hypotonia (muscle weakness and low muscle tone) that improves with age; feeding problems and poor weight gain in infancy; rapid and excessive weight gain between ages 1 and 6; narrow face with almond-shaped eyes and a small mouth with downturned corners; undescended testicles and small penis in males; scant or no menstrual periods in females; delayed puberty; overall developmental delay before age 6, including mild to moderate mental retardation or learning problems; and compulsive eating and preoccupation with food.

Because the condition can recur in

families, genetic testing is recommended for families at risk. The most challenging aspect of treating a child with PWS is weight management.

Precancerous

The term used to describe a condition that could become cancerous if left untreated.

Preconception counseling

See GENETIC COUNSELING.

Preeclampsia

A complication of pregnancy, also known as toxemia of pregnancy, in which the woman's blood pressure rises to an abnormal level. Symptoms include a headache, abdominal pain, nausea, and vision problems (such as blurred vision and blind spots). Sudden weight gain (more than 2 pounds in a week) due to swelling or fluid retention can also occur. One in 10 pregnant women develops preeclampsia, typically after the 20th week of a first pregnancy.

The cause of preeclampsia is not known. The only cure is delivery of the baby. When the condition is mild, doctors often recommend rest and allow the pregnancy to continue with careful monitoring of both the woman and the fetus. Various tests, such as a NONSTRESS TEST, may be performed to evaluate the health of the fetus and to determine whether an early delivery is required.

In about one pregnancy in 1,000, preeclampsia can progress to a more serious condition called ECLAMPSIA, in which seizures and coma may occur. Eclampsia must be treated in a hospital to protect the lives of both the woman and the fetus.

Pregnancy

The period from conception to birth, usually lasting about 40 weeks. Pregnancy causes numerous physiological changes in a woman, including cessation of menstrual periods, enlargement of the breasts, pigmentation changes in the skin, and progressive enlargement of the abdomen as the fetus grows. Each of the three stages of pregnancy, or trimesters, lasts about 3 months. See PRENATAL CARE.

Pregnancy tests

Tests on a woman's blood or urine that doctors use to detect a pregnancy. Over-the-counter HOME PREGNANCY TESTS that evaluate a urine sample are available at drug stores; if used correctly, they are nearly as accurate as those performed by a doctor. All of these tests involve the detection of a hormone called HUMAN CHORIONIC GONADOTROPIN (HCG) in the woman's urine or blood. HCG is produced in large quantities by the developing placenta during the first few weeks of pregnancy.

Pregnancy, multiple

A pregnancy in which there is more than one fetus. Multiple pregnancies carry an increased risk of complications, such as high blood pressure, PREECLAMPSIA, and POLYHYDRAMNIOS. Preterm labor is common; about half of all multiple births occur before the 37th week of pregnancy because the fetuses can grow too large for the uterus, which triggers uterine contractions. Women pregnant with multiple fetuses will undergo frequent ultrasound examinations to monitor fetal growth. See also MULTIPLE BIRTHS and TWINS.

Prehypertension

A condition that puts a person at risk of developing hypertension. A person is considered to have prehypertension if he or she has blood pressure readings that are consistently between 120/80 mm Hg and 139/89 mm Hg. See also BLOOD PRESSURE; HYPERTENSION.

Preleukemia

See MYELODYSPLASTIC SYNDROME.

Premature birth

The delivery of a baby before or during the 37th week of pregnancy. Smaller and more fragile than full-term babies, premature infants often must be closely monitored in neonatal centers, where they sleep in incubators that carefully control oxygen, temperature, and humidity. Because they are not fully developed, they are at increased risk of having breathing and liver problems, low blood sugar levels, and infection and bleeding.

Specific causes of premature birth include TOXEMIA OF PREGNANCY, diabetes, thyroid disturbances, PLACENTA PREVIA, fetal abnormalities, multiple pregnancies (such as twins), and infectious diseases, such as syphilis. Sometimes labor is induced before a pregnancy is full term because the mother's health makes it safer for the baby to be delivered than to continue the pregnancy. But despite being at risk for numerous diseases and disorders, most premature babies grow up to be normal and healthy. See PRETERM LABOR.

Premature ejaculation

Ejaculation that occurs before both partners have had an opportunity to fully enjoy the sexual experience. The cause of premature ejaculation is usually not physical and treatment is often successful, especially when the partner is involved. Treatment focuses on helping the man learn to control his ejaculation reflex.

Premenstrual syndrome

Physical and mental changes that some women experience each month as their menstrual period approaches. Also called PMS. See MENSTRUATION, DISORDERS OF.

Prenatal care

Health care provided to pregnant women. Prenatal care also involves education about pregnancy, labor, delivery, and parenting and the promotion of adequate nutritional support. Prenatal care ideally begins before the woman becomes pregnant and continues with monthly visits until 28 weeks of gestation, then every 2 to 3 weeks until 36 weeks' gestation, and then weekly until the baby is born. Prenatal care makes possible the early detection and treatment of problems and helps ensure a healthy pregnancy. See also PRENATAL TESTING.

Prenatal testing

Tests and procedures to help ensure that a pregnancy produces a healthy baby while maintaining the mother's health. Routine maternal blood tests are used to check blood type, Rh factor, and immunity to hepatitis B and German measles (rubella) and to rule out the presence of anemia and syphilis. Testing for HIV is recommended for women who are at high risk. Urine tests are given regularly to detect diabetes and the protein albumin, which, if elevated, can be a sign of PREECLAMPSIA (a condition of pregnancy in which blood pressure is raised).

All women are offered the option of "triple screen" blood tests between the 15th and 20th weeks to evaluate the risk of DOWN SYNDROME or a NEURAL TUBE DEFECT in the fetus. One test measures the level of alpha-fetoprotein (AFP), a protein produced by the developing fetus. The other tests measure two hormones produced by the placenta: human chorionic gonadotropin (HCG) and estriol (a form of estrogen). Glucose screening is done between the 24th and 28th weeks to test for GESTATIONAL DIABETES.

Most pregnant women are screened for group B streptococcal bacteria in the reproductive and urinary tracts; some infected women can transmit the infection to the baby during delivery. Group B strep infections can cause serious complications such as pneumonia in newborns.

Ultrasound (see ULTRASOUND SCANNING) is an imaging procedure that helps a doctor evaluate the size, health, and position of the fetus. A test called a biophysical profile is used to evaluate fetal muscle tone, breathing, heart rate, movement, and the quantity of amniotic fluid. Screening for suspected genetic disorders may be done when a fetus is at risk. The most common genetic tests used during pregnancy are AMNIOCENTESIS and CHORIONIC VILLUS SAMPLING (CVS). Two tests commonly used to monitor a baby's heart rate for possible problems are the contraction stress test and the nonstress test.

Prepuce

A covering of skin, usually referring to the FORESKIN on the penis.

Presbyopia

Age-related, progressive loss of the ability to focus on close objects. Presbyopia worsens gradually until approximately age 65 years, when the eyes have lost almost all of their ability to focus on close-up objects. Presbyopia is usually treated with glasses. See FARSIGHTEDNESS.

Pressure points

Areas on the body at which relatively light pressure can compress an artery against an underlying bone. Pressure is applied to slow or stop bleeding from a wound.

Pressure sores

Open sores that develop on the skin from sustained pressure on a part of the body; also known as bedsores or decubitus ulcers. Pressure sores occur when a person sits or lies in the same position for an extended time. The pressure squeezes blood vessels, reducing the flow of blood and nutrients to the skin. Pressure sores most often occur on the buttocks, tailbone, shoulder blades, heels, and ankles. If left untreated or if they become infected, bacteria can enter the bloodstream and lead to SEPSIS, which can be fatal.

The first step in the treatment of pressure sores is to reduce the pressure on the area. Open sores must be kept clean, rinsed, and covered with a dressing. Antibiotics may be required to combat infection. Severe pressure sores require surgery to remove dead tissue. Pressure sores can be prevented by good hygiene and by regularly changing the position of people who use wheelchairs or are confined to bed.

Preterm labor

Labor that occurs before or during the 37th week of pregnancy. Preterm labor can threaten the life of the fetus. The warning signs of preterm labor include vaginal bleeding, watery vaginal discharge, abdominal cramps that may be accompanied by diarrhea and fever, pressure in the pelvis, low backache, and uterine contractions or tightening. Any of these signs should be reported to the doctor or midwife immediately.

The diagnosis of preterm labor is made by examining the cervix. If it has begun to open or shorten, the doctor may order an ultrasound to estimate the size and age of the fetus and determine its position in the uterus. The mother may be asked to monitor the contractions for a few days, noting any increase in frequency or severity. The cervix will be examined frequently to detect changes that indicate LABOR has begun, such as dilation (opening) or effacement (thinning).

The doctor may stop preterm labor if neither the mother nor the baby is in danger of infection, bleeding, or other medical complications. Bed rest and extra fluids given by mouth or by intravenous drip are sometimes enough to stop contractions; if labor can be stopped, the mother may be able to remain at home. In some cases, preterm labor has advanced too far to be stopped, while in other cases, medical problems for either the mother or fetus make premature delivery necessary. See PREMATURE BIRTH.

Priapism

Persistent, painful erection of the penis without sexual desire or arousal. Priapism is a rare but serious condition caused by blood trapped in the penis. The condition primarily affects young men. Priapism can result from prolonged sexual activity, injury or infection in the genitals, certain medications, blood disease (leukemia, sickle cell anemia), cancer in the pelvis, a pool of clotted blood in the pelvis, or a tumor on the spine affecting the nerves that control erections. Prompt treatment is necessary to prevent severe, permanent injury to the penis. Immediate treatment consists of pain medication, drugs to reduce blood pressure, drawing blood from the penis through a needle, or injecting medication into the penis.

Primary

A term denoting a disease or disorder that originates in a specific organ or tissue. For example, primary lung cancer arises in the lung, whereas metastatic lung cancer arises from a cancer that originates elsewhere and spreads to the lung.

PRK

See PHOTOREFRACTIVE KERATECTOMY.

Proctitis

Inflammation of the rectum. In some cases, proctitis is related to ulcerative colitis (inflammation of the lining of the colon). When the rectum is the only part of the colon to be inflamed, proctitis is more likely to be the result of a SEXUALLY TRANSMITTED DISEASE (STD). Itching and pain in the rectum and around the anus and sometimes bleeding are the primary symptoms of proctitis caused by an STD. The treatment of proctitis depends on its underlying cause. Doctors generally prescribe anti-inflammatory drugs for proctitis. Treating STDs promptly is essential.

Progesterone

A female sex hormone produced by the ovaries. Progesterone prepares the endometrium (lining of the uterus) for a fertilized egg. The hormone is vital to a successful pregnancy and a healthy fetus as it promotes the normal growth and functioning of the placenta (the organ that develops in the uterus and nourishes the fetus). Progesterone is also produced in small amounts by the adrenal glands in men and women and in the testicles in men.

Prognosis

A prediction concerning the probable course of a disease and the chances of recovery and survival.

Prolactin

A hormone made in the pituitary gland that stimulates production of breast milk. See BREAST-FEEDING.

Prolapse

Displacement of all or part of an organ from its normal position. There are various types of prolapse. See UTERUS, PROLAPSE OF THE and MITRAL VALVE PROLAPSE.

Prophylactic

A drug, procedure, or device used to prevent disease. The term prophylactic is also used to refer to a CONDOM.

Prostaglandins

Hormonelike substances manufactured in the body that produce a wide range of effects, including pain and inflammation in damaged tissue.

Prostate gland

A walnut-sized organ located just below the bladder and in front of the rectum in males. The gland produces fluids that form part of SEMEN, the fluid released during ejaculation. Muscular tissue in the prostate also has a role in ejaculation. The prostate gland consists of two main parts; the inner part produces the secretions that keep the lining of the urethra moist, and the outer part produces the secretions that mix with sperm.

Prostate, cancer of the

A malignant tumor of the PROSTATE GLAND, which is part of the male reproductive system. Prostate cancer is the second most common cancer among men, after skin cancer, and the second most common cause of cancer deaths among men, after lung cancer. The exact cause is not known, but age is a factor: prostate cancer is rare in men younger than age 50. Heredity also plays a role: men whose fathers or brothers have had the disease, particularly when young, are at higher risk. It is twice as common among blacks as among whites, and blacks tend to develop it at a younger age. Diet (especially a high-fat diet) may also play a role.

In most cases, prostate cancer progresses slowly. As a result, early detection increases the chances for long-term survival. In its early stages, when the tumor is small and confined to the prostate, it causes no symptoms. The symptoms appear only as the tumor enlarges and spreads outside the prostate, first to nearby organs (the bladder, urethra, seminal vesicles), and later to distant parts of the body, particularly the bones. Symptoms can include blood in the urine; pain or difficulty urinating; the need to urinate frequently, particularly at night (see NOCTURIA); inability to achieve or maintain erections (see ERECTILE DYSFUNCTION); and persistent pain in the pelvis, lower back, or upper legs.

Because prostate cancer causes no symptoms in the early stages, it is usually detected during a routine medical examination. Physicians use two basic methods to screen for prostate cancer: a digital rectal examination (in which the doctor uses a gloved finger to feel the prostate for abnormalities) and the PROSTATE-SPECIFIC ANTIGEN (PSA) TEST. The PSA test checks the blood for PSA, a protein released by prostate cells. High levels of PSA can indicate prostate cancer. If an abnormality is found in either test, a sample (biopsy) of prostate tissue is needed to determine whether cancer is present. If cancerous cells are found, further tests are performed to determine the stage of the cancer. The choice of treatment options includes watchful waiting (since prostate cancer tends to progress slowly), surgery to remove the pro-

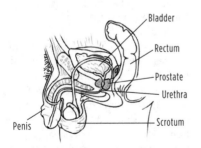

Anatomy of the prostate

The prostate gland surrounds part of the urethra, just beneath the bladder. Sperm formed in the testicles go to the prostate gland, which bathes them with fluids, then stores and nourishes them in sacs called the seminal vesicles (at the base of the prostate) before releasing them into the urethra during ejaculation.

state and surrounding lymph nodes, radiation therapy to kill cancer cells (including BRACHYTHERAPY), and hormone therapy to slow the growth of the tumor or shrink it. Chemotherapy is used for men whose disease has spread outside the prostate.

Early detection of prostate cancer offers the best chance for successful treatment. Some current guidelines recommend that all men older than 50 have a rectal examination and PROSTATE SPECIFIC (PSA) TEST; for blacks and for whites who have a family history of prostate cancer, the age to start screening is 45.

Prostate, enlarged

Noncancerous swelling of the PROSTATE GLAND. An enlarged prostate is also known as benign prostatic hyperplasia (BPH), which is usually a result of aging. Benign prostatic hyperplasia develops first in the portion of the prostate surrounding the urethra, narrowing this urinary passage. Signs include slowed or delayed start of urination, a weak urine stream, pain during urination, blood in the urine, difficulty emptying the bladder, frequent urination, repeated urinary tract infections, increased urination at night, a strong sudden desire to urinate, and leaking of urine (see INCONTINENCE, URINARY). Sexual functioning is usually not affected. In severe cases, the ability to urinate may be lost because of blockage to the urinary tract by the enlarged prostate. The inability to urinate may develop slowly, leading to kidney damage and kidney failure, or it can occur suddenly and be very painful. Complete blockage is a medical emergency.

An enlarged prostate is usually diagnosed with a digital rectal examination (in which the physician inserts a finger into the rectum to examine the prostate). Additional tests may be performed, for example, to determine the rate of urine flow or the amount of urine left in the bladder after urination or to visually inspect the prostate and bladder (cystoscopy). A blood test for prostate cancer, the PSA (prostate-specific antigen) test, is often recommended.

Severity of symptoms and the problems they pose for the person are key factors in determining treatment. Treatment options include annual monitoring for men with no or minor symptoms or medication to relax the muscles of the urethra for easier urination or to lower prostate hormone levels, which can reduce the size of the gland and decrease symptoms. Surgery may be recommended for men with incontinence or severe symptoms that do not respond to medication.

Prostatectomy

Surgical removal of all or part of the PROSTATE GLAND. Prostatectomy is performed to eliminate the symptoms of an enlarged prostate (see PROSTATE, ENLARGED) or to treat cancer of the prostate (see PROSTATE, CANCER OF THE), particularly in its early stages.

Transurethral incision of the prostate (TUIP) is the least extensive and invasive procedure and is used to treat urinary difficulties in men whose prostate is only slightly enlarged. Transurethral resection of the prostate (TURP) is similar to TUIP, but it is more extensive, removing more of the prostate. Radical prostatectomy is major surgery that removes the whole prostate gland.

Prostate-specific antigen (PSA) test

A blood test used to detect and monitor prostate cancer (see PROSTATE, CANCER OF THE). PSA is a protein normally found in the blood of adult men. Its level is increased in some prostate disorders, including prostate cancer. Monitoring PSA levels over time can help detect prostate cancer in its early stages, when the chances of successful treatment are highest. The test can also be used to evaluate the effectiveness of treatment for prostate cancer.

Prostatitis

Inflammation of the PROSTATE GLAND. Prostatitis can be caused by a number of microorganisms, such as bacteria normally found in the intestinal tract, those that cause certain SEXUALLY TRANSMITTED DISEASES, and those that cause bladder and urinary tract infections.

Symptoms may come on suddenly and severely (acute prostatitis) or be long-standing and mild, with periodic flare-ups (chronic prostatitis). Symptoms can include fever and chills along with pain in the lower back, abdomen, testicles, or the area between the scrotum and anus. Other symptoms include pain or burning during urination, ejaculation, or bowel movements; increased urge to urinate; and blood in the urine or semen. In severe cases, the man cannot urinate, and urine must be drained from the bladder through a thin rubber tube (catheter).

Bacterial prostatitis is treated with antibiotics during a 4- to 16-week period. Nonbacterial prostatitis may require only a 2-week course of medication. Men with prostatitis are also advised to drink large amounts of fluid to help clear the urinary tract of infectious microorganisms and to avoid foods and beverages that can irritate the urethra, such as caffeine, alcohol, spicy food, or chocolate.

Prosthesis

An artificial or manufactured substitute for a missing or nonfunctioning body part. Prostheses can include artificial legs, arms, teeth, eyes, and joints.

Protease inhibitors

A drug class used to treat AIDS (acquired immunodeficiency syndrome). Protease inhibitors work by suppressing the ability of HIV (human immunodeficiency virus) to reproduce. Protease inhibitors are always used in combination with other AIDS drugs and sometimes with other protease inhibitors. It is important for protease inhibitors to be taken exactly as prescribed, because drug resistance can develop very quickly in HIV. People with AIDS should never use protease inhibitors alone, and they should never miss doses or days of therapy.

Proteins

Complex organic compounds found in every living cell. Proteins are made up of chains of AMINO ACIDS containing carbon, hydrogen, oxygen, and nitrogen. Protein is necessary in the diet to provide the body with adequate amino acids for building proteins. Proteins are the main component of muscles, organs, and glands. The cells of muscles, tendons, and ligaments are maintained with protein.

Proteinuria

The presence of protein in the urine. Proteinuria indicates that the kidneys may not be functioning properly.

Proton pump inhibitors

Antiulcer drugs used to treat peptic ulcers, ESOPHAGEAL REFLUX (in which stomach acid backs up into the esophagus, causing painful heartburn), and diseases in which too much acid is released into the stomach. Proton pump inhibitors block the production of stomach acid by inhibiting the proton pump, the system that gastric cells use for making stomach acid. Proton pump inhibitors are usually taken before meals.

Protozoa

The simplest single-celled organisms classified as animals. Some protozoa can infect the body and cause diseases such as DYSENTERY and sleeping sickness.

Pruritus

The medical term for itching. Pruritus ranges from a mild urge to scratch to an overwhelming, unbearable itch. Common causes of pruritus include insect bites; allergic contact dermatitis (such as poison ivy); irritants such as chemicals, detergents, soaps, or wool; dry skin; and allergic reactions to food or drugs. Pruritus that occurs all over the body without skin lesions can be a sign of diabetes, liver disease, kidney failure, thyroid disorders, cancer, or psychological problems.

In most cases, pruritus responds to treatment. Scratching should be avoided because it can damage the skin and worsen the itching. Mild, soapless cleansers should be used. In cases of persistent or severe pruritus, it is important to consult a dermatologist for diagnosis and treatment. Doctors may prescribe medications such as topical corticosteroids.

Pseudo-obstruction

Dilation or enlargement of the colon that mimics a mechanical obstruction in the absence of an actual blockage. This condition typically develops after abdominal surgery or in people who are severely ill. (See also ILEUS, PARALYTIC.) Most people with pseudo-obstruction are successfully treated with bed rest, insertion of a NASOGASTRIC TUBE for suction, and administration of intravenous fluids to prevent dehydration and shock. If the enlargement continues, perforation (a hole or erosion) of the intestine is a risk. Sometimes the pseudo-obstruction can be relieved by colonoscopy. Surgery is also sometimes required. See SMALL-BOWEL TRANSPLANT.

Pseudogout

A form of arthritis caused by crystals of calcium pyrophosphate dihydrate (CPPD) in one or more joints. Pseudogout is distinguished from true GOUT by the difference in the composition of the crystals. Pseudogout usually involves large joints such as the knees, wrist, and ankles, while gout (which results from uric acid crystals) typically involves the first joint of the big toe. In pseudogout, the CPPD crystals in the joint cause severe inflammation and produce symptoms such as pain, swelling, and localized redness.

Symptoms may be relieved with nonsteroidal anti-inflammatory drugs (NSAIDs) or corticosteroid injections into the joint.

Pseudohermaphroditism

A condition in which a baby's genitals are ambiguous and the sex of the baby is not clearly identifiable. People with HERMAPHRODITISM are born with genitals of both sexes, while people with pseudohermaphroditism have the genitals of one sex. A priority in the early care of a child with pseudohermaphroditism is accurately determining the gender as soon after birth as possible. A specialist in treating hormonal problems in infants, such as an endocrinologist, should test and evaluate the child to make the correct identification of sex. Once the sex is identified, hormones may be used to treat the child. Reconstructive surgery can also be performed.

Pseudomembranous colitis

Inflammation of the mucous lining of the colon that develops as a complication of antibiotic use. Overuse of antibiotics results in the death of bacteria that normally reside in the colon and control the growth of other organisms. When these protective bacteria are no longer present, an overgrowth of the bacteria *Clostridium difficile* (*C. difficile*) may develop. The *C. difficile* bacteria produce a toxin that causes inflammation, which can result in severe watery diarrhea. Necrosis (death of tissue cells) and toxemia (the presence of poisons in the bloodstream) can occur in severe cases. An antibiotic is prescribed to fight the infection. Severe pseudomembranous colitis can be life-threatening and normally requires hospitalization.

Psittacosis

A rare bacterial disease that infects the lungs and is transmitted from birds to humans. The infection is caused by a strain of the *Chlamydia* bacterium that is carried by parrots, pigeons, poultry, and other birds. Humans become infected by inhaling dust particles or feathers contaminated with infected birds' droppings, by handling infected live birds or carcasses, and by bite wounds from infected birds.

In humans, the symptoms may resemble mild influenza, but they can vary in severity and include high fever, chills, sore throat, severe headache, loss of appetite, nausea, and vomiting. Psittacosis is diagnosed after a physical examination, a history of contact with birds, and by laboratory evaluation of respiratory secretions. It is usually treated successfully with antibiotics. See also AVIAN FLU.

Psoriasis

A chronic, noncontagious skin disorder characterized by scaling. Scaling occurs when cells in the epidermis (outer layer of skin) form too rapidly and pile up on the surface of the skin. The most common type of psoriasis is psoriasis vulgaris, consisting of red plaques (patches of thick raised skin) with silvery scales. Other varieties include pustular psoriasis (in which there are puslike bumps); erythrodermic psoriasis (red scaly areas involving the entire body); guttate psoriasis (characterized by red, teardroplike spots); and inverse psoriasis (in which there are smooth red plaques in the skin folds). In one in ten people, PSORIATIC ARTHRITIS (painful arthritis affecting the fingers, toes,

and spine) precedes or follows psoriasis of the skin.

Usually psoriasis is characterized by raised red or pink plaques covered by thick, silvery scales. While psoriasis can affect any skin area, lesions most commonly appear on the scalp, elbows, knees, lower back, palms, soles, armpits, and genitals. The onset varies widely, from gradual and mild to swift and severe. Lesions vary from small patches of dandrufflike scaling to major eruptions covering large areas of skin. Moderate to severe cases lead to painful cracking or splitting of the skin. Widespread psoriasis often causes emotional discomfort and embarrassment. Psoriasis is diagnosed through a thorough examination of the skin and nails. A skin biopsy may also be necessary.

Treatment is based on the type of psoriasis, its severity, the extent of skin areas involved, and a person's responsiveness to initial treatments. Bath treatments and moisturizers are soothing but must be combined with more potent remedies. The first line of treatment is topical medication applied to the skin. Topical treatments for psoriasis include corticosteroid creams, lotions, and ointments; synthetic forms of vitamin D3; coal tar; anthralin; topical retinoids; and salicylic acid.

If topical medications do not work, phototherapy (treatment with light) is tried. Ultraviolet light slows the rapid growth of skin cells and is used when psoriasis has not responded to topical treatments.

Psoriatic arthritis

A specific type of arthritis that develops in the joints of some people who have PSORIASIS. Symptoms, which can be mild and appear gradually or come on suddenly, may include restricted range of motion and discomfort in one or more joints, stiffness, pain, throbbing, swelling, or tenderness. The joints closest to the ends of the fingers and toes and the knees and elbows are most often affected. There may be morning stiffness and tiredness.

Diagnosis is made on the basis of clinical history, physical examination, blood tests, X rays, and laboratory testing of fluid drawn from the affected joints. Treatment of mild psoriatic arthritis may include the use of aspirin, ibuprofen, or other nonsteroidal anti-inflammatory drugs (NSAIDs). Physical therapy, exercise programs, applying heat, soaking in warm water, and the use of splints may also be recommended. In severe cases, medications including methotrexate, sulfasalazine, etretinate, puva, and gold compounds, by injection or orally, may be prescribed.

Psychiatry

The branch of medicine that studies, diagnoses, and treats mental illness. A psychiatrist is a physician who specializes in the treatment of mental disorders. Since psychiatrists are physicians, they can diagnosis mental disorders and separate them from other disorders (for example, Tourette syndrome or stroke), prescribe medications, and perform psychotherapy.

Psychoanalysis

See PSYCHOTHERAPY.

Psychogenic

A symptom or illness that arises from psychological causes, such as stress, interpersonal conflicts, or family issues, rather than a physical disease.

Psychological counseling

See PSYCHOTHERAPY.

Psychology

The branch of science that studies the mind, mental and emotional processes, and behavior. Psychology investigates learning, memory, perception, motivation, emotion, language, personality, social behavior, intelligence, child development, and mental illness. A psychologist is a nonphysician professional who specializes in the study of human behavior.

Psychopharmacology

The study and use of medications to control psychological states, particularly in the treatment of mental illness. Most psychopharmacological agents affect chemicals in the brain known as neurotransmitters, which convey signals from one brain cell to another. By raising or lowering the levels of certain neurotransmitters, medications can change how the brain reacts, often eliminating or reducing the symptoms of mental illness.

Psychopharmacological agents that act in similar ways are grouped into broad categories, including ANTIDEPRESSANTS, ANTIPSYCHOTIC DRUGS, STIMULANTS, and ANTIANXIETY DRUGS.

Psychosis

A severe mental illness in which a person loses touch with reality, experiences unusual perceptions (hallucinations), and holds false beliefs called delusions. Psychotic disorders include SCHIZOPHRENIA (an illness involving delusions, hallucinations, abnormal speech, and strange behavior) and delusional disorder (in which a person has a persistent belief that seems very real to him or her but is not shared by others).

Psychosomatic

Relating to a physical symptom or illness that originates in, or is worsened by, mental or emotional factors.

Psychotherapy

Also called talk therapy; the treatment of emotional problems, behavioral issues, or mental illnesses through verbal communication. A psychotherapist is a professional who uses techniques such as re-education, suggestion, retraining, and exploration of the emotions to treat emotional problems and mental illness. There are three fundamental approaches to psychotherapy: behavior therapy, psychodynamic psychotherapy, and humanistic therapy. Behavior therapy aims to improve the person's functioning, whether the origin of the problem is understood or not. Psychodynamic psychotherapy was developed originally from the ideas of Sigmund Freud, who invented psychoanalysis, and is based on the theory that understanding the self, particularly the emotional past and the hidden feelings of the unconscious mind, is key to resolving emotional problems or illnesses. Humanistic therapy (also known as existential therapy or gestalt theory) focuses on the person's immediate feelings, rather than thoughts or behaviors, and works toward increasing the person's self-awareness.

Psychotropic drugs

See ANTIPSYCHOTIC DRUGS.

Pterygium

A pinkish, triangular thickening of the membrane that lines the eye (con-

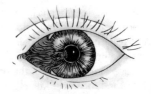

Accumulated tissue
Thickening of tissue on the conjunctiva (outer membrane covering the eye), called pterygium, may become red and inflamed, or it may interfere with tearing, causing dry eye.

junctiva) that can grow and cover part of the cornea (the clear outer layer of the eye). It usually grows on the inner corner of the eye and may grow large enough to interfere with vision if it covers the cornea. These growths are most common in people between ages 20 and 40 years who live in sunny climates, making exposure to sunlight a likely cause. The growth can be removed surgically for cosmetic reasons, because of discomfort, or if vision is obscured.

Ptosis

Drooping of one or both upper eyelids. See EYELID, DROOPING.

Puberty

The period of life in which a child makes the physical transition into adulthood. Sexual characteristics develop and sexual organs mature, making reproduction possible. Puberty is triggered when the pituitary gland and hypothalamus in the brain signal the body to begin producing sex hormones. In girls, the ovaries produce estrogen (the female sex hormone) and other hormones; in boys, the testicles produce testosterone (the male sex hormone) and other hormones.

The physical changes of puberty

usually begin between ages 8 and 13 in girls and between 9 and 14 in boys and progress at different rates for each person. After age 10, girls begin a period of rapid growth. Girls normally double their 10-year-old weight by age 18. Because estrogen adds body fat, while testosterone builds muscle, girls acquire a larger proportion of fat to muscle and bone than do boys. The earliest visible sign of female puberty is the appearance of breast buds. Soon afterward, pubic hairs start to appear.

About 2 to 2-1/2 years elapse between the start of puberty and a girl's first period. During this time, breasts grow fuller and more pubic hair appears. Underarm hair begins to grow, and sweat glands under the arms cause an increase in perspiration and body odor. The nipples may become more apparent and pubic hair is almost fully grown. A girl usually gets her first menstrual period between the ages of 11 and 14.

Puberty is later in boys, making them temporarily smaller than girls the same age. Because testosterone builds muscle, boys have a larger proportion of muscle and bone to fat than girls. The enlargement of the testicles and scrotum is the first visible sign of puberty in boys. Soon afterward, sweat glands under the arms cause an increase in perspiration and body odor. The next manifestations are usually the appearance of pubic hair, a deepening voice, and the first ejaculation. Testicles continue to grow, and the penis becomes thicker and longer. Pubic hair eventually begins filling in, and the penis and scrotum darken. Hair grows on the chin and under the arms. Boys normally experience a great gain in height toward the end of puberty.

Public health

The area of medicine concerned with assessing, safeguarding, and improving the health of an entire population or community. The public health discipline seeks to prevent the spread of disease; protect against environmental hazards such as air and water pollution and toxic waste; and prevent injuries through such measures as automobile seat belt laws and workplace safety regulations.

PUBS

See PERCUTANEOUS UMBILICAL CORD BLOOD SAMPLING.

Puerperium

Medical term for the 6 weeks following childbirth. During this period, a woman's body begins to return to normal from the physical changes of pregnancy and childbirth. Internal organs, including the uterus and cervix, shrink back to normal size and hormones return to pre-pregnancy levels.

Pulmonary

Describes diseases, conditions, disorders, or structures related to the lungs.

Pulmonary disease, chronic obstructive

See CHRONIC OBSTRUCTIVE PULMONARY DISEASE.

Pulmonary edema

A life-threatening condition involving the accumulation of fluid in the lungs caused by increased pressure in the small blood vessels of the lungs (capillaries) or leakage of fluid from damage to the tissue lining the capillaries and airways. In pulmonary edema, pressure in the veins of the lungs increases, forcing fluid from the capillaries into the alveoli (air sacs of the lungs). This can also result from damage to the capillaries that causes them to leak fluid. The excess fluid in the air sacs interferes with their normal function of exchanging oxygen and carbon dioxide.

Pulmonary edema may be caused by or be a complication of heart conditions, including a heart attack, disease of the mitral or aortic valves, and impaired cardiac function. Other associated disorders include kidney failure, infection, toxic inhalation, pulmonary embolism, aspiration of water into the lungs in near-drowning incidents, and abuse of medications or illegal drugs.

The symptoms may include shortness of breath and a sensation of being unable to take in enough air. Wheezing and coughing that sometimes brings up blood may be accompanied by feelings of anxiety and restlessness. Perspiration may be excessive, and the skin may be pale.

Pulmonary edema is a medical emergency requiring urgent evaluation and treatment. Diuretic medications are given to remove excess fluid, and morphine is given to relieve congestion and anxiety. If a heart disorder is involved, appropriate treatment and medication are prescribed. In severe cases, oxygen is given to restore the blood oxygen level.

Pulmonary embolism

The sudden blockage of an artery in the lung, usually by a blood clot that has traveled through the bloodstream. A pulmonary embolism may also be caused by tumor tissue, piece of fat, an air bubble, or, in pregnancy, by amniotic fluid. In most cases, other unblocked arteries can deliver sufficient blood to the affected area of the lung to prevent death of lung tissue. When a large blood vessel is blocked or when there is underlying lung disease, the amount of blood may be inadequate to prevent lung tissue death, a condition called PULMONARY INFARCTION.

If the blockage in the lungs is small, there may be no symptoms, but there is usually some degree of shortness of breath and chest pain. The chest pain may be experienced as sharp, stabbing, burning, and aching or as a dull, heavy sensation. Often, the chest pain is worsened by breathing deeply or coughing. Pain may also occur in the shoulder, arm, neck, jaw, or other areas of the body. Other symptoms include a cough that begins suddenly and sometimes produces blood or blood streaks in the sputum. The pulse may be irregular or weak. If the source of the pulmonary embolism is a clot in the lower extremities, there may be pain and swelling in one or both legs.

A pulmonary embolism is most commonly diagnosed with a lung scan or spinal CT scan. A lung perfusion scan involves a small amount of radioactive material that is injected into a vein and travels to the lungs, where it outlines the blood supply of the lung and can reveal an obstruction of a blood vessel. Lung ventilation scans, performed with the perfusion scan, reveal the areas where air is being exchanged and compare these areas with the pattern of blood supply to the lung. With these combined scans, a pulmonary embolism will show normal ventilation with decreased blood supply.

Pulmonary embolism requires emergency medical treatment and hospitalization. Treatment requires anticoagulant therapy, which is done to inhibit the formation of more clots. Anticoagulant therapy includes intravenous infusions of heparin or injections of low-molecular-weight heparin followed by warfarin taken orally. Thrombolytic therapy may be used to dissolve a large, life-threatening embolism (see THROMBOLYTIC DRUGS) using medication such as streptokinase or tissue plasminogen activator (TPA), which dissolves clots.

Ongoing anticoagulant therapy with medications that inhibit blood clotting can substantially reduce the rate of recurrence. Surgery may be recommended.

Pulmonary fibrosis

A disease in which lung tissue has become scarred and thickened from inflammation. Pulmonary fibrosis is also known as interstitial lung disease or interstitial fibrosis of the lung. Pulmonary fibrosis causes the permanent loss of the affected lung tissue's capacity to absorb oxygen into the blood. The extent of the scarred tissue determines the level of disability experienced by the person who has the disease. The condition can be the result of several diseases and conditions, particularly those that involve abnormalities of the immune system. Other causes include infections that affect the lungs, including tuberculosis, and exposure to mineral dusts (such as silica, carbon, metal, and asbestos) or organic dusts (such as molds and bird droppings).

People who have pulmonary fibrosis have similar symptoms regardless of the cause, although the symptoms may range from very mild to moderate to extremely severe. In the early stages, the symptoms may be barely noticeable and would not necessarily prompt a person to seek medical care. One of the earliest symptoms is a dry cough and breathlessness during exercise. The course of pulmonary fibrosis is unpredictable. Symptoms can develop gradually or follow a rapidly progressive course.

Pulmonary fibrosis may be diagnosed with a blood test, chest X ray, and pulmonary function tests given during both rest and exercise. BRONCHOSCOPY, lung biopsy, and CT (computed tomography) scans may be used.

CORTICOSTEROIDS may be administered, sometimes in combination with other medications, to treat inflammation associated with pulmonary fibrosis and can reverse the disease in certain cases. Oxygen therapy may be prescribed to help with breathing. In severe cases or if other lung diseases are present, lung transplantation may be recommended.

Pulmonary function tests

A series of tests that measure the lungs' capacity to hold air, move air in and out, and exchange oxygen and carbon dioxide. Pulmonary function tests are commonly used to evaluate lung disorders. The results of the tests are compared with normal standards based on a person's age, height, weight, and sex, and are expressed as a percentage of the predicted value.

Pulmonary hypertension

See HYPERTENSION, PULMONARY.

Pulmonary hypertension, primary

Abnormally high blood pressure in the pulmonary artery. Primary pulmonary hypertension is a rare disorder of unknown cause. The disorder develops in response to increased resistance to blood flow in the lung's arterial blood vessels. The increased workload of pumping blood against this resistance causes the right side of the heart to become enlarged and eventually leads to heart failure and respiratory failure.

Progressive shortness of breath on exertion is the primary symptom. Other symptoms include hyperventilation, chest pain under the sternum, sensations of weakness and fatigue, dizziness, light-headedness when standing upright, fainting, and coughing up blood.

Because there is no known cure, the goal of treatment is to control the symptoms. Vasodilators may be beneficial to some people. See also CHRONIC OBSTRUCTIVE PULMONARY DISEASE.

Pulmonary infarction

The death of lung tissue from an insufficient blood supply to a part of the lungs. Pulmonary infarction may be associated with PULMONARY EMBOLISM. The disorder can also be caused by congenital heart disease associated with severe pulmonary hypertension or sickle cell disease. The symptoms develop over a period of several hours and include coughing, blood-stained sputum, sharp chest pain with breathing, and fever. They may be experienced for several days, becoming milder with the passage of time.

Pulmonary infarction can be diagnosed by a chest X ray or other scanning technique that reveals a lesion on the lung and a collection of fluid, or PLEURAL EFFUSION, on the side in which the infarction has occurred.

Blood test results may reveal abnormalities that indicate lung tissue death. Small areas of dead tissue may heal spontaneously by absorption, leaving narrow scars, or they may reabsorb entirely, leaving normal lung tissue. Larger areas of dead tissue may be irreversible.

Pulmonary insufficiency

Breathing dysfunction resulting in impairment in the oxygen and carbon dioxide exchange required for body function; also referred to as respiratory insufficiency. Pulmonary insufficiency results in reduced oxygen levels or elevated levels of carbon dioxide, which cause respiratory acidosis, a condition affecting acid-base balance of the body. Pulmonary insufficiency can progress to respiratory failure.

The leading cause is cigarette smoking. The condition is associated with lung diseases including chronic obstructive pulmonary disease (COPD), emphysema, chronic bronchitis, and pulmonary fibrosis. Acute conditions such as pulmonary edema (fluid in the lungs) and pneumonia can also cause pulmonary insufficiency.

The primary symptom is shortness of breath that occurs when a person is at rest and persists for a period ranging from several months to years. A respiratory rate faster than 20 breaths per minute is another sign of pulmonary insufficiency. A physical examination by a doctor can reveal rapid, labored breathing, excessive use of chest muscles during inhalation, and abnormal breath sounds or inadequate air exchange.

Treatment is based on supportive care, smoking cessation, and low-flow oxygen therapy if needed. Complications include enlargement of the heart and heart failure.

Pulmonary rehabilitation

Programs designed to offer education, therapeutic exercise, and functional activities for people with lung disorders and diseases such as EMPHYSEMA, chronic bronchitis, and PULMONARY FIBROSIS.

Pulse

The rhythmic expansion and contraction of an artery that results from the beating of the heart. The normal adult pulse rate at rest ranges from 60 to 100 beats per minute, although exercise, illness, injury, and stress can produce much faster rates. Pulse rates lower than 60 beats per minute are referred to as BRADYCARDIA; rates higher than 100 beats per minute are referred to as TACHYCARDIA.

Puncture wounds

Injuries in which an object penetrates the skin or a body part. Puncture wounds often do not bleed heavily but, although they might close up right away, they can be very dangerous because they are susceptible to infection. A puncture wound through a shoe is particularly prone to serious infection. Medical care is essential for preventing infection and protecting against tetanus.

Pupil

The opening in the center of the eye through which light passes. The iris, the colored area encircling the pupil, contains muscles that adjust the size of the pupil in response to the amount of light and focusing needed. The iris opens (dilates) the pupil to allow more light to enter or to focus on far objects. The pupil contracts to restrict light coming in and to focus on near objects.

Pus

A thick, yellow-to-white fluid that consists of white blood cells, cell debris, and dead tissue cells. Pus forms in infected tissue of body structures and is produced by the inflammatory process (see INFLAMMATION).

Pustules

Also called pimples, elevations of the skin containing pus that result from inflamed hair follicles. Pustules are formed when hair follicles or sweat pores become blocked by an oil called sebum, which promotes the multiplication of bacteria that are normally present in the hair follicles. The increase in bacteria causes inflammation, irritation, and redness at the site of the blocked follicle. When the follicle ruptures, its contents are spread into surrounding skin, which causes the inflammation to spread. See also ACNE.

Pyelography

An X ray of the urinary system made with a dye that highlights the kidneys and ureters (the tubes that carry urine from the kidneys to the bladder).

Pyelonephritis

For symptom charts, see ABDOMINAL PAIN, page viii, and BACKACHE, page x.
Inflammation of the kidney caused by a bacterial infection. Pyelonephritis is usually associated with a URINARY TRACT INFECTION that has spread to the kidneys. Initial symptoms of acute pyelonephritis begin

suddenly and may include backache (especially tenderness in the middle and lower back), a high fever with chills, side pain, nausea, and vomiting. Some people may also experience frequent urges to urinate and find it difficult and painful to urinate. These symptoms require immediate medical attention as the infection can spread from the kidneys to the bloodstream. There is also a risk of permanent kidney damage.

Chronic pyelonephritis may cause symptoms that are mild and temporary, including side pain or abdominal pain.

Mild cases of pyelonephritis in healthy people are generally treated with oral antibiotics. In severe cases, hospitalization and treatment with intravenous fluids and antibiotics may be necessary.

Pyloroplasty

See VAGOTOMY.

Pyuria

The presence of white blood cells or pus in the urine. Pyuria is usually the sign of a urinary tract infection (see URINARY TRACT INFECTIONS) or an infection of the kidney, such as PYELONEPHRITIS.

Q fever

A zoonosis, or disease transmitted by animals, that is caused by a bac-

terium. Q fever occurs in domestic and farm animals without causing symptoms. In humans, Q fever causes symptoms in only half of people infected. Symptoms include a sudden high fever, chills, severe headache and fatigue, loss of appetite, and muscle pain. Infection of the connective tissue that surrounds the lungs' air sacs can cause chest pains. Other possible symptoms include sore throat, dry cough, abdominal pain, vomiting, or diarrhea. Q fever is almost never fatal, but prolonged infection can progress to hepatitis or endocarditis.

Q fever may be misdiagnosed as the flu. Blood tests can confirm the diagnosis. Treatment includes oral antibiotics such as tetracycline in adults and chloramphenicol in young children.

Quadriplegia

See PARALYSIS.

Quarantine

The isolation of a person or persons to limit the spread of a known or suspected infection with a contagious disease. Quarantine may be imposed on people who have been exposed to serious contagious diseases, as well as those who have acquired a contagious infection or who are believed to have been infected. See also EPIDEMIC; INFECTIOUS DISEASE.

Quickening

The first movements of a fetus that a pregnant woman feels. Women usually feel quickening for the first time during the 16th week of their first pregnancy. In subsequent pregnancies, quickening can occur as early as the 14th week.

R

Rabies

A life-threatening disease that affects the central nervous system. Rabies is caused by a virus that is found in the saliva of infected warm-blooded animals and is usually transmitted to humans and domestic pets by the bites of infected animals. Untreated, the disease is almost always fatal.

Whenever a person has been bitten by a warm-blooded animal, there is a possibility of exposure to rabies. Fox, raccoon, and rat bites have a very high risk of rabies. As an immediate first-aid procedure, the site of the animal bite should be thoroughly washed with soap and hot water as soon as possible. A doctor should be notified, or the person who has been bitten should visit the nearest hospital emergency department at once; prompt medical attention is essential to preventing death.

The time between the biting incident and the appearance of the first signs of rabies is usually 3 to 7 weeks, but the range extends from 4 days to 2 years. The first symptoms of rabies are often similar to those of any viral infection, including high fever and general malaise. Within 2 to 3 days of these symptoms, rabies infection causes pain followed by tingling at the site of an animal bite. The skin becomes sensitive to changes in temperature, there is excessive production of saliva with drooling, and there are severe muscle spasms in the mouth and throat. The infected person also experiences dramatic mood swings between rage and calm and, ultimately, has seizures. Untreated, rabies causes complete paralysis, as well as heart or respiratory failure within 7 to 25 days following the start of symptoms.

The course of treatment involves the use of a passive antibody injected directly into the wound. A vaccine is also injected, usually at five intervals, over a 28-day period. Treatment is usually effective if started promptly.

Rabies immune globulin, human

An immunizing agent. Rabies immune globulin is used along with rabies vaccine to prevent infection caused by the rabies virus. It works by providing antibodies needed to neutralize the rabies virus. The effects of rabies immune globulin will last long enough to provide protection until the body can produce its own antibodies against the rabies virus.

Rabies immune globulin is given to people who have been bitten, scratched, or licked by an animal known or suspected to have rabies. Because its purpose is to prompt the body to create its own antibodies, rabies immune globulin is given only once.

Rad

The unit used to measure the amount of ionizing radiation absorbed during X-ray procedures. See X RAYS.

Radial keratotomy

A surgical procedure to correct near-sightedness by making small incisions in the clear outer covering (cornea) of the eye in a spokelike (radial) pattern. The incisions penetrate almost all the way through the cornea, which flattens in the center and becomes steeper in its outer, downward-sloping portion. This change shifts the way light rays are bent as they pass through the cornea, allowing them to focus on the retina and correcting the nearsightedness.

Radial keratotomy is generally effective in reducing mild to moderate amounts of nearsightedness. Side effects and complications may include glare in night vision, sensitivity to light, fluctuation of vision during the day, overcorrection or undercorrection, severe scarring of the cornea, infection, the growth of blood vessels in the incisions, perforation of the cornea, and an increased risk of rupture of the cornea. Radial keratotomy has become a less popular procedure in recent years, particularly since the introduction of LASIK.

Radiation

The emission of high-energy, penetrating waves used to diagnose and treat various medical conditions. In medicine, radiation generally refers to ionizing radiation, which produces immediate chemical effects on human tissue. Ionizing radiation includes X rays, gamma rays, and particle bombardment such as neutron beams, electron beams, and protons. Radiation is used as a diagnostic tool in the form of X rays. It is also used therapeutically to treat cancer in the form of X rays, cobalt, and radium.

Radiation therapy, which is targeted to specific tissues being treated, uses much higher levels of ionizing radiation. Radiation is also used in nuclear medicine. The diagnostic uses of radiation include newer X-ray technologies such as CT (computed tomography) SCANNING and PET (positron emission tomography) SCANNING.

Radiation sickness

Also known as radiation poisoning; symptoms and illness that result from exposure to excessive doses of ionizing radiation. Radiation sickness may be caused by a single exposure to radiation at a very high level or by ongoing exposure to lower levels over time. Radiation sickness caused by long-term exposure is generally delayed and can result in cancer and premature aging. The severity of radiation sickness depends on the amount of radiation, the type of radiation, the duration of the exposure, and the areas of the body that have been exposed.

Radiation therapy

Also known as radiotherapy; treatment of malignant (cancerous) tumors and benign (not cancerous) conditions using X rays or radionuclides. Radiation therapy is the use of high-energy radiation to destroy or shrink malignant or benign cells by carefully regulating the dose and by targeting to the treatment site.

Radiation therapy may be the primary treatment, or it may be combined with other treatments before or after surgery. When it is used before surgery, the goal is to shrink a cancerous tumor. After surgery, radiation may be used to stop the growth of remaining cancer cells.

While radiation therapy is not physically disfiguring (as radical surgery can be), there may be unpleasant side effects that occur during or immediately after treatment. These side effects are usually mild but may be severe for some people. Typically, the symptoms are temporary and usually improve within 3 to 6 weeks.

Radiation therapy, interstitial

See BRACHYTHERAPY.

Radiculopathy

Damage to the nerve roots that enter or leave the spinal cord. Radiculopathy may be caused by problems such as disk prolapse (see SLIPPED DISK), spinal arthritis, or thickening of the meninges (the membranes that cover the brain and spinal cord). Symptoms include severe pain and sometimes loss of feeling in the area supplied by the affected nerves. There may also be weakness, paralysis, and wasting of the muscles supplied by the nerves. Treatment of the underlying disease is required. Analgesics and physical therapy provide some relief of symptoms.

Radioactivity

The spontaneous emission of radiation. Radioactivity is caused by the disintegration of the nuclei of atoms when they emit electromagnetic rays called X rays and gamma rays.

Radioisotope scanning

A nuclear medicine technique that uses radioactive isotopes injected into the bloodstream to visualize internal organs. Radioactive isotopes are substances that give off beta or gamma rays, which are similar to X rays. Radioisotope scanning allows for the observation and study of the size, shape, and location of organs or bones. The procedure can be used to evaluate organ function or to locate sites of disease, structural abnormalities, abscesses, or tumors. Radioiso-

tope scanning may also be used to monitor and evaluate ongoing treatment for a disease or condition.

Radiology

A branch of medicine concerned with the use of radiant energy in the diagnosis and treatment of disease. Radiology is the scientific discipline of medical imaging with the use of X rays, nuclear medicine, MRI (magnetic resonance imaging), and ultrasound scanning. A radiologist is a physician who is trained in the use of radiant energy, specifically X rays and radionuclides, radiation physics, and biology.

Radionuclide scanning

See NUCLEAR MEDICINE.

Radiopharmaceuticals

Drugs used to diagnose or to treat certain medical conditions. Radiopharmaceuticals are used by nuclear medicine specialists to study how a particular organ is working and to detect tumors or cancer that may be present. Radiopharmaceuticals are radioactive. Given in very tiny, safe amounts, they expose a person to about the same amount of radiation as an X ray does.

Some radiopharmaceuticals are used in larger amounts to treat certain kinds of cancer or other diseases. The radiopharmaceuticals are preferentially taken up in the cancerous area of an organ, where they destroy the cancerous tissue.

Radon

A colorless, gaseous, radioactive element produced by the disintegration of radium, uranium, lead, zinc, and iron ore. Radon is thought to cause an increase in lung cancer when found in microscopic particles in environmental airborne dust. It is odorless, colorless, tasteless, and not irritating to the lungs, which is why it is important for people to get their homes tested for radon. It is believed that 11 percent of lung cancer cases are related to radon. Radon is used in radiation therapy.

Rape

Any form of sexual intercourse that is forced on a person without consent. Rape is a crime of aggression and violence and is not a form of healthy sexual relations. Abnormal brain chemistry and abnormal early sexual experiences are each thought to play a role in the behavior of rapists.

Being treated for rape is complicated because rape is a crime. Injuries must be treated at the same time that evidence is collected. Someone who has been raped should be examined by a physician before washing or showering, so samples of the rapist's blood, hair, or semen can be obtained for use as evidence of the crime. In addition to injuries due to physical force, the physical effects of rape can include a sexually transmitted disease or, for women, pregnancy. The doctor can prescribe hormones that reduce the risk of pregnancy. Medications are also available to reduce the risk of acquiring a sexually transmitted disease.

Rape has profound psychological effects on victims, who may need to seek psychological counseling. See also DATE RAPE.

Rash

A flat or raised skin eruption characterized by changes in skin color or texture. Symptoms of rashes vary widely. Redness is common, and many are crusted or blistered. While some rashes cause no physical pain, many cause itching, swelling, and inflammation. Even otherwise symptom-free rashes can be cosmetically disturbing and lead to emotional distress. Rashes are due to a wide variety of causes, including allergic reactions (commonly to drugs or poisonous plants) and bacterial or viral infections. Rashes usually respond well to simple home remedies such as applying cool compresses and soothing lotions and taking over-the-counter antihistamines. However, when rashes are persistent, cause severe discomfort, or are accompanied by fever, it is important to consult a doctor.

Raynaud disease

A condition in which the arteries carrying blood to the fingers or toes constrict on exposure to cold or during emotional upset. The fingers or toes turn chalky white, and they may also sting or feel cold and numb. The skin may turn blue and then red when normal blood flow is restored. Unlike RAYNAUD PHENOMENON, Raynaud disease is an exaggerated version of a normal reflex that restricts blood flow to the extremities, and the disease is usually more of a nuisance than a disability.

Prevention is the best approach to Raynaud disease. This includes protection against the cold and avoiding tobacco use (nicotine constricts blood vessels in the hands and feet). Medications may also be prescribed to prevent blood vessel spasms.

Raynaud phenomenon

A condition in which the arteries carrying blood to the fingers or toes constrict on exposure to cold or during emotional upset. The nose and ears may also be affected. The fingers or toes turn chalky white, and they may also sting or feel cold and numb.

The difference between Raynaud phenomenon and RAYNAUD DISEASE is that Raynaud phenomenon occurs as a result of an underlying condition, such as a rheumatic disease (for example, scleroderma), exposure to certain chemicals (for example, vinyl chloride), or long-term use of vibrating equipment, such as jackhammers. Raynaud disease is independent of any underlying condition.

RDIs

See REFERENCE DAILY INTAKES.

Reactive airway disease

A group of lung and lower airway disorders characterized by wheezing, a high-pitched whistling sound. Causes of reactive airway disease include the chronic condition asthma, bronchial infections such as bronchiolitis and bronchitis, colds (see COLD, COMMON), congenital lung defects, a tumor, cystic fibrosis, inhalation of a foreign object, and pneumonia. Besides wheezing, other symptoms of reactive airway disease include chest tightness or pain, straining of chest muscles while breathing, and rapid breathing. In severe reactive airway disease, a lack of oxygen may cause the skin to grow bluish or gray.

Although wheezing is sometimes clearly audible, most often, the physician must listen to the lungs with a stethoscope to detect wheezing. The doctor may also order blood tests, chest X rays, and sputum or phlegm cultures. Devices such as a spirometer

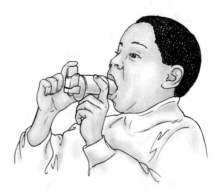

Child using an inhaler
A child with a reactive airway disease such as asthma may use an inhaler to take bronchodilators to open clogged passageways in the lungs or corticosteroids to fight inflammation. These drugs are often taken with a device called an inhaler. Some inhalers have a spacer, which makes the device easier to use properly. The child needs to learn to shake the inhaler, exhale, and close the lips around the spacer.

or a peak flow meter may be used to measure lung function.

Treatment of reactive airway disease varies according to its underlying cause. If wheezing is caused by a foreign body, the object must be removed by a doctor. If the cause is a congenital lung defect or tumor, surgery may be necessary. Medications may include bronchodilator drugs, corticosteroids, and allergy medications. Bronchodilators relax the muscles around airways and open bronchial tubes.

Reagent

A substance used to produce a chemical reaction to detect, measure, or produce other substances.

Receptor

A nerve cell that responds to a stimulus in the environment by producing nerve impulses. The term "receptor" may also refer to the area on the surface of a cell to which a chemical must bind to have its effect.

Recombinant DNA

Altered DNA (deoxyribonucleic acid) created by the insertion of a portion of DNA from another source. Recombinant DNA has been altered by chemical, biological, or enzymatic means to enable the foreign DNA that is placed in the host DNA to be replicated along with the host DNA.

Recombinant DNA is currently used to develop substances of medical value, as in gene therapy, or of economic value, as in the genetic engineering of food plants. In one example, the human gene that controls the production of human insulin is transferred and cloned in bacteria. The bacteria cells become factories that produce human insulin.

Reconstructive surgery

Any surgical operation to restore function to body structures that are defective or damaged. Reconstructive surgery focuses on congenital defects, such as cleft lip and palate, and deformities caused by injury, disease (for example, the loss of a breast to cancer surgery), or aging.

Rectal bleeding

Bleeding from the rectum can be a sign of disease. Often, rectal bleeding results from a minor problem such as hemorrhoids. But it may be caused by a more serious disorder such as COLITIS, CROHN DISEASE, or CANCER. Any rectal bleeding requires prompt medical attention. Regular screening tests are also recommended to detect rectal bleeding that may not be visible. A FECAL-OCCULT BLOOD TEST to detect hidden traces of blood in the feces should be done yearly after age 50 to check for colon and rectal cancer.

Rectal examination

A digital examination of the rectum to check for cancer. In the examination, the doctor inserts a gloved finger into the rectum to check for growths and to evaluate the prostate gland in men.

Rectal prolapse

A condition in which the end of the rectum bulges or protrudes out of the anal canal. Rectal prolapse occurs when the muscles supporting the perineum (the area between the anus and genital organs) become stretched or weakened. This condition is most common in older people and is usually the result of straining to defecate. Other causes may include weakness of the pelvic muscles, loss of control of the anal sphincter, a neurological condition, or a genetic predisposition. If the condition becomes permanent, surgery may be recommended but is not always successful.

Rectocele

A weakness in the back wall of the vagina causing a woman's rectum to bulge into the vagina. Rectoceles are usually caused during childbirth by the stretching of the pelvic muscles that support the vagina, rectum, and bladder.

Symptoms may include pressure or aching in the vagina and a feeling of pressure or discomfort during a bowel movement. Constipation can also occur, because stool can collect in the area where the rectum presses into the vaginal wall.

A doctor can easily diagnose a rectocele during a routine pelvic examination. Minor symptoms can be relieved by practicing Kegel exercises—alternately contracting and relaxing pelvic floor muscles. In severe cases, surgery may be recommended.

Rectum

The last segment of the large intestine, or colon, which connects with the anus. Food that has been fully processed in the small and large intestines is stored as stool, or feces, in the colon, then moved into the rectum by muscular contractions.

Three folds of membrane extending across the rectum (transverse folds) act like valves to control the movement of feces through the rectum until the urge to defecate occurs. When feces distend the walls of the rectum, the pressure causes nerve impulses to pass to the brain, which sends messages to the muscles in the anus to relax and allow passage of the stool. See also COLON; DIGESTIVE SYSTEM.

Rectum, cancer of the

Cancer that originates in the rectum, the lower part of the large intestine just below the colon. Colon and rectal cancers are often jointly called colorectal cancer. Most cancers of the large intestine grow slowly; therefore, colorectal cancer can often be cured with early detection and treatment.

Warning signs include blood in the stool or a sudden change in bowel habits. Any abrupt or persistent, unexplained constipation or diarrhea after years of regularity is cause for concern. Any blood in the stool or changes in bowel habits require immediate medical attention. Rectal discomfort, bloating, rumbling, and an

urgency to pass stool are other symptoms.

There may be no symptoms until the cancer causes an intestinal obstruction (see INTESTINE, OBSTRUCTION OF) or the intestine ruptures. Rupture can lead to peritonitis (a life-threatening inflammation of the peritoneum, the lining of the abdominal cavity).

Cancer in the rectum may narrow the passageway for stool, causing bowel movements to be thinner in shape or potentially blocking the passage of stools. Left untreated, cancer can spread to nearby organs.

Tests commonly ordered to determine the cause of symptoms include a lower gastrointestinal (GI) series (an X-ray procedure also called a barium enema) and SIGMOIDOSCOPY or COLONOSCOPY.

When cancer is not advanced, surgery is the best treatment. If the tumor is located in the upper part of the rectum, the surgeon cuts out the diseased portion of the rectum and rejoins the colon to the remaining healthy rectal tissue. When cancer occurs lower in the rectum, it may be necessary to remove the rectum and anus. In these cases, a permanent colostomy is created to form an artificial exit for feces. See also COLON, CANCER OF THE.

Red eye

A term used to describe inflammation of the eye that causes the eye to have a red appearance. Depending on its cause, red eye may be accompanied by pain, tearing, tenderness, or changes in vision. Since red eye can have a variety of causes, the eye needs to be examined by a medical professional to determine the underlying disease. Possible causes include infection in the membrane covering the eye and eyelid (CONJUNCTIVITIS), inflammation and infection in the eyelid (STYE, CHALAZION, or BLEPHARITIS), infection of the tear sac (DACRYOCYSTITIS), injury (eye injury), a foreign body, GLAUCOMA, allergy, environmental irritants, or inflammation of the eyeball.

Reduction

A manipulative procedure for realigning displaced broken bone ends or "reducing" the dislocated bones of a joint to normal angles. Reduction is the technical term for the repositioning of bones. When surgery is required to treat a fracture or joint, the technique is called open reduction. After reduction, sometimes a rod, pins, a plate, screws, or special bone cement is used to hold the reduced bone fragments in place. If a hip, shoulder, or other joint becomes dislocated as a result of trauma, reduction involves setting the displaced bones by manipulating them into their proper position without surgery. This is called closed reduction.

Reference daily intakes

RDIs; a set of dietary references for protein, vitamin, and mineral intakes used to identify amounts per serving on food labels. RDIs, which replaced the term "US RDAs" (recommended daily allowances), have been used by the US government since 1996. Intakes for all other nutrients are referred to as Daily Reference Values (DRVs).

Referred pain

Pain felt in a part of the body other than its original source. Referred pain occurs because at times differ-

ent parts of the body are supplied by the same nerve or nerve root. When nerve impulses reach the brain, they are misinterpreted as coming from the other area.

Reflex sympathetic dystrophy

Also known as reflex sympathetic dystrophy syndrome or RSDS, a chronic condition characterized by severe burning pain accompanied by swelling, excessive sweating, and extreme sensitivity to touch, pressure, motion, or temperature change.

Reflex sympathetic dystrophy syndrome is a nerve disorder that most commonly follows an injury or an illness, such as a heart attack. It is especially common after trauma, such as a gunshot wound. Reflex sympathetic dystrophy most commonly develops between the ages of 20 and 60 and affects the arms or legs. The pain described by people with this condition is typically severe and out of proportion to any original injury. Pain continues to worsen over time. A visible symptom of RSDS is warm, red, dry skin that later turns bluish, cold, and sweaty.

Diagnosis of reflex sympathetic dystrophy is based mainly on observation of symptoms. Doctors may also conduct a test to detect the temperature changes that are typical of this condition. X rays or bone scans are also useful in making the diagnosis.

Early treatment gives the best results. If treatment is started within 3 months, complete recovery is possible. A variety of drugs are prescribed for RSDS, including anti-inflammatory drugs, corticosteroids, antidepressants, anticonvulsants, calcitonin, and opioids. Most people also require at least one sympathetic nerve block, in which doctors inject numbing anesthetic into nerves. Other options include TENS (transcutaneous electrical nerve stimulation) and physical or occupational therapy.

Reflex, primitive

Involuntary muscular responses to sensory stimuli seen in infants. Primitive reflexes govern the infant's movements and disappear as the baby's neurological system matures. Physical examination of newborn babies includes the attempt to elicit various reflexes, because the absence of normal primitive reflexes can indicate neurological disorders.

In adults, primitive reflexes can occur as a result of diseases that affect brain function, such as ALZHEIMER'S DISEASE, STROKE, or brain damage from trauma.

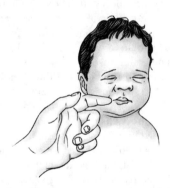

Rooting reflex
In the first 3 to 6 months of life, a baby has automatic primitive reflexes, probably related to feeding or protecting himself or herself, even before neurological development is complete. These reflexes will gradually disappear as the child gains conscious control over muscle movements. Rooting reflex is the name for the reflex in which stroking a baby's cheek causes him or her to turn toward the finger and open his or her mouth, searching for a breast or bottle.

Reflux

See ESOPHAGEAL REFLUX.

Refractive surgery

An operation that can improve or correct the ability of the eye to focus by permanently changing the shape of the cornea (the clear outer layer of the eye). Refractive surgery may eliminate the need to wear glasses or contact lenses or reduce the strength of the correction. Various types of refractive surgery can be used to correct nearsightedness (difficulty seeing distant objects), farsightedness (difficulty seeing close objects), and astigmatism (tilted, distorted vision due to an irregularly shaped cornea). See RADIAL KERATOTOMY; LASIK; PHOTOREACTIVE KERATOTOMY.

Regional anesthesia

See ANESTHESIA, REGIONAL.

Regional enteritis

See CROHN DISEASE.

Regression

A return to an earlier, less mature developmental stage in the face of stress. Regression helps provide comfort during stress and conflict and is considered a defense mechanism.

Regurgitation

The forceful, involuntary ejection of stomach or esophageal contents through the mouth. (See also VOMITING.) The backflow of blood through a defective heart valve is also known as regurgitation.

Rehabilitation

The process of using therapeutic measures and education to physically restore the health or ability of a person who is disabled, has undergone surgery, or has been injured or ill. Rehabilitation focuses on helping a person regain the physical abilities that have been lost or impaired.

Rehydration fluid, oral

A preparation designed to treat dehydration due to diarrhea. Watery diarrhea can rapidly cause a loss of body fluids and crucial body salts. Left untreated, this depletion can lead to shock. Young children and older people are particularly at risk. Oral rehydration fluid is available over-the-counter at pharmacies. It contains water, salts, and glucose. Homemade preparations can also be used. Doctors advise drinking rehydration fluid at half-hour intervals until pale-colored urine is passed. Medical attention is necessary if diarrhea continues longer than 2 days or if it is especially severe.

Reimplantation, dental

Replacing a tooth torn from its socket in an injury to the mouth. If the tooth is properly preserved until a dentist can be seen, the tooth can often be saved by being reimplanted into the gum by the dentist. It is recommended that the tooth be kept in milk. If milk is not available, it may be placed in cool water or wrapped in a clean wet cloth.

Reiter syndrome

A form of inflammatory arthritis transmitted by sexual contact and the organisms that cause dysentery; it occurs in people who have a genetic susceptibility to it. Typically, the first symptom in men is a penile discharge. Subsequent symptoms for men or women include painful joints, often in the knee, heel, or fingers. An eye inflammation called conjunctivitis and a skin rash similar in appearance to psoriasis may follow. An episode of Reiter syndrome may last a few weeks or several months. The symptoms may appear once or return. The joints are rarely damaged permanently. When severe, Reiter syndrome can cause tenderness and pain in the joints and is generally treated with pain-relieving medication such as NONSTEROIDAL ANTI-INFLAMMATORY DRUGS (NSAIDs), including aspirin and ibuprofen.

Relapsing fever

A disease that is transmitted to humans when they are bitten by ticks or lice. Relapsing fever is characterized by a high fever that recurs intermittently and lasts 3 to 5 days each time it occurs. Between bouts of illness, there are intervals of recovery varying in length from several days to more than a week. In the United States, the disease is always tick-borne and is generally limited to the western regions of the country.

The parasites that cause relapsing fever are called *Borrelia* spirochetes. Carried in insect vectors and transmitted to humans, these parasites enter the bloodstream and travel to internal organs, particularly the spleen, liver, and brain. The most prominent symptoms occur within 3 to 11 days after exposure and include sudden chills with high fever, rapid heartbeat, severe headache, vomiting, muscle and joint pain, and delirium.

Possible complications include abortion (miscarriage) in a woman who is pregnant, exacerbated asthma, inflammatory rashes on the skin and mucous membranes, and severe inflammation of the eyes that may lead to blindness. Heart failure may also occur. Death from relapsing fever is rare, but young children, pregnant women, older people, and people who are malnourished or debilitated are more vulnerable to severe disease.

Relapsing fever is treated with oral tetracycline or erythromycin, given intravenously in severe cases. Supportive treatment may include replacing fluids and restoring electrolyte balance.

Relaxation techniques

Methods of reducing the symptoms of stress and anxiety by eliminating tension held in the body. Relaxation techniques lower heart and breathing rate, decrease oxygen consumption, and reduce the levels of chemicals in the blood that rise in response to stress.

Some relaxation techniques are similar to MEDITATION as practiced in Eastern and Western spiritual traditions. Exercise disciplines such as T'ai chi and yoga are also used for relaxation. Research has shown that relaxation techniques, combined with medication, are effective for treating stress-related diseases, such as migraine headaches and high blood pressure.

REM sleep

Rapid eye movement sleep. Throughout the night, people move through different stages of sleep. These stages include the activity of REM sleep, as well as the four stages of NREM (non-rapid eye movement) sleep: transitional sleep, light sleep, and two stages of deep or delta sleep. Dreams occur during REM sleep, when the body becomes still except for eye movement and brain activity speeds up. Brain functions slow during more restful NREM sleep.

Remission

Disappearance of the signs and symptoms of a disease. A remission may be temporary or permanent.

Renal

Pertaining to or around the kidneys.

Renal cell carcinoma

A type of malignant kidney tumor that occurs only in adults; also known as hypernephroma. Renal cell carcinoma is the most common form of cancer of the kidney and forms on the edge of the kidneys. A history of smoking increases the risk substantially.

As the tumor enlarges, it grows into healthy kidney tissue, causing symptoms such as persistent fever, loss of appetite, and weight loss. Renal cell

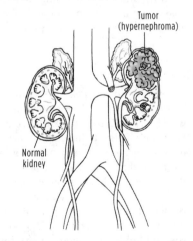

Tumor
(hypernephroma)

Normal
kidney

Kidney tumor
A hypernephroma is a slow-growing kidney tumor that often gives no early warning signs. Symptoms may include pain between the ribs and hip, weight loss, fatigue, or a mass on the kidneys that a doctor discovers.

carcinoma spreads much more slowly than many other kinds of cancer. It is unusual for the cancer to result in kidney failure before it is diagnosed. Bleeding from the tumor may produce red or cloudy urine.

Early detection of renal cell carcinoma is crucial. It can be cured if the tumor is discovered and removed at an early stage. Urine samples will be obtained for analysis. Diagnostic tests may include intravenous PYELOGRAPHY, ULTRASOUND SCANNING, CT (computed tomography) SCANNING, and MRI (magnetic resonance imaging) of the kidney.

If renal cell carcinoma is diagnosed, the affected kidney is removed. The remaining healthy kidney can usually compensate for the missing one. See KIDNEY CANCER.

Renal colic

Painful, intermittent, and severe spasms on one side of the back usually caused by one or more kidney stones.

Renal diet

A diet prescribed in cases of chronic kidney (renal) failure. In individuals with kidney damage, the kidney may be less efficient at eliminating waste in the urine. Consequently, these waste products, normally cleared by the kidneys, build up in the blood. In such cases, doctors recommend a renal diet, which limits the intake of protein, potassium, sodium, phosphorus, and fluids, to lessen the work for the kidneys.

Bread, cereal, pasta, and rice are the main sources of calories in a renal diet. Special flours and bread that are protein-free and low in potassium and phosphorus are used. Protein intake is restricted, and usually milk, meat, and eggs supply the limited amount needed. Depending on potassium and phosphorus restrictions, a small amount of vegetables and fruits are permitted. Because renal diets may not provide all the necessary nutrients, doctors may recommend supplementation with electrolytes and vitamins.

Renal transplant

See KIDNEY TRANSPLANT.

Renal tubular acidosis

A condition that produces an acidic imbalance as the result of the inability of the kidneys to excrete adequate amounts of the acid normally generated by chemical processes in the body. The normal pH balance of the body is slightly alkaline. In renal tubular acidosis, the pH balance is tipped toward acidic. Acidity causes problems such as calcium loss from the bones. The dissolved calcium accumulates in the bloodstream and is excreted by the kidneys, resulting in abnormal bone structure (called osteomalacia), impaired growth in children, skeletal deformities, and muscle weakness.

Renal tubular acidosis may be caused by several factors including autoimmune disorders; a condition called hypercalciuria, which is an excess of calcium in the urine; recreational drug use; genetic disorders; and heredity, which is the most common cause in children. There may be no symptoms, or symptoms may include fatigue, weakness, confusion, diminished alertness, an increased respiratory rate, dehydration, nausea, and muscle pain.

Alkaline medications, including sodium bicarbonate and potassium citrate, may be given to correct the acidic pH in the body and to increase lowered potassium levels. Thiazide diuretics may also be necessary to increase the reabsorption of bicarbonate.

Renal vascular hypertension

High blood pressure caused by disorders of the blood vessels that supply the kidneys with blood. About 20 percent of the blood pumped from the heart passes through the kidneys. The blood enters through the renal artery (a major branch of the aorta), is filtered by the kidneys, and returns to the heart via the renal vein.

Renal vascular hypertension is caused by a narrowing of the renal artery, most commonly from atherosclerosis and less commonly from conditions such as fibromuscular dysplasia or vasculitis, atherosclerosis, preeclampsia and eclampsia, or fibromuscular dysplasia.

Intravenous pyelography, ultrasound scanning, MRI scanning, and an arteriogram (an X ray of an artery) may be needed to diagnose the condition.

Medication may be prescribed to control high blood pressure in people who have renal vascular hypertension. To prevent progressive kidney failure and to improve high blood pressure conditions, surgery may be indicated in some cases.

A more recently developed treatment called percutaneous transluminal angioplasty (PCTA) has been successful in treating renal artery stenosis and improving high blood pressure. In this procedure, a catheter with a deflated balloon at its tip is threaded through an artery in the thigh, then guided upward into the narrowed renal artery. Sometimes a stent is placed to help keep the artery open. See ANGIOPLASTY, BALLOON.

Renin

An enzyme released into the blood by the kidney in response to stress. Renin reacts with the liver to produce angiotensin, which eventually causes constriction of the blood vessels and an increase in blood pressure. It is estimated that 10 to 15 percent of people with high blood pressure have too much renin in their blood. The overproduction of renin can occur from a condition called renal (kidney) hypertension. See RENAL VASCULAR HYPERTENSION.

Repetitive strain injury

An injury that occurs when repeated movements of one part of the body damage the tendons, nerves, muscles, and other soft tissues. The muscles and tendons in the arms are most commonly affected by the condition. People who engage daily in jobs requiring repetitive movements of the fingers, hands, arms, and shoulders are particularly vulnerable to RSI. Those jobs include typing on a keyboard, using a computer mouse, playing a musical instrument, and working on an assembly line. Carpal tunnel syndrome, tendinitis, tenosynovitis, and certain other disorders that cause muscle and tendon pain are sometimes included in the classification of repetitive strain injuries.

Typically, the symptoms of RSI develop gradually and may be experienced only when a person is performing repetitive movements. Pain, aching, tingling, coldness, numbness, tightness, burning, or restricted movement may be felt. Sometimes, there is swelling in the affected area. Clumsiness or loss of strength and coordination in the hands may be another symptom.

A physician can diagnose RSI by taking a medical history, including asking the person about lifestyle factors that may contribute to the condition, and by physical examination. X rays and blood tests may be necessary to rule out rheumatoid arthritis and other similar disorders. NONSTEROIDAL ANTI-INFLAMMATORY DRUGS (NSAIDs) are often recommended to relieve pain and reduce swelling. Physical therapy and splinting of the affected parts may help.

When symptoms are apparently related to a person's job, an occupational doctor or nurse can offer advice about posture changes and special equipment to help prevent RSI. When RSI is diagnosed early and a person makes an effort to avoid its cause, a complete recovery can be expected.

Reproduction, sexual

Production of a child through the fertilization of a woman's egg with a man's sperm.

Reproductive system, female

The group of organs and structures, both internal and external, involved in a woman's capacity to have sexual intercourse, produce eggs (reproductive cells), become pregnant, and give birth.

A woman's external genital area is called the vulva, located between her thighs and encompassing all the structures that surround and protect the entrance to her internal reproductive organs. The mons pubis is the hairy mound of tissue that covers the pubic bone of the pelvis. Under the mons pubis there are two sets of labia (or lips) that cover the opening into her body. The outer labia majora are covered with hair; the inner labia minora are hairless. The clitoris, a small button of tissue that lies at the point where the two labia minora meet at the top, is extremely sensitive and can become erect during sexual arousal. The urethral opening, from which urine leaves a woman's body, lies just below the clitoris. Below the urethral opening is the opening to the vagina, the entrance into the internal reproductive organs.

Internally, the vagina is the muscular canal that leads into the uterus from the outside of the body. It accommodates the male penis during sexual intercourse, and it is the birth canal during childbirth. At the point where the vagina enters the uterus, a hard, round organ called the cervix forms the lower end (or neck) of the uterus. The cervix is actually doughnut shaped, with an opening in the middle through which menstrual fluids can pass; the opening of the cervix widens to permit childbirth.

The uterus lies inside the protective framework of the pelvis. It is a hollow organ with muscular walls; the inner walls are lined with tissue (endometrial tissue) richly supplied with blood vessels. In the event of pregnancy, a fertilized egg will develop into a fetus inside the uterus.

Extending from either side of the uterus are two fallopian tubes. These passages carry eggs from the ovaries to the uterus. The ovaries contain many eggs, present in a woman's body from birth. Each of these eggs lies in a tiny cavity called a follicle. Within the follicle, the female hormones estrogen and progesterone are produced. These hormones, together with hormones produced in the brain, regulate the reproductive cycle that releases one egg each month for possible fertilization. See also MENSTRUATION.

Reproductive system, male

The group of organs involved in a man's capacity to produce sperm (male reproductive cells), have sexual intercourse, and fertilize an egg (female reproductive cell) to produce offspring.

The penis and the testicles are the visible male reproductive organs. The testicles, also known as testes, are two glands lying in a pouch of skin (called the scrotum) between a man's thighs. Each testicle produces sperm (male reproductive cells) and secretes the male hormones called androgens, including testosterone. The testicles continually produce millions of sperm in densely packed tubules. These tubules lead to another structure called the epididymis, located on the back of each testicle. Sperm move from the testicles into the epididymis, where they mature.

During sexual arousal, sperm travel from the epididymis into a long tube called the vas deferens, which passes up into the body into the seminal vesicles—two sacs that lie just behind the bladder. In the seminal vesicles, fluid (called seminal fluid) is added to the sperm to produce the liquid called semen. Semen moves into the urethra, a tube that leads from the bladder to the outside of the body.

As the semen passes into the urethra, it receives additional fluids from the prostate gland, a small gland that surrounds the urethra just under the bladder. Muscular tissue in the prostate also has a role in the ejaculation of semen from the body.

The penis, extending from between the testicles, is composed of tissue that can become engorged with blood during sexual arousal; the engorgement causes the penis to lengthen and become erect. Semen passes through the urethra in the erect penis and is propelled out of the body by strong contractions during a sexual orgasm, a process called ejaculation.

Resection

Surgical removal of all or part of an injured or diseased organ.

Resident

A medical school graduate who is undergoing postgraduate training in a supervised training program. In a teaching hospital, residents are overseen by an attending physician.

Respiration

The total process by which the body takes in oxygen from the environment, transports it in the blood to body cells, uses it to create energy, and gets rid of the waste products of cell function in the form of carbon dioxide in exhaled air. Respiration is often thought to be synonymous with breathing, but breathing is only the mechanical, or external, part of the respiratory function.

Respirator

An apparatus that modifies the air inhaled through it. A respirator may be a face mask worn by a firefighter, for example, to block the inhalation of dust particles or other undesirable items, such as smoke. A respirator may also be a life-supporting device (ventilator) that supplies oxygen or a mixture of oxygen and carbon dioxide given to someone who cannot breathe independently.

Respiratory distress syndrome

Respiratory failure produced by an illness or injury that causes an accumulation of fluid in the lungs, a condition called pulmonary edema. Respiratory distress syndrome is a medical emergency that can progress to extreme difficulty in breathing and results in a life-threatening deficiency of oxygen in the blood.

It is sometimes caused by sepsis (severe, widespread infection in the body). The syndrome occurs when the lungs' small air sacs and capillaries are damaged, which allows blood and fluid to leak into the spaces between the air sacs and ultimately into the air sacs themselves.

Symptoms such as shortness of breath develop rapidly, generally within 24 to 48 hours of the illness or injury. The skin may develop a mottled appearance or a bluish coloration, and the person may be disoriented or unconscious.

A doctor can detect wheezing or crackling sounds in the lungs when examining the chest with a stethoscope. Analysis of blood gases usually reveals a decreased oxygen level in the blood. Chest X rays may indicate fluid accumulating in lung and airway spaces normally filled with air.

Immediate medical attention is es-

sential to preserve life. A person who has respiratory distress syndrome must be treated promptly in a hospital's intensive care unit. The underlying cause requires treatment, and low oxygen levels urgently require oxygen therapy.

Supportive care includes providing intravenous fluid and intravenous feedings to prevent dehydration and malnutrition. Lung infections, such as bacterial pneumonia, commonly occur and need antibiotic therapy.

See also CARDIOPULMONARY RESUSCITATION (CPR).

Respiratory failure

A condition in which impairment of the breathing system results in an increase in carbon dioxide and a decrease of oxygen in the blood. Respiratory failure may be chronic or acute and can be caused by any of a number of lung diseases and disorders of the lung, including respiratory distress syndrome, lung infections, medication overdoses, and structural injuries or abnormalities of the lungs and chest wall. The condition results in an inadequate amount of oxygen to meet the vital needs of organs and has a high mortality rate. This deprivation of oxygen can cause a range of symptoms, including personality changes, headache, confusion, cardiac arrhythmia, loss of consciousness, and coma. Pulmonary hypertension (see HYPERTENSION, PULMONARY) and heart failure (see HEART FAILURE, CONGESTIVE) may eventually occur.

The goal of treatment is to maintain sufficient delivery of oxygen to the lungs, usually by means of oxygen therapy, and to restore the normal exchange of oxygen and carbon dioxide in the bloodstream. Bronchodilators and antibiotics may be prescribed.

Respiratory function tests

See PULMONARY FUNCTION TESTS.

Respiratory system

The group of organs that brings oxygen from the air into the bloodstream and expels the waste products, including carbon dioxide. The organs of the respiratory system accomplish the physical process of breathing to bring air into the body and then expel it, as well as the more complex biochemical process of respiration to fuel the cells of the body with oxygen. See also BREATHING PROBLEMS; LUNG.

Respiratory therapy

A program of evaluation, treatment, and care for people with breathing problems and chronic lung conditions, including asthma and emphysema. Respiratory therapy may also provide life-support treatment in emergency medical situations to treat heart failure, drowning, or shock. This form of therapy includes the use of devices that provide oxygen or medication that is inhaled as a mist or gas.

Respiratory tract infection

Infectious disease of any of the organs or structures involved in breathing. When the infections affect the upper area of the respiratory system, they are generally referred to as common colds (see COLD, COMMON). Lower respiratory tract infections may involve the larger airways in the lungs, causing bronchitis, or the smaller airways in the lungs, producing bronchiolitis. Viral or bacterial infections of the deeper parts of the lungs can cause pneumonia.

Treatment depends on the cause. Since there are no effective medications currently available to treat viral infections, treatment for these infections is usually limited to supportive therapies to ease discomforts. Bacterial respiratory infections usually require antibiotics.

Respite care

A variety of services that offer caregivers temporary relief from their responsibilities of caring for disabled or older people. Respite care is offered through in-home and community services, such as home health care, adult day care, and temporary, short-term institutional care.

Restless leg syndrome

Also known as RLS, a condition characterized by unpleasant, restless sensations in the legs and an irresistible impulse to move them. People with RLS may experience tingling, twitching, fidgeting, aching, prickling, or burning of the legs when they lie in bed or sometimes even when they sit down. These sensations are usually worse at night and can lead to insomnia. Sensations are relieved by activity, such as walking. Many people with RLS also experience periodic limb movements in sleep (PLMS). Treatment includes care for any preexisting underlying condition and sometimes use of medications, such as anticonvulsants, benzodiazepines, opioids, levodopa, and dopamine agonists. See also SLEEP DISORDERS.

Reticulocyte

An immature red blood cell that has developed beyond the stage in which a nucleus is present.

Retina

The light-sensitive membrane that forms the inner layer of the back of the eye and contains the nerve receptors for vision. Light that has passed into the eye reaches the retina as an inverted image. The retina is a complex structure, a ten-layered membrane lined with two kinds of light-sensitive cells. Rod cells—so-called because of their shape—perceive shape and movement. Cone cells are sensitive to both light and color and have a role in visual acuity, or sharpness of perception. Because the retina has many more rods than cones, the eye can perceive light in darkness, but it sees color best in bright light. Rods and cones—also called photoreceptors—respond to light focused on the retina by translating the stimulus into electrochemical nerve signals.

Retinal artery occlusion

Blockage of a blood vessel that carries blood to the retina. The blockage usually results from a fat deposit or a blood clot that cuts off the blood supply to the retina, damaging the affected portion. The principal symptom of retinal artery occlusion is sudden blurring or blindness in one eye. Emergency treatment consists of massaging the eyeball, with the hope of dislodging the blockage before the retina is permanently damaged by the loss of blood. Carbon dioxide gas may be given to widen the artery and move the clot or fat deposit, thereby reducing the size of the affected area of the retina. Anticoagulant drugs are given to dissolve blood clots and restore normal blood flow. Even with treatment, some or all vision in the eye may be lost because of irreversible damage to the retina.

Retinal artery occlusion can be a sign of increased risk of stroke. The condition is most likely to occur in older people as a result of underlying disease, such as diabetes mellitus, type 1 and type 2; high blood pressure (hypertension); or abnormally high pressure within the eye (glaucoma).

Retinal detachment

Separation of the RETINA from the underlying tissues. Retinal detachments are usually caused by a tear or hole in the retina. Eye fluids leak through the opening and accumulate under the retina, lifting it off the tissues that support it. A retinal detachment is painless, but it causes major

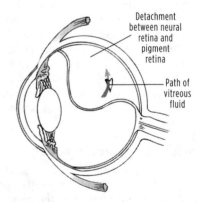

Detachment between neural retina and pigment retina

Path of vitreous fluid

Leaking fluid

As a result of aging or trauma, the neural retina can break and the vitreous body can become more liquid. The vitreous fluid passes under the neural retina and separates it from the adjacent pigment retina, causing the serious condition called retinal detachment.

changes in vision. These include bright flashes of light, particularly off to the sides of the visual field; a sudden increase in floaters (translucent shapes that move through the field of vision); blurred vision; or the sensation that a thick curtain is being pulled across the eye. Retinal detachment is an emergency that may lead to blindness and requires immediate medical attention.

Treatment depends on the extent of detachment. If the retina has a scar or hole but is not completely detached, it can be repaired with a laser (photocoagulation) or by using a cold probe in a procedure called cryopexy.

If the retina has a large detachment, more extensive surgery is needed.

Retinal hemorrhage

Bleeding from small blood vessels in the surface of the retina. Retinal hemorrhage is usually caused by extremely violent force to the eye; it is a common sign of shaken baby syndrome, a type of severe child abuse. The condition can also result from falls from at least 50 feet, serious motor vehicle accidents, certain abnormalities of the nervous system and blood vessels, infection, high-altitude mountaineering and, rarely, as a complication of normal childbirth and general anesthesia.

Retinal tear

See RETINAL DETACHMENT.

Retinal vein occlusion

Blockage of a blood vessel that carries blood away from the retina. The blockage is usually caused by a diseased arterial wall compressing the venous wall at a crossing point or by a blood clot. Retinal vein occlusion

impairs sight if swelling or ischemia (poor blood flow) occurs in the center of the retina. Often the blood and fluid are absorbed naturally, and vision may return to normal. If the blood persists, the change in vision may be permanent. Laser therapy may treat any persistent swelling of the retina.

Retinitis

Inflammation of the retina.
See RETINOPATHY.

Retinitis pigmentosa

Progressive degeneration of the retina leading to poor vision in dim light, loss of vision to the sides, and reduced central vision. The disease takes its name from the darkly pigmented appearance of the retina in an eye examination. In many cases, blindness eventually results. No treatment is known. Wearing sunglasses to block ultraviolet light and taking antioxidants such as vitamin E may delay progression of the disease.

Retinoblastoma

See EYE TUMORS.

Retinoids

A group of compounds that are structurally related to retinol and function like vitamin A. Retinoids are used in the treatment of various skin diseases and digestive ailments.

Retinol

See VITAMIN A.

Retinopathy

Abnormality of the retina, which can be caused by many different conditions. In its most severe form, retinopathy can result in the abnormal growth of blood vessels and scar tissue in the retina and a retinal detachment, resulting in extreme distortion of vision or blindness. Less severe forms of the disease can be treated surgically. It can also cause the arteries in the eyes to narrow and bleed, damaging the retina and causing visual disturbances. Retinopathy can be caused by premature birth, hypertension, and diabetes mellitus, type 1 and type 2 (see RETINOPATHY, DIABETIC).

Retinopathy of prematurity

An eye disease in extremely premature infants. In this disorder, the developing blood vessels of the light-sensitive retina become damaged. Vision problems ranging from nearsightedness to blindness can result.

In many infants, retinopathy heals on its own. Other times, surgery is necessary. Damaged blood vessels can be repaired with either cryotherapy (freezing) or laser surgery. Surgery does not always completely correct the problem.

Retinopathy, diabetic

Progressive damage to the retina as a result of diabetes. Diabetic retinopathy develops as a long-term complication of both type 1 (insulin-dependent) and type 2 (non-insulin-dependent) diabetes (see DIABETES MELLITUS, TYPE 1; DIABETES MELLITUS, TYPE 2). About half of those who have had diabetes for 10 years or longer develop some degree of diabetic retinopathy. The disease can lead to severe or complete vision loss, and it is a leading cause of blindness in the United States.

This initial stage of the disease is known as background (or nonproliferative) diabetic retinopathy. It causes no pain, and, although the changes in the retina are visible to a specialist during an eye examination, they lead to only subtle changes in vision. Vision changes noticeably if bleeding and fluid leakage occur in the macula, the central portion of the retina, which is responsible for sharp, central vision. This macular edema, as it is known, causes blurred vision.

Vision also changes noticeably if proliferative diabetic retinopathy develops. The lack of oxygen in the retina prompts the growth of new blood vessels, which are abnormally weak and rupture easily. Blood leaking into the vitreous (the clear jelly-like substance in the center of the eye) blocks the passage of light and impairs the person's vision. The formation of scar tissue may pull the retina away from the back of the eye and cause RETINAL DETACHMENT, which is a medical emergency that can lead to blindness.

Controlling the blood sugar level and the hypertension that often accompanies diabetes are the best measures for delaying or preventing the start of diabetic retinopathy. In addition, every person who has diabetes should undergo a thorough eye examination at least once a year to detect any retinal changes in the earliest stages. If macular edema develops, it is treated with laser photocoagulation.

Retractor

An instrument used to hold the sides of a surgical incision open or hold back the surrounding organs and tissues so the surgeon has access to the area being operated on.

Retropubic suspension

A surgical procedure for women to correct stress incontinence (urine leakage when coughing or sneezing) caused by a cystourethrocele, a weakness in the tissues supporting the bladder and urethra. Surgery is indicated only when Kegel exercises, hormone replacement therapy, and other treatments have not been effective in correcting the pelvic support problems that cause urine leakage.

Retrovirus

An infectious particle that consists of RNA (ribonucleic acid) genetic material, instead of DNA (see DE-OXYRIBONUCLEIC ACID). Retroviruses contain proteins, which can attach to cell membranes and allow the retrovirus to enter and infect the cell. The virus that causes AIDS (acquired immunodeficiency syndrome) is a retrovirus, as is the virus that causes T-cell leukemia (see LEUKEMIA; T CELL).

Rett syndrome

A rare, pervasive developmental disorder in children. An affected child's head is of normal circumference at birth, followed by a gradual slowing of head growth. Rett syndrome occurs in four stages. In stage one, children appear to develop normally for their first 6 to 18 months. Development slows and eventually comes to a halt in stage two. In stage three (between 9 months and 3 years), the child begins to lose previously acquired speech and motor skills. There may also be a loss of interest in social activities. Stage four sees a gradual return of learning, but at a slower rate. Most children with Rett syndrome are mentally retarded and may have problems with coordination and walking. Treatment options are limited. Most people with Rett syndrome will need some degree of custodial care.

Reye syndrome

A very rare childhood disorder that is potentially fatal to children under 18; it is strongly associated with taking aspirin, but the exact cause remains unknown. In Reye syndrome, a child's brain and liver swell, following a viral infection (such as influenza or chickenpox) or an upper respiratory tract infection. A third of cases occur in children who have chickenpox. To avoid risk, children under 18 should be treated for fever with ibuprofen or acetaminophen instead of aspirin.

The onset of symptoms begins 3 to 7 days after the start of a viral illness, when an affected child begins to vomit forcefully every 1 to 2 hours over a 24- to 36-hour period. There may be a headache and changes in consciousness ranging from lethargy and sleepiness to agitation and anger. Additional symptoms include confusion, disorientation, delirium, hallucinations, and a rapid heartbeat. If the disorder progresses, brain swelling and injury can eventually lead to a seizure or coma.

A child showing the symptoms of Reye syndrome should be brought immediately to a hospital emergency department. Hospitalization is mandatory for children diagnosed with Reye syndrome. Fluids lost during vomiting need to be replaced intravenously. Children must be monitored for brain swelling, and medications may be administered to control it. By increasing a child's breathing rate, a ventilator (mechanical breathing device) can also help control pressure on the brain. A blood transfusion or kidney dialysis may be required. In some cases, surgery may be performed to reduce pressure on the brain.

There is no cure for Reye syndrome. Prospects for recovery often depend on the seriousness of the case and the effectiveness of the treatments. If the disorder is treated promptly, a child can recover completely in 5 to 10 days.

Rh immune globulin

A blood protein used as a treatment if a person with Rh-negative blood is exposed to Rh-positive blood; also known as RhoGAM. (See RH INCOMPATIBILITY.) Rh immune globulin is also used to treat a bleeding disorder known as immune thrombocytopenic purpura.

Rh incompatibility

A potentially life-threatening condition that can develop when a mother with Rh-negative blood has a baby with Rh-positive blood. Rh-positive and Rh-negative indicate the presence or absence of an inherited blood characteristic known as the Rh factor (named after the rhesus monkey, the species in which the factor was originally identified). If Rh-positive blood mixes with Rh-negative blood, the Rh-negative blood develops antibodies to the Rh factor and attacks it. Such a situation can arise when a woman with Rh-negative blood is carrying a fetus with Rh-positive blood. Small amounts of blood from the fetus leak across the placenta during pregnancy and birth and stimulate an antibody response (Rh isoimmunization) in the mother that attacks the baby's blood cells. Usually the disease occurs in a subsequent pregnancy, after the woman develops antibodies to the Rh factor.

Rh incompatibility is now almost entirely preventable. Early in pregnancy the mother's Rh blood group is established with a simple blood test (see BLOOD GROUPS). If she has Rh-negative blood, she is given an injection of Rh immune globulin during the 28th week of pregnancy to destroy any Rh-positive fetal red blood cells in her bloodstream and prevent the mother from forming Rh antibodies. This injection has no risk, even if the fetus proves to have Rh-negative blood. If the newborn has Rh-positive blood, another injection of Rh immune globulin is given within 72 hours of birth to eliminate any fetal blood cells that may have entered the mother's bloodstream during labor.

In rare cases in which antibody sensitization in the mother has already occurred, the fetus is given blood transfusions in the uterus to replace the Rh-positive blood with Rh-negative blood. The baby is then delivered before it reaches full term.

Rheumatic fever

An inflammatory illness that occurs as a delayed complication of group A *Streptococcus* infection of the upper respiratory tract. The illness, which is not contagious, can occur within 3 to 35 days after a person has had strep throat but received no treatment for it. Rheumatic fever produces inflammatory lesions in the connective tissue of the heart, joints, tissues below the skin, and central nervous system. Complications of rheumatic fever following a single episode of the illness are unusual, but they may include valvular heart disease, congestive heart failure, and persistent arthritis.

A child with rheumatic fever has a high temperature, a lack of appetite, and general malaise. He or she is often pale and sweaty. Symptoms may include painful joint swelling and the joints may become reddened and hot to the touch. If the heart is affected without involvement of the joints and the infection is mild, there may be only mild symptoms including fatigue, poor coloring, and general malaise.

In severe infections, the principal symptom is breathlessness, especially with exertion or when the person is in a lying position. This requires emergency medical attention because without treatment heart failure can occur. Also, a rash of reddish circles with pale centers may appear on the front and back of the trunk.

Rheumatic fever may be suspected in a person with the typical symptoms combined with a history of strep throat. Blood samples and a culture of the throat are generally taken for analysis in a laboratory.

All cases of rheumatic fever are treated with antibiotics to combat any remaining bacteria from the original strep throat infection and to prevent ongoing or recurrent infection. Anti-inflammatory corticosteroid medication may be necessary to treat very severe cases in which the heart is seriously affected.

Rheumatism

A common term, now considered medically obsolete, that may be used to indicate a variety of conditions characterized by soreness, stiffness, or pain in the muscles or joints. Spe-cific diseases that may be referred to as rheumatism are rheumatic fever, osteoarthritis, myositis, bursitis, and rheumatoid arthritis.

Rheumatoid arthritis

A type of joint inflammation in which several parts of the body may be affected. In this more serious, systemic form of arthritis, the immune system develops antibodies that create a gradual and chronic inflammation of the thin membrane lining the joints. The inflammation eventually spreads to other parts of the joints and weakens the bones that are linked together by the joints.

Usually the small joints are affected, primarily the knuckles and toe joints of the hands and feet. Other joints, including the wrists, knees, ankles, and neck, are sometimes affected. The inflammation may also involve the eyes, heart, lungs, blood vessels, and other tissues just beneath the skin. Rheumatoid arthritis is characterized by morning joint stiffness, fatigue, muscle aches, low-grade fever, and weight loss.

Rheumatoid arthritis is diagnosed by clinical symptoms and findings along with blood tests such as the erythrocyte sedimentation rate (ESR) and the rheumatoid factor (RF), both of which indicate a generalized inflammation in the body. X rays may also show changes in the joints typical of rheumatoid arthritis.

The use of NONSTEROIDAL ANTI-INFLAMMATORY DRUGS (NSAIDs), such as aspirin, ibuprofen, and naproxen, and heat applications may help control pain. Exercises may be recommended by a physical therapist. In active cases of rheumatoid arthritis, medications that interrupt the process that produces the disease may be prescribed. These include penicillamine, gold compounds, sulfasalazine, and methotrexate. Chemotherapy drugs may be given to reduce the blood levels of antibodies. In early stages, surgical removal of the inflamed membrane covering the joint (a procedure called a synovectomy), may be considered.

Rheumatoid arthritis, juvenile

See JUVENILE RHEUMATOID ARTHRITIS.

Rheumatology

The medical science that is concerned with rheumatoid diseases, or diseases that affect the joints, muscles, bones, and associated fibrous tissues. A rheumatologist is an internist or pediatrician who has received additional training and experience in this medical science.

Rhinitis

Inflammation of the mucous membrane lining the nose that may result from a number of causes, including the common cold (see COLD, COMMON), allergies, irritation of the nose from air pollutants, and the side effects of medications such as over-the-counter nasal decongestant sprays.

The most common symptoms of rhinitis are a stuffy nose, nasal obstruction (blockage of nasal passageways), and postnasal drip (the sensation of mucus dripping from the back of the nose into the throat). The cause is often a cold, which is an infection with a virus.

Chronic rhinitis may be caused by continual exposure to chemicals in the workplace (such as house paint or photo-developing solutions), environmental pollutants, or ongoing contact with irritants such as chlorine in a swimming pool.

Allergic rhinitis (hay fever) is the result of an exaggerated response to inhaling (breathing in) a foreign substance such as pollen, mold, tobacco smoke, animal dander, or components of household dust, specifically dust mites. The allergic response causes a release of many chemicals, including histamine (a body chemical released during an allergic reaction), which increases blood flow to the nasal membranes, causing nasal congestion and an excess production of mucus.

Vasomotor rhinitis is nasal inflammation caused by the expansion of the abundant supply of blood vessels in the nose. The expansion may be from sensitivity to temperature changes, stress, or environmental irritants such as smoke or smog.

Rhinitis is diagnosed by examination and evaluation by a doctor. The treatment depends on the cause of rhinitis. If the condition is caused by the common cold, the doctor may recommend one or more medications such as a decongestant. Treatment on the inside of the nose, possibly with injections of one of the corticosteroids, and efforts to eliminate possible irritants, may be recommended.

Rhinoplasty

See NOSE RESHAPING.

Rhythm method

See NATURAL FAMILY PLANNING.

Rib

Any one of the oval, curved bones that form most of the skeleton of the chest. There are 12 pairs of ribs, each of which joins a vertebra in the spine. See SKELETAL SYSTEM.

Rib, fractured

A broken rib bone that may be caused by forceful trauma, such as a fall or a blow to the chest, or by the pressure of intense coughing or sneezing. Symptoms include pain that intensifies when a breath is taken, tenderness and shallow breathing, and bruising at the site of the injury. In most cases, a fractured rib will heal naturally within 3 to 8 weeks. A physician should be notified if the person has a high temperature, a cough develops, or thick or bloody sputum is coughed up. Emergency medical care should be sought when there is difficulty breathing or an increase in pain, or if the person has nausea, vomiting, or abdominal pain.

Riboflavin

Vitamin B2, an important nutrient in the metabolism of carbohydrates, fats, and protein. See VITAMIN B.

Ribonucleic acid

See RNA.

RICE (first aid)

An acronym or abbreviation for the first aid techniques used to minimize bleeding and swelling of an injured joint on an arm or leg. RICE stands for:

- *REST* The person should lie quietly while medical assistance is sought.

- *ICE* An ice pack or cold compress may be used to minimize swelling of the injured area.

- *COMPRESSION* A snug bandage may be used to reduce swelling and bleeding.

- *ELEVATION* The person's feet should be elevated about 12 inches

higher than the head, to keep blood flowing to the brain.

Rickets

A disease affecting the bones in the skeleton, characterized by inadequate calcium and phosphate in the bones. Rickets is usually caused by a severe deficiency of vitamin D; it occurs mainly in infancy and childhood if milk or vitamin D–fortified beverages are not consumed and exposure to sunlight is limited. Symptoms include bowlegs and knock-knees, nodular enlargements on the bones, muscle pain, profuse sweating, chest deformities, spinal curvature, and enlargement of the skull, liver, and spleen. The bones may be tender when touched. Treatment is with a diet rich in calcium, vitamin D, and phosphorus. Adequate exposure to sunlight is also beneficial.

Rigor mortis

The temporary stiffening of the muscles of the body after death. Rigor mortis typically sets in from 3 to 7 hours after death, and it generally disappears between 3 and 4 days later, when decomposition begins.

Ringing in the ears

See TINNITUS.

Ringworm

A fungal skin infection characterized by ring-shaped, red, scaly patches. See also TINEA.

RNA

Ribonucleic acid. A molecule consisting of a nucleic acid found in all living cells and in many viruses. RNA is the nucleic acid that carries the flow of genetic instructions from the DNA (deoxyribonucleic acid) to the rest of the cell. RNA occurs in several forms defined by their functions, including messenger RNA, transfer RNA, and chromosomal RNA. RNA reads the chemical GENETIC CODE of the DNA that defines each gene. In order for a cell to make a protein, the DNA dictates the genetic code to a strand of messenger RNA, which then moves outside the cell nucleus to the cytoplasm where RNA directs the production of protein according to the genetic code.

Rocky Mountain spotted fever

An infection in humans that is transmitted by microscopic parasites called *Rickettsiae*; also known as tick fever. Wood or dog ticks are the vector of infection, transmitting the disease from rodents to humans. *Rickettsia rickettsii*, the bacteria that cause Rocky Mountain spotted fever, attack the endothelium (cells that line the walls of small blood vessels). Within 1 to 2 days of being bitten by an infected tick, a person may experience a loss of appetite and general malaise, followed by headache, chills, muscle and joint pain, light sensitivity, and pain at the back of the eyes.

A rash of small red spots typically appears on the ankles and wrists 2 to 3 days after the fever begins. The rash then spreads to the limbs, trunk, and occasionally the face. As the rash progresses to large sores, Rocky Mountain spotted fever is easily distinguishable from the other diseases it resembles, such as measles.

If not treated, Rocky Mountain spotted fever can be fatal. Prompt treatment with chloramphenicol and tetracyclines for a minimum of 10 days is usually effective.

Root canal treatment

A therapeutic procedure to treat an infection of the soft inner core (the dental pulp) in the tooth. The pulp or nerve is the soft tissue inside the natural crown and root portions of the tooth.

Rosacea

A skin disease characterized by varying degrees of facial redness due to enlargement and dilation of blood vessels beneath the skin surface; also known as adult acne. Common signs of rosacea are redness, pimples, and the appearance of spidery small blood vessels on the face. Often people have only one or two symptoms. Usually, chronic inflammation and redness affect the forehead, cheeks, chin, and nose. Redness first appears to be a blush or sunburn but gradually becomes more noticeable and does not go away.

A serious complication of rosacea is rhinophyma, a swollen, bright red nose caused by oil glands that enlarge and lead to a buildup of excess tissue. Eye problems are another possible complication. In about half of the people affected, there may be redness, burning, tearing, and irritation of the eyes.

Rosacea is a treatable (but not curable) disorder that often goes undiagnosed. It may be mistaken for acne or sunburn. A dermatologist can diagnose rosacea by observing the appearance of the skin. Early diagnosis is essential because rosacea can become progressively worse without treatment.

Treatment is tailored to the individual. When topical antibiotics such as metronidazole prove ineffective, oral antibiotics including tetracycline, minocycline, erythromycin, or doxycycline may be prescribed. Isotretinoin is an option but can cause serious side effects, including birth defects.

Roseola infantum

A benign infectious disease, usually caused by human herpesvirus 6 (HHV-6), that typically affects infants and young children between the ages of 6 months and 3 years. Roseola infantum is characterized by a high fever and a rash, which breaks out as the fever lessens.

Diagnosis of roseola infantum is generally made by ruling out other possible causes of the fever and confirming when the rash breaks out and the fever resolves. The symptoms are treated to make the infant or child more comfortable, but there is no medical treatment for the illness, which improves on its own within a week.

Rotator cuff disease

A defect in the muscles at the back of the shoulder. The rotator cuff is the muscle group attached to the shoulder blade. Defects in the rotator cuff may be due to injury, strain, or overuse that causes tears in the muscle. Painful arc syndrome, left untreated, can lead to rotator cuff disease.

The symptoms of rotator cuff disease are stiffness, pain with movement, and restriction of movement. Left untreated, the tears may cause muscle tissue loss. In some cases, gentle stretching and strengthening exercises may help restore normal use of the muscle. In more severe cases, surgery may be recommended.

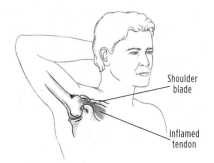

Shoulder inflammation
A tendon in the rotator cuff area may become inflamed when it rubs against the long end of the shoulder blade, which projects over the shoulder joint.

Rotator cuff tendinitis

Inflammation of the muscles and tendons that connect the upper arm bone to the shoulder blade. Rotator cuff tendinitis may be caused by repetitive stress on the muscles. It may also occur if the tendons become pinched under the shoulder bones, which may occur when inflammation or bone spurs narrow the tendon space. It can occur with repetitive elevation of the affected arm. See also TENDINITIS.

Rotavirus

An infectious virus that is the most common cause of infectious diarrhea in children. Most infected children develop symptoms such as nausea, vomiting, diarrhea, and low-grade fever. Although fever and vomiting disappear after a few days, diarrhea may continue for several more days. Diarrhea and vomiting can make the body lose too much fluid, leading to dehydration, a potentially serious problem that may require hospitalization. A child suspected of being dehydrated should be seen by a doctor.

Warning signs include dry lips, tongue, and skin; sunken eyes; fewer tears when a child cries; a sunken soft spot on a baby's head; and less frequent urination.

A child who has rotavirus should drink adequate fluids. Commercially prepared electrolyte solutions can be used to speed up the rehydration process.

Roundworms

A type of worm that lives in the intestines of humans and other mammals. In the adult stage, a roundworm can be almost 10 inches long and as thick as a pencil; The females produce eggs in the intestines, which pass out of the body in the feces.

A light infestation of roundworms can cause mild abdominal pain. In more severe infestations, the larvae can migrate to organs including the liver, lungs, and eyes, where they may cause allergic reactions, including asthma, and serious complications, including vision loss. The infestations are cured by medications that destroy or paralyze the worms or break down the roundworms' attachment to the intestinal wall so they can be eliminated in the feces.

Rubella

A contagious viral infection, also called German measles. Symptoms of rubella usually appear within 16 to 18 days after exposure. About half the people who become infected get a rash. The disease in an infected person is contagious from 10 days before the rash appears up to 15 days after the rash appears. Other symptoms may include mild fever, aching joints, headaches, general malaise, runny nose, and reddened eyes.

Sometimes rubella is mild and the person has no symptoms. Fatigue, swollen glands, and soreness in the joints may occur in children. These symptoms may or may not appear in adolescents and adults.

Symptoms of rubella must be clinically differentiated from other infections, including measles and scarlet fever. Blood tests are generally used to identify antibodies to the virus and confirm a diagnosis of rubella. The rash commonly lasts up to 3 days, and the fever lasts from 1 to 5 days.

A safe and effective vaccine can prevent rubella. The rubella vaccination is commonly given in combination with vaccines against measles and mumps, and is called the MMR (measles-mumps-rubella) vaccine. The MMR vaccine is routinely given to children, but may also be administered to adults who have not received it previously.

Complications of rubella are rare but may include arthritis, bleeding, encephalitis, and middle ear infections. Rubella is most dangerous when it occurs in a woman who is pregnant.

Rubeola

See MEASLES.

Runner's knee

A sports injury (see SPORTS INJURIES) caused by mechanical malfunctions of the knee during running activities, resulting in a softening of the cartilage in the kneecap. The cartilage of the kneecap relies on intermittent compression to release waste products and receive nutrients from the knee joint's synovial fluid. If the kneecap shifts to the side or does not track smoothly in its thighbone groove during running, portions of its cartilage may not be able to release waste and receive nutrients normally. The result is a deterioration of the cartilage. Symptoms include pain around and under the kneecap, which may be experienced after sitting for some time with the knees bent. The pain may be worsened while running downhill or descending stairs.

When runner's knee is first detected, activities that stress the knee area should be decreased to allow healing. Exercises to build strength in the hip and thigh muscles will not stress the kneecap and may help recondition the knee. Running shoes that provide extra support may be helpful.

A physical examination by a doctor specializing in sports medicine should rule out other possible knee, hip, ankle, and foot problems. If more conservative measures are not successful, injections of corticosteroids or arthroscopic surgery may be considered.

Rupture

A break or tear in an organ or tissue. A rupture in the muscles of the groin can cause a hernia, which may require surgery. When inflammation causes a rupture in an intestine, it is a life-threatening emergency.

S

Sac

Any structure or body organ shaped like a bag or pouch.

Sacroiliitis

An inflammation of the sacroiliac joint, which is one of a pair of joints in the lower back near the pelvis. Sacroiliitis produces an aching pain in the lower back and may be a symptom of a variety of conditions or diseases. When the pain occurs on both sides of the lower back, it can be caused by ANKYLOSING SPONDYLITIS, REITER SYNDROME, PSORIATIC ARTHRITIS, RHEUMATOID ARTHRITIS, or JUVENILE RHEUMATOID ARTHRITIS. When there is pain on one side, sacroiliitis may be due to GOUT, OSTEOARTHRITIS, or an infection. Sacroiliitis is diagnosed by X rays and blood tests. Treatment is with NONSTEROIDAL ANTI-INFLAMMATORY DRUGS (NSAIDs), such as ibuprofen and aspirin, or if the joint is infected, antibiotics.

Sacrum

A triangular bone in the lower spine. The sacrum lies just above the last bone of the spine, the coccyx or tailbone, and below the lumbar spine. The sacrum joins with the hip bones at the sacroiliac joints to form the rear of the pelvis.

SAD

See SEASONAL AFFECTIVE DISORDER.

Saddle block

See ANESTHESIA, SPINAL.

Safe sex

Also called safer sex; the exercise of precautions while participating in sexual activity in order to decrease the risk of transmitting or acquiring sexually transmitted diseases (STDs). Safe sex behaviors may also include precautions to avoid undesired pregnancy (see CONTRACEPTION). Physicians recommend the use of male or female latex condoms during sexual intercourse. In order to be effective, condoms must be in place before the beginning and until the end of sexual activity and must be used during every encounter. Other safe sex measures include abstinence and a faithful, monogamous sexual relationship.

Saline

A solution of salt in purified water. Saline is 0.9 percent sodium chloride in water that can be mixed with medication for injection or administered intravenously to replace lost sodium and chloride to the blood. Saline can also be used as a plasma substitute for the temporary maintenance of living tissue such as a tooth that has been knocked out or to moisten dry eyes or nasal passages.

Saliva

The watery mixture of secretions from glands in the mouth. Saliva is a clear, alkaline, somewhat sticky fluid secreted by the SALIVARY GLANDS. Saliva is made up of water, mucus, and enzymes.

Salivary glands

Three pairs of glands in the mouth that secrete saliva into the mouth. Saliva is a clear fluid that helps clean the teeth and gums, moistens food for swallowing, and adds an enzyme (chemical accelerator) to chewed food that converts complex starches into sugars. There are three major pairs of salivary glands: the submandibular glands lie toward the back of the mouth close to the sides of the jaw; the sublingual glands are located at the base of the tongue; and the parotid glands are in the back of the mouth. The parotid glands are the largest of the three pairs. From the salivary glands, which contain tiny saliva-secreting sacs, a network of ducts carry the saliva into the mouth.

Salmonella

A strain of bacteria that can be present in food or water without affecting the appearance, smell, or taste. *Salmonella* is the most frequently reported cause of food-borne illness in the United States and has been known to exist for more than 100 years. Infections with *Salmonella* may involve only the intestinal tract, or they may spread to the bloodstream and to other areas of the body. The bacteria are usually transmitted by the oral-fecal route, and the source of infection is usually the ingestion of food or water contaminated by fecal matter.

The symptoms of *Salmonella* infection can occur within 8 to 72 hours of ingesting contaminated food or water. These symptoms, which may persist from 4 to 7 days, include severe headaches, chills, abdominal cramps, diarrhea, nausea, vomiting, mild fever, and muscle aches. *Salmonella* infection is diagnosed by testing a stool specimen for the presence of the bacteria.

When severe, the infection may spread to the bloodstream and cause serious conditions, including MENINGITIS and even death. Such cases require hospitalization, prompt antibiotic treatment, isolation, and supportive medical care. Young children, older people, and people with impaired immune systems are most at risk for severe infections. Antibiotics should be avoided in mild cases because they may delay the elimination of the bacteria from the intestines.

Salpingectomy

Surgery in which one or both fallopian tubes (the tubes that transport an egg from an ovary toward the uterus) are removed. Salpingectomy is usually performed to treat an ECTOPIC PREGNANCY (one that develops outside the uterus) or a chronic pelvic inflammation that has damaged a fallopian tube. This treatment is usually used only when a fallopian tube is irreversibly destroyed by disease. See PELVIC INFLAMMATORY DISEASE.

Salpingitis

A condition occurring when infectious agents invade the uterus and spread to the fallopian tubes, ovaries, and surrounding tissues. Acute salpingitis, a type of pelvic inflammatory disease, causes lower abdominal pain and tenderness and often a high fever. Chronic salpingitis causes recurring discomfort in the lower abdomen, sometimes with a low-grade fever and a backache. Menstrual periods may be heavy in both acute and chronic infections.

Salpingitis is most commonly caused by sexually transmitted infections. Salpingitis can also occur after an intrauterine device (see IUD) is inserted, or after a MISCARRIAGE, abortion, D AND C, ENDOMETRIAL BIOPSY, HYSTERECTOMY, or other procedure that requires inserting instruments into the uterine cavity. It is most common among young, sexually active women. Treatment usually includes antibiotics for the infection and aspirin or acetaminophen for pain.

Salpingo-oophorectomy

Surgical removal of the ovaries and fallopian tubes. This procedure is used to treat cancer of the ovary and some cases of pelvic inflammatory disease. The fallopian tube is usually removed with its adjacent ovary, because the tube is typically damaged by the same condition that affects the ovary. The surgery involves an incision into the abdomen.

In menstruating women, the removal of both ovaries dramatically reduces hormone levels and induces menopause immediately.

Salt

Any compound formed by a base and an acid; sodium chloride (common salt). Common salt, or table salt, is only one of many salts. See SODIUM.

Sarcoidosis

A chronic, multisystem, autoimmune disorder that can affect many body systems, but most commonly involves the lungs or lymph nodes. Sarcoidosis is characterized by the appearance in affected tissues of small, round lumps of dead tissue. These lumps, called granulomas, usually heal and disappear on their own, even without medical treatment. When the granulomas do not resolve, the affected tissues remain inflamed, and scarring develops. The disease is caused by an immune system disorder that occurs for no known reason.

Sarcoidosis varies in severity among individuals and may affect any part of the person's body. Some people have few or no symptoms. Other people experience many intermittent symptoms, or even severe progressive disease. Fatigue and general malaise are the most common initial symptoms. Pulmonary symptoms are also common and include cough and shortness of breath. A skin rash may suddenly appear on the face, arms, or shins. Inflammation of the eyes occurs in about 15 percent of cases. The disorder can cause an irregular heart rate, and lead to the implanting of a pacemaker.

Sarcoidosis can be difficult to diagnose and is sometimes misdiagnosed as TUBERCULOSIS (TB). A preliminary diagnosis is generally based on a medical history, a physical examination, and a chest X ray, which reveals abnormalities in about 90 percent of cases.

An affected person should avoid cigarette smoke and exposure to dust and chemical irritants that might cause further damage to the lungs. People with active symptoms usually benefit from taking CORTICOSTEROIDS.

Sarcoma

A type of cancerous tumor arising in a number of tissues, including bones, cartilage, connective tissues, muscles, the inner layer of the skin, fibrous tissues, fat, blood vessels, nerves, the linings of the chest and abdominal cavities, and the coverings of the lungs, abdominal organs, and heart. Although sarcomas can arise almost anywhere in the body, they most commonly occur in the fat or muscle of an arm or leg. The most common symptom is soreness or swelling that progressively worsens.

Treatment may include surgery, RADIATION THERAPY, and CHEMOTHERAPY. Some sarcomas may be very aggressive, with a strong tendency to spread elsewhere in the body, particularly to the lungs. Because of this tendency to metastasize (spread), surgery to remove the primary cancer completely is performed whenever possible. In some cases, successful surgical removal of a sarcoma can restore normal functioning. About half of all people with sarcomas achieve long-term survival.

SARS

See SEVERE ACUTE RESPIRATORY SYNDROME (SARS).

Saturated fats

Fats that come from meats, poultry, dairy products, and solid vegetable fats that are mostly hard at room temperature. The exceptions are coconut and palm kernel oils, which remain liquid at room temperature. Saturated fats (along with trans-fatty acids) are the fats most responsible for high cholesterol levels and an increased risk of heart disease. See FATS AND OILS.

Scabies

A parasitic infestation that causes intense itching and a rash. In scabies, small mites burrow into the skin to lay eggs. Scabies is usually spread through close contact with an infested person.

The first symptom of scabies is intense itching, especially at night. The early rash may be composed of small red bumps, like pimples. Eventually, the burrows made by the mites appear as thin red marks on the skin. In severe cases, the skin becomes crusty, scaly, and thickened. Scabies is most common between the fingers; in the armpits; on the waist, elbows, wrists, ankles, and feet; and in the areas around the breasts, buttocks, and genitals.

Scabies is usually diagnosed through a physical examination, taking special care to inspect skin crevices. Diagnosis can be confirmed by removing a mite from its burrow and identifying it under a microscope. Scabies is treated with prescription creams (scabicides) containing ingredients such as permethrin or lindane. Itching is controlled with lotions and antihistamines. Family members and others in close contact with the affected person must also be treated.

Scalds

Burns caused by hot liquids or hot vapors. Scalds are burns that result from contact with moist heat. Scalds are usually not as deep as those created by contact with flames, but they can produce deep burns. If the clothing of a person is saturated with scalding, hot liquid, the clothes should be removed quickly but carefully. In the case of small scalds, cold water will stop further tissue damage and lessen pain, but ice should never be placed directly on the wound. If the person is scalded over a large area of his or her body, the person may be in a state of shock, and emergency medical care must be sought at once.

Scalp

The tough skin that covers the skull above the face and ears that is usually covered with hair. The scalp has five layers of tissue with an extensive blood supply. Scalp hair, which helps prevent heat from leaving the body, grows faster than any other hair on the body—an average of about ½ inch every month. Underlying muscles loosely attach the scalp to the skull.

Scalpel

A very precise surgical knife used to cut tissue in operations. A plasma scalpel is a device that uses a high-temperature gas jet for cutting rather than a blade.

Scarlet fever

An infection caused by group A *Streptococcus* bacteria (see GROUP A STREPTOCOCCUS INFECTION) that occurs in a small number of people following an initial streptococcal infection of the throat (strep throat) or skin. Scarlet fever was once considered serious, and it commonly occurred in children between the ages of 2 and 10 years. For unknown reasons, scarlet fever is less common at the current time, despite a constant level in the number of streptococcal infections. The bacteria that cause scarlet fever are spread by direct contact with infected persons or by airborne droplets in the coughs, sneezes, and exhalations of an infected person.

Scarlet fever causes a characteristic bright red rash that begins under the arms and on the neck, chest, armpit, inner thighs, and groin area as small red spots that gradually become elevated and spread over the body. Within a few days, the redness fades and a finely textured rash, sometimes referred to as a sandpaper rash, develops. In addition to the rash, symptoms of scarlet fever may include sore throat, fever, vomiting, a red and swollen tongue, chills, headache, and general malaise.

The illness is diagnosed by a physical examination combined with a throat culture that tests positive for group A *Streptococcus*. The infection is treated with antibiotics, usually penicillin, and acetaminophen for fever and discomfort. Given proper treatment, scarlet fever is usually easily cured within a week or less.

Schistosomiasis

A parasitic disease (also known as bilharziasis) that is a major health problem in many tropical countries. Schistosomiasis is caused by a flat-bodied worm, or fluke, called a schistosome, which is carried by snails and migrates through fresh water to penetrate a person's skin. The infestation producing schistosomiasis can cause bleeding and the formation of scar tissue inside the bladder, intestines, or other organs, including the liver and lungs.

The disease may occur 4 to 6 weeks after an initial infection, and symptoms can include fever, cough, abdominal pain, diarrhea, and allergic reactions. If the infection is untreated, complications may include colon polyps with bloody diarrhea, liver problems, inflammation of structures of the urinary system including the kidneys, and lesions in the central nervous system. Schistosomiasis is diagnosed by microscopic identification of parasite eggs in the stool or urine. The disease is treated with worm-combating medications.

Schizophrenia

A severe mental illness characterized by persistent, bizarre disturbances in thought, communication, perceptions, emotions, and behavior. Schizophrenia is considered a psychosis because people with the disease become detached from reality.

Because schizophrenia is a severe illness that often leaves the individual incapable of functioning, hospitalization may be required to prevent harm to the person during disease episodes. Medications known as antipsychotics or neuroleptics are used to control symptoms. Stopping medication usually results in a return of symptoms. Behavior therapy or psychotherapy can be helpful.

Sciatica

Pain that radiates along the sciatic nerve that extends from the lower back down into the buttocks and down along the back of the leg past the knee. Sciatica is usually caused by pressure on the nerve from a herniated or ruptured disk. Pain ranges from merely irritating to severe and debilitating. It usually affects only one side. Treatment includes physical therapy and medication, such as NONSTEROIDAL ANTI-INFLAMMATORY DRUGS (NSAIDs), oral CORTICOSTEROIDS, or epidural corticosteroid injections. In some cases, surgery is necessary.

Scleritis

Inflammation of the white (sclera) of the eye. Symptoms can include severe eye pain, red discoloration, blurred vision, sensitivity to light, excessive tearing, or rarely, a protrusion of the eyeball. Fifty percent of patients with scleritis have an associated systemic disease—frequently an autoimmune disease such as RHEUMATOID ARTHRITIS, lupus, or INFLAMMATORY BOWEL DISEASE. Less commonly, scleritis is the result of infection, such as from TUBERCULOSIS or LYME DISEASE. Scleritis is a serious condition that can lead to perforation of the eyeball. Treatment usually consists of oral corticosteroid or NONSTEROIDAL ANTI-INFLAMMATORY DRUGS (NSAIDs) and medical management of any underlying disease.

Scleroderma

A chronic autoimmune disease of the connective tissue. Scleroderma is a relatively rare disease that involves symptoms that are most apparent when they affect the skin. If the skin is unaffected, the person may have internal organ abnormalities affecting the heart, lungs, gastrointestinal tract, and kidneys.

There are two classifications of scleroderma. The localized form, which occurs more frequently in children, generally affects only a few areas of skin or muscle tissue. This rarely develops into the systemic form of the disease. Progressive systemic sclerosis can involve many body tissues and organs. The skin, esophagus, gastrointestinal tract, blood vessels, muscles, joints, lungs, kidneys, heart, and other internal organs may be affected.

One or more of the following symptoms may be experienced with scleroderma: swelling of the hands and feet; extreme sensitivity to cold in the extremities; stiff, aching joints and possible structural abnormalities of the joints; thickening and hardening of the skin; dry mucous membranes; and problems involving the digestive system, gastrointestinal tract, the mouth, the face, or the teeth.

It may be difficult to confirm a diagnosis as many symptoms of scleroderma are the same or similar to those associated with other connective tissue diseases, including rheumatoid arthritis, lupus, and polymyositis. A program of treatment for scleroderma is entirely dependent on the symptoms and their severity. CORTICOSTEROIDS, immunosuppressive drugs, and medications to treat high blood pressure may be prescribed.

Sclerosis

The hardening of a body part, often as a result of inflammation. Sclerosis is often used to describe changes in the circulatory system (such as those that occur in ATHEROSCLEROSIS).

Scoliosis

An abnormal curvature of the spine found in infants, young children, adolescents, and some adults. The spinal curve in scoliosis may have an "S" or a "C" shape. What causes scoliosis in most young people is unknown. Genetic, hormonal, and metabolic factors may have a role. Most cases of scoliosis are mild and painless. In severe cases, the spine rotates in addition to curving so that the ribs on one side of the body become prominent.

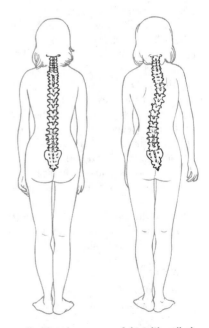

Healthy spine   **Spine with scoliosis**

Spinal curvature

Scoliosis may involve twisting of the vertebrae in the area of the curve. There may also be two areas of curvature (an "S" shape) or a single curve (a "C" shape).

There may be constant back pain and breathing problems.

If signs of scoliosis are noted, the child should see the doctor. Diagnosis is based on a physical examination and sometimes X rays to pinpoint the size of the curve. At a certain level of curvature, bracing of the back may be recommended to prevent a worsening of the condition.

When the curve is most severe, surgical treatment may become necessary. The most common surgical procedure connects the vertebrae in the curve with solid bone and holds them there with metal devices.

Scorpion stings

Painful wounds made by a scorpion, a type of arachnid with a venomous stinger in its tail. Most scorpion bites cause local reactions similar to a bee sting and are not life-threatening. However, the sting of the bark scorpion *(Centruroides sculpturatus)* of the southwestern United States can be fatal, especially to children. Several hours after the sting, symptoms include seizures, labored breathing, muscle spasms, nausea, tingling, and numbness. Treatments include applying cold packs to the sting area and taking mild painkillers. People with more severe symptoms may require emergency treatment.

Scotoma

An area of lost or diminished vision within a person's visual field.

Scratch test

An approach to allergy testing performed to identify the allergen that produces symptoms in an affected person. Scratch tests are also called skin prick testing and involve introducing a drop of allergen extract into the skin using a small sharp instrument that causes a small break in the skin.

Screening

The testing of apparently healthy people to detect a specific disease or disorder at an early, treatable stage. Screening is the cornerstone of preventive medicine and includes testing for problems such as high blood pressure, high cholesterol, and certain types of cancer. Doctors recommend periodic blood pressure measurements, cholesterol tests, dental checkups, eye examinations, and skin examinations. In addition, women are advised to have Papanicolaou smears (see PAP SMEAR), clinical breast examinations, and mammograms (see MAMMOGRAM). Prostate and testicular examinations are recommended for men. Other screening tests a doctor may order include blood tests, bone density measurements, URINALYSIS, electrocardiograms (see ELECTROCARDIOGRAM), COLONOSCOPY, and tests for SEXUALLY TRANSMITTED DISEASES.

Screening tests for newborns

Tests for specific disorders in newborn infants, in which symptoms may not develop before irreversible damage has been done and for which early treatments is effective. These tests are performed on all babies born in most states within the United States. The baby's heel is pricked to obtain blood for laboratory analysis.

Babies in all 50 states are routinely screened for PKU (phenylketonuria), a digestive disorder that can cause brain damage and mental retardation, and HYPOTHYROIDISM, a hormone deficiency that can retard growth and mental development. Most states also screen for galactosemia, a metabolic disorder that can cause death or blindness and mental retardation. Screening can also be done for SICKLE CELL ANEMIA, an inherited blood disease that can cause severe pain and even death; CYSTIC FIBROSIS, a chronic respiratory disease; congenital adrenal hyperplasia, a disease in which certain hormones are deficient; and biotinidase deficiency, an enzyme deficiency that can cause death.

Scrotum

The pouch of delicate skin and connective tissue that hangs below the penis and contains the testicles. The scrotum has oil-secreting glands and fine pubic hairs on its surface. See REPRODUCTIVE SYSTEM, MALE.

Scurvy

A condition caused by a prolonged lack of VITAMIN C (ascorbic acid) in the diet. Foods rich in vitamin C include citrus fruits, such as oranges and lemons, sweet peppers, and leafy green vegetables. The symptoms of scurvy include fatigue, muscle weakness, joint and muscle aches, and a rash on the legs. Gums swell and bleed easily, and teeth eventually loosen.

Today scurvy is rare in the United States and other countries where fresh produce is readily available. Treatment of this disease is with supplements of vitamin C.

Seasickness

See MOTION SICKNESS.

Seasonal affective disorder

A form of recurring DEPRESSION that begins in the fall or winter and re-solves in the spring or summer. Seasonal affective disorder is commonly abbreviated SAD. In addition to the fall or winter onset of low mood, symptoms include lack of energy, loss of interest in work and other important activities, declining sexual interest, craving for carbohydrate foods (such as pasta, rice, potatoes, and pastry), increased appetite and weight gain, lengthened sleep time, and movement that is slow, sluggish, and lethargic. Light therapy is an effective treatment. Antidepressant medication can also be effective.

Seat belts

Safety belts worn in vehicles to protect drivers and passengers in case of accidents. Seat belts are designed to hold the driver and passengers in place during an accident, preventing them from being hurled forward and injured by the force of the crash. When properly used, seat belts include both lap and shoulder belts.

Sebaceous cyst

See EPIDERMAL CYST.

Sebaceous glands

Oil-producing glands in the skin. The sebaceous glands secrete sebum, the fatty acid that lubricates the skin. In teenagers, hormonal changes stimulate the sebaceous glands to produce excess sebum, which can lead to clogged pores and acne. As a person grows older, the sebaceous glands become less active, and the skin becomes drier.

Seborrheic dermatitis

A chronic, benign (not cancerous) skin condition characterized by red, greasy skin covered with yellowish or white flaky scales. Inflammation occurs in areas having the greatest number of sebaceous (oil-producing) glands in the skin. Seborrheic dermatitis may begin in infancy as cradle cap, return in adolescence when the sebaceous glands become more active, and persist throughout life. Seborrheic dermatitis commonly affects the scalp (as dandruff), the area between the eyebrows, the sides of the nose, the area behind or just inside the ears, the chest, and the groin.

Treatment is with over-the-counter dandruff shampoos containing ingredients such as coal tar, salicylic acid, selenium sulfide, sulfur, and zinc pyrithione. A doctor may prescribe a stronger shampoo that contains ketoconazole or recommend topical corticosteroids.

Seborrheic keratosis

A brown, black, or flesh-colored benign (not cancerous) skin lesion that has a waxy, wartlike appearance. Seborrheic keratoses are a common feature of aging and are most common on the chest or back. Although they are not a serious health problem, if growths become large or irritated, bleed easily, or are unsightly, they can be removed surgically.

Secondhand smoke

See PASSIVE SMOKING.

Secretion

The body's release of chemical substances, such as estrogen or adrenaline, into the bloodstream.

Sedation, conscious

See CONSCIOUS SEDATION.

Sedatives

Drugs used to cause drowsiness or sleep; antianxiety drugs. Sedatives are intended to cause various degrees of relaxation. Sedatives can reduce anxiety in doses that do not promote sleep. Sedatives include several classes of drugs and are used to treat INSOMNIA, anxiety, and EPILEPSY.

Examples of classes of sedatives include benzodiazepines, used to reduce anxiety; barbiturates, used to treat epilepsy; and hypnotic drugs, used to induce sleep.

Seizure

A sudden episode of uncontrolled electrical activity in the brain. Seizures may cause a series of involuntary muscle contractions, behavioral changes, sensory abnormalities, or a temporary lapse in consciousness. Seizures are often but not always a sign of EPILEPSY, a neurological disorder characterized by repeated seizures, caused by abnormal electrical activity in the brain. About half of all seizures have no known cause. In other cases, seizures are linked to infection and fever (see SEIZURE, FEBRILE), trauma, substance abuse, or other medical problems.

Types of seizures

There are more than 30 different types of seizures. Seizures are divided into two main categories: partial seizures and generalized seizures.

PARTIAL SEIZURES Partial seizures start in just one part of the brain. Frequently these seizures are identified by the part of the brain with which they are associated (for example, partial frontal lobe seizures). In a simple partial seizure, a person remains conscious but experiences symptoms related to the part of the brain in which the abnormal impulses develop. In temporal lobe epilepsy, these may include unexplainable sensations of joy or anger or unusual thoughts or feelings. Sometimes what starts in a localized area of the brain expands and a complex partial seizure results, in which a person experiences a change in or loss of consciousness. People who have this type of seizure may engage in unusual repetitive behavior (such as blinks or twitches) called automatisms.

Partial seizures (especially complex partial seizures) are often preceded by auras. An aura is an unusual sensation that is a warning sign of an impending seizure. An aura may consist of a strange feeling, abnormal perceptions, or visual disturbances such as seeing stars or flashes. When there is no loss of consciousness, an aura is actually a simple partial seizure in which a person maintains consciousness.

GENERALIZED SEIZURES Unlike partial seizures, generalized seizures are caused by abnormal neuronal activity in multiple parts of the brain. These seizures may cause convulsions, massive muscle spasms, falls, and loss of consciousness. There are many different kinds of generalized seizures. In absence seizures (formerly called petit mal), a person seems to be staring into space and may have jerking or twitching muscles. Tonic seizures cause stiffening of the muscles, and clonic seizures cause repeated jerking movements. A person having an atonic seizure loses muscle tone and may fall down.

Tonic-clonic seizures (formerly called grand mal seizures) cause stiffening, jerking, and a loss of consciousness.

Treatment

Correct treatment depends on the accurate diagnosis of the underlying cause of seizures. Mild seizures, such as absence seizures, require no immediate first aid treatment. However, it is important to see the doctor for medical evaluation. First aid for tonic-clonic seizures involves laying an affected person on his or her side, loosening their clothing, removing any sharp and hard objects, and not restraining the person or putting anything in his or her mouth. Anyone who has this type of seizure must be evaluated by a physician as soon as possible. If the seizure lasts for longer than 5 minutes or if there are repeated seizures, emergency medical attention is required.

Antiepileptic drugs are the first line of treatment for epileptic seizures. When seizures cannot be adequately controlled with medication, doctors consider surgical alternatives.

Seizure, febrile

A seizure experienced by a child with a high fever. A febrile seizure generally follows a rapid rise in body temperature. The affected child experiences a tonic-clonic (or grand mal) seizure, characterized by jerking of the arms and legs, stiffening of the body, and a loss of consciousness that lasts from 30 seconds to 5 minutes.

Other possible symptoms of a febrile seizure include incontinence, clenched teeth or biting of the cheek or tongue, difficulty or absence of breathing, and bluish skin color. Following the seizure, the child usually goes to sleep.

Although their symptoms appear alarming to parents, most febrile seizures have no lasting effect on a child and are rarely associated with EPILEPSY. Febrile seizures do not lead to brain damage.

When first-time febrile seizures occur, the child should be evaluated by a doctor as soon as possible. The physician will conduct tests to make sure that a first-time seizure does not have a more serious underlying cause, such as MENINGITIS or ENCEPHALITIS.

In the past, children who experienced febrile seizures were treated with anticonvulsant drugs to prevent epilepsy. But doctors have discovered that in most instances the long-term risks of anticonvulsants, such as possible damage to the developing brain, outweigh any benefits. Consequently, treatment consists primarily of aggressive early treatment of fever.

Selective serotonin reuptake inhibitor drugs

Selective serotonin reuptake inhibitor (SSRI) drugs are antidepressants such as fluoxetine that work by blocking the reuptake of a chemical transmitter called serotonin into nerve cell endings. This activity keeps the concentration of serotonin in the brain higher, which reduces symptoms of DEPRESSION and other psychological disorders.

In addition to the treatment of depression, SSRIs are also used to treat OBSESSIVE-COMPULSIVE DISORDER, generalized anxiety disorder (see ANXIETY DISORDERS), PANIC DISORDER, social anxiety disorder, and bulimia nervosa, an eating disorder.

Selenium

A trace mineral found in soil and food. Selenium is an essential mineral believed to be closely associated with VITAMIN E. Selenium is also one of the antioxidants that protect cells from certain chemical reactions associated with aging, heart disease, and cancer.

Self-mutilation

A mental illness in which a person feels, for emotional reasons, compelled to cut, burn, or do other forms of painful harm to his or her body. Self-mutilation is not a suicide attempt, but people who mutilate themselves are at greater risk for suicide. The disorder also carries the risk of infection from using dirty instruments. Self-mutilation is often accompanied by mood disorders such as DEPRESSION and anxiety and requires evaluation by a psychiatrist or other mental health professional. Medication and psychotherapy may be useful for controlling mood.

Semen

The thick fluid that is internally secreted and discharged from the penis upon ejaculation. Semen contains millions of sperm, which can travel from the vagina and within the uterus into a fallopian tube and fertilize an egg. When semen is released by the penis into the vagina during sexual intercourse, pregnancy may result.

Semen, blood in the

See HEMATOSPERMIA.

Seminoma

The most common form of testicular cancer. See TESTICLE, CANCER OF THE.

Senses

Taste, smell, touch, hearing, and vision. Senses provide people with information about the world around them. The senses receive sensory material from the environment, such as light, sound, odors, and vibrations.

Sensitization

A person's first exposure to an allergen or other foreign substance, such as an infectious agent. Sensitization leads to an immune response that can produce the symptoms of allergies, a process also called allergic sensitization. When the sensitized person is exposed to the same allergen subsequently, he or she will have a more immediate and stronger allergic reaction to it.

Sensitization may also refer to the body process that is mimicked by immunization, which involves exposing a person to an antigen that provokes an immune response. The goal is to increase immunity and set the stage for a more vigorous secondary immune response when a person is later exposed to the same antigen. The mechanism used for immunization is what protects the person after he or she is exposed to an infectious agent.

Sepsis

A system-wide response to bacterial infection of a wound or tissues, which may lead to the rapid multiplication of bacteria and an accumulation of bacterial toxins in the bloodstream. See also SEPTIC SHOCK.

Septal defect, atrial

A hole in the septum (wall) between the atria (two upper chambers of the heart). Because of the defect, blood is shunted from the left atrium to the right when the heart fills with blood. This increases blood flow to the lungs, forcing the right ventricle (a lower chamber) of the heart and the lungs to work harder. Over time this can lead to abnormal enlargement of the right ventricle and pulmonary hypertension (high blood pressure in the lungs). Fluids in the lungs and cardiac arrhythmia (abnormal heartbeat) may also follow. People with atrial septal defects are also at increased risk for blood clots traveling to the brain, resulting in STROKE.

As a rule, it is best to surgically repair an atrial septal defect sooner rather than later, before permanent damage occurs. The patient without other heart problems can anticipate a normal life expectancy.

Septal defect, ventricular

A hole in the septum (wall) between the ventricles (two lower chambers)

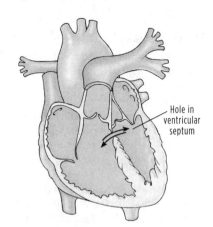

Hole in ventricular septum

Ventricular septal defect
A hole in the septum between the two ventricles allows deoxygenated blood to mix with oxygenated blood.

of the heart. Because of the defect, blood that does not normally flow between the ventricles can flow from the left ventricle to the right as the ventricle contracts, increasing blood flow in the right side of the heart. If the hole is large enough to substantially increase blood flow, the right ventricle and the lungs must work harder to compensate. Over time this can lead to abnormal enlargement of the right ventricle and pulmonary hypertension (high blood pressure in the lungs). Fluid accumulation in the lungs and cardiac arrhythmia (abnormal heartbeat) may also follow. The defect also increases the risk of a blood clot's traveling to the brain, resulting in a stroke.

Many small ventricular septal defects close on their own and cause no symptoms except for a murmur (the sound of abnormal blood flow). If the defect is large or fails to close, it can be repaired surgically if the operation is done before any permanent damage occurs.

Septic shock

An inflammatory response that is caused by toxins produced by bacteria—commonly staphylococci, meningococci, or *E. coli* organisms—which damage tissues and trigger a dramatic drop in blood pressure. Septic shock is a life-threatening condition that requires emergency medical treatment.

Septic shock develops from the condition called bacteremia, in which bacteria enter the bloodstream. The first symptom is usually a decrease in mental alertness. Blood pressure drops, and the skin and extremities become warm to the touch, which is the opposite of the anticipated effect of lowered blood pressure. The heart beats at an abnormally rapid rate, and breathing rate increases dramatically. Fever or even low body temperature often develops.

As septic shock progresses, the extremities become cool and pale. Organ failure can occur involving the kidney, lungs, and liver. Blood clots may form in the blood vessels, and heart failure may occur.

Septic shock must be diagnosed and treated early to prevent death. Once organ failure starts, the condition often becomes irreversible even with treatment.

Septicemia

A systemic illness caused by the spread of bacteria or their toxins into the bloodstream; also known as blood poisoning. The bacteria move quickly through the blood to other organs, causing spiking fevers and chills, fast heartbeat, rapid breathing, a seriously ill appearance, and a feeling of impending doom.

If the septicemia is untreated, the result is SEPTIC SHOCK, which causes low blood pressure and body temperature and mental confusion. Death occurs in more than half of the people who develop septic shock, even with antibiotic therapy.

Septum

A wall or partition that divides one section of a body part or cavity from another. An example is the septum in the nose, a piece of cartilage that divides the nasal passages.

Septum, deviated

A deformity of the septum, the structure that separates the nostrils and is composed of bone and cartilage covered by a layer of mucous membrane. A deviated septum is the condition in which a portion of this bone is crooked or curves to one side.

Rarely, a deviation in the septum may obstruct air flow and make breathing through the affected nostril difficult. The reduced flow of air can encourage growth of bacteria and trap pollen.

A deviated septum is diagnosed by a physical examination of the nose. If the deviation causes health problems or recurrent disease, surgery may be recommended.

Septum, perforated

An opening or hole in the surface of the septum, the wall inside the nose that separates the two nostrils. The condition can cause bleeding, crusting, and whistling in the nose. If the perforation is severe and causes health problems, the hole may be surgically repaired. A perforated septum is one of the potential consequences of cocaine abuse.

Serotonin

A chemical that functions primarily to transmit signals between the nerve cells of the human brain. Abnormally low levels of serotonin are associated with DEPRESSION, OBSESSIVE-COMPULSIVE DISORDER, and eating disorders. Serotonin is also known as 5-hydroxy-tryptamine (5-HT).

Serum

The clear fluid portion of blood. Serum does not contain blood cells. It is essentially similar in composition to blood plasma, but lacks fibrinogen and other substances used in the coagulation (clotting) process. Serum contains many proteins, including

antibodies formed as part of the immune response to protect against infection.

Severe Acute Respiratory Syndrome (SARS)

A serious form of pneumonia thought to be caused by a virus that does not respond to standard antibiotic treatment. Symptoms of severe acute respiratory syndrome (SARS) include high fever, shortness of breath, a dry cough, and difficulty breathing. The illness can be fatal.

Sex

Another term for male or female gender; also a commonly used synonym for sexual intercourse and many other forms of sexual activity. See also SEX EDUCATION; SEXUAL INTERCOURSE.

Sex change

The surgical and medical process used to change a person's sex from male to female or female to male. Sex change is performed as treatment for gender-identity disorder, in which an individual acts and presents himself or herself as a member of the opposite sex and feels profoundly uncomfortable with his or her physical sex.

Sex chromosomes

Chromosomes associated with the determination of sex and gender.

In mammals, the sex chromosomes consist of the female X chromosome and the male Y chromosome. Females have two X chromosomes; males have an X and a Y.

Sex education

Also called sexuality education. Courses given to children and adolescents by a school or community group to provide an opportunity for young people to learn about sexuality and how it can affect their lives. A comprehensive sex education curriculum typically incorporates topics related to human sexuality including growth and development, human reproduction, anatomy, physiology, masturbation, sexual response, sexual orientation, contraception, and abstinence.

Sex hormones

The hormones that influence sexual differentiation and development and enable the reproductive cycles to function properly. Sex hormones are secreted by the ovaries in females and the testicles in males at an early stage of fetal development. They trigger the hypothalamus to secrete the hormones appropriate to the sex of the fetus.

The major female sex hormones, estrogen and progesterone, are produced mainly by the ovaries. The male sex hormones, known as the androgen hormones, include testosterone, which is produced by the testicles. Follicle-stimulating hormone (FSH) and luteinizing hormone (LH) are sex hormones produced by the pituitary gland in both men and women.

Sex therapy

A directive approach to treating sexual problems that focuses on the problems themselves rather than only on their roots in the individual's personality. Problems treated in sex therapy may include erectile dysfunction (impotence), premature ejaculation, and lack of orgasm. Sex therapy is most often conducted with both partners.

Sexual abuse

See ABUSE, SEXUAL.

Sexual addiction

A condition characterized by a preoccupying desire to repeatedly engage in sex that is driven by a deep-seated, compulsive need, with only brief tension release after orgasm.

Sexual assault

See ASSAULT, SEXUAL.

Sexual desire, inhibited

An absence of normal sexual fantasies and desire for sexual activity that causes significant distress or difficulty in relationships. The lack of desire may be lifelong (primary), or it may appear after a period of normal sexual activity (secondary). The inhibition may apply to all forms of sexual expression with all partners, or it may hold true for only one particular activity or for one partner.

Inhibited sexual desire is the most common sexual dysfunction. The cause can be physical or psychological. Inhibited sexual desire is often a natural result in persons who were abused sexually or raped as children. Treatment consists of sex therapy to resolve relationship difficulties. Medication and psychotherapy can also be helpful for individuals with DEPRESSION or for resolving the emotional effects of abuse or rape.

Sexual dysfunction

Any impairment in sexual response that causes emotional distress and prevents an individual or couple from experiencing satisfaction as a result of sexual activity.

Sexual dysfunctions are classified into four groups. In sexual desire disorders (see SEXUAL DESIRE, INHIBITED), there is an abnormal absence of sexual fantasies and desire for sexual activity.

Disorders of sexual arousal are commonly referred to as frigidity in women and impotence in men (see ERECTILE DYSFUNCTION).

Sexual pain disorders consist of pain during intercourse (dyspareunia; see INTERCOURSE, PAINFUL) and an involuntary spasm of the vagina that prevents entry (see VAGINISMUS). Orgasm disorders refer to the inability to reach climax following sufficient foreplay or stimulation (see ORGASM, LACK OF). The causes of sexual dysfunction can be physical, psychological, or a combination of both. Treatment of sexual dysfunction depends on the cause. It can include changing medications, and counseling that focuses on sexuality (see SEX THERAPY).

Sexual intercourse

The penetration of a woman's vagina by a man's penis. The penis must be erect or semierect to enter the vagina. Once inside, the penis ejaculates or releases a thick fluid called semen.

Sexually transmitted diseases

A large group of disease syndromes that are transmitted by sexual contact and sexual activities; also known as STDs.

Any person who is sexually active is susceptible to STDs, and it is estimated that 1 in 5 people in the United States is a carrier. These diseases are transmitted by contact with infected body secretions, including semen, blood, and vaginal fluids. Several pathogens can infect these secretions and be sexually transmitted to cause

STDs. These include bacteria, including those that cause GONORRHEA, SYPHILIS, and chlamydia viruses, which are responsible for many STDs including herpes simplex, human papillomavirus, strains of hepatitis, molluscum contagiosum, cytomegalovirus, and HIV and AIDS; protozoa, such as those causing trichomoniasis; fungi; and ectoparasite infestations, including crab lice.

An infected person may not have symptoms of an STD. Most people who are infected with HIV have no symptoms, making the infection difficult to diagnose. If there are STD symptoms, they may include sores, pain, and itching in the genital area for both men and women. In addition, men may experience a discharge from the penis, painful urination, and swelling and pain in the testicles. Women may notice a vaginal discharge or change in usual vaginal secretions. If an STD has progressed to pelvic inflammatory disease, there may be lower abdominal pain and painful sexual intercourse.

Treatment of STDs depends on the infective pathogen involved. Bacterial STDs, including gonorrhea, chlamydia, syphilis, and chancroid, are treated with antibiotic therapy and can be cured with treatment.

Outpatient surgery may be recommended to treat genital warts and sometimes provides an effective cure. There are new medical approaches to control the progress of HIV and AIDS, and there is increased success with treating associated illnesses, but there is no cure for hepatitis.

Seeking immediate medical treatment when an STD is suspected can prevent severe infection and longterm consequences. Abstaining from sexual activity until a doctor has determined that the infection is no longer contagious helps prevent reinfection and halts the spread of STDs.

Shaken baby syndrome

A severe and potentially fatal form of child abuse in which the abuser violently shakes a baby. The signs of shaken baby syndrome range from subtle to severe. A shaken infant may exhibit symptoms such as poor feeding, vomiting, lethargy, or irritability. In some children, there may be telltale marks on the upper arms or whatever part of the body was grasped when the baby was shaken. Severe shaking can lead immediately to respiratory difficulty, a seizure, or loss of consciousness.

Shaken baby syndrome can be difficult to diagnose. Often there are no visible external injuries.

In addition to the care of a pediatrician or family physician, a shaken baby may require treatment by a neurologist, neurosurgeon, or ophthalmologist. In addition to treatment of the original injury, follow-up care is necessary. The long-term consequences of shaken baby syndrome include mental retardation, severe motor dysfunction, seizure, and blindness. Shaken baby syndrome is a form of abuse, and reporting the case to the local child protective agency is mandatory (see ABUSE, CHILD).

Shigellosis

An infectious disease caused by a genus of bacteria called *Shigella* that causes diarrhea in humans. Shigellosis, also known as dysentery, is transmitted by contact with an infected person's diarrheal stools and occurs most commonly when basic personal hygiene, including hand washing, is not practiced.

Shigellosis can also be acquired by ingesting food or water that has become contaminated.

Infected people develop diarrhea, fever, and stomach cramps within 1 or 2 days of exposure. The diarrhea may be bloody and become so severe that hospitalization becomes necessary. Children younger than 2 years may have high fever and seizures.

Correct antibiotic therapy kills the *Shigella* bacteria and shortens the length of the illness. In rare cases, REITER SYNDROME is a complication of shigellosis.

Shin splints

An injury common to runners that involves one of the muscles in the lower leg pulling on the shinbone (tibia), which sometimes results in tiny tears in the muscle. Usually the anterior tibial muscle located on the front of the shin is affected. Shin splints cause pain along the front or inner side of the shin, depending on the muscle involved. Stretching can make the pain worse.

The pain of shin splints may be felt at the start of a run or jog and decrease gradually as the workout continues, or it may be felt throughout the activity. When the pain is intense and localized on the shin bone, medical attention should be sought to rule out the possibility of a stress fracture or other bone or muscle lesions.

Stopping the exercise that caused the pain is generally recommended the first 2 to 3 days after symptoms appear, depending on the individual. The pain may be treated by applying ice before and after training.

NONSTEROIDAL ANTI-INFLAMMATORY DRUGS (NSAIDs), such as aspirin and ibuprofen, may help. Taping or splinting the affected area is sometimes beneficial. Physical therapy may be prescribed.

Shingles

A painful rash that is a second outbreak of the varicella-zoster virus, the virus that causes chickenpox; also known as herpes zoster. Shingles is due to reactivation of the virus that remains dormant in the body after causing the initial chickenpox infection.

Shingles is characterized by a rash and blisters that typically occur on one side of the body following the path of a nerve. The rash often wraps around part of the chest or back. Blisters near an eye require evaluation by an ophthalmologist because if there is any eye involvement, permanent eye damage can result.

Shingles usually heal within a few weeks. However, in some older people or those people with weakened immune systems, an agonizing condition called postherpetic neuralgia can result.

Doctors recommend seeking medical treatment at the first sign of itching, burning, and tingling. The virus that causes shingles can be passed on only to people who have not had chickenpox. Primary treatment of shingles, with antiviral drugs such as acyclovir, is most effective when begun within 3 days of developing the rash. Applying cool compresses and soothing lotions may help relieve the itching and burning.

Shock

See SHOCK, PHYSIOLOGICAL.

Shock therapy

See ECT (ELECTROCONVULSIVE SHOCK THERAPY).

Shock, anaphylactic

A life-threatening type of allergic reaction affecting the entire body. Anaphylactic shock occurs when a person has been sensitized to a substance and the immune system has been triggered to recognize that substance as a threat. If the sensitized person encounters the substance again, the body reacts with a sudden, severe reaction affecting all body systems. Symptoms include hives; itching; swelling of the eyes, lips, tongue, hands, and feet; wheezing, coughing, and breathing problems; blue or red skin; and dizziness, confusion, rapid pulse, nausea and vomiting, diarrhea, and abdominal cramps. Symptoms usually develop rapidly.

Anaphylactic shock can occur in response to any allergen. Although anaphylactic shock occurs infrequently, it is life-threatening. To prevent it, people with known allergies should avoid the suspect allergens, and people with histories of allergic reactions to insect bites or stings may be instructed to carry an emergency kit containing injectable epinephrine.

Shock, electric

Injury caused by exposure of skin or internal organs to electric current. Electric current can cause injury in three ways: by causing cardiac arrest, by damaging muscle tissue, or by burning the skin.

Symptoms of electric shock may include fatigue, broken bones, headache, impaired hearing, heart attack, hyperventilation, muscle pain, breathing problems, vision loss, and unconsciousness.

First aid for electric shock includes shutting off the electric current, if possible. If turning off the power source is not possible, a dry, nonconducting object such as a broom, wooden chair, rubber doormat, or rug can be used to push the person away from the source of the electrical current. A person should never touch an individual who is still in contact with the electrical source. Once away from the source of the current, the person's breathing should be checked, and CARDIOPULMONARY RESUSCITATION (CPR) should be started.

Shock, insulin

A condition in which an abnormally low blood sugar (glucose) level results in unconsciousness; also called HYPOGLYCEMIA. Insulin shock occurs when excessive insulin is released into the bloodstream by the pancreas; it is most likely to occur in a person who takes insulin for diabetes. Symptoms may progress rapidly, and a person experiencing an insulin reaction can progress quickly from feeling nervous, hungry, apprehensive, and confused to sweating profusely to loss of consciousness or seizure.

First aid measures for insulin shock include providing the person with some kind of carbohydrate or sugar, such as orange juice, candy, or carbonated drinks made with sugar if he or she is able to swallow. If the person does not recover promptly or if they cannot take anything orally, emergency medical assistance should be sought.

Shock, physiological

A condition occurring when insufficient blood flows through the body. Physiological shock is characterized by very low blood pressure, a decreased amount of urine, and cell or tissue damage. Symptoms of physiological shock include irritability or lethargy; bluish lips and fingernails; chest pain; cool, clammy skin; cold hands and feet; dizziness or feeling faint; nausea and vomiting; rapid pulse; shallow breathing; excessive thirst; unconsciousness; weakness; and confusion.

If physiological shock is suspected, emergency medical aid should be sought immediately. Physiological shock is a life-threatening condition and can progress rapidly without emergency intervention.

Shock, septic

See SEPTIC SHOCK.

Short stature

A term applied to individuals who are among the shortest 5 percent of people for their age and sex. Short stature may be a symptom of a medical condition, such as delayed or precocious puberty, HYPOTHYROIDISM, or skeletal dysplasia, or it may represent a normal inherited trait. People of short stature can sometimes benefit from growth hormone medication.

Shortness of breath

See BREATH, SHORTNESS OF.

Shoulder, dislocated

An injury in which the ends of the bones that form the shoulder joint are forced from their normal positions. A dislocated shoulder is usually caused by a blow, a fall, or other trauma. An injured shoulder that is visibly out of position, misshapen, swollen, difficult to move, and intensely painful probably has been dislocated or broken. Numbness can indicate nerve damage. Medical attention should be sought immediately. A dislocated shoulder is diagnosed by physical examination and X ray and treated by a procedure called reduction, followed by at least 2 weeks of arm immobilization in a sling.

Shunt

An abnormal or surgically created passage between two usually unconnected body channels or cavities.

Sick building syndrome

A set of symptoms characterized by fatigue, headaches, eye irritation, dizziness, and respiratory complaints that affect people who work in modern airtight office buildings. Although the exact cause of the syndrome remains unknown, it is believed to be long-term exposure to low concentrations of airborne pollutants such as mold. Doctors may recommend antihistamines, analgesics, and other medications to control symptoms.

Sick sinus syndrome

A group of signs and symptoms caused by inadequate function of the heart's natural pacemaker. In the healthy heart, a region known as the sinus node initiates the heartbeat. If the sinus node malfunctions, the heart may beat too slowly, pause for too long between beats, skip beats, or fire too rapidly. If it stops functioning altogether, another part of the heart's electrical system takes over the sinus node's role, but usually at a heart rate that is substantially lower than normal.

The leading sign of sick sinus syndrome is bradycardia, a slow heartbeat, less than 60 beats per minute, accompanied by episodes of tachycardia with heartbeat over 100 beats per minute. Palpitations (uncomfortably rapid heartbeats) may also occur, or the person may sense both fast and slow heartbeats. When the heartbeat drops below 50 beats per minute, fainting spells, chest pain from insufficient blood supply to the heart, dizziness, shortness of breath, unusual fatigue, disturbed sleep, muscle aches, or confusion may arise. If sick sinus syndrome continues untreated, it may lead to heart failure as the heart cannot supply sufficient blood to the body.

In its mild form with no symptoms, sick sinus syndrome requires no treatment. Treatment begins only when the syndrome becomes advanced and symptoms are distressing or dangerous. The usual treatment consists of surgically implanting a pacemaker, an electronic device that controls heartbeat, and prescribing antiarrhythmic medications to prevent abnormally rapid heartbeat rhythms. See also AR-RHYTHMIA, CARDIAC.

Sickle cell anemia

An inherited, chronic blood disorder that alters the shape of red blood cells and causes them to function abnormally; also known as sickle cell disease. The cause of the disease is an abnormality in hemoglobin, the pigment in red blood cells that transports oxygen. After they give up their oxygen, molecules of the abnormal hemoglobin, called hemoglobin S, tend to clump into rods that deform the normally round red blood cells into sickle shapes. Unable to squeeze through small blood vessels because of their shape, the sickle cells block blood flow, causing tissue and organ damage and pain. In addition, the sickle cells have a life span of only 10 to 12 days versus 120 days for normal red blood cells. The body cannot replace them fast enough, resulting in anemia, an ongoing decline in red blood cells.

The clinical manifestation of sickle cell anemia varies from one person to another. Some people have mild symptoms, while others have severe manifestations of the disease. Blockage of blood vessels by sickle cells cause many of the symptoms.

Children with sickle cell anemia do not usually show evidence of the disease until they reach 4 months of age. One of the first signs results from blockage of small blood vessels in the hands and feet, which causes them to swell painfully. Growth and development tend to be slower than normal, and puberty is delayed.

Chronic anemia causes fatigue, pale skin, weakness, and breathlessness after mild exercise. Because the bone marrow expands to increase red blood cell production, the bones thin, making them vulnerable to fracture. The rapid breakdown of red blood cells may cause the skin and sclera (whites of the eyes) to take on a yellow color (jaundice). Vision deteriorates if the retinas (light-sensitive tissue at the back of the eyes) receive too little oxygen, and visual impairment can result. Some children have strokes when sickle cells clog blood vessels in the brain. Sickle cells can collect in the lungs, producing an illness resembling pneumonia.

Many with the disease experience crises when sickle cells cut off blood flow to a part of the body. Practically any organ or joint can be affected. Crises cause severe pain that lasts from a few hours to several weeks. They can be brought on by any situation that increases the demand for oxygen, such as extremely high altitudes or infection.

Over time, sickle cell anemia can harm the internal organs. The liver and the spleen are commonly affected. The liver may malfunction, and the spleen may become scarred, cease to function, and have to be removed surgically. The heart often enlarges as a way of compensating for the decrease in oxygen flowing into the body and may set the stage for heart failure later in life.

There is no cure for sickle cell anemia. In the past, the disease resulted in premature death. With current therapies, however, approximately 50 percent of people with sickle cell anemia survive to their mid-40s.

The goal of treatment is to prevent crises and reduce symptoms when they occur. People with the disease are advised to avoid extremely high altitudes (for example, flying in unpressurized airplanes or mountaineering), stress, extreme fatigue, strenuous exercise, dehydration, and sources of infection (such as crowded public spaces during flu season). Infants and young children are commonly prescribed penicillin to prevent infection.

Sickle cell trait

Inheritance from one parent of one copy of the gene that causes sickle cell anemia. Inheritance from both parents is required for full-blown sickle cell anemia. In the United States, 1 in 12 black people are carriers of the sickle cell trait. Most experience no symptoms, but conditions that greatly increase the oxygen demands on the body, such as extremely high altitudes or extreme cold, may produce a crisis. See SICKLE CELL ANEMIA.

Side effect

An unwanted drug effect; an adverse drug reaction. Most drugs produce unintended effects or side effects in addition to the intended action, although most people do not experience these side effects. Most side effects are predictable and range from mild to very serious.

SIDS

See SUDDEN INFANT DEATH SYNDROME.

Sigmoid colon

The lowest section of the colon, or large intestine, before the rectum. This section of the colon gets its name from its S shape. The sigmoid colon connects to the descending colon above and the rectum below.

Sigmoidoscopy

A procedure in which the interior of the large intestine is examined by using a flexible, lighted tube called a sigmoidoscope. Sigmoidoscopy is a type of endoscopy that allows a doctor to view, photograph, and videotape the inside of the lower part of the large intestine without surgery. This procedure is used to look for early signs of cancer and other abnormalities in the rectum and sigmoid colon (the last part of the colon).

SIL

Squamous intraepithelial lesion. A system for classifying cervical dysplasia, abnormal cells on the cervix. Squamous intraepithelial lesion refers to abnormalities in the squamous cell

layer that covers the cervix. The classification system is used to describe abnormal PAP SMEAR results.

Low-grade changes, or LSIL, describes mild cellular change. This classification includes both mild dysplasia and changes seen in women infected with human papillomavirus, a sexually transmitted disease that can cause venereal warts and is often a precursor of cancerous cells. Moderate or severe dysplasia and carcinoma in situ of the cervix (where the cancer has not penetrated beyond the surface layer of the cells) are classified as high-grade or severe, or HSIL.

Silicosis

Permanent scarring of the lungs that is caused by long-term exposure to and inhalation of silica (quartz) dust. Silicosis is an occupational lung disease that is caused by inhaling the primary constituent of sand, which is silica. It occurs among miners who work in coal, lead, copper, silver, and gold mines and foundry workers.

Symptoms begin to appear after 10 to 30 years of working in an environment in which there is continual exposure to the dust. The scarring of lung tissue decreases the lungs' flexibility and produces difficulty breathing. This eventually interferes with the ability of the lungs to transfer oxygen into the blood.

Mild cases of silicosis do not cause breathing difficulties. Coughing that produces sputum is a common early symptom. More severe silicosis results in severe shortness of breath.

Lung damage associated with silicosis adds strain to the heart and may lead to TUBERCULOSIS and heart failure (see HEART FAILURE, CONGESTIVE).

The illness cannot be cured, but elimination of exposure to silica dust can halt its progress in some cases. Breathing problems may be improved with treatments used for chronic obstructive pulmonary disease (COPD), including courses of medications that keep airways open and free of secretions.

Single-photon emission computed tomography

See SPECT.

Sinus

A cavity or channel, usually within a bone, such as the air-containing spaces in the bones of the nose, lined with mucous membranes. There are numerous sinuses in the bones of the skull.

Sinus, facial

Any of the air-containing spaces in the bones of the face. There are four

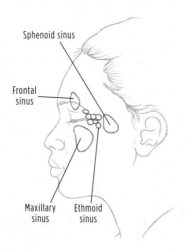

Facial sinuses
The nasal bones of the skull contain air chambers that surround and drain into the nose.

pairs of facial sinuses: the frontal sinuses in the bone of the forehead, just over the eye sockets; the maxillary sinuses in the cheekbones under the eyes; the ethmoid sinuses on either side of the bridge of the nose; and the sphenoidal sinuses directly over the bridge of the nose. The sinuses are lined with mucous membrane that helps trap particles in the air inhaled through the nose; the mucus drains into the nose.

Sinus bradycardia

An unusually slow heartbeat brought on by normal causes, such as deep relaxation or excellent fitness, or by abnormalities of the conduction systems, such as sick sinus syndrome. Sinus bradycardia requires no treatment unless it causes symptoms.

Sinus tachycardia

A fast heartbeat originating in the sinus node, the heart's own pacemaker. Sinus tachycardia is normal during exercise or when a person experiences anxiety. It may also be caused by shock, hypotension (low blood pressure), hypoxia (insufficient oxygen supply), congestive heart failure, or fever.

Sinusitis

For symptom chart, see HEADACHE, page xxii.

An inflammation and infection of the moist air cavities, called sinuses, located around the nose, behind the cheeks, and in the forehead above the eyes. Sinusitis is considered acute when it lasts for fewer than 30 days and chronic when it persists for more than 30 days. Sinusitis may be caused by an infection with bacteria, fungal infections, or allergic reactions. In rare instances, a dental infection is associated with sinusitis. Swelling and tenderness in the affected sinus or sinuses is usually the first sign of sinusitis. Headache is a common symptom, and there may be a discharge of yellow or green mucus from the nose. Pain behind and between the eyes accompanied by a severe headache may also occur. Fever, chills, and malaise may indicate spread of the infection.

Sinusitis is treated by methods to improve nasal drainage and control infection. Steam inhalation and saline nasal washes may be used to promote drainage of the sinuses. For adults, medications to constrict swollen membranes and open up the sinuses may be prescribed or recommended, either in topical form or to be taken orally. About 90 percent of all sinus infections are caused by viruses and do not require antibiotics. However, a course of oral antibiotic therapy of at least 10 to 12 days' duration is generally prescribed for a bacterial sinus infection. When sinusitis does not respond to antibiotics, functional endoscopic sinus surgery (see FESS) may be necessary for adult patients.

Sjögren syndrome

A disease in which the salivary glands and the lacrimal glands (which produce tears) are progressively destroyed by malfunction of lymphocytes (white blood cells that fight infection) and plasma cells (white blood cells that produce antibodies). The glands producing moisture in the vagina may also be involved. Tissues and structures of the skin, respiratory tract, gastrointestinal tract, the sweat glands, liver, kidneys, lungs, and thyroid glands may also be affected. This syndrome may be involved in RHEUMATOID ARTHRITIS, systemic lupus erythematosus (see LUPUS ERYTHEMATOSUS, SYSTEMIC), polymyositis, or SCLERODERMA.

While there is currently no cure for Sjögren syndrome, there may be relief for most of its major symptoms, which include dry mouth, a burning sensation in the mouth and throat, a hoarse and weak voice, cracks on the tongue and lips, and swelling of the salivary glands. Smell and taste may be diminished. Yeast infections and dental decay can result. Increasing fluid intake and using sugarless gum and hard candy can be helpful for keeping the mouth moist.

Early diagnosis and treatment of the symptoms are important for avoiding complications.

Skeletal system

The bones of the body that together form a structural framework and protect internal organs and soft tissues. Bones are attached to one another at a juncture called a joint, with tough fibrous bands known as ligaments. The skeletal muscles are attached to bone with connective bands called tendons. Together, the bones, muscles, and joints form a moving structural system known as the musculoskeletal system. The typical human body has 206 individual bones forming the skeleton.

Skeleton

The bones of the body. See SKELETAL SYSTEM.

Skier's thumb

A sprain of the ligament that is attached to the joint of the thumb and controls the bending and straightening motions as well as side-to-side movements of the thumb. Skier's thumb results in instability of the thumb and a loss of function. There may be pain and swelling in the area. The ability to bring together the ends of the thumb and forefinger may be limited. X rays may indicate a complete rupture of the ligament. If the thumb joint is sufficiently stable, a thumb cast or brace may be worn for 3 to 6 weeks to immobilize the joint and allow healing. If the ligament is completely ruptured, surgery is usually necessary to reconnect the torn ends of the ligament.

Skin

The protective outer tissue covering the body. The skin holds in body fluids, helps regulate body temperature, and forms the first line of defense against infection and injury to internal body structures and tissues. The skin is also a vast sensory organ, filled with nerve endings that register touch, pressure, heat, and cold.

Skin allergy

A skin reaction that is caused by exposure to an allergy-causing substance. (See also CONTACT DERMATITIS.) Skin allergy occurs in response to a substance that may cause no apparent rash or inflammation the first time a person is exposed to it. But, on subsequent occasions, after the skin has become allergic to the substance, further exposure produces an eruption.

Symptoms of skin allergy vary from person to person but often include redness, itching, inflammation, or scaling. A dermatologist can help people avoid allergens by identifying the substances that cause reactions. Treatments to control symptoms may include applying cool compresses, soothing lotions, and topical CORTICOSTEROIDS and taking antihistamines. Taking oatmeal baths may relieve itching. Scratching should be avoided to allow a rash to heal.

Skin cancer

The most common form of cancer in the United States. Skin cancer is linked to cumulative exposure or chronic exposure to the ultraviolet rays of the sun. While the risk of nonmelanoma skin cancers increases with cumulative exposure to the sun, melanoma—the most serious type because it spreads to other organs—is linked to intermittent intense sun exposure, genetic factors, and moles. To detect skin cancer, doctors recommend regular self-examination. It is important to consult a doctor upon finding any new skin growth; a change in the surface or color of a mole; a spot or bump that is getting larger, scaling, oozing, or bleeding; a sore that does not heal within 3 months; or itchiness or pain in a lesion.

Types of skin cancer

There are three main types of skin cancer: BASAL CELL CARCINOMA, SQUAMOUS CELL CARCINOMA, and malignant melanoma (see MELANOMA, MALIGNANT). Basal cell and squamous cell carcinomas are often referred to as nonmelanoma skin cancers to differentiate them from melanoma, which is by far the most serious of the three. Most skin cancers occur on areas of the skin that are frequently exposed to sunlight.

Basal carcinomas rarely spread and typically are cured by surgical removal. Squamous cell carcinomas if caught early usually respond to local surgery; however, they can spread and in cases of advanced disease, death may occur. Malignant melanomas are the most dangerous type of skin cancer. If caught early, melanomas can be cured by surgery. Treatment depends on the depth of the lesion, and if the melanoma has spread. CHEMOTHERAPY and immunotherapy are useful for nonlocalized disease.

Skin graft

A plastic surgery technique to repair damaged skin, usually as a result of a serious burn or in reconstructive surgery. In a skin graft, a portion of skin is separated surgically from its original place on the body and moved to a new location. Skin grafts are commonly taken from an inconspicuous area, like the buttocks or upper part of the thigh, and transplanted to a site on the same individual (called an autograft). The graft can also be made between different individuals (allograft) or between different species (xenograft). After the graft is made, the transplanted skin receives its blood supply from the new site.

Skin patch

A small, adhesive device applied to the skin like a bandage that releases a measured dose of a drug into the bloodstream over 24 hours.

Skin tag

A small, soft, flesh-colored growth that protrudes from the skin; also known as a cutaneous papilloma.

Skull

The bony framework of the head. The skull contains 22 separate bones. Eight bones form the cranium, which houses the brain. Fourteen bones form the facial skull. The facial bones also have immovable joints, except for the two temporomandibular joints on either side of the lower jaw.

There are four tiny bones that are not part of the skull itself, but are within it. The hyoid bone, sometimes called the hyoid cartilage, is suspended by ligaments from the skull at the back of the tongue. It anchors the muscles of the tongue. Three small bones, also called the auditory ossicles, are in the middle ear. Named for their shapes—the hammer (malleus), anvil (incus), and stirrup (stapes)—these bones conduct sound waves into the inner ear.

Skull, fractured

A break in the cranial (skull) bones. A fractured skull may involve visible damage to the cranial bones, including heavy bleeding; but a skull fracture can be hidden by the hair. Symptoms of a skull fracture can in-

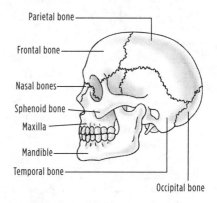

Parietal bone

Frontal bone

Nasal bones

Sphenoid bone

Maxilla

Mandible

Temporal bone

Occipital bone

Cranium and face
The bones of the skull comprise the cranium, which houses the brain, and the facial skeleton, which provides the structure for the face. These bones interlock to form a strong, yet somewhat flexible framework.

clude bruising or discoloration behind the ear or around the eyes; blood or clear fluid leaking from the ears or nose; unequal-sized pupils; or deformity of the skull, including swelling or depressions. Other symptoms may include loss of consciousness, memory lapses or amnesia (loss of memory), blurred vision, confusion, irritability, and headache.

A fractured skull is a medical emergency, and medical assistance must be sought to prevent brain damage or death.

SLE

See LUPUS ERYTHEMATOSUS, SYSTEMIC.

Sleep

The body's rest cycle, including a state of natural unconsciousness. Sleep is characterized by a mostly unmoving body posture and diminished sensitivity to external stimuli. Sleep is triggered by complex hormonal activity that responds to cues from the body and the environment. The sleep-wake cycle is controlled by the body's internal clock.

Most sleep—about 80 percent—is dreamless and is known as nonrapid eye movement (NREM) sleep. During NREM sleep, breathing and heart rate are slow and regular, blood pressure is low, and the sleeper is relatively still. Rapid eye movement (REM) sleep is associated with dreaming, which occurs during three to five periods of REM sleep each night at intervals of 1 to 2 hours. REM sleep is characterized by irregular breathing and heart rate, as well as by involuntary muscle jerks. Periods of REM sleep are variable in length.

Sleep apnea syndrome

A group of sleep disorders involving repeated episodes when a person stops breathing while asleep. Sleep apnea syndrome may be caused by a momentary blockage or obstruction in the throat or upper airway, or it may occur as the result of a dysfunction in the area of the brain that controls breathing.

Snoring is the most common symptom of sleep apnea and may be associated with intermittent gasping, choking, and absence of breathing that awaken the person in a state of anxiety. Episodes when breathing stops during sleep can last more than 10 seconds and may occur as many as 60 times per hour. These events may be experienced 30 to 300 times during a single night and can be serious if the oxygen supply to the blood and brain decreases while the level of carbon dioxide in the body increases. Over

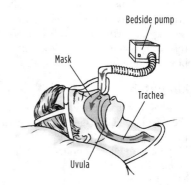

Snoring and sleep apnea

Doctors may prescribe continuous positive airway pressure (CPAP) to treat sleep apnea syndrome. To be treated with CPAP, the person wears a mask to bed that pumps air into the nose during sleep. The force of the air opens the airway so that air can enter the trachea (windpipe) and lungs.

time, severe sleep apnea may result in headaches, debilitating sleepiness during daytime hours, and diminished mental ability. Heart failure (see HEART FAILURE, CONGESTIVE) and pulmonary insufficiency can eventually develop.

When the syndrome is determined to be caused by blockage in the throat and upper airways, the first line of approach to treatment involves lifestyle changes. The affected person is advised not to smoke or drink, to lose weight if overweight, and to avoid tranquilizers, sleeping pills, and other sedating medication.

If sleep apnea is caused by a dysfunction in the section of the brain that controls breathing, the affected person may need to use an artificial breathing device while sleeping. Also, a dentist can design a custom device worn during sleep that reduces sleep apnea and snoring.

If these lifestyle changes and procedures do not eliminate the risks associated with sleep apnea, a treatment technique called continuous positive airway pressure (CPAP) may become necessary. The device is worn like a small oxygen mask over the nose and delivers a mixture of air under pressure through the nose. CPAP maintains regular breathing during sleep by keeping the airway open.

Sleep disorders

A host of disorders including IN-SOMNIA, NARCOLEPSY, RESTLESS LEG SYNDROME, parasomnia, and SLEEP APNEA SYNDROME. Problems sleeping can affect a person's energy level, and his or her overall health. Difficulty getting to sleep or remaining asleep are symptoms of this common problem, which can be short and self-limiting or persist for years.

Sleepwalking

A disorder characterized by periods of sitting up, moving about, or engaging in other complex activities (such as dressing or eating) while still asleep. Injury from a fall, walking through a window, wandering outside, or bumping into obstacles is a serious risk of sleepwalking. This risk is heightened if sleepwalking includes frantic actions such as running. Contrary to popular belief, a sleepwalker may be awakened without risk.

Slipped disk

A common back disorder in which the rupture of the backbone disk through its protective cartilage covering creates painful pressure on spinal nerves. A slipped disk may also be called a herniated disk or disk prolapse. It usually occurs in the lower back but may also take place in the cervical, or neck, region.

When the herniated, or slipped, disk exerts pressure, irritates, or pinches the spinal nerves, it can produce numbness, weakness, and pain that can be severe. If the sciatic nerve is pinched, the pain and numbness can radiate from the lower back down into the buttocks, into the back of the thigh and calf, and even into the foot. This type of pain is called SCIATICA. If left untreated over time, a slipped disk can damage the spinal nerves by constant pressure on the nerve root.

MRI (magnetic resonance imaging) is commonly used to diagnose disk problems. The first line of treatment for a slipped disk may include a brief period of bed rest during the acute phase and taking NONSTEROIDAL ANTI-INFLAMMATORY DRUGS (NSAIDs) such as aspirin or ibuprofen. Prescriptions for muscle relaxant and painkilling medications may be given. It may be necessary to wear a back brace or a cervical collar. Applications of heat or cold may be advised. When the pain subsides, physical therapy, including exercise, may be prescribed to help strengthen weakened back muscles and restore mobility of the back. If pain, numbness, and disability persist, surgery to remove the herniated disk to relieve pressure on the spinal nerves may become necessary.

Small cell carcinoma

A form of lung cancer. Small cell carcinoma, also known as oat cell carcinoma, is characterized by cells that are small and round or oval and look like oat grains when seen under a microscope. It is the most aggressive type of lung cancer and is usually found in people who smoke or used to smoke. Common symptoms include a chronic cough, blood in the sputum, wheezing, repeated episodes of pneumonia, fever, weakness, weight loss, and chest pain. Advanced disease may also include hoarseness, shortness of breath, enlarged lymph nodes in the neck, pain in the arm and shoulder, difficulty swallowing, and drooping eyelids.

CHEMOTHERAPY and RADIATION THERAPY are commonly used to treat the disease. Surgery is rarely recommended in cases of small cell lung cancer because the tumor typically spreads throughout the body even at an early stage.

Small-bowel resection

A surgical procedure performed under general anesthesia in which part of the small intestine is removed. A small-bowel resection is performed to treat serious intestinal disorders, such as cancer, obstruction, or INFLAMMATORY BOWEL DISEASE.

Small-bowel series

A series of X rays using the contrast medium barium to examine the small bowel (intestine). A small-bowel series can reveal the causes of MALABSORPTION SYNDROME or detect the presence of CROHN DISEASE or a tumor. The test is typically performed, as necessary, in conjunction with an upper gastrointestinal (GI) series.

Small-bowel transplant

Surgical procedure to treat chronic intestinal failure. Small-bowel transplantation is considered for people who have intestinal failure and cannot tolerate tube feeding. Immunosuppressive drugs given after surgery increase the chances for a successful transplant and a return to normal eating. Serious risks include infection and organ rejection. Because of the risks, the procedure is performed less frequently than kidney, heart, or liver transplants.

Smallpox

An acute infectious disease that is caused by a virus. Due to the availability of an effective vaccine and a worldwide vaccination campaign, smallpox has not existed as a naturally acquired infection since 1977. The World Health Organization declared the disease officially eradicated throughout the world in 1980. When smallpox existed as a significant health threat, it was a contagious infection for those in very close quarters, characterized by a rash of small blisters filled with clear fluid. The virus causing smallpox was readily transmitted via exposure to the respiratory secretions of infected people, through direct contact with the lesions of the skin and mucous membranes, or by contact with materials such as clothing and bed linens that had been contaminated.

The symptoms of smallpox included fever, chills, headache, nausea, vomiting, and severe muscle aches. By the fourth day of illness, the fever decreased and the characteristic rash appeared.

There are no medications known to be effective against the disease. Smallpox virus has been identified as a possible agent of terrorism, or a bioweapon.

Smear

A small amount of body tissue or fluid spread on a glass slide for examination under a microscope.

Smell

The perception of odors and scents through stimulation of the olfactory (pertaining to smell) nerve in the upper portion of the nose. When special sensory cells in the nose are stimulated by tiny molecules in substances in the environment, the thin, sensitive fibers in the olfactory nerve convey these smell sensations to the olfactory bulb, located at the front of the brain, behind the nose. Common treatments to correct the loss of the sense of smell include surgery to open the nasal passages or medications to reduce nasal inflammation.

Smoke inhalation

See INHALATION, SMOKE.

Smoking cessation

A process of ending dependence on nicotine, the addictive drug in tobacco products. Since nicotine is highly addictive, withdrawal from it is often unpleasant, causing an intense craving for cigarettes (or other tobacco products), difficulty concentrating, irritability, hunger, constipation, and trouble sleeping. Because tobacco use is the single greatest cause of disease and premature death in America today (over 430,000 deaths a year), doctors strongly encourage quitting smoking.

Numerous medications for smoking cessation now exist, and should be tried since they can dramatically increase success rates. The "first-line" products include a variety of nicotine-replacement products ("gum," skin patches, inhaler, nasal spray, and lozenge) and oral medication. Some are available without prescription. Persons using nicotine replacement therapy must not smoke while using the medication, and should continue treatment at least 6 to 8 weeks for optimal success. Abstinence that lasts 3 months or more strongly indicates success.

Smoking, tobacco

Puffing or inhaling the smoke of cigarettes, cigars, or pipes. The primary active substance in tobacco smoke is nicotine, a highly addictive substance that has both stimulant and depressant effects. Smoking is the leading cause of preventable death and disability in the United States. One in five deaths in the United States every year is caused by tobacco.

When tobacco smoke is inhaled, nicotine enters the bloodstream and reaches the brain. There it stimulates the release of the hormone epinephrine (adrenaline), resulting in increased insulin production, a sudden release of sugar into the blood, and a quick burst of energy. Nicotine promotes memory and alertness, enhances certain cognitive skills, reduces appetite, and decreases stress. As the nicotine level in the blood drops and the epinephrine and sugar subside, the person feels depressed and fatigued. This effect induces the smoker to smoke again.

Nicotine also promotes the release of the brain chemical dopamine, which affects the nerve pathways controlling pleasure and reward. A similar action is seen with the use of cocaine, marijuana, alcohol, narcotics, and other abused drugs, and it explains nicotine's powerful potential for addiction.

Smoking and health

While a smoker is smoking, the heart rate increases from 10 to 20 beats per minute, and blood pressure rises from 5 to 10 millimeters of mercury as blood vessels constrict, causing the heart to work harder. Smoke also contains carbon monoxide, which displaces oxygen in the blood and reduces the oxygen supply to the heart and other organs. Over time these effects can result in severe damage to the heart and circulatory system. In addition, smoking increases the tendency of blood to clot, which contributes to the two to three times increased risk of stroke found in smokers and also makes certain kinds of heart attacks more likely. In addition to the damage done to the heart by nicotine, of the more than 4,000 chemicals in tobacco smoke, at least 63 are cancer-causing (carcinogenic).

Smoking is the leading cause of cancer of the mouth, pharynx (throat), larynx (voice box), and lungs. Smoking is also linked with cancer of the stomach, urinary bladder, esophagus, cervix, and kidney.

Smoking has a role, too, in the development of 85 percent of emphysema and chronic bronchitis cases. Women who smoke enter menopause earlier than nonsmokers, and smokers who are pregnant increase the risk of stillbirth and low birth weight in their newborns. Smoking may also cause sexual problems, particularly erectile dysfunction (impotence) in men, because of impaired blood flow to the genitals, and it can contribute to high blood pressure (hypertension).

Secondhand or passive smoke also poses serious health risks, including an increased risk for lung cancer and heart disease in people exposed to it. Children raised in households with smokers are at higher risk of asthma and other disorders.

Treatment

When a person stops smoking, the negative health consequences of the addiction begin to reverse themselves. Within as little as 2 or 3 days, ex-smokers notice a sharpening of taste and smell, for example. Within a few months, lung function increases and shortness of breath eases, circulation improves, walking and exercise become easier, and the risk of respiratory infections drops. Over the next several years, the increased chance of cancer and heart disease from smoking decreases. After 5 years of not smoking, the risk of heart disease falls to that of a person who has never smoked. After 10 to 15 years of nonsmoking, the risk of lung cancer and heart disease, the two biggest killers, is no higher in an ex-smoker than in someone who has never smoked.

Snakebite

Injury caused when the flesh is pierced by the fangs of a snake; reptile bite (see BITES, REPTILE).

Snoring

Noisy sounds produced during sleep because of an obstruction to the free flow of air through the passages at the back of the mouth. Snoring affects up to 60 percent of the adult population.

Snoring may be caused by poor muscle tone in the tongue and throat or by overly relaxed muscles resulting from deep sleep, alcohol intake, narcotics, or sedatives. The relaxed muscles cause the back of the tongue or the top of the throat to collapse and obstruct the airway. An extended soft palate or a long uvula can intensify snoring. Colds, sinus infections, and allergies can block the nasal passages and contribute to the mouth breathing that often causes snoring. Deformities of the nose, such as a deviated septum (see SEPTUM, DEVIATED), may also have a role. Children with large tonsils or adenoids and children with asthma may be more prone to snoring.

Extremely loud snoring can be a symptom of obstructive sleep apnea (see SLEEP APNEA SYNDROME).

Sodium

A mineral needed by the body for normal function. Sodium controls the volume of fluid outside the cells and helps to maintain acid-base balance. Sodium helps to maintain the electrical system within the nervous tissue, thereby maintaining function of nerves and muscles. The amount of sodium in the body is controlled by the kidneys.

Sodium occurs naturally in most foods and drinking water, and it is easily absorbed. Sodium is also added to many food products. Adults should consume a maximum of between 1,100 and 3,300 milligrams of sodium per day; but since a single teaspoon of table salt contains 2,300 milligrams of sodium, it is easy to consume too much.

Soft-tissue injury

Any injury to the muscles, tendons, or ligaments generally caused by overuse or physical trauma. Soft-tissue injuries include muscle strains and sprains, bruises, pulled muscles, tendinitis, fibrositis, and carpal tunnel syndrome.

Solar plexus

A network of interconnected nerves in the abdomen that lies behind the stomach and between the adrenal glands. Also called the celiac plexus, the solar plexus sends out nerve branches to the stomach, intestines, and most other abdominal organs.

Soluble fiber

See FIBER, DIETARY.

Solvent abuse

See INHALANTS.

Somatic

Having to do with the body. Somatic is an adjective referring to the body as distinct from the mind.

Somatization disorder

A mental illness characterized by frequent complaints about physical symptoms that have no discernible physical cause and that arise from emotional conflict or anxiety.

Treatment consists of developing a relationship with one doctor to prevent repeated unnecessary testing, reassuring the patient that follow-up will control symptoms, encouraging discussion about causes of stress, and teaching new ways of dealing with stress.

Somatoform disorders

A group of closely related mental illnesses characterized by distressing physical symptoms that lack a physical cause and arise instead from emotional conflict or anxiety. Examples include hypochondriasis (an excessive concern with the possible symptoms and signs of illness), body dysmorphic disorder (a disabling preoccupation with an imagined or exaggerated physical defect), pain disorder (frequent, persistent complaints about pain lacking a physical cause), somatization disorder (frequent, persistent complaints about symptoms with no physical cause), and conversion disorder (symptoms affecting voluntary motor or sensory neurologic function).

Sore throat

Pain in the throat caused by inflammation of the tissue lining the throat passage. The medical term for sore throat is pharyngitis. A sore throat can become more painful when a person speaks or swallows. It is sometimes a symptom of infection that may have originated elsewhere in the body.

The most common cause of a sore throat is a viral infection, such as the viral infections that cause the common cold (see COLD, COMMON), flu, or mononucleosis. Bacterial infections such as *Streptococcus* (the bacterium that causes strep throat), or *Staphylococcus* (a common bacterium that can release toxins into the bloodstream) are less common but still important causes of sore throat.

A doctor can identify and evaluate a sore throat by observing the red, swollen tissue lining the throat. If the condition has persisted for more than a few days, the doctor may also use a swab to collect a sample of throat cells and secretions to be examined in a laboratory.

Sore throats caused by a cold or flu or by localized irritation usually pass when the infection disappears or when the irritants are avoided. A sore throat that persists needs medical attention. Antibiotics are prescribed only for bacterial infections.

Soy

A type of bean used in many food products that may have significant health benefits. In laboratory tests, a chemical in soybeans has been of benefit in limiting the growth of cancer cells. A number of studies in humans have demonstrated that soy protein lowers total cholesterol and LDL (low-density lipoprotein) cholesterol without lowering HDL (high-density lipoprotein) cholesterol, the "good" cholesterol.

Spasm

An involuntary muscle contraction. Muscle cramps (see CRAMP) are sudden, painful spasms caused by an excessive and prolonged contraction of the muscle fibers. Spasms may be due to overuse, muscle stress, or dehydration. Exercise-related cramps usually occur during or immediately after workouts, due to muscle fiber damage and a buildup of chemicals such as lactic acid. Minor spasms do not require treatment. However, a person with an unexplained, persistent, or painful spasm should seek a doctor's care.

Spastic colon

See IRRITABLE BOWEL SYNDROME.

Spastic paralysis

Also known as spastic paraplegia, a neurological disorder characterized by increased rigidity of the muscles (spasticity) and weakness or paralysis of the lower body. The progress of spastic paralysis, which can be caused by a genetic disorder, varies from person to person. Although some medications may reduce spasticity, there is no specific treatment to slow degeneration of affected nerves. Supportive measures include physical therapy and walking aids. Other causes of spastic paralysis include infections, multiple sclerosis, and spinal cord tumors.

Spasticity

A condition characterized by stiff or rigid muscles. In spasticity, certain muscles are continuously contracted. This can interfere with movement, gait, or speech. Spasticity is usually caused by damage to part of the brain or spinal cord that controls voluntary movement. Possible causes of damage include stroke, cerebral palsy, multiple sclerosis, and spinal cord or brain injury.

Symptoms include clonus (a series of rapid muscle contractions), hyper-tonicity (increased muscle tone), exaggerated deep tendon reflexes, fixed joints, muscle spasms, and scissoring (involuntary crossing of the legs). Treatment includes medication (such as baclofen, clonazepam, and diazepam) and physical therapy (for example, range-of-motion exercises and muscle stretching). In some cases, surgery is necessary.

Specialist

A doctor who focuses on a certain part of the body or on specific diseases. For example, cardiologists are specialists in heart disorders. Specialists have many years of training in their areas of specialty or subspecialty.

Specimen

A sample of a body fluid or tissue for laboratory analysis.

SPECT

Single-photon emission computed tomography. SPECT is a nuclear scanning technique that is similar to CT (computed tomography) SCANNING because a specialized cameralike device receives signals and feeds them into a computer. The computer then transmits the results to a monitor that displays cross-sectional or two-dimensional images. SPECT is used to evaluate brain disease and abdominal disease.

Speculum

An instrument used to hold open a body passageway such as the vagina for an examination such as a pelvic examination or a procedure.

Speech disorders

A group of disorders that result in ineffective or impaired communication due to difficulty speaking. The most common cause of speech problems in children is mental retardation. Other potential causes include attention deficit/hyperactivity disorder (ADHD), autism, cerebral palsy, cleft palate (see CLEFT LIP AND PALATE), dental problems, hearing loss, learning disabilities, palate disorders, Tourette syndrome, and vocal cord injuries. Adults can also develop speech disorders as a result of stroke, ALS (amyotrophic lateral sclerosis), Parkinson disease, or multiple sclerosis.

Early evaluation and treatment of speech disorders are best. A child can quickly fall behind if speech and language development is delayed. It is especially important to evaluate children who are at high risk because of problems such as cerebral palsy or chronic ear infections. Treatment of a speech disorder depends on its underlying cause.

Speech therapy is the primary treatment for many types of speech disorders, such as stuttering and articulation deficiencies. Depending on the results of evaluation, different services may be recommended.

Cleft palate is a common cause of speech disorders. Surgery to repair a cleft palate generally takes place when a child is aged 6 to 12 months.

Speech mechanism

The structures involved in the production of sound that is modified into spoken language. The production of speech sounds begins with air that is pushed out of the lungs and passes up through the trachea into the larynx (voice box). The larynx is a hollow organ, located between the pharynx and the trachea, and constructed of several pieces of cartilage. The largest

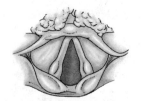

Open vocal cords

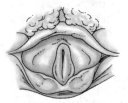

Closed vocal cords

How speech is produced

The vocal cords remain open while air is inhaled and exhaled, and close on exhalation. Sounds are produced when air vibrates through the folds.

of these is the thyroid cartilage, commonly called the Adam's apple, which lies at the front of the throat and projects slightly outward. The cricoid cartilage is just below it, connecting the thyroid cartilage to the trachea. At the back, on top of the cricoid cartilage, are two projections called the arytenoid cartilages. The vocal cords (also called vocal folds) stretch across the larynx, suspended from the thyroid cartilage in front and the arytenoid cartilages at the back. At rest, the vocal cords lie apart, forming an opening (called the glottis) through which air passes for breathing.

For speech production, the vocal cords contract and become taut, so that they vibrate as air passes between them to produce sound. Changes in the tightness of the cords produce changes in the pitch of the sound, and changes in the size of the larynx and other chambers in the throat and head alter the volume.

Speech therapy

Treatment to help people overcome problems with oral communication. Speech therapy is the primary treatment for many types of speech disorders, such as stuttering and articulation deficiencies. Different types of speech therapy are recommended for different problems. Speech therapy is usually conducted by a speech-language pathologist, a professional who is trained at the master's or doctoral level to evaluate speech disorders and prepare plans to improve speech.

Sperm

The male reproductive cell, which is produced in great numbers in the testicles beginning at puberty; also called spermatozoa. The production of sperm is triggered by the male sex hormone testosterone and gonadotropin hormones produced in the pituitary gland. A single sperm has an enlarged head, which contains the cell nucleus and genetic material. A tail on the cell propels the highly mobile sperm. Sperm cells exit a man's body in a fluid called semen, during the process of ejaculation. An ejaculation can contain 500 million sperm. (See REPRODUCTIVE SYSTEM, MALE.) As a result of sexual intercourse, a single sperm may join with an egg in the process of fertilization, which may result in pregnancy.

Sperm count

A laboratory test to determine the number of sperm cells in a sample of semen (the thick, white fluid expelled from the penis at sexual climax). A sperm count varies from 20 to 250 million sperm cells per milliliter of semen.

Sperm motility

A laboratory test to determine the ability of sperm cells to move (motility) or be motile. Normally, about 50 percent of sperm are motile. Sperm cells that move poorly or not at all are generally incapable of fertilizing a female egg cell and causing pregnancy.

Spermatocele

A noncancerous mass that develops in the small coiled tubules (epididymis) on the back of the testicle. A spermatocele is filled with fluid and dead sperm cells and is usually painless. It requires medical treatment only if it grows large enough to cause discomfort or difficulty.

Spermicides

Chemical agents that kill sperm or make them unable to fertilize an egg. Spermicides are used as a form of birth control and are most effective when combined with another birth control method, such as a condom, diaphragm, or cervical cap. See CONTRACEPTION, OTHER METHODS.

SPF

See SUN PROTECTION FACTOR.

Sphincter

A ring of muscle fibers that narrows a passage or closes an orifice. For example, sphincters control the opening and closing of the bladder and anus. A sphincter acts as a valve, regulating inflow or outflow. A sphincter can function automatically or can be partly under voluntary control, as with the bladder.

Sphincterotomy

Surgical cutting of a sphincter muscle, typically the one that is located at the junction of the intestine with the bile and pancreatic ducts. Endoscopic sphincterotomy (also known as endoscopic retrograde sphincterotomy, or ERS) is a useful treatment for certain abnormalities of the bile ducts, pancreas, and gallbladder. ERS developed as an extension of the diagnostic procedure ERCP (endoscopic retrograde cholangiopancreatography). ERCP combines the use of X rays and endoscopy to examine the stomach, duodenum, bile ducts, and pancreas. In endoscopy, a slim, flexible, lighted tube is used to view, photograph, videotape, and take a sample of tissue for study. ERS permits the treatment of problems diagnosed through ERCP. Many times, the term ERCP is also used to refer to the treatments performed in ERS.

Sphygmomanometer

An instrument used to measure blood pressure in the arteries. A sphygmomanometer allows a doctor or nurse to determine both the systolic and diastolic pressures in an artery. The average blood pressure measurement for a healthy adult is 120/80 millimeters of mercury.

Spina bifida

A birth defect in which there is incomplete closure in the spinal column. (See also BIRTH DEFECTS; NEURAL TUBE DEFECT.) There are three major types of spina bifida: spina bifida occulta, meningocele, and myelomeningocele. In spina bifida occulta, the mildest form, there is an opening in the vertebrae of the spinal column but no apparent damage to the spinal cord. Meningocele, the rarest form, is the presence of a cyst protruding through the open part of the spine; this can be removed by surgery.

In myelomeningocele, the most severe form of the condition, a portion of the spinal cord itself protrudes through the back. Tissues and nerves may be covered by skin or exposed. Surgery is performed in the first 48 hours of life to drain spinal fluid and protect children against hydrocephalus, an accumulation of fluid in the brain. If hydrocephalus occurs, it is controlled by shunting (the implantation of a shunt or drain to relieve fluid buildup).

Children with myelomeningocele may continue to need operations throughout childhood. They may also

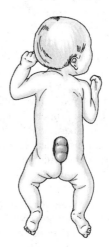

Baby with spina bifida
Spina bifida ("divided spine") is one of the most commonly occurring severe birth defects in the United States. A flattened mass of nervous tissue along the spine is exposed in spina bifida.

need training to manage bowel and bladder function and help with mobility skills. Crutches, braces, or wheelchairs may be required. Children who also have a history of hydrocephalus can experience learning problems. Adequate folic acid intake (400 mg daily) in women of childbearing age and during the first month after conception is important in the prevention of spina bifida.

Spinal anesthesia

See ANESTHESIA, SPINAL.

Spinal cord

A ropelike elongation of nerve tissue that extends down the back from the brain and is enclosed within the bones of the spine. The brain and spinal cord are the two main structures of the central nervous system, which controls and coordinates all of the body's functions and activities.

Running about 18 inches down the back, the cord is housed in the column of individual bones called vertebrae. Within this bony spinal column, the nerve tissue is further protected by an extension of the meninges, the three layers of membrane that protect the brain, and a cushioning layer of cerebrospinal fluid between the inner two layers.

Spinal fusion

A major surgical procedure sometimes considered to treat severe, persistent back pain, such as that caused by a slipped disk. Spinal fusion is accomplished by joining two or more adjacent bones of the spine, or vertebrae; by using bone fragments obtained from the person undergoing the surgery; or by using bone tissue from a bone bank or a synthetic bone material.

Spinal injury

Injuries affecting the bone or cartilage that make up the spine, as well as injuries that damage or destroy the spinal cord, which is made up of nerve pathways that transmit impulses between the brain and the body. See BACK PAIN; SLIPPED DISK.

Spinal cord injuries usually lead to some degree of permanent disability. When the spinal cord is injured in the cervical, or neck area, the injury may cause death if the nerves that control breathing are damaged. Spinal cord injuries in the neck area can also result in complete paralysis and general numbness in both the arms and the legs (quadriplegia).

The symptoms of spinal cord damage in a person who has been injured include an inability to move the legs and a lack of physical sensation, or numbness. The person should not be moved, and emergency medical attention should be sought immediately. Spinal cord injuries are diagnosed by X rays, myelograms, CT (computed tomography) SCANNING, or MRI (magnetic resonance imaging) scanning.

Spinal stenosis

A narrowing of the bony spinal canal formed by the vertebrae and the intervertebral disks. Spinal stenosis is caused by arthritis in the joints of the spine, which enlarges the joints and narrows the spinal canal. This narrowing can compress and pinch the nerves that travel through the lower spine into the legs. Symptoms include aching in the lower back and sometimes a sharp pain that extends into both buttocks, the thighs, and, at times, the calves and feet. Rest usually relieves the discomfort.

Anti-inflammatory medication and physical therapy are usually the initial treatments offered for spinal stenosis. A back support brace, such as a lumbar corset, may be beneficial. In severe and persistent cases, surgical decompression of the lower back area, called lumbar laminectomy, may be considered.

Spinal tap

See LUMBAR PUNCTURE.

Spine

The column of bones and cartilage that extends down the back, supporting the head and torso and enclosing the spinal cord.

Each of the individual bones of the spine is called a vertebra. Altogether, the spine contains 33 vertebrae: seven in the neck (cervical vertebrae), 12 in the upper back (thoracic vertebrae), five below the ribs in the lower back (lumbar vertebrae), five fused into a single unit called the sacrum, and four fused into a single unit called the coccyx (tailbone). Each vertebra is a uniquely shaped, asymmetrical bone. It is a ring enclosing a central canal. Winglike projections extend from the back of the ring. The spinal cord passes through the canal. Nerves branching off of the spinal cord pass between the vertebrae.

A cushion of fibrous cartilage with a gelatinous center lies between all of the vertebrae except the first two below the skull and those in the sacrum and coccyx. These flexible cushions, called disks, allow the spine a range of movement and flexibility.

Spinocerebellar degeneration

An inherited disease characterized by progressive dysfunction of the cerebellum, spinal cord, and peripheral nerves. See FRIEDREICH ATAXIA.

Spirometry

A test that measures the function of the lungs. Spirometry helps doctors evaluate the lungs' capacity to take in air, the amount of air the lungs can hold, the amount of air exhaled by the lungs, and the rate of speed (airflow) of exhalations.

Spleen

An organ in the upper left side of the abdomen, next to the stomach and pancreas, that filters old or damaged red blood cells out of the bloodstream and produces some infection-fighting agents.

The largest structure in the lymphatic system, the spleen is composed of lymph tissue that produces antibodies (proteins that can destroy certain foreign microorganisms), phagocytes (cells that can ingest some

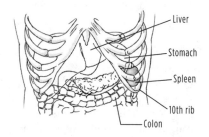

Location of the spleen
The spongy, purple spleen lies in the upper part of the abdominal cavity, just under the rib cage on the left side of the body.

microorganisms), and lymphocytes (a type of white blood cell).

The spleen is soft and spongy, which makes it vulnerable to injury, especially when it enlarges. It can be removed, because other organs in the lymphatic system can take over its many activities.

Splenectomy

The surgical removal of the spleen. A splenectomy is performed in patients whose spleen has been injured in an accident, when a person has leukemia, LYMPHOMA, or other diseases that cause the spleen to enlarge beyond its normal size.

Splenomegaly

An abnormal enlargement of the spleen. Causes may include portal hypertension (increased blood pressure in the portal vein, which carries blood from the intestines to the liver); cirrhosis (a severe liver disease); hemolytic anemia (see ANEMIA, HEMOLYTIC); malignant lymphoma; leukemia; systemic lupus erythematosus; malaria; infections (such as mononucleosis); and hypersplenism. The signs of splenomegaly are pain in the upper left side of the abdomen and a feeling of abdominal fullness. Treatment depends on the underlying cause of splenomegaly. In severe cases, removal of the spleen (see SPLENECTOMY) may be necessary.

Splinters

Sharply pointed fragments that enter the skin. Most splinters can be removed with tweezers and a needle. To avoid infection, instruments must first be sterilized by cleaning them in rubbing alcohol. Deeply embedded splinters require removal by a physi-

cian. A splinter in an eye should not be removed by anyone other than a physician. Instead, both eyes should be covered loosely and the person with the injury should be taken to an ophthalmologist or hospital emergency department.

Spondylitis

A condition involving inflammation of one or more vertebrae. Spondylitis is another term for the chronic inflammatory disease called ankylosing spondylitis, which affects the vertebral joints of the spine and the joints between the spine and the pelvis, eventually causing them to fuse together.

Spondylolisthesis

A condition in which one vertebra in the spine slips forward on the vertebra below it and becomes out of alignment with the other spinal vertebrae. The misaligned vertebra puts pressure on nearby spinal nerves. In most cases involving adults, the forward movement of the upper vertebra is minimal and there is no risk of continual slippage that would cause the upper vertebra to become disconnected from the vertebra below it.

Common symptoms include stiffness and pain across the small of the back that extends into the buttocks and possibly into the leg and foot. Numbness and weakness of the foot may also be experienced. The condition is aggravated with activity and relieved with rest. Tightness of the hamstrings is common.

Treatment involves reducing symptoms by strengthening the back muscles. Physical therapy exercises to strengthen the back and abdomir muscles may help stabilize the spine. Medication may be prescribed to control pain and ease associated muscle spasms. Bed rest at short intervals may be beneficial. Surgery becomes necessary only if conservative treatment fails.

Spondylolysis

A defect in a vertebra in the lower back, typically the last vertebra at the bottom of the spine, an area called the lumbar spine. The defective area of this vertebra is the bony ring that protects the spinal cord and connects the vertebral bone to the facet joints at the top and bottom of each vertebra. In spondylolysis, the back part of the vertebra and the facet joints are connected only by soft tissue. It is believed that this can be caused by an incompletely healed stress fracture of the vertebra affected. There is usually a lump of hardened tissue in the area where the stress fracture did not completely heal. This tissue may press on the nerve roots at the bottom of the spine, causing pain that extends down into the legs. The condition first appears in childhood and is common among young football players, gymnasts, and ballet dancers.

Spondylolysis can result in a condition called SPONDYLOLISTHESIS, in which one vertebra slips forward on the vertebra below it.

Spondylosis

A term referring to various degenerative diseases of the spine.

Sporotrichosis

A chronic fungal infection caused by that is found on rose or barﻪshes and on sphagnum moss r mulches, as well as in the soil. Often called gardener's disease, it occurs when open cuts or sores on the skin make contact with the mold, which is spread via lymphatic fluid and forms small, round masses of tissue on the skin's surface or deep within the skin. If the infection is not treated, these nodules break down into inflamed, pus-filled cavities in the skin or become open sores. If the infection spreads through the bloodstream, other areas of the body may be affected, particularly the joints.

The lesions caused by sporotrichosis may be easily misdiagnosed as spider bites. A swabbed culture from an active lesion offers a definitive diagnosis. The oral antifungal medication itraconazole is generally used to treat skin infection. If the lungs or bloodstream are involved, amphotericin B is administered.

Sports injuries

The group of conditions and disorders of the musculoskeletal system that are caused by participation in athletics or other forms of exercise. Sports injuries may involve injury to the bones, joints, muscles, ligaments, and tendons. See also RICE; TENDINITIS.

Sports medicine

The field of medical study and practice that involves injuries to the body from sports and athletic activities that usually involve musculoskeletal injuries.

Sprain

A forcible wrenching or twisting of a joint that may involve severe stretching or tearing of attached ligaments. A sprain does not involve dislocation of the joint, but may cause injury to surrounding blood vessels, muscles, tendons, or nerves. Sprains generally produce significant swelling and pain, as well as bruising if blood vessels are ruptured. The pain may prevent joint movement. Sprains are treated initially by RICE (rest, ice, compression, and elevation). After the pain subsides, exercises are prescribed to regain function.

Sprue

See CELIAC DISEASE.

Spur

An abnormal, spike-shaped outgrowth of bone tissue, often found on the bottom of the back of the heel. Bone spurs may be tender when gentle pressure is applied and usually cause sharp pain when weight is placed on the foot. Over time, if a protective bursa (a fluid-filled sac that acts as a cushion) develops over the spur, the bursa may become inflamed, causing swelling and increased pain. Favoring the sore heel may alter the gait and contribute to back pain. When bursitis is associated with a heel spur, the foot should be rested and protected from pressure by a special pad. NONSTEROIDAL ANTI-INFLAMMATORY DRUGS (NSAIDs) or localized corticosteroid injections may be recommended. Surgery may become necessary if the condition persists and is painful. See OSTEO-ARTHRITIS.

Sputum

Mucus and other matter coughed up and expectorated (spat) from the mouth. The analysis of sputum is an important component in the diagnosis of certain diseases, especially TU-BERCULOSIS. Doctors also use sputum cultures to select appropriate antibiotic therapy for the treatment of tuberculosis, pneumonia, and bronchitis.

Squamous cell carcinoma

The second most common type of skin cancer. The two other common types are basal cell carcinoma and malignant melanoma (see MELANOMA, MALIGNANT). Squamous cell carcinoma arises from the epidermis (the outer layer of skin). It is more aggressive than basal cell cancer and more likely to spread to other locations such as nearby lymph nodes. Left untreated, tumors may even spread into internal organs and become incurable. Squamous cell carcinoma is slow growing and, when properly treated, has a very high cure rate (more than 95 percent). The principal risk factor for developing squamous cell cancer is chronic sun exposure. Any new growth that changes color, ulcerates, bleeds, or does not heal can be an indication of squamous cell carcinoma and the person should seek medical attention. Squamous cell carcinoma usually develops from a red, scaly, precancerous skin lesion known as actinic keratosis. Actinic keratoses usually occur on sun-damaged parts of the body, such as the face, scalp, ears, and backs of the hands.

If a doctor suspects skin cancer, he or she will take a complete medical history; examine the size, shape, color, and texture of the lesion in question; ask about the history of the growth; check the rest of the body; and perform a skin biopsy.

In the early stage of the disease, squamous cell carcinoma in situ (Bowen disease) can be removed by topical chemotherapy, cryosurgery (freezing with liquid nitrogen), or electrodesiccation (burning with an electric current delivered through a probe) and curettage (scraping). However, most squamous cell carcinomas must be surgically removed.

If there is a suspicion that the cancer has spread, nearby lymph nodes are removed and studied under a microscope. For large cancers, skin grafting and reconstructive surgery are often necessary. Radiation therapy may be considered when surgical removal is not feasible.

SSRI drugs

See SELECTIVE SEROTONIN REUPTAKE INHIBITOR DRUGS.

St. John's wort

An herbal remedy used to treat mild to moderate DEPRESSION, anxiety, SEASONAL AFFECTIVE DISORDER, and sleep disorders. St. John's wort is thought to work by reducing the rate at which brain cells reabsorb the neurotransmitter serotonin, low levels of which are associated with depression. However, it is not considered as effective against depression as are prescription medications.

Stapedectomy

A surgical procedure to treat hearing loss caused by otosclerosis, an inherited disorder of the middle ear. Stapedectomy is performed through the ear canal under local anesthesia. Stapedectomy is a well-established surgical procedure with a high rate of success, but improvement in hearing may vary from one person to another.

Staphylococcal infections

The group of infections caused by bacteria of the *Staphylococcus* genus,

commonly known as staph. Staphylococcal bacteria produce illness directly by causing infection or indirectly by making products, such as toxins, that are responsible for food poisoning and toxic shock syndrome. Some species of staphylococcal bacteria can be present on the skin and in the nose of a healthy person without causing problems; others can cause fatal illness. People who have diabetes or weakened immune systems are particularly vulnerable to staph infections.

To prevent staph infections, it is important to avoid eating foods that have not been properly refrigerated. Common foods affected include milk, eggs, meats, poultry, and potato salad. If a person has a staph infection, it should start to clear up after 1 day; if not, medical attention should be sought.

Staph infections are treated with antibiotics, but the bacteria have the capacity to develop resistance to these medications. For this reason, it is important to take the recommended dosage for the prescribed length of time.

Status asthmaticus

An intense and continuous asthmatic state. Status asthmaticus does not respond to the usual treatments for asthma and can produce severe shortness of breath that results in exhaustion and collapse. This extreme asthmatic state, which has become increasingly prevalent in children, requires immediate and aggressive treatment. See ASTHMA.

STDs

See SEXUALLY TRANSMITTED DISEASES.

Stem cell

A cell with the ability to divide indefinitely and give rise to the specialized cells that make up tissues and organs. Stem cells are found in humans at every stage from embryo to adult. In the embryo, they occur as the inner mass of cells in the early developmental stage known as the blastocyst. Since these cells eventually develop into every tissue and organ in the human body, they are called pluripotent (from Latin and meaning many-powered). Pluripotent cells taken from human embryos may have the potential to grow into cell lines in the laboratory, which could then be used for cell therapy (methods of treating disease by replacing diseased cells with healthy ones grown from stem cells).

Stenosis, valvular

A narrowing, stiffening, or obstruction, particularly of one or more heart valves. In the healthy heart, four valves act like gates that open to allow blood to flow from one area to another, then close to prevent backward movement. Valvular stenosis limits blood flow. Symptoms depend on which valve is affected.

Aortic stenosis

Aortic stenosis affects the valve connecting the heart to the aorta (the body's main artery). Because the narrowing partially blocks the aortic valve, blood flow to the body is reduced, and the heart must work harder to compensate.

Aortic stenosis may exist in a mild form for years before symptoms appear. Symptoms include fatigue, abrupt fainting spells, shortness of breath with exercise or at night, angina (chest pain), and swelling in the ankles. Medications may be used to treat the symptoms of aortic stenosis. These include angiotensin-converting enzyme (ACE) inhibitors, anticoagulants, and diuretics, which remove salt and fluid from the body. Once symptoms of aortic stenosis become severe, surgery to repair or replace the valve (see HEART VALVE SURGERY) is needed.

Mitral stenosis

The mitral valve connects the atrium (upper chamber) and the ventricle (lower chamber) on the left side of the heart. Stenosis of the mitral valve impairs blood flow from the atrium to the ventricle when the atrium contracts. Mild forms of mitral stenosis produce no symptoms or only symptoms that become noticeable as the disease worsens with age. Symptoms include breathlessness with little or no exercise, constant fatigue, frequent bronchitis, chest pain, and palpitations (uncomfortably rapid heartbeat).

The symptoms of mitral valve stenosis can be treated with medications. Diuretics are used to drain excess fluid from the lungs, and digoxin is used to slow a rapid heartbeat. Surgery to repair or replace the valve is also an option.

Pulmonary stenosis

Blood flows from the right ventricle through the pulmonic valve to the pulmonary artery, which leads to the lungs. Pulmonary stenosis limits the flow of blood into the lungs. Possible symptoms include fatigue, shortness of breath with exercise, light-headedness, and loss of consciousness. In severe cases, pulmonary stenosis leads to swelling in the arms, legs, and abdomen and to an enlarged liver.

Untreated pulmonary stenosis usually causes death before age 30. The treatment is open-heart surgery to replace the pulmonic valve or balloon valvotomy to restore normal blood flow.

Tricuspid stenosis

Blood returning from the body flows into the right atrium, through the tricuspid valve, and into the right ventricle. Tricuspid stenosis limits the blood flow from the right atrium to the right ventricle. Possible symptoms include general weakness and pain in the upper right abdomen. Shortness of breath, fluid retention, and fatigue may also occur.

Tricuspid stenosis that causes symptoms is rare, commonly occurs in conjunction with other valve problems, and is usually caused by congenital heart disease or rheumatic fever. Treatment often depends on the severity of the associated valve disease. Surgery may be needed to repair the damaged valve.

Stent

A small, cylindrical tube of wire mesh inserted into a passageway such as a section of diseased artery to hold it open. The stent is put into place with a catheter, a thin tube threaded into a vein and guided to the site of the diseased artery.

Stereotactic surgery

Also known as stereotaxic surgery; guided brain surgery. Stereotactic surgery is performed through a tiny hole in the skull and guided by CT (computed tomography) SCANNING.

This procedure may be performed in people with advanced Parkinson disease (a progressive, degenerative disease of the nervous system characterized by muscle rigidity, weakness, and tremor), for whom medications are no longer effective. It can also be used to remove deep brain tumors or abscesses.

Sterility

The condition of being free from live bacteria or other pathological microorganisms. Sterility in medicine applies to maintaining a state of cleanliness in medical settings that prevents the transmission of infectious agents, either directly or indirectly. See also STERILIZATION.

In popular language, the terms sterility or being sterile are sometimes used to refer to people who are unable to conceive or deliver a child; the medical term for this condition is infertility.

Sterilization

The use of physical or chemical procedures for the purpose of destroying all disease-causing microorganism life, including bacterial endospores (organisms that reproduce asexually) that may be resistant to such procedures.

Sterilization, female

See TUBAL LIGATION.

Sterilization, male

See VASECTOMY.

Sternum

The breastbone; the long bone in the front wall of the chest. The sternum joins with the collarbones (clavicles) at the top, and seven pairs of ribs are attached to it. The sternum is extremely strong to protect the heart from injury.

Steroids

See ANABOLIC STEROIDS; ANDROGENS; and CORTICOSTEROIDS.

Stevens-Johnson syndrome

See DRUG ERUPTION.

Stiff neck

Limited mobility of the neck, often because of a simple muscle spasm. A more chronic and serious stiff neck may be caused by osteoarthritis, osteoporosis, or slipped or degenerative disks in the cervical spine. Stiffness upon waking or exposure to extremes of cold can also contribute to a stiff neck. Possible trauma to the neck includes WHIPLASH injuries.

Muscle spasms in the neck can also produce stiffness in the area. A stiff neck can be a symptom of MENINGITIS when fever, headache, sensitivity to light, and vomiting are also present. It is important to have a stiff neck evaluated and diagnosed by a doctor before self-help treatment is attempted. Recommended treatment may depend on the cause of the condition.

Still disease

A rare disease, also known as JUVENILE RHEUMATOID ARTHRITIS (JRA), that affects children from 2 to 5 years of age.

Stillbirth

The birth of a dead baby after the 28th week of pregnancy. Stillbirths can have many causes, the most common being severe birth defects. Other causes include a lack of oxygen to the fetus as a result of placental abruption or a knot in the umbilical cord.

Stimulants

Drugs that temporarily increase the rate of activity or function of all or part of the body. Some stimulants affect specific organs, such as the heart, lungs, or brain. Most stimulants, however, help to activate the central nervous system.

Stings, marine

Injury caused by a marine animal. Marine stings can be very painful and quite toxic. Marine animals known to sting include the jellyfish, sea anemone, Portuguese man-of-war, stingray, sea urchin, and spiny fish, some of which, even after they are dead, can inject venom through their tentacles into the skin of swimmers. Marine stings can cause an acute stinging or burning sensation, rash, blistering, physiological shock, and allergic reactions. Death rarely occurs except when the person drowns as a result of shock.

First aid measures include the removal of all tentacles by someone who is wearing gloves, to prevent being stung themselves. The area of the sting should be washed with seawater followed by vinegar or rubbing alcohol. Hydrocortisone cream should be applied, and medical attention should be sought.

Stokes-Adams syndrome

Fainting, sometimes accompanied by a seizure, caused by a heart rhythm disorder. The heart rate falls so low that the body and brain receive insufficient oxygen. Stokes-Adams syndrome can be caused by some heart medications (for example, beta blockers, calcium channel blockers, and digoxin), heart disease, certain neuromuscular conditions (such as muscular dystrophy), and connective tissue diseases that affect the heart, including systemic lupus erythematosus. To treat Stokes-Adams syndrome, medications that affect the heart rhythm should be stopped. A pacemaker, an electronic device that controls heartbeat, can also be implanted in the chest to maintain a normal heart rate.

Stoma

A surgically created opening in the body. For example, stoma is commonly made in the abdominal wall to allow stool to pass from the body into a bag. Stomas are used in the treatment of digestive diseases, such as ulcerative colitis, CROHN DISEASE, or colorectal cancer. (See COLITIS; COLON, CANCER OF THE.)

Stomach

A major organ of the digestive system, located in the upper left side of the abdomen. The stomach receives swallowed food from the esophagus and breaks it down further by means of acidic secretions and churning action. From the stomach, the food passes into the small intestine.

Specialized cells in the lining of the stomach walls chemically promote digestion in several ways. Some cells secrete hydrochloric acid, which provides the right chemical environment for another secretion called pepsin and kills microorganisms that may be in the food.

Stomach cancer

Cancer that originates in the stomach. At first, the symptoms of stomach cancer may mimic those of peptic ulcer disease. These include vague indigestion, loss of appetite, and discomfort after eating. In more advanced cases, there may be abdominal pain, weight loss, difficulty swallowing, frequent vomiting, and abdominal swelling. Signs of internal bleeding can appear. These include anemia, vomiting with blood, and melena (blood in the stool). Melena makes the stool black, sticky, and strong-smelling.

If a person older than age 45 has a sudden case of indigestion, it is important to see a doctor. Early diagnosis and treatment of stomach cancer offer the best chance for a cure. Diagnosis of stomach cancer is made through tests, such as gastroscopy (visual examination of the esophagus, stomach, and duodenum using a lighted viewing tube called a gastroscope) and an upper gastrointestinal (GI) series (an X-ray procedure also called a barium swallow).

When stomach cancer is diagnosed at an early stage, it can be surgically removed. A gastrectomy (surgical removal of all or part of the stomach) is performed to treat some cases. When stomach cancer is advanced, surgery may still be recommended to relieve symptoms and prevent obstruction. CHEMOTHERAPY and RADIATION THERAPY may also alleviate symptoms and slow the course of the disease.

Stomach pumping

Also known as gastric lavage or stomach flushing, the washing out of the stomach.

Stomach pumping is usually done

in a hospital emergency department. In the procedure, the doctor repeatedly introduces water or saline into the stomach through a tube and then suctions the fluids out along with any poisonous substances that have been ingested. Possible complications include inhaling any liquids or poisons, pneumonia, and bleeding.

Stomach stapling

A common type of surgery for obesity. Its purpose is to reduce stomach size and slow the rate at which the stomach empties. Stapling is performed only on people who are at least twice their ideal body weight who have been unable to lose weight in supervised weight loss programs.

Stomach stapling is performed in a hospital under general anesthesia and takes 2 to 3 hours. Stapling reduces the volume of food that the stomach can hold. Although stomach stapling is one of the most effective methods of weight loss, the surgery carries a high risk for complications including death. See also BARIATRIC SURGERY.

Stool

Excrement passed from the anus in a bowel movement. See FECES.

Stool softeners

Drugs used to treat constipation. Stool softeners are a type of laxative (see LAXATIVES) used to promote the formation and passage of soft, formed stools without straining.

Strabismus

Misalignment of the eyes so they point in different directions; also known as crossed eyes. In esotropia, the most common form of strabismus in infants, one eye turns inward. Accommodative esotropia mostly affects children who are farsighted (have difficulty focusing on close objects). Trying to focus the eyes for vision at short distances causes the eyes to cross. In exotropia one eye turns outward. Exotropia is most likely to be obvious when a person is trying to focus on a distant object or when he or she is tired, ill, or daydreaming.

Strabismus in children often needs to be treated very early, even in infancy, in order to reduce the risk of permanent vision loss in the misaligned eye. For accommodative esotropia, eyeglasses may be sufficient to solve the problem. The power in the glasses allows the accommodative reflex to relax, resulting in less turning in of the eyes.

Many cases of strabismus require surgical repair. In children, the operation is done under general anesthesia in a hospital; in adults, local anesthesia in an outpatient clinic may be an option. Depending on the individual case, surgery may be performed on one or both eyes.

Strain

A modestly pulled or stretched muscle. Strains are usually confined to muscle but may also involve tendons or ligaments. Some muscle fibers may be damaged by a strain. Sudden, strenuous movements, often occurring during sports activities, are most frequently the cause.

The symptoms of a strain may include pain, swelling, and bruising, as well as some loss of function or strength. Severe strains may produce painful muscle spasms. Strains usually heal independently within 2 to 3 days with the aid of RICE and taking over-the-counter NONSTEROIDAL ANTI-INFLAMMATORY DRUGS (NSAIDs). If a strain persists for more than a few days, a doctor should be consulted.

Strapping

A preliminary treatment for heel pain that has been diagnosed as caused by a mechanical problem in the foot. Strapping, or wrapping adhesive tape to exert pressure and hold the heel in place, for example, is considered an effective approach to testing the potential of orthotics therapy (the use of custom-made shoe inserts) for individual cases of foot pain. Generally, if strapping reduces foot pain significantly within the first 24 to 72 hours, an orthotic device is prescribed for ongoing treatment. Joints can also be strapped.

Strawberry nevus

See HEMANGIOMA.

Strength training

The activities and exercises devoted to building muscle by challenging muscle tissue and forcing it to adapt to stress. Weight lifting and resistance training, often using machines that can be adjusted to an individual's needs and requirements, are the basic elements of strength training.

Strengthening exercises

See EXERCISE, STRENGTHENING.

Strep throat

An inflammation of the section of the throat located between the tonsils and the larynx, or voice box. Strep throat is usually caused by an infection with group A streptococcal bacteria. The illness is spread via direct person-to-person contact with infected nasal secretions or saliva. Not all patients have symptoms, and the bacteria can exist in the throat of a healthy person without producing symptoms. Others may have such mild symptoms that they do not seek medical attention.

When symptoms of strep throat appear, they may include a sore, reddened throat, difficulty swallowing, a fever that comes on suddenly, tender and swollen glands in the neck, malaise, nausea, loss of appetite, and sometimes a rash.

Diagnosis is generally based on the finding of streptococcal bacteria in a throat culture. Most symptoms improve within a week with or without the use of antibiotics. However, antibiotic treatment is needed to prevent the serious associated complications of strep throat including middle ear infection, sinusitis, abscesses on the tonsils, rheumatic fever, scarlet fever, impairment of kidney function, and mastoiditis (inflammation of the bone behind the middle ear).

Streptococcal infections

Infections caused by the *Streptococcus* genus of bacteria. There are several classified groups within this genus, each one responsible for a different group of infections: group A *Streptococcus* and group B *Streptococcus* are the two principal groups responsible for many common infections, as well as severe illnesses. Group D *Streptococcus*, *Streptococcus pneumoniae*, and the viridans group of streptococci are three other groups within this genus of bacteria that can cause infection.

Group A *Streptococcus* usually causes mild illness and is responsible for the skin infection impetigo and most cases of pharyngitis, an inflammation of the part of the throat between the tonsils and the voice box. Strep throat is a common form of pharyngitis.

Infections that are termed invasive group A streptococcal disease include two potentially fatal infections. Streptococcal toxic shock syndrome causes a dramatic drop in blood pressure and organ failure. The second, necrotizing fasciitis (also known as "flesh-eating disease"), is a severe, painful inflammation of the fibrous sheath that encloses and connects the muscles, causing tissue death in surrounding muscle, fat, and skin. The invasive group A streptococcal diseases can be treated with many different antibiotics.

Surgery may be required to treat necrotizing fasciitis. Early treatment reduces the risk of death.

Group B streptococcal bacteria are the most common cause of life-threatening infections in newborns, including sepsis and MENINGITIS. They are also a common cause of newborn pneumonia. Group B bacteria in women can affect the urinary and genital tracts. Diagnosis of these infections is especially important to pregnant women because the infection can spread to the newborn during childbirth. Bladder infections, womb infections, and stillbirth can also occur in pregnant women with group B streptococcal infections. Among adults, blood infections, skin or soft tissue infections, and pneumonia are the most common diseases caused by group B streptococcal bacteria. Cultures of blood or spinal fluid are taken to identify these bacteria,

and the infections are successfully treated with antibiotics, usually penicillin.

Group D streptococcal bacteria can produce complications in the human digestive tract. Bacteria in this group are also associated with diseases or conditions including septicemia, endocarditis, and appendicitis. There are two divisions of group D streptococcal bacteria: one is a cause of urinary tract infections, and the other has proven to be resistant to many common antibiotics. Most group D streptococcal infections are successfully treated with antibiotics.

Streptococcus pneumoniae bacteria cause pneumonia, meningitis, and middle ear infections. *Streptococcus viridans* bacteria inhabit the mouth and are responsible for a significant percentage of tooth decay.

Stress

The physical and psychological reaction to a challenging or adverse stimulus. Stress is part of life, and some degree of it is necessary to maintain normal alertness. There are two basic types of stress: a short, intense experience known as the fight-or-flight response, and a less intense, longer-term response mobilizing the body's resources for endurance in meeting a challenge.

Stress can have physical causes or emotional causes. Stress can in turn trigger, exacerbate, or worsen a variety of physical diseases. Asthma and migraine headaches occur more often during periods of stress. Once the cause of stress is known, steps can be taken to reduce or manage it. See also POSTTRAUMATIC STRESS DISORDER.

Stress fracture

A small crack or break in a bone that is caused by repeated jarring or pressure to the bone. Stress fractures may occur in the feet and upper part of the shinbones as a result of overuse, improper form, or repetitive impact. The symptoms include gradually increasing pain and localized tenderness that are relieved with rest. Stress fractures are not usually visible on X rays, though they can be seen on a bone scan or MRI scan. Diagnosis may be made after a doctor's physical examination and the taking of a medical history that includes details of athletic or aerobic activities. The only treatment for stress fractures is a period of rest, usually for about 6 to 8 weeks, sufficient to allow complete healing.

Stress testing

See CARDIAC STRESS TESTING.

Stress ulcer

A type of peptic ulcer that may develop following a major illness, serious injury, burn, or shock. See PEPTIC ULCER DISEASE.

Stridor

Shrill wheezing and noisy, hoarse breathing that is most common in young children with a respiratory infection. Stridor occurs when their upper airways narrow, usually due to swelling and an increase in mucus from a respiratory tract infection. (However, narrowing can also occur without stridor.) Very often, the cause of stridor is CROUP, an inflammation of the larynx and trachea that makes breathing noisy and difficult.

A child whose stridor is caused by croup has a distinctive cough that sounds like the bark of a seal. A physician should see any young child with stridor as soon as possible.

Stroke

Damage to part of the brain caused by an interruption to its blood supply or leakage of blood outside of vessel walls.

There are several different causes of stroke. Most strokes are ischemic; that is, they are caused by reduced blood flow to the brain when blood vessels are blocked by a clot or become too narrow for blood to pass through. Brain cells are consequently deprived of oxygen and die. Strokes can also be hemorrhagic, which describes a stroke that occurs when blood vessels are damaged or ruptured (see HEMORRHAGE, CEREBRAL; HEMORRHAGE, SUBARACHNOID).

Stroke symptoms most commonly affect only one side of the body. Changes in brain function depend on the location and extent of injury to the brain. Symptoms may range from very mild abnormalities to severe problems such as paralysis. Common symptoms of a stroke are weakness, numbness, tingling, decreased sensation, cognitive decline, impaired vision, an inability to recognize or identify stimuli, problems with swallowing, loss of coordination, loss of memory, vertigo, personality changes, DEPRESSION, changes in consciousness (such as sleepiness, apathy, stupor, or loss of consciousness), paralysis, and lack of control over the bladder or bowels. Language difficulties following a stroke may include difficulty speaking or understanding speech, slurred speech, and problems with reading or writing. When the symptoms of a stroke last for less than 24 hours and are followed by complete recovery, the episode is known as a transient ischemic attack. This can be a warning signal of a future stroke.

A stroke is a life-threatening condition for which immediate emergency treatment is required. Hospitalization is necessary, and treatment may include lifesaving interventions and supportive measures. Diagnostic tests may include MRI (magnetic resonance imaging), CT (computed tomography) SCANNING, angiography, ultrasound, functional MRI, and magnetic resonance angiography (MRA). (See BRAIN IMAGING.) An ELECTROCARDIOGRAM (ECG) or echocardiogram may be used to detect any heart problem that may have contributed to the development of a stroke.

There is no cure for a stroke. The goal of treatment is to prevent the spread of the stroke, control symptoms, and maximize an affected person's ability to function. Surgery may be required to remove a blood clot or to repair damage. Possible medications include CORTICOSTEROIDS, diuretics, anticonvulsants, blood thinners, and analgesics. Outcomes vary widely. Even with prompt treatment, death may occur.

Stuffy nose

See RHINITIS.

Stuttering

A speech disorder characterized by speech that is interrupted by stopping and frequent repetition or prolongation of sounds. Tics, eye-blinks, or tremors of the lips and face may accompany stuttering.

Between the ages of 2 and 4, many children normally appear to stutter as they develop complex language skills. Most outgrow the trait around age 5 when they begin school. A child who continues to stutter after age 5 or a younger child whose stuttering significantly interferes with his or her speech should see a doctor. A hearing test may be recommended. A speech therapist may be asked to do an evaluation. See also SPEECH DISORDERS.

Stye

A small abscess occurring on the edge of the upper or lower eyelid or in the eye's corner. A stye, also called a hordeolum, is caused by a bacterial infection, which is usually due to staphylococcal bacteria, of the glands at the base of the eyelid. The surrounding area may be red and swollen and painful or itching. The stye may range from the size of a pinhead to the size of a pea. Styes usually drain without treatment.

Self-care of a stye may include applying warm, moist compresses. If a stye forms a whitehead without opening up or gets worse over time, it may need to be drained by a doctor.

Subarachnoid hemorrhage

See HEMORRHAGE, SUBARACHNOID.

Subclinical

A term describing a disease or condition that is in its early stages and is so mild that it produces no symptoms.

Subconjunctival hemorrhage

Bleeding under the external membrane of the eye (conjunctiva). A subconjunctival hemorrhage looks like a bright red patch on the white of the eye and produces no pain. Subconjunctival hemorrhages disappear on their own in 1 to 2 weeks and require no treatment unless bleeding elsewhere in the body is present.

People may have an increased risk for developing subconjunctival hemorrhage if they are taking aspirin or other blood thinners. Persons who develop subconjunctival hemorrhages without an identifiable cause should be checked for high blood pressure and possible bleeding disorders.

Subconscious

Mental activity that occurs just below the level of normal conscious awareness. In the psychoanalytic theory of Sigmund Freud, the subconscious level lies between the conscious and the unconscious.

Subcutaneous

A medical term meaning beneath the skin.

Subdural hemorrhage

Bleeding into the space between the two outer membranes (called the dura mater and the arachnoid) of the three membranes covering the brain. Blood leaking from the outermost membrane, the dura mater, is caused by ruptured blood vessels, usually small veins. The blood seeps slowly into the space between the two membranes and collects there, forming a blood clot, or subdural hematoma. Subdural hemorrhage is usually caused by a blow to the head or other head injury. Symptoms may include drowsiness, confusion, persistent headache, listlessness, imbalance, vomiting, and weakness or numbness on one side of the body. Over a few days or several weeks, these symptoms may appear. Prompt medical attention is essential.

Diagnostic tests may include a CT (computed tomography) scan or MRI (magnetic resonance imaging). If a subdural hematoma is detected, surgery to remove the clot may be recommended, depending on the size. If the clot is small, the blood is usually gradually absorbed and does not present further problems.

Subglottic stenosis

A condition produced by lesions that narrow the channel in the area of the lower throat directly below the vocal cords. The narrowing may be present at birth or appear later in life. When the condition is congenital, the symptoms may include noisy breathing, hoarseness, a barking cough, or a weak or unusual cry. If the lesion causes minimal obstruction, there may be no symptoms until an infection of the respiratory tract causes inflammation in the area and further narrows the air passage.

Some young children outgrow the condition by the time they reach 3 or 4 years of age. Others may require periodic dilation of the trachea with tracheal dilators. In some instances, tracheotomy (a surgical opening to insert a tube into the trachea to keep the airway open) may be necessary.

When subglottic stenosis is acquired, it is considered a more serious medical condition. It may be caused by infection, chemical irritation, or a foreign body in the throat, but it is most often caused by prolonged intubation beginning at birth or shortly thereafter. Tracheotomy and other surgical treatments are more often required when subglottic stenosis is acquired.

Subluxation

The partial dislocation of a joint. The most common joints affected by subluxation include the shoulder, elbow, kneecap, and the neck. See DISLOCATION, JOINT; SHOULDER, DISLOCATED.

Sucrose

A disaccharide sugar composed of two simple sugars (monosaccharides). Sucrose—better known as table sugar—is made of fructose and glucose. Like other sugars, sucrose is a carbohydrate that serves as a source of energy for the body. Whether eaten as pure sugar or as an additive to foods such as breakfast cereal or desserts, sucrose provides empty calories, meaning calories with no other nutrients.

Sudden infant death syndrome

The sudden and unexpected death of an apparently healthy infant while asleep; also called SIDS. SIDS is the leading cause of death of infants in the first year; the highest incidence comes between ages 1 and 4 months.

Placing a sleeping infant on his or her back is of primary importance to prevent SIDS, especially in the first 6 months of life when SIDS is most common. Contrary to popular belief, choking is no more common in infants lying on their backs than in those lying in another position. Tight-fitting, firm mattresses in cribs that meet current safety standards are recommended. A baby's head should not be covered while sleeping.

Home monitors are sometimes used by parents to monitor any sounds of choking or labored breathing, but medical research has not confirmed that monitors help prevent SIDS. An infant who stops breathing or turns blue requires emergency medical care.

Suffocation

Severe oxygen deprivation that leads to a life-threatening deficiency of oxygen in the blood. Episodes involving suffocation may injure the lungs and reduce the amount of oxygen delivered to vital organs. Permanent damage to the brain and heart may also occur. Survival generally depends on how quickly breathing and lung function are restored and how soon oxygen reaches the vital organs of the person who is suffocating.

Visible foreign objects obstructing airflow should be removed from the mouth or throat if possible. Mouth-to-mouth resuscitation should be started immediately for a person who does not appear to be breathing. If the person does not have a heartbeat, CARDIOPULMONARY RESUSCITATION (CPR) should be given.

A person who is suffocating should be taken to a hospital emergency department by trained emergency personnel. Resuscitation efforts should continue during travel to the hospital. In a hospital setting, efforts will be made to provide oxygen to the bloodstream.

Strategies such as mechanical hyperventilation to reduce cerebral swelling are used to prevent or minimize brain damage in a person who has survived an episode of suffocation.

Sugar

A carbohydrate that serves as a major source of energy for the body. When consumed in their natural forms, sugars are consumed along with fiber, minerals, and vitamins. (See also CAR-

BOHYDRATES.) Refined sugar (table sugar) provides calories with no other nutrients.

Suicide

A self-inflicted death that results from a person's intended, direct, and conscious effort to kill himself or herself. Suicide is particularly common among people with mental or emotional disorders, particularly DEPRESSION, MANIC-DEPRESSIVE ILLNESS, SCHIZOPHRENIA, and substance-abuse disorders. When an individual survives a suicide attempt, the initial need is for immediate medical care to treat the physical consequences such as a brain injury or damage to organs. Once the person's physical condition is stable, psychotherapy can begin.

Suicide prevention programs aim to help people who are contemplating suicide before they actually commit a lethal act. Suicide prevention hotlines, for example, are 24-hour telephone services in which trained volunteer counselors answer calls from people thinking about killing themselves.

Suicide, threatened

Direct or indirect threats or attempts to commit suicide. Many people who commit suicide talk about it before making an attempt. Because most suicides are preventable, suicide threats or attempts should always be taken seriously (see also DEPRESSION). Any attempted suicide must be treated as a medical emergency; help must be sought as quickly as possible.

Sulfa drugs

Antibiotics used to treat bacterial and some fungal infections. Sulfa drugs are medically known as sulfonamides.

Sulfa drugs work by interfering with the metabolism of bacteria, thereby killing them. Because sulfa drugs concentrate in the urine before being excreted, they are often used to treat urinary tract infections.

Ophthalmic sulfa drugs are used to treat infections of the eye. They are available as eye drops or ointments.

Sulfonamides and phenazopyridine are combination drugs made up of sulfa drugs and a urinary pain reliever, used to treat infections of the urinary tract and to relieve the associated pain, burning, and irritation.

Sulfonamides and trimethoprim are found in a combination used to treat several infections. Sulfadiazine and trimethoprim are used to treat urinary tract infections; the combination is also used to treat bronchitis, middle ear infection, and traveler's diarrhea.

Erythromycin and sulfisoxazole is a combination antibiotic used to treat ear infections in children.

Sulfonamides

See SULFA DRUGS.

Sun protection factor

A measurement of the effectiveness of sunscreen in blocking ultraviolet B (UVB) light. Protection from the sun is essential in the prevention of skin cancer and other skin damage. Doctors recommend sunscreens with a sun protection factor (SPF) of at least 15.

Sunburn

Tender, red, swollen skin due to overexposure to the ultraviolet rays of the sun. Sunburns can also be caused by sun lamps or tanning beds. Initial symptoms of pain and redness are often followed by itching and blistering.

Most sunburns respond to treatment. Applying cool compresses and taking cool baths can relieve some of the heat and discomfort. Helpful medications include over-the-counter oral ibuprofen for discomfort and 1 percent topical hydrocortisone cream. The person with sunburn must drink enough fluid to prevent dehydration.

To prevent sunburn, doctors recommend applying a sunscreen with a sun protection factor (SPF) of at least 15 before going outdoors, using a broad-spectrum sunscreen that provides ultraviolet A (UVA) and ultraviolet B (UVB) protection, and wearing protective clothing.

Sunscreens

Substances that block the effects of harmful rays from the sun. Sunscreens are lotions or oils spread on the skin to prevent sunburn, a cause of early wrinkling and skin cancer. Chemical sunscreens protect against sunburn by absorbing damaging ultraviolet (UV) light, while physical sunscreens protect against sunburn by reflecting, scattering, or blocking the UV rays.

The choice of a sunscreen involves selecting a product with a suitable SPF (sun protection factor) rating. The number of the rating is a comparison of the amount of time it takes to produce sunburn on protected skin to the amount of time needed to cause sunburn on unprotected skin. SPF 2 means that if it takes 10 minutes to produce sunburn on unprotected skin, it will take 20 minutes on skin protected with a lotion rated SPF 2. If the same person uses a product

rated SPF 15, it will take 150 minutes, or 2-½ hours, to develop that sunburn. Sunscreens rated SPF 15 or higher are recommended as effective protection, but people should limit their exposure to the sun even when using sunscreen protection.

Sunstroke

See HEAT STROKE.

Superinfection

A second infection that occurs in addition to a previous infection. Superinfections are often caused by a different microbial agent than the one that caused the first infection. This new infectious agent may have originated from a source outside the body or from within the body. If the initial infection was treated with antibiotics, the microorganism causing the superinfection may be resistant to the treatment used.

Superinfections can produce life-threatening illness. Influenza, for example, can progress to pneumonia from a superinfection of a more virulent strain of bacterial pneumonia, such as *Pseudomonas* pneumonia.

Suppository

A cylinder-shaped capsule containing a drug and an inactive material, such as cocoa butter, that dissolves once inside the body. Tiny suppositories are inserted into body cavities such as the rectum or vagina. Drugs administered by suppository include antifungal drugs, local anesthetics, laxatives, CORTICOSTEROIDS, antibiotics, and drugs to prevent vomiting and nausea.

Suprarenal glands

Another name for the adrenal glands.

Surfactant

A fatty substance that is secreted by cells lining the alveoli (the lungs' air sacs) and that coats the alveoli. Surfactant helps the air sacs expand, stretch, and maintain flexibility as a person inhales and exhales air. It also lowers the surface tension in the air sacs so pressure is evenly distributed among them.

Several diseases and disorders may contribute to inadequate production of surfactant and the consequent loss of elasticity in the lungs. The immature lungs of premature infants may not make enough surfactant to prevent collapse of the alveoli. This can lead to respiratory distress in the newborn. Corticosteroid therapy may be given to the mother during labor before delivery to increase the infant's surfactant levels. Surfactant may also be given directly to infants to reduce the risk of respiratory distress.

Surgery

The specialty in medicine that focuses on diseases, injuries, or conditions best managed or treated by procedures that involve opening, manipulating, and repairing a part of the body. Also, the word "surgery" is used to refer to a specific procedure or operation, such as bypass surgery. A surgeon is a physician specially trained to perform operations that involve the cutting of body tissue.

Suture

A surgical stitch to repair an incision, tear, or wound. Various materials are used for sutures, including silk, wire, and synthetic materials. Some sutures must be removed; others dissolve.

Swallowing difficulty

Problems with passing food or liquid from the mouth to the stomach, a condition medically termed dysphagia. Normally when a person eats or drinks, the chewed food or liquid is swallowed by a sequence of several mechanical events. The tongue pushes the material to the back of the throat where muscle contractions quickly move it along. It passes from the back of the throat to the esophagus, the tube connecting to the stomach. Muscles at the top and bottom of the esophagus open and close quickly to propel food into the stomach. Difficulty swallowing can be painful and disturbing. The causes of the condition vary; however, most are not medically serious and can usually be treated effectively.

There are generally two categories of conditions that may cause difficulty swallowing. The most common category, called esophageal dysphagia, is produced by a narrowing of the lower esophagus. It is often caused by stomach acid that backs up into the esophagus (see ESOPHAGEAL REFLUX), which can cause inflammation and scarring of the lower esophagus. Tumors or an abnormal band of tissue constricting the lower esophagus may also narrow the channel. The narrowing of the esophagus can create a sensation of food being lodged in the base of the throat and may be accompanied by pressure or pain in the chest.

Another condition, called oropharyngeal dysphagia, is the weakening of throat muscles that may be caused by age or by a stroke or neuromuscular disorder. The weak muscles in the throat make it difficult to pass food from the mouth into the throat, resulting in coughing or a choking sensation or the feeling that food is going down the windpipe. Other possible causes of difficulty swallowing include the formation of a small pouch, called a diverticulum, in the back of the throat or esophagus.

For some people, difficulty swallowing is not based on any structural impediments and may be triggered only by specific kinds of swallowing—such as attempts to swallow pills, tablets, or capsules. Stress can trigger muscle spasms or the sensation of a lump in the throat.

Tests to evaluate the condition may include a barium swallow, which involves drinking a barium solution to coat the inside of the esophagus so it can be imaged and observed. Endoscopy is a procedure for viewing the esophagus, which involves passing a thin, flexible tube called an endoscope down the throat.

If difficulty swallowing is determined to be caused by gastroesophageal reflux, medications to reduce stomach acid may be prescribed. If there are spasms of the esophagus, muscle relaxants may be prescribed. If the condition is caused by a narrowing of the esophagus, a procedure called esophageal dilatation may be performed via endoscope.

Swedish massage

A widely practiced form of massage therapy. Swedish, or European-style, massage features long, soothing strokes, kneading, pressing, and light pounding movements as a method to get blood moving and to loosen tight muscles.

Swimmer's ear

An infection in the ear canal, often caused by swimming in polluted water. The medical term for the condition is otitis externa. This condition usually begins with a blocked feeling and itching of the ear. These feelings may progress to intense pain caused by swelling of the tissue in the ear canal pressing against surrounding bone. There may also be tenderness just outside the ear canal, swollen glands in the neck, and a discharge from the ear, which may be a yellow, foul-smelling pus or a milky liquid. The discharge may block the ear canal and impair hearing.

Ear drops containing a corticosteroid and an antibiotic are usually prescribed to treat swimmer's ear. Fungus infections are generally treated with repeated cleaning and medications; rarely are antibiotics prescribed.

Swimmer's shoulder

Tendinitis or tears of the rotator cuff muscle caused by a strain on the shoulder joint produced by the constant motion of a person swimming. Swimmer's shoulder can be prevented by resting the shoulder regularly between swims and stopping a swim at the first sign of shoulder pain. Proper swimming technique may help prevent swimmer's shoulder. Weight lifting with lighter weights and increased repetitions may help condition the shoulders. Physical therapy is generally recommended for treating swimmer's shoulder. Cortisone injections into the area may be recommended.

Sympathectomy

The use of chemicals or surgery to deaden sympathetic nerves leading to a painful body part. The surgical division of sympathetic nerve pathways is most often performed to improve circulation for those with diseases such as ATHEROSCLEROSIS, claudication, Buerger disease, and Raynaud phenomenon.

Sympathetic nervous system

The division of the autonomic nervous system (which controls unconscious, automatic body functions) that directs the body's responses to stress or danger (the so-called fight-or-flight response). This activity consumes stored energy in the body. Typical sympathetic activity includes widening the air passages in the lungs, increasing heart rate and opening the pupils wider.

Symptom

An indication of a disorder, disease, or condition that is felt by a person before seeking medical evaluation or advice.

Syncope

A loss of consciousness caused by a temporary deficiency of blood supply to the brain. See FAINTING.

Syndrome

A number of symptoms occurring together that characterize a specific disease. Examples include carpal tunnel syndrome, Down syndrome, and Reye syndrome.

Synovectomy

The surgical removal of the membrane, called the synovial membrane, that lines the inside of a movable joint. Synovectomy is performed, usually through an arthroscope, to treat recurrent synovitis, which is an inflammation of the synovial membrane. The surgery may be performed to treat the early stages of RHEUMATOID ARTHRITIS when the synovial membrane of only one joint is badly inflamed.

Synovitis

An inflammation of the synovial membrane, a condition that often accompanies RHEUMATOID ARTHRITIS. The synovial membrane is a layer of cells that lines the inner surfaces of movable joints. The membrane produces the viscous fluid that bathes and lubricates the joint as it moves, thus helping the joint remain limber and flexible. When disease causes inflammation and swelling of the synovial membrane producing synovitis, the function of the joint is severely impaired. Treatment consists of bed rest, acetaminophen for pain, crutches, and possible traction.

Synovitis, toxic

A childhood disorder that causes inflammation in the hip joint. Toxic synovitis is most common between the ages of 3 and 6 and more frequently affects boys than girls. Although its exact cause remains unknown, toxic synovitis is most likely connected to a viral infection. A limp and hip pain (usually on one side of the body) are the most common symptoms of toxic synovitis. Often an affected child has a viral illness, such as a cold or flu. There may also be a low-grade fever of up to 101° F and associated pain in the knee or thigh of the affected leg. Symptoms usually disappear within 1 to 4 weeks.

The primary treatment for toxic synovitis is bed rest. A family physician or pediatrician may also prescribe anti-inflammatory drugs.

Synovium

A layer of cells that form a membrane to line the inner surfaces of a joint. The synovial membrane secretes synovial fluid that fills and lubricates the joint space. This fluid is essential to proper functioning of the joint and aids in the movement of joints, supplies nutrients and oxygen to the joint tissues, destroys foreign matter in the blood and tissues of a joint, and fights infection.

Syphilis

A serious bacterial infection and usually one of the sexually transmitted diseases (STDs) or, infrequently, a nonvenereal infection that may be transmitted to the newborn by the infected mother or acquired through a contaminated blood transfusion. Both forms of syphilis are spread by direct contact with the skin sore that usually occurs as a result of the infection.

Symptoms and diagnosis

There are three stages to syphilis. The first symptom of the primary stage is a single small sore called a chancre that is firm, round, and painless. The sore appears at the site where the bacterium entered the body. If the person does not get medical treatment during this stage, the infection progresses to a second stage.

Secondary stage syphilis occurs as a rash on one or more areas of the skin that appears when the chancre is fading or several weeks thereafter. This rash can take any one of a number of different forms.

The latent stage of untreated syphilis begins when the symptoms of the secondary stage disappear. There are no symptoms or signs of infection, but the bacteria can remain active in the body and begin to damage internal organs, including the brain, nerves, eyes, heart, blood vessels, liver, bones, and joints.

First- and second-stage syphilis infections are diagnosed by microscopic detection of the bacterium in infectious sores. An accurate and inexpensive blood test can also identify antibodies to the bacteria soon after the infection occurs. It is recommended that all pregnant women have this blood test. A person who has tested positive should refrain from sexual activity until the results of at least two follow-up blood tests are negative. Diagnosis of third-stage syphilis may require an examination of spinal fluid.

A baby's symptoms of syphilis may include skin sores, profuse nasal discharge that may be bloody, slimy patches in the mouth, inflammation of the bones in the arms and legs, a swollen liver, anemia, jaundice, or a small head. If untreated, an infected baby may have seizures and is at risk for retardation. The infection can also cause the baby's death.

Treatment and risk factors

If a person has had syphilis for less than a year, a single injection of penicillin will completely cure the infection. Repeated doses are required when a person has had the disease for longer than a year. Babies born with congenital syphilis require daily penicillin treatment for 10 days.

People who have been diagnosed with primary stage syphilis and are receiving medical treatment for the infection must abstain from sexual contact until the sores have healed. The person should also notify all sex partners to seek medical attention. A person who has had syphilis remains susceptible to reinfection if exposed again.

Systemic

Affecting organs and tissues throughout the body rather than a specific organ or body part. For example, systemic disorders such as diabetes mellitus or hypertension can affect the entire body.

Systemic lupus erythematosus (SLE)

See LUPUS ERYTHEMATOSUS, SYSTEMIC.

Systolic blood pressure

The force blood exerts against the arteries when the heart is contracting. Systolic blood pressure is the first of two numbers in a blood pressure measurement, for example, 120/80. The lower number is a measurement of diastolic blood pressure. See BLOOD PRESSURE.

T cell

A type of white blood cell that orchestrates the immune system's response to certain types of infection and to malignant cells; also known as a T lymphocyte. Developed in the thymus, T cells act directly to fight diseases or organisms, such as bacteria; to stimulate B lymphocytes or helper T cells; and to suppress some B lymphocyte functions.

A count of a person's T cells can be helpful in the diagnosis of immunodeficiency or lymphocytic diseases. Some diseases may result in greater than normal T-cell levels, while others are linked with lower than normal T-cell levels. AIDS (acquired immunodeficiency syndrome) is known to damage T-cells, and following T-cell levels is an important part of treatment planning and monitoring for people with HIV infections.

Tachycardia

An abnormally rapid heartbeat. In an adult, tachycardia refers to a heartbeat in which an abnormal focus in the upper region of the heart sporadically triggers a rapid heart rate. Symptoms include palpitations (uncomfortably rapid heartbeat), shortness of breath, chest pain, light-headedness, and fainting. Tachycardia is classified and treated by its point of origin in the heart (see TACHYCARDIA, PAROXYSMAL SUPRAVENTRICULAR; TACHYCARDIA, VENTRICULAR). Tachycardia may be caused by exercise, stress, congenital heart defects (those present at birth), CARDIOMYOPATHY (impaired heart muscle function), MYOCARDITIS (inflammation of the heart muscle), or kidney failure.

Tachycardia, paroxysmal supraventricular

An abnormally rapid heartbeat that begins in the upper region of the heart and occurs sporadically. In adults the heartbeat can rise to between 150 and 250 beats per minute; in children it may go even higher. The person is aware of an uncomfortably rapid heartbeat and may experience feelings of anxiety and doom, shortness of breath, chest tightness, fainting, and dizziness and may appear pale.

If symptoms are mild, using a technique called the Valsalva maneuver may interrupt the attack. This consists of holding the breath and straining or coughing while leaning the upper body forward. Splashing cold water on the face is helpful in some cases. Medications may be prescribed to control heart rhythm.

In some cases, applying an electric shock to the heart (see CARDIOVERSION) restores a normal heartbeat. A minimally invasive technique called radiofrequency ablation (see ABLATION THERAPY) can be used to alter the heart's electrical pathway permanently and prevent future episodes.

Tachycardia, ventricular

An abnormally fast heartbeat that originates in the ventricles (lower chambers) of the heart. Ventricular tachycardia requires urgent medical attention and may be life-threatening. Sustained ventricular tachycardia tends to deteriorate into ventricular fibrillation, in which the heart flutters rapidly and inefficiently rather than pumping. Ventricular fibrillation results in death within minutes unless a normal heart rhythm is restored.

In most cases ventricular tachycardia is associated with heart disease. It can also be caused by congenital heart defects (those present at birth),

CARDIOMYOPATHY (impaired heart muscle function), MYOCARDITIS (inflammation of the heart muscle), and kidney failure. Symptoms include shortness of breath, dizziness, fainting, chest pain, and palpitations (uncomfortably rapid heartbeat). In some cases, the heart will stop beating suddenly (cardiac arrest), and the person collapses.

The most common treatment for ventricular tachycardia is medication with drugs known as antiarrhythmics. If this approach fails, a normal heartbeat may be restored with cardioversion (an electrical shock to the chest). If episodes of ventricular tachycardia continue after cardioversion, a device called an implantable cardioverter defibrillator (ICD) can be placed surgically in the chest. See also ABLATION THERAPY.

Tachypnea

Abnormally fast, deep breathing. Tachypnea can upset the balance of gases in the blood by decreasing the levels of carbon dioxide in the bloodstream. Tachypnea can be a symptom of many diseases and disorders.

Stress, anxiety, overexertion, and nervousness are common causes of tachypnea. Diseases and conditions including ASTHMA, CROUP, PNEUMONIA, PULMONARY EMBOLISM, KETOACIDOSIS, PULMONARY FIBROSIS, CHRONIC OBSTRUCTIVE PULMONARY DISEASE (COPD), interstitial pneumonia, BRONCHIOLITIS, PNEUMONITIS caused by exposure to chemicals, PULMONARY EDEMA, and RESPIRATORY DISTRESS SYNDROME all can produce tachypnea. Severe pain or fear may produce tachypnea. It is sometimes associated with an overdose of medications.

Treatment is generally aimed at controlling the cause of the symptom. If there is a question as to what is causing tachypnea or if there is severe pain, medical attention should be promptly sought.

Talipes

The name for clubfoot. A congenital deformity in which the foot is twisted out of shape or position. Clubfoot may take many forms. A heel that is turned inward or outward can cause an individual to walk on the side of the foot; or a raised heel may cause a person to walk on his or her toes. The classic clubfoot is a deformity in which the heel is both raised and twisted. Treatment may include special shoes, braces, physical therapy, or surgery.

Talk therapy

Any method for treating mental or emotional problems that relies principally on verbal interaction between the person and a professional therapist. See GROUP THERAPY; PSYCHOTHERAPY.

Tall stature

Extreme growth in height that begins in childhood or adolescence; also known as gigantism. Unusually tall stature may be caused by the pituitary gland overproducing growth hormone, usually due to a pituitary tumor. The excess pituitary hormone causes all parts of the body to grow extremely large. The condition differs from acromegaly in that it occurs before full maturation and the bones of the arms and legs are affected.

If a child or adolescent seems to be growing at an exceptional rate, a doctor should be consulted. CT (computed tomography) SCANNING or MRI (magnetic resonance imaging) can detect and locate the presence of a pituitary tumor. Radiation therapy or surgery may be recommended to eliminate the tumor. Medications are sometimes prescribed to control a pituitary tumor. In most cases, treatment can restore normal levels of growth hormone.

Tamponade

Accumulation of so much fluid inside the pericardium (sac surrounding the heart) that it prevents the heart from pumping sufficient blood to the body. Tamponade is caused by pericarditis (inflammation of the pericardium), which can be caused by TUBERCULOSIS, a tumor, an ANEURYSM (ballooning) of the major artery that carries blood into the body, injury to the pericardium in surgery or in an accident, HYPOTHYROIDISM (an underactive thyroid gland), radiation therapy of the chest, systemic lupus erythematosus (see LUPUS ERYTHEMATOSUS, SYSTEMIC), or a viral infection.

Tamponade is a medical emergency that requires immediate attention. The excess fluid can be removed by means of a needle inserted through the chest wall into the pericardium. In some cases surgery to repair or remove the pericardium is required.

Tapeworm infestation

Infestation by worms that are carried in immature forms by animals, especially cattle, pigs, and fish. Tapeworm infestation occurs in humans after eating undercooked, infested animal products, such as beef, pork, and fish. The larvae enter a person's intestines and within 2 months grow into adult tapeworms that attach to the intestinal wall.

Symptoms of tapeworm infestation are generally mild. In some cases, segments of a tapeworm may detach and be eliminated in the feces. Rarely, fish tapeworms cause anemia. APPENDICITIS and inflammation of the bile duct, called CHOLANGITIS, can be complications of tapeworm infestation.

Diagnosis is accomplished by microscopic identification of the tapeworms' eggs from a stool culture. Anthelmintic medications can destroy or paralyze the worms, loosening their attachment to the intestinal wall and allowing them to be passed out of the body in the stool.

Tarsal tunnel syndrome

A condition produced by compression of a nerve that passes through a narrow passage behind the ankle bone located on the inner side, running down into the heel and foot. The cause may be an injury to the ankle, including a sprain or fracture, or a growth such as a cyst or tumor that presses against the nerve. Symptoms may include pain, numbness, tingling, or burning sensations anywhere along the bottom of the foot.

The discomforts of tarsal tunnel syndrome can be relieved by the use of orthotics, corticosteroid injections, or surgery to release the compressed nerve.

Tartar

The calcified bacterial plaque (see PLAQUE, DENTAL) that forms from mineral salts in the saliva and accumulates on and adheres to the surfaces of the crowns and roots of the teeth.

Taste

One of the five senses. Taste belongs to the body's chemical sensing system. It is closely related to smell, for flavors are recognized mainly through the sense of smell. There are approximately 9,000 taste buds (tiny clusters of cells that sense flavors from foods) on the surface of the tongue. Taste buds in different parts of the tongue sense the four basic tastes: salty, sweet, bitter, and sour.

Tattooing

Permanent discoloration and inscriptions from pigment applied to the skin and then forced into the skin with needles. Many health-related risks are associated with unsanitary tattooing methods, including both localized infection and blood-borne illnesses such as HEPATITIS and HIV (human immunodeficiency virus). Today the preferred method of tattoo removal is laser surgery, which removes tattoos without scarring.

Tay-Sachs disease

A progressive neurological genetic disorder characterized by the accumulation of a fatty substance in the nerve cells of the brain. The most common form of the disease affects infants, who appear healthy at birth and seem to develop normally for the first few months of life. However, they lack the enzyme hexosaminidase A (hex A), which is necessary for the ongoing breakdown of a substance called ganglioside GM2 and other fatty substances in the brain and nerve cells. As their nerve cells gradually become clogged with fatty material, babies with Tay-Sachs disease gradually become unable to smile, crawl, or turn over, and they lose the ability to grasp or reach with their hands. Eventually they become deaf, blind, and unable to swallow. Their muscles weaken and become paralyzed. There is no cure for Tay-Sachs disease. Treatment is limited to making the child as comfortable as possible. Children with Tay-Sachs disease usually die by age 5. Tay-Sachs disease occurs most frequently among descendents of central and eastern European (Ashkenazi) Jews.

Potential parents can have a blood test to measure the quantity of hex A in their blood. Prenatal diagnosis of Tay-Sachs disease can be accomplished using either AMNIOCENTESIS or chorionic villus sampling (see CHORIONIC VILLI).

TB

See TUBERCULOSIS.

Tear duct, blocked

Blockage or narrowing of the tube that normally drains tears from a child's eyes. Many babies are born with the condition, usually because the membrane covering the ducts at birth fails to disappear. In older babies and children, blocked tear ducts most often result from an inflammation such as CONJUNCTIVITIS. In newborns who have blocked tear ducts, tears flow heavily from the eyes rather than draining normally through ducts into the nose and throat. There may also be some discharge of mucus or pus. When tear duct obstruction is caused by infection, there may be redness, pain, and swelling in the eyes, in addition to excessive tears.

If a bacterial infection has blocked the child's tear ducts, the pediatrician will prescribe an antibiotic. Otherwise, massaging the lower eyelid and clearing away discharge generally can relieve the problem.

Blocked tear ducts in newborns usually clear up on their own or with massage by age 1. When blockages fail to respond to treatment, surgery may be necessary.

Tears

A liquid that lubricates the eyes, keeps them clean and moist, and helps prevent infection. The majority of tears are produced in the lacrimal glands, which are located in the upper eyelids, and other glands in the conjunctiva, and they spread across the eye in a film with each blink. Excess tears drain away through a duct that leads to the nose. Inadequate tear production results in DRY EYE; excess production or inadequate drainage, in tearing.

Teeth

Hard structures set into the jaw and upper mouth that chew food and help form speech sounds. Each tooth has three parts. The visible crown extends up from the line of the gum. The root, which represents most of the tooth's bulk, is bound into the bone by a tough, fibrous membrane. The neck is the narrow region between the crown and root. The surface of the crown is covered with enamel, which is the hardest substance in the body and insensitive to touch or pain. Below the enamel lies the main part of the tooth called the dentin, which is less hard than the enamel and sensitive. The core of the crown, neck, and root is filled with a fibrous pulp richly supplied with

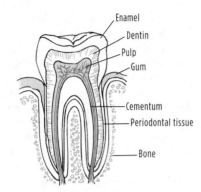

Structure of a tooth

Enamel covers the surface of the tooth to the gum line. Dentin is the underlying hard part of the tooth, extending all the way through the root. It is covered below the gum by cementum, a substance harder than bone but softer than enamel. Under the dentin, the pulp contains nerves and blood vessels.

nerves and blood vessels through the root canal. The tooth is partially encased in a bony socket. See also DENTAL EXAMINATION.

Teeth, care of

Caring for the teeth involves brushing the teeth at least twice daily with a fluoride toothpaste, and dental flossing at least once a day using the technique recommended by a dentist or dental hygienist.

Teething

The gradual emergence of teeth in a baby or young child. Baby teeth start breaking through the gums at between 5 and 9 months of age. The two bottom front teeth usually come in first. Although the rate at which children teethe varies greatly, most have all 20 baby teeth by the age of 2-1/2. See also TOOTH ERUPTION.

Temperature

The degree of heat in the body. A normal body temperature is about 98.6°F (37.0°C) but can range anywhere from 97.8°F (36.5°C) to 99.0°F (37.2°C). See also FEVER.

Temporal arteritis

See ARTERITIS, GIANT CELL.

Temporal lobe epilepsy

See EPILEPSY, TEMPORAL LOBE.

Temporomandibular joint disorder (TMJ)

Also known as TMJ syndrome; see CLICKING JAW.

Tendinitis

The painful inflammation of the strong fibrous structures, called tendons, that connect muscles to bones. Tendinitis is usually caused by the tendon being irritated by overuse or injury or injured by repeated or prolonged pressure that produces friction between the tendon and bone tissue. Tendinitis most commonly occurs in joints such as the ankle, knee, and shoulder. The symptoms include localized tenderness, possible swelling, and pain during an increased pace of activity. Diagnosis is made on the basis of physical examination and occasionally an MRI (magnetic resonance imaging). Treatment may include rest, support, elevating and icing the affected area after the activity, physical therapy, and the use of NONSTEROIDAL ANTI-INFLAMMATORY DRUGS (NSAIDs) to relieve pain and control inflammation and swelling. In serious cases, cortisone injections may provide relief.

Tendon

A fibrous cord that anchors a muscle in place, often to a bone or to cartilage. Tendons are strong but flexible connective tissue. They are made of dense masses of parallel elastic fibers, a structure that allows them to stretch in order to protect the muscles and ligaments from strain. Contraction of the muscle causes the tendon to pull on the bone or tendon to which it is attached, moving that part of the body. The tendons in the hands, wrists, and feet are enclosed in fibrous capsules and bathed in a fluid that helps the tendons move smoothly.

Tendon release

A surgical procedure for treating TRIGGER FINGER or other conditions involving restraint or binding of a tendon and its associated tissues. Tendon release is generally considered only when immobile joints are unresponsive to less invasive treatments, such as taking the NONSTEROIDAL ANTI-INFLAMMATORY DRUGS (NSAIDs) aspirin or ibuprofen.

Tendon repair

The surgical reattachment of tendons that have been completely torn apart or severed as a result of excessive physical effort or injury. Tendon repair should be performed as soon as possible for the best results.

Tennis elbow

An overuse sports injury (see SPORTS INJURIES) resulting in inflammation, strain, or minor tears in the tendons of the forearm muscles near the elbow. Tennis elbow is caused by repeated stress on this area of the arm, particularly the stress produced by sudden twisting movements of the forearm during a backhand tennis swing. The condition is also seen in electricians and carpenters. Extensor muscles in the forearm are attached to tendons that connect to the outer bump of the elbow. The usual symptoms are tenderness when pressure is placed on the outer elbow, along with pain felt on the outer, bony bump of the elbow joint. Aching in the muscles at the outer side of the forearm often accompanies the pain in the soft tissues surrounding the elbow joint. Attempting to grasp objects may intensify the pain, and sometimes it becomes difficult to fully straighten the elbow.

When tennis elbow is mild, the best treatment may be limiting or stopping entirely activity using that arm until the pain goes away. Anti-inflammatory medications and ice may help relieve symptoms. Physical therapy exercises may be recommended to help strengthen surrounding muscles. In some cases, corticosteroid injections or surgery may be considered.

Tenolysis

The surgical procedure for releasing a tendon from surrounding adhesions. When a tendon is restricted, normal mobility is impaired. Tenolysis restores this function.

Tenosynovitis

An inflammation of the sheath of tissue and membrane that surrounds a tendon and aids in moving joints. Tenosynovitis often accompanies tendinitis. Most commonly affected are the tendons connecting muscles to bones in the shoulder, elbow, wrist, fingers, hip, knee, or ankle. It is caused by injury or inflammation of a tendon or, in rare cases, by infection.

Tenosynovitis is sometimes associated with rheumatoid arthritis, and in some cases, the cause is unknown. The condition may be caused by a bacterial infection, especially if there has been a puncture wound. This is a more medically serious form of tenosynovitis. If a joint feels hot as well as inflamed, emergency care should be sought, because this is an indication of infectious involvement in the SYNOVIUM of the joint. The infection can cause permanent impairment to the affected tissues if not treated immediately with antibiotics.

Sometimes the inflammation causes the affected tissues to become visibly swollen as a result of fluid accumulation. There may be localized tenderness, difficulty moving a joint or straightening a finger, and severe or disabling pain with passive movement. There may be a crackling sound when the affected joint is moved.

The first line of treatment in the absence of infection is generally rest and stopping the activity that caused tenosynovitis. A resumption in activity tends to cause the condition to return. Ice may be applied, and painkilling and anti-inflammatory medications may become necessary to control pain and inflammation. If the symptoms are in the foot, a short-leg walking cast for 4 to 6 weeks may be helpful. In some cases, when more conservative approaches have failed, injections of a corticosteroid or surgery may be considered.

TENS

Transcutaneous electrical nerve stimulation. TENS is a type of therapy for pain relief. It uses electrical impulses to interfere with pain signals to the brain. With this technique, small electrodes are placed on an area where there is pain to transmit electrical impulses. TENS can be used along with other pain management strategies to relieve back or neck pain, arthritis pain, a pinched nerve, FIBROMYALGIA, headache, menstrual cramps, SCIATICA, or SHINGLES. Transcutaneous electrical nerve stimulation must be prescribed by a doctor.

Teratogen

An agent or factor that produces abnormalities or deformities in a fetus. Teratogens usually fall into three categories: drugs and chemical agents; infectious agents; and radiation. Teratogens have different effects, depending on the stage of the pregnancy.

Teratoma

An abnormal growth, usually found in an ovary or testicle, formed from tissue that is not normally found in those organs. Teratomas can be benign or malignant and can consist of a mixture of tissues including cells from the epithelium, bone, hair, teeth, cartilage, or muscle.

Terminal care

Care for a person with a limited time left to live. In terminal care, the emphasis shifts from finding a cure to maximizing the quality of the person's remaining life. Medical treatment consists primarily of relieving symptoms and pain. See also HOSPICE.

Termination of pregnancy

See ABORTION, ELECTIVE.

Testicle

One of the pair of oval glands that produce sperm, the male reproductive cells, and the male sex hormone testosterone. Also called testes, the testicles are located in the groin in a sac of skin called the scrotum. The male hormones secreted in the testicles, including testosterone, influence male characteristics, such as facial hair and a lower voice, sexual desire, and sexual function. These secretions are known collectively as androgen hormones. Muscle fibers originating from the groin surround the testicles. See REPRODUCTIVE SYSTEM, MALE.

Testicle self-examination

A procedure for a man or boy to check his own testicles for cancer. Since testicular cancer often develops without symptoms, regular self-examination is a preventive measure that can catch the disease early, when it is most curable. (See TESTICLE, CANCER OF THE.) Physicians recommend that males between the ages of 15 and 40 examine their testicles every month. The man or boy should seek medical attention if an area feels bumpy and hard or if one of the testicles is swollen. Pain and swelling in the scrotum can indicate an infection.

Testicle, cancer of the

Also called testicular cancer; a malignant tumor that begins in the testicle. Testicular cancer is rare, but it is the most common malignancy in men between 18 and 34 years old. The disease is highly curable, particularly when detected and treated early.

Symptoms and types

The most common sign of testicular cancer is painless enlargement of the testicle. The enlargement occurs gradually and may in time cause a sensation of heaviness or aching in the testicle and scrotum. Often, a hard lump can be felt. If the cancer has spread beyond the testicle, there may be pain in the back or discomfort in the abdomen. Certain rare testicular cancers can cause enlargement of breast tissue.

A number of different kinds of malignant tumors can appear in the testicle. The vast majority are germ cell tumors, so named because they arise in the tissues that produce the sperm, or germ cells. Seminomas are the most common type of germ cell tumor. The others are known as nonseminomas. Malignancies can also begin in the supportive tissues of the testicle; these tumors are known as stromal tumors. Stromal tumors are much less common than germ cell tumors. In men older than age 50, cancer is less likely to originate in the testicle than to have spread from elsewhere in the body.

Diagnosis and treatment

In addition to a physical examination, a doctor suspecting a man has testicular cancer may prescribe an ultrasound examination, which visualizes the organ by bouncing sound waves off it. The blood may also be tested to screen for certain proteins and other substances that can indicate cancer. If the lump looks and feels suspicious, the next step is to remove it and examine the tissue for cancer cells in the laboratory. In most cases, the entire testicle along with the tubule (vas deferens) that carries sperm cells from the testicle to the prostate gland is removed through an incision in the groin and then examined in the laboratory.

Once a tumor of the testicle has been identified as cancer, follow-up tests are performed to see if the disease has spread. CT (computed tomography) SCANNING involves the use of rotating X rays to create a series of images from many angles to examine the lymph nodes in the groin and abdomen.

Follow-up treatment after removal of the testicle depends on the type of cancer and the degree to which it has spread. Early-stage cancer is usually treated with postsurgical radiation of the lymph nodes in the groin and the back of the abdomen. Seminomas are very sensitive to X rays; the dose of radiation needed to kill them is lower than for most other cancers.

Complications depend on treatment. When only one testicle is removed, a man retains his ability to have erections and to father children. Radiation and chemotherapy produce temporary infertility; fertility usually returns within 2 years after treatment.

Testicle, ectopic

A testicle that has strayed from the normal path of descent during development and lies in an abnormal position outside the scrotum. This condition differs from cryptorchidism, in which the testicle stops somewhere along the path of normal descent. An ectopic testicle is most often found under the skin in the groin.

An ectopic testicle is usually treated surgically. The testicle and its blood supply are moved into the scrotum; more than one surgery may be needed to position the testicle correctly. In some cases, the ectopic testicle dies and must be removed.

Testicle, pain in the

Aches or pains that begin in the testicles, the glands contained within the scrotum, which is the skin-covered pouch between the legs in a man. Sometimes, the discomfort radiates into the lower abdomen. Usually such aches and pains are not cause for alarm. However, severe pain from one side that comes on suddenly, particularly if accompanied by nausea or vomiting, requires immediate medical attention. It can arise from torsion of the testicle, a condition in which the normal blood supply to the testicle is cut off. Untreated torsion can cause the testicle to die and may require it to be removed. Other causes of pain in the testicle are injury, dilated veins in the scrotum, hernia, or a stone in the lower end of the tube connecting the kidney to the bladder. Cancer is rarely a cause of pain in the testicle.

Testicle, retractile

A phenomenon found among boys before puberty in which one or both testicles are pulled up out of the scrotum during cold weather, excitement, or physical activity. The condition requires no treatment since a retractile testicle moves into normal position during puberty.

Testicle, torsion of the

A twisting of the testicle on its blood supply, which blocks blood flow. Torsion usually affects only one testicle, and it typically causes sudden, severe pain accompanied by nausea and vomiting. The testicle quickly swells, the skin of the scrotum (the pouch between the legs containing the testicles) turns red, and the pain radiates into the abdomen. The condition is most common in adolescents and young men between 12 and 20 years of age. Immediate medical treatment is needed to prevent the death of the tissues in the testicles. In most cases, surgery is required to untwist the testicle and to attach it with surgical stitches to the wall of the scrotum; this prevents the condition from occurring again.

Testicle, undescended

Failure of one or both testicles to descend into the scrotum (the protective pouch that hangs behind the penis) before birth. Known as cryptorchidism, the condition is common in premature infants and also occurs in some full-term babies. In most cases, the testicles descend into the scrotum within the first 3 months of life, and no treatment is required.

If cryptorchidism does not resolve on its own, surgery may be needed to locate the undescended testicle and move it into the scrotum. Treatment is usually successful. Untreated cryptorchidism is likely to leave the man unable to father children in adulthood.

Testosterone

The primary male reproductive hormone, one of the androgen hormones, produced primarily within the cells inside the testicles. Testosterone circulates within the bloodstream and is critically important to the maintenance of male reproductive and sexual development and function. It has an important role in a man's bone and muscle growth, as well as in typical male physical characteristics, including facial hair, deepening of the voice, and increased muscle mass.

Tetanus

A bacterial disease that affects the nervous system. Tetanus, sometimes called lockjaw, is now a rare disease because of widespread immunization. The bacteria that cause the disease are found throughout the environment and are often seen in soil contaminated with animal manure. A person can contract tetanus by bacterial contamination of an open wound on the skin or mucous membrane. When the bacterium, *Clostridium tetani*, contaminates a wound, it produces a toxin called tetanospasmin, which attaches to nerves around the wound area. Inside the nerves, the toxin is transported to the brain or spinal cord, interfering with the normal activity of the nerves, especially those that signal muscle activity.

A cut or puncture injury susceptible to tetanus infection may be too minor to warrant medical evaluation, even after it has been contaminated. Symptoms of tetanus usually appear within 3 to 8 days after contamination, but may take as long as 3 weeks. More heavily contaminated wounds tend to produce earlier symptoms. Typically, the first sign of tetanus is muscular stiffness of the jaw, a symptom called trismus, which is why the disease is known as lockjaw. The jaw stiffness is often followed by stiffness of the neck, difficulty swallowing or chewing, rigidity of abdominal muscles, spasms, profuse perspiration, and fever.

Complications from untreated tetanus can be severe, including spasm of the vocal cords or respiratory muscles that interferes with breathing, hypertension, abnormal heart rate, coma, systemic infection, clotting in the blood vessels of the lungs, pneumonia, and, ultimately, death. Mortality rates are highest among young children, people who are older, and intravenous drug abusers.

If a person has a wound and has not had a tetanus toxoid booster within the previous 10 years, a single booster injection is given on the day the injury occurred, when possible. A booster may also be given if a wound is at high risk for tetanus and the last booster was administered more than 5 years before infection. If a person has not been previously immunized and has a high-risk wound, he or she may be given tetanus immune globulin.

Tetanus infections are usually treated in an intensive care unit of a hospital. Antibiotics are given to destroy the tetanus bacteria, and antitoxin is administered to neutralize the toxin produced by the bacteria.

Tetany

An abnormal condition characterized by spasms of the arm and leg muscles. Tetany, a potentially life-threatening condition, is caused by a severe lowering in the calcium level, which may be due to a lack of VITAMIN D, HYPO-PARATHYROIDISM (underactivity of the parathyroid glands), alkalosis (an abnormal state caused by excessive vomiting, hyperventilation, exposure to high altitudes), or the ingestion of alkaline salts. Tetany can also cause spasms of the larynx, resulting in breathing difficulties. Acute tetany may lead to respiratory obstruction requiring a tracheostomy.

Tetracyclines

A class of antibiotics used to treat bacterial infections. Tetracyclines are used for many diseases, including ROCKY MOUNTAIN SPOTTED FEVER,

typhus fever, and tick fevers; upper respiratory infections; PNEUMONIA; pelvic infection, GONORRHEA, and URINARY TRACT INFECTIONS. Tetracyclines are also used to treat severe acne; TRACHOMA, a chronic eye infection; and CONJUNCTIVITIS ("pink eye"). Tetracyclines are often prescribed for people who are allergic to penicillin. A woman who is pregnant should not take tetracycline. There are several different types of tetracyclines, including doxycycline, minocycline, oxytetracycline, and tetracycline.

Tetralogy of Fallot

A congenital defect of the heart, characterized by four abnormalities that result in inadequately oxygenated blood being pumped throughout the body.

Tetralogy of Fallot involves four defects in the structure of the heart: ventricular septal defect (a hole in the wall between the right and left ventricles), narrowing of the pulmonary valve, displaced aorta, and a thickening of the wall of the right ventricle.

Babies born with the defect have various symptoms, including difficulty feeding; failure to gain weight; slow growth; poor general development; bluish skin color, especially when agitated; and shortness of breath made worse by exercise.

Treatment includes surgery to correct the defects in the heart, usually between ages 3 and 5. In severe cases, surgery may be performed earlier.

Thalassemia

A group of genetic blood disorders that affect the production of one of the protein chains that forms the hemoglobin molecule. Thalassemia exists in two types—alpha thalassemia and beta thalassemia—each of which is subdivided into three subtypes. Thalassemia minor, also called trait, is associated with a very mild anemia that cannot be corrected with iron supplements but has no other symptoms. Thalassemia intermedia causes moderately severe hemolytic anemia (see ANEMIA, HEMOLYTIC) and requires regular medical care and occasional blood transfusions. Thalassemia major is a serious disease characterized by the inability to create enough normal hemoglobin to survive, calling for regular blood transfusions.

Alpha thalassemia affects the formation of fetal and adult hemoglobin. Infants with alpha thalassemia major or intermedia suffer severe oxygen deprivation and are born with massive fluid accumulation.

Beta thalassemia minor, or trait, is associated only with mild incurable anemia, which may cause slight fatigue. A person with thalassemia trait is not at risk for developing a more severe form of the disease.

Beta thalassemia major is characterized by some or all of the following signs and symptoms: severe anemia; jaundice; enlarged spleen; fatigue; listlessness; reduced appetite; enlarged, fragile bones; facial malformations; growth problems; and increased susceptibility to infection. Children with untreated thalassemia major will die of severe anemia.

People with thalassemia major require blood transfusions every 3 to 4 weeks to survive, while those with thalassemia intermedia may need only occasional transfusions. A side effect of regular transfusions is a buildup of excess iron in the organs of the body. Excess iron buildup is treated with deferoxamine, a medica-

tion that binds with iron and allows it to be excreted. The only cure for thalassemia is a bone marrow transplant.

Thallium

A radioisotope used in nuclear medicine that emits gamma rays and closely resembles potassium. Thallium 201 is used as a diagnostic imaging aid to evaluate the blood flow and viability of the heart muscle. When injected intravenously into the person to be scanned, the radioisotope enters healthy tissue quickly. Areas with poor blood flow and decreased blood supply, as well as tissue that has died because of insufficient blood supply, take up the thallium much more slowly and show up as "cold spots" on a nuclear scan.

Therapy

See PSYCHOTHERAPY.

Thiamin

A nutrient that is essential for energy production from carbohydrates and for nerve and muscle function. See VITAMIN B.

Thiazolidinediones

A class of oral drugs for the treatment of DIABETES MELLITUS, TYPE 2. They work by increasing the sensitivity of tissues to insulin. They restore the blood sugar level to normal without producing low blood sugar. Examples of this drug type include pioglitazone HCl and rosiglitazone maleate.

Thoracentesis

A procedure in which fluid is removed from the space around the lungs; also known as a pleural tap. Thoracentesis is performed to relieve the symptoms associated with fluid accumulation and to analyze the fluid for diagnostic purposes. In the procedure, which is performed under local anesthesia, the doctor uses a fine needle to draw out the fluid.

Thoracic outlet syndrome

A complex condition characterized by pain and abnormal sensations in the hand, arm, shoulder, or neck. The thoracic outlet is located at the top of the rib cage, between the chest and neck. Compression of the nerves, veins, or arteries in this area may cause pain, numbness, tingling, muscular weakness, and atrophy. Inadequate blood flow may lead to bluish discoloration and swelling in the arm and hand. An affected person can also develop RAYNAUD DISEASE. Thoracic outlet syndrome may be caused by poor posture or anatomical abnormalities. The primary treatment is physical therapy. In some cases, surgery is necessary to correct the problem.

Thoracotomy

A surgical procedure to open the chest (thorax). A thoracotomy is usually performed to allow a surgeon to operate on a diseased heart, lung, or other chest cavity organ.

Thorax

The medical name for the chest, the region of the body that lies between the neck and the diaphragm muscle and is encased by the ribs. The main structures in the thorax are the heart, lungs, esophagus, aorta, and pulmonary arteries.

Thrill

A vibration felt by doctors when examining the chest by touch (palpation). Thrill can be a sign of abnormal blood flow in the heart caused by a defective valve.

Throat

The pharynx; muscular, membrane-lined passage that carries air from the nose to the trachea (windpipe) and food from the mouth to the esophagus. The throat is subdivided into the nasopharynx, (which lies above the soft palate), the oropharynx (between the soft palate and larynx), and laryngopharynx (which is behind the larynx and is continuous with the esophagus).

Throat cancer

A malignant tumor originating in the cells that cover the mucous membrane lining the throat. Throat cancer is also known as cancer of the pharynx. This cancer tends to penetrate the mucous membrane and muscle layers, spreading into surrounding tissue as it grows. It can spread to lymph nodes (see LYMPH NODE) in the neck and into the bloodstream and be carried to the lungs and other organs. Cancers near the mouth tend to remain localized unless they are not successfully treated. Cancers near the nose and in the lower throat may spread early before symptoms appear.

A tumor growing in the pharynx can interfere with hearing, smell, taste, speech, and swallowing. Symptoms may include a mild, persistent sore throat or cold lasting for longer than 2 weeks, persistent cough, sudden hoarseness, or a change in the sound of the voice. The person may also experience difficulty swallowing, painful swallowing, coughing up blood with phlegm, blood in the saliva, a white patch in the mouth, ear pain or a blocked feeling in the ear, a hard lump in the throat or a lymph node in the neck, and swollen lymph nodes in the neck. A tumor located directly behind the nose may cause partial hearing loss, nasal obstruction, nosebleeds, ringing in the ears, and pain or pressure in the middle ear.

Abnormal growths in the throat may be visible to a doctor using mirrors or a lighted viewing tube, called a fiberoptic scope. All lesions, growths, or tumors are biopsied, or a test for the EPSTEIN-BARR VIRUS is done. If cancer is present, imaging scans can help establish how widespread it is. If the cancer has not spread beyond the lymph nodes, surgery can remove the abnormal growth entirely, and the cancer will go into remission.

If the cancer is in the area of the throat behind the nose, the person typically receives high-dose radiation to the head and neck, possibly after chemotherapy to shrink the tumors. If the growths are small and in the area of the throat near the mouth, they may be treated with radiation alone to avoid disfigurement and other complications. If the cancer does not respond to radiation treatments, surgery may become necessary. Tumors in the lower throat usually require surgery.

Laser surgery may be used to treat some throat cancers. This approach may be less risky and offer greater preservation of voice function and swallowing ability.

Thrombectomy

A surgical procedure performed with a catheter to remove a thrombus (blood clot) that has formed in a blood vessel and is blocking blood flow through it.

Thrombocytopenia

A shortage of platelets, blood cells that have a key role in clotting. Symptoms include profuse blood loss after injury or surgery, a measleslike rash known as purpura (usually on the lower legs), nosebleeds, swollen joints, blood in vomit or feces, and heavy menstrual flow. Widespread bleeding, particularly in the digestive system or brain, can be life-threatening.

Thrombocytopenia is classified as idiopathic or secondary. Idiopathic thrombocytopenia usually arises from the body producing antibodies against its own platelets, which then attack and destroy them. Secondary thrombocytopenia is a complication of another disease. Possible causes include viral or bacterial infections, systemic lupus erythematosus, chronic lymphocytic leukemia, sarcoidosis, cancer of the ovary, and some medications (see LEUKEMIA, CHRONIC LYMPHOCYTIC; LUPUS ERYTHEMATOSUS, SYSTEMIC; OVARY, CANCER OF THE; SARCOIDOSIS).

Thrombocytopenia is a common, temporary complication of bone marrow transplant (see BONE MARROW TRANSPLANT, ALLOGENEIC; BONE MARROW TRANSPLANT, AUTOLOGOUS).

In children, idiopathic thrombocytopenia often resolves without treatment. In adults, the idiopathic form of the disease can be treated with CORTICOSTEROIDS (prednisone) or thrombopoietin, a substance that promotes the production of platelets. When medication does not work, the spleen may be removed surgically to reduce bleeding. Secondary thrombocytopenia is treated with therapy aimed at the underlying disease or by changing medication. People who have undergone a bone marrow transplant receive platelet transfusions until platelet production by the transplanted marrow becomes sufficient.

Thrombocytosis

An increase in platelets, the blood elements that have a key role in clotting. In most cases, thrombocytosis is a physiological reaction to another condition, such as cancer, surgery (typically splenectomy), trauma or injury, severe infection, inflammatory disorders such as RHEUMATOID ARTHRITIS, iron-deficiency anemia (see ANEMIA, IRON-DEFICIENCY), or recovery from THROMBOCYTOPENIA (an abnormally low number of platelets). This kind of reactive thrombocytosis is usually temporary, and the person is free of symptoms. In older patients, however, it may lead to blood clots that precipitate a heart attack or stroke. See MYELOPROLIFERATIVE DISORDERS for more information about the disease and its treatment.

Thromboembolism

Blockage (embolism) of a blood vessel by a thrombus (blood clot) that has formed elsewhere in the body and has been carried through the bloodstream.

Thrombolytic drugs

Drugs used to dissolve blood clots and to open blood vessels. Thrombolytic drugs are used in the treatment of blood clots within blood vessels in the heart and lungs and in clotting associated with hip replacement. Thrombolytic drugs are also used to prevent clotting when tubes are placed in the body. If given within 3 to 6 hours after a heart attack, the drugs help to increase survival.

Thrombophlebitis

Inflammation of a vein because of the formation of a blood clot (thrombus); also known as phlebitis. Thrombophlebitis usually develops in the veins of the legs and less commonly in the arms. If it affects the superficial veins, it can be treated with medications, such as analgesics to stop pain and anti-inflammatory drugs to reduce swelling. Support stockings help in some cases, as do elevating the leg and applying warm compresses. Thrombophlebitis affecting a deep vein is a more serious condition known as deep vein thrombosis. See THROMBOSIS, DEEP VEIN.

Thrombosis

The formation or presence of a blood clot inside a cavity of the heart or a blood vessel.

Thrombosis, deep vein

A blood clot in a large vein. Deep vein thrombosis usually occurs in the leg, less often in the arm or pelvic veins. The blood clot blocks the vein and prevents the flow of blood back to the heart, causing the blood to back up and resulting in swelling and pain or tenderness. There is a risk that a portion of the blood clot can break free, travel through the bloodstream, and lodge in the lungs, brain, heart, or other organ, where it can cause serious damage and even death. In most cases, deep vein thrombosis resolves through natural healing, as the blood clot dissolves and normal blood flow is restored. Hospitalization for initial treatment is usually required. Anticoagulants (such as heparin or warfarin) or antiplatelet drugs (such as aspirin) are used to prevent further clotting and prevent clots from traveling through the bloodstream.

Thrombus

A blood clot that forms within a cavity of the heart or a blood vessel.

Thrush

A yeast infection of the moist surfaces of the mouth caused by *Candida* fungi, especially *Candida albicans*. It is very common in babies and newborns, who can contract the fungus during delivery when the mother has a vaginal yeast infection. The symptoms tend to appear within 7 to 10 days of infections that occurred during childbirth and delivery.

In adults thrush is much less common and is frequently found in people who have a compromised immune system, such as those with HIV infections. Thrush occurs when the normally occurring yeast organisms become overgrown because of certain conditions, such as when a person is taking antibiotics, an irritation of gums and other oral tissues caused by dentures, or a condition that affects the immune system.

Thrush causes creamy, white, curdlike patches to appear inside the mouth, particularly on the tongue, roof of the mouth, back of the throat, and around the lips. The white material on the surface of the patches covers red, inflamed areas that may bleed slightly with contact. The corners of the mouth may be red, moist, and cracked. In infants, the diaper area may be examined to check for diaper rash caused by *Candida*.

Thrush generally flares up and then heals on its own, but it may cause chronic infections in people with impaired immunity, chronic illness, or malnourishment. In rare cases, the fungus that causes thrush can affect tissue in the esophagus and cause difficulty swallowing, which is a medical emergency.

Diagnosis of thrush is usually made by a physical examination of the mouth. Patch scrapings may be tested in a laboratory if the preliminary diagnosis is in question. Thrush is treated with antifungal medication.

Thymus

A two-lobed organ of lymphatic tissue located under the top of the sternum (breastbone) near the end of the trachea (windpipe). The thymus is central to the immune system and the development of white blood cells. One type of white blood cell, the T cell, is produced in the red bone marrow and matures in the thymus, from which its name derives.

Thyroglossal cyst

An abnormality present at birth that produces a swelling in the neck. In a developing fetus, a small channel between the thyroid gland and the tongue is meant to close as the fetus grows. If this channel or parts of it remain in place or remain open when the infant is born, an abnormal channel between the thyroid gland and the tongue is created. A cyst can form around the channel, and the cyst causes swelling. If the thyroglossal cyst becomes infected, it can lead to formation of a thyroglossal fistula (abnormal passage between the cyst and the neck). Because of the chance of repeated infections, a cyst or fistula should be surgically removed.

Thyroid cancer

A cancerous tumor that develops in one or both lobes of the thyroid, the butterfly-shaped gland located below the Adam's apple at the front of the neck. Thyroid cancer is rare and affects women more than men.

The follicular cells of the thyroid gland produce and store THYROXINE and the protein thyroglobulin. Thyroxine controls the breakdown of complex molecules to supply the body with energy in a process known as metabolism. Thyroxine also regulates the buildup of cells and tissues from less complex molecules.

The most prevalent form of thyroid cancer develops in the follicular cells and is called papillary carcinoma, or papillary adenocarcinoma. This is a slow-growing cancer that is usually present in only one of the lobes of the thyroid.

Follicular carcinoma, or follicular adenocarcinoma, is the second most common form of thyroid cancer. Like papillary carcinoma, it develops in the follicular cells. This type of thyroid cancer is considered more aggressive than papillary carcinoma and tends to grow into the blood vessels and spread from there to the lungs and bones, as well as to other body parts early in the course of the disease.

Symptoms

A mass or a slow-growing lump in the neck is one of the symptoms of thyroid cancer. Other symptoms include neck pain or a persistent cough that is resistant to treatment.

In some cases, a swollen lymph node may indicate the possibility of thyroid cancer. A hoarse voice may result from pressure on the nerve to the voice box caused by a tumor on the thyroid. If a thyroid tumor obstructs the windpipe, there may be difficulty swallowing or breathing.

Diagnosis and treatment

During a physical examination, the neck will be felt to determine the size and condition of the thyroid gland and to check for the presence of nodules on the gland. The lymph nodes in the neck will also be examined for enlargement. If thyroid disorders including cancer are suspected, a doctor may order further diagnostic tests, particularly if a nodule is found on the thyroid gland. The most conclusive diagnostic test for thyroid cancer is fine-needle aspiration of a thyroid nodule.

Thyroid scanning allows a doctor to determine the spread of thyroid cancer. The doctor may request ultrasound scans to differentiate benign growths such as cysts and cystic tumors from cancerous growths such as solid tumors, CT (computed tomography) SCANNING to view the thyroid from different angles, or MRI (magnetic resonance imaging) to produce computer-generated images of cross-sectional views of the thyroid.

Surgery is the main approach to the treatment of thyroid cancer. A surgeon removes all of the thyroid, including the cancerous cells and possibly other noncancerous parts of the thyroid. In most cases involving cancer, the entire thyroid gland and the lymph nodes in the area must be surgically removed. Radioactive iodine treatments may be used to destroy cancerous thyroid tissue remaining after surgery.

When all of the thyroid gland is removed, thyroid hormone medication is taken orally for the rest of the person's life. This hormone therapy reestablishes normal metabolism.

Thyroid function tests

Diagnostic procedures that measure the performance of the thyroid gland. These tests detect HYPERTHYROIDISM (overactivity of the thyroid gland) or HYPOTHYROIDISM (underactivity of the thyroid gland), and the tests include blood tests and THYROID SCANNING procedures.

Thyroid gland

A gland in the endocrine system, located under the larynx (voice box) and wrapped around the top of the trachea (windpipe). The thyroid gland consists of two lobes, one on each side of the windpipe, joined by a piece of tissue called the isthmus.

The thyroid tissue has two types of cells capable of secretion called follicular cells and parafollicular cells (or C cells). Most of the thyroid is made up of follicular cells, which are arranged in the form of hollow follicles supported by a loose fibrous tissue richly supplied with blood vessels. The

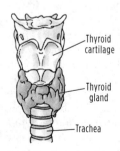

Thyroid cartilage

Thyroid gland

Trachea

Location of thyroid
The thyroid gland wraps around the top of the trachea (windpipe) in the neck. Levels of the hormones secreted by the thyroid are controlled by the thyroid-stimulating hormone released by the pituitary gland, which in turn is controlled by the hypothalamus.

follicles produce a number of hormones. Two of these, thyroxine and triiodothyronine, are iodine-based compounds that regulate body metabolism (the chemical activity in cells that releases energy from nutrients or uses energy to create other needed components, such as proteins). Insufficient thyroid hormone production is known as HYPOTHYROIDISM; an overproduction of thyroid hormones causes HYPERTHYROIDISM.

Thyroid nodule

A localized swelling in the thyroid gland. Thyroid nodules affect a small segment of the population, usually without symptoms. In rare instances, a thyroid nodule is an indication of THYROID CANCER.

As thyroid nodules are generally painless, the swelling may not be noticeable to the person with the nodule or by visual examination. The nodules are often discovered during routine physical examination. Benign thyroid nodules tend to be smooth, firm, and easily detected upon palpation of the neck. Cancerous nodules are usually hard. If the cancer has spread, the lymph nodes in the neck may be swollen. Further testing, including ultrasound and thyroid scans and biopsies, may be ordered to clarify a diagnosis of thyroid nodules.

If a thyroid scan reveals a cold nodule, and further tests indicate that the nodule may be cancerous, the nodule will be surgically removed. Benign thyroid nodules are usually monitored regularly.

Thyroid scanning

A diagnostic procedure that generates an image of the thyroid gland. Thyroid scanning is one of several thyroid function tests. The test is performed to determine the size, structure, and function of the thyroid gland and to diagnose the cause of an overactive thyroid.

Thyroid scanning is performed by injecting iodine tagged with a radioisotope into the person being tested. The thyroid gland absorbs the radioactive iodine, which highlights the gland on a scan.

Thyroidectomy

Surgical removal of most or all of the thyroid gland. Thyroidectomy is performed to treat thyroid cancer. It is generally followed with daily doses of thyroxine to prevent symptoms of HYPOTHYROIDISM (underactivity of the thyroid gland).

Thyroiditis

Inflammation of the thyroid gland. Thyroiditis occurs in several different forms. The most common form of thyroiditis is HASHIMOTO THYROIDITIS. In Hashimoto thyroiditis, the thyroid becomes less efficient at converting iodine into the thyroid hormone THYROXINE.

In DE QUERVAIN DISEASE, a less common form of thyroiditis, the gland is tender and painful and swells rapidly. The thyroid releases excessive amounts of thyroid hormone into the blood, causing HYPERTHYROIDISM (overactivity of the thyroid gland). The feelings of illness caused by de Quervain disease may require bed rest. One of the NONSTEROIDAL ANTI-INFLAMMATORY DRUGS (NSAIDs) may be recommended to reduce the inflammation in the gland. When the symptoms are prolonged, the medication cortisone may be prescribed.

Thyroid-stimulating hormone

See TSH.

Thyrotoxicosis

The general term for severe HYPERTHYROIDISM (overactivity of the thyroid gland). Thyrotoxicosis refers to the group of symptoms and physical changes associated with severe hyperthyroidism, regardless of the cause. Thyrotoxicosis is characterized by nervousness, weakness, difficulty sleeping, increased appetite, restlessness, increased perspiration, muscle cramps, fatigue, excessive thirst, atrophy of muscles, tremor, menstrual irregularities, bulging eyes, unexplained weight loss, diarrhea, an intolerance to heat, an increased heart rate, and palpitations.

Thyrotoxicosis may be associated with goiter and is sometimes a complication of GRAVES DISEASE. It can be fatal if congestive heart failure (see HEART FAILURE, CONGESTIVE) or PULMONARY EDEMA occur.

Thyrotropin-releasing hormone

See TRH.

Thyroxine

The principal metabolic hormone secreted by the thyroid glands; also known as T4. Thyroxine is produced in the thyroid gland by a synthesis of iodine with the amino acid tyrosine. The thyroid gland requires dietary iodine to produce thyroxine.

Thyroid hormone regulates the metabolism of glucose and fat by the liver and increases the release of cholesterol by the liver. It also regulates carbohydrate metabolism and the synthesis and breakdown of protein. In the digestive system, the hormone promotes the contractions of the smooth muscles and regulates the secretion of digestive juices. Thyroxine aids in the normal development, tone, and function of the muscles associated with the skeleton and the heart. Bone growth and regulation of the growth of the nervous system involve thyroxine; it also regulates the rate of oxygen use by the cells and the generation of body heat. Thyroxine is involved in fertility and the secretion of milk from the breasts of a lactating woman.

TIA

Also known as TRANSIENT ISCHEMIC ATTACK; a temporary loss of function in an area of the brain resulting from a reduced blood supply to the brain. A TIA is often a warning sign of an impending STROKE and requires evaluation by a doctor.

Tic

A repetitive, rapid, sudden, and involuntary movement, spasm, or twitch that usually affects muscles in the face, neck, or shoulders, including the throat and voice. A person with a tic experiences the movement as irresistible but can suppress it for a limited period of time. Tics tend to worsen during periods of stress or focused concentration and usually disappear during sleep. The action in a tic can be simple (for example, repeating a single word, grunting, or grimacing) or complex (for example, repeating phrases or sentences, jumping, or stamping the feet). Tics can be precipitated or worsened by medication. Tics are also a principal feature of the neurological disorder known as TOURETTE SYNDROME. The underlying cause of tics is unknown.

Tic douloureux

See TRIGEMINAL NEURALGIA.

Tietze syndrome

See COSTOCHONDRITIS.

Tinea

A general term for a group of related skin infections caused by different species of fungi; or a fungal skin infection characterized by ring-shaped, red, scaly, or blistery patches. Fungi thrive in warm moist areas and cause tinea infections such as jock itch (tinea cruris) in the groin area and athlete's foot (tinea pedis) between the toes. Other locations of tinea include the body (tinea corporis), the face (tinea faciei), and scalp (tinea capitis). Tinea versicolor is a fungal infection characterized by a rash consisting of white or brown patches on the trunk.

The most common symptoms of tinea are itching, redness, and a circular lesion with inflamed, spreading borders and a clear center. However, symptoms vary according to the site of the infection and its severity.

To obtain proper treatment, it is essential to distinguish tinea from other skin problems such as DERMATITIS or PSORIASIS. Diagnosis is made through evaluating the appearance of the skin and tests such as a skin scraping.

Simple cases of tinea respond well to treatment with antifungal creams or powders. Severe infections require oral antifungal medications. Possible complications of tinea include secondary bacterial infections, which must be treated with antibiotics.

Tinea versicolor

A fungal infection of the skin. Tinea versicolor is characterized by a rash consisting of scaly white and tan patches on the upper arms, chest, and back. The majority of people who develop the infection are teenagers or young adults. See TINEA.

Tingling

An abnormal, prickling feeling in the skin. Tingling may be a sign of damage or irritation to nerves in the affected area. It can also be a sign of poor circulation. It is a different problem than numbness, which suggests instead that the nerve is indeed damaged. A brief tingling sensation, as when a person's hand or foot "falls asleep," is not a cause for concern. However, a persistent tingling or pins and needles sensation may be caused by medical problems such as nerve injury; lack of blood supply; diabetes mellitus, type 1 and type 2; thyroid problems; VITAMIN B$_{12}$ (cyanocobalamin) DEFICIENCY; CARPAL TUNNEL SYNDROME; TRANSIENT ISCHEMIC ATTACK; STROKE; or MULTIPLE SCLEROSIS.

Tinnitus

The sensation of persistent or intermittent ringing, hissing, tinkling, whistling, roaring, buzzing, chirping, or other abnormal sounds in the ears or head in the absence of external sound. The tones may be single or multiple. The sensation can cause minimal discomfort or be severe and extremely disturbing. The condition, often described as ringing in the ears, is sometimes associated with hearing impairment. Subjective tinnitus is the term for head sounds heard only by the person with the condition. Objective tinnitus, caused by abnormalities in blood vessels around the outside of the ear or by muscle spasms, produces clicking or crackling sounds inside the middle ear that may be audible to others.

Most instances of tinnitus are due to damage to the microscopic endings of the hearing nerve in the inner ear. The damage may be associated with advancing age or exposure to loud noise. Temporary tinnitus may result from a small plug of earwax, OTOSCLEROSIS (hardening of the middle ear bones), allergies, ear or sinus infections, other diseases or conditions, or injuries.

Finding the specific cause of tinnitus may require extensive testing under the supervision of an otolaryngologist and an audiologist. The audiologist may perform a complete hearing evaluation, including audiometry and other hearing tests.

If there is also hearing loss, a hearing aid set at a low level can reduce the level of sound and temporarily eliminate it for some individuals. A device called a tinnitus masker can be combined with a hearing aid or worn separately to produce a low-level, pleasant, neutral sound that can reduce or eliminate the perception of tinnitus.

When tinnitus is related to temporomandibular joint disorder, or TMJ (see CLICKING JAW), treatment of the condition may help eliminate the head noise.

Tissue

Any group of similar cells arranged to perform a particular function. The body consists of four types of tissue. Epithelial tissue forms the skin and mucous membranes that line organs and structures such as the respiratory system, the blood vessels, stomach, vagina, and intestine. Connective tissue, such as fat and tendons, supports and protects structures in the body. Muscle tissue, which has three distinct varieties (skeletal, smooth, and cardiac) helps move the limbs and forms much of the heart, lungs, and other internal organs. Nerve tissue, which makes up the cells called neurons, receives and conducts electrochemical impulses.

Tissue-typing

A laboratory test for identifying compatible tissue in prospective organ donors and recipients. Tissue-typing helps reduce the chances of organ rejection by closely matching the immune system of the donor to that of the recipient.

TMJ syndrome

Also known as temporomandibular joint disorder; see CLICKING JAW.

Tobacco chewing

Using tobacco that is not smoked but is placed in the mouth. When tobacco is chewed or placed between the cheek and gum, nicotine mixes with the saliva and enters the bloodstream through the mucous membrane lining the mouth. Smokeless tobacco produces the same nicotine drug response as tobacco smoking, but without the need to inhale smoke into the lungs. It is every bit as addictive as smoked tobacco.

While smokeless tobacco reduces the risk of cancer of the respiratory tract associated with smoking, it poses serious health risks of its own. An increased risk of cancer of the mouth, particularly in the cheek and gum, is associated with smokeless tobacco. It is also linked to a higher in-cidence of cancer of the larynx, esophagus, and pancreas.

Tobacco smoking

See SMOKING, TOBACCO.

Tocopherol

See VITAMIN E.

Toe

One of the five digits of the foot, similar in skeletal structure to the finger. The toe consists of skin and connective tissue enclosing two or three joined bones called phalanges, which are connected by tendons to muscles in the foot and lower leg. The phalanges join at hinge joints, which are moved by tendons that flex or extend the toe.

Toenail, ingrown

See INGROWN TOENAIL.

Toilet training

Various methods for helping a child gradually achieve bowel and bladder control. Most children are not ready for toilet training until age 2, although it is also normal to begin a little later.

Tongue

The muscular, flexible organ on the floor of the mouth that functions in taste, chewing, swallowing, and speaking. The tongue is formed by internal bands of striated muscle. External muscle attached to the bones of the mouth hold it in place. Taste buds located on the surface of the tongue detect sweet, salty, bitter, and acidic flavors and stimulate the salivary glands beneath the tongue to produce saliva. See TASTE.

Tongue cancer

A malignant tumor on the tongue that begins as a small lump or a thick, firm white patch. In time, the lump or patch becomes an ulcer with a firm, raised rim and a sensitive center that may bleed readily. This is a SQUAMOUS CELL CARCINOMA, meaning that when viewed under the microscope, the cells of the cancer are relatively flat, like skin cells. If left untreated, tongue cancer may spread throughout the mouth to the gums, floor of the mouth, lower jaw, and neck. Eventually, it can spread into other organs of the body, often the lungs. If the tumor enlarges, the tongue can become stiff and rigid. A large tumor can block the throat, interfering with normal speaking, swallowing, and breathing. It is one of the more serious forms of cancer that can occur in the mouth. Tongue cancer occurs most often in people who use tobacco, consume large amounts of alcohol, or wear dentures. A dentist often detects the first signs of tongue cancer during a routine dental examination. A growth on the tongue that may be painless and lasts more than 10 to 20 days, becomes worse, or spreads rapidly should be examined by an otolaryngologist (a specialist in disorders of the ear, nose, and throat and related structures).

Treatment is generally determined by an oncologist (cancer specialist), based on the stage or spread of the disease. Radiation therapy, chemotherapy, or surgery to remove the tumor may be recommended. A small tumor on the tongue may be removed with little effect on the tongue's function or the appearance of the mouth.

Tonometry

A test that measures pressure within the eyes. Tonometry is used to test for GLAUCOMA, a disease in which rising pressure inside the eyeball may impair vision.

Tonsillectomy

Surgical removal of the tonsils as a treatment for severe, recurrent tonsillitis or for tonsils that obstruct the airway. A tonsillectomy is most commonly performed on children who are 6 or 7 years old. Generally, if a child gets tonsillitis with high fever three or more times a year, the doctor will recommend a tonsillectomy.

The operation is also sometimes recommended when an abscess (collection of pus) develops on the tonsils or when a child has difficulty swallowing due to inflamed tonsils. Obstructed breathing due to enlarged tonsils may indicate the need for tonsillectomy. Such children will snore loudly and have obstructive SLEEP APNEA SYNDROME. In adults, tonsillectomy is usually performed only as a biopsy for cancer in the area of the tonsils or adenoids.

In those with tonsillitis, the adenoids (clusters of tissue above the soft palate) may become inflamed with tonsillitis and may sometimes be removed at the same time as the tonsils, a procedure called ADENOIDECTOMY.

Tonsillitis

An inflammation of the tonsils, the two small masses of tissue at the back of the mouth, on both sides of the throat. Tonsillitis may occur intermittently and is caused by an infection, most commonly from viruses or the

Streptococcus bacteria. The tonsils help filter out and fight bacteria and viruses that enter the body through the mouth and nose. When the tonsils become overwhelmed by infectious organisms, they become inflamed. Tonsillitis is a common childhood illness, most often affecting children between the ages of 5 and 15 years.

Tonsillitis causes the tonsils to swell and become redder than usual. The throat is usually sore, and the voice may be changed somewhat as a result of the swelling caused by tonsillitis. Swallowing may be uncomfortable or painful. The lymph nodes (see LYMPH NODE) in the neck may become swollen and tender. There may be fever, chills, coughing, headache, and foul-smelling breath. A white or yellow coating or white specks may appear on the tonsils within a few days of the onset of infection. If the infection becomes severe, a child may experience ear pain and have difficulty breathing.

Antibiotics are prescribed to treat bacterial infections; symptoms usually disappear within 2 or 3 days. However, if an antibiotic is taken for strep throat, the entire course of medication should be taken, even if the symptoms are gone. In severe, recurrent, or resistant cases of tonsillitis, removal of the tonsils is recommended (see TONSILLECTOMY).

Tonsils

Small oval masses of lymphatic tissue in the mouth and throat (pharynx). Technically, there are three pairs of tonsils; they are located at the base of the tongue (lingual tonsils), in the throat just behind the tongue (palatine tonsils), and close to the opening of the nasal cavity into the pharynx (pharyngeal tonsils; also known as adenoids). Tonsils are large in children, shrinking slowly after age 3. The pharyngeal tonsils disappear completely by adulthood, and the palatine tonsils decrease to the size of almonds. The tonsils filter and destroy infectious material entering the body through the mouth and nose. See TONSILLITIS; TONSILLECTOMY.

Tooth abscess

An accumulation of pus that is enclosed in the bone tissue at the tip of the root in a tooth. The cause of a tooth abscess is usually a bacterial infection in the pulp. The infection may originate in untreated tooth decay or in dead pulp tissue inside the tooth.

A tooth abscess causes persistent toothache or throbbing pain at the site. Biting and chewing often cause extreme pain. The side of the face may swell. In response to the infection, glands in the neck may become swollen and tender and there may be a fever.

If a tooth abscess is the result of a completely infected permanent tooth located in the back of the jaw, or a primary tooth, the dentist may extract the tooth. In many cases, if enough tooth structure remains, the tooth can be saved by performing root canal treatment.

Tooth decay

The decalcification and disintegration of the structure of a tooth from plaque (see PLAQUE, DENTAL) and acid-producing food deposits on the teeth. The acids dissolve the hard mineral enamel covering the surface of the teeth, creating a small hole, or cavity (see CAVITY, DENTAL), in the enamel.

Tooth eruption

The emergence of the primary teeth and the permanent teeth as they appear above the gum line. Tooth eruption of the primary teeth generally begins with the bottom central incisors (the front teeth) when an infant is 6 months old and is completed when the second molars come in at the age of about 24 months. The primary teeth typically erupt in a fairly regular sequence from the front of the mouth to the back. They are shed in about the same sequence, with the first teeth to erupt being the first to be shed, usually starting at about the age of 6 or 7 years. At that age, the heavier, larger permanent teeth, which have developed within the gum below the primary teeth, usually begin to erupt. By the time a child is 11-½ or 12 years old, he or she has often shed all the primary teeth and acquired most of the permanent teeth, with the exception of the second and third molars (wisdom teeth).

Some pain may be experienced with the normal eruption of teeth. Over-the-counter painkillers, such as acetaminophen, may be taken to manage the discomforts of erupting teeth until a dentist can be consulted. Aspirin should never be given to children younger than 18 years of age, because of the risk of their developing REYE SYNDROME, a rare but potentially fatal illness.

Tooth extraction

The removal of a tooth. Tooth extraction is generally performed by a dentist or oral surgeon because of tooth decay, advanced gum disease (see PERIODONTAL DISEASE), severe fracture, dental impaction, overcrowding, or malocclusion (irregular alignment).

Toothache

Pain experienced in a tooth or teeth. If the discomfort increases or continues during a 4- to 6-week period, a dentist should be seen for an evaluation. When a toothache is transitory, periodic, and associated with sensitivity to hot or cold food or drinks, the cause may be minor gum recession, which exposes the cementum on the surface of the root and causes sensitivity. If sharp pain is experienced when biting down, or if there is lingering pain after exposure to hot or cold substances, the cause may be a loose filling, a crack in the tooth, or TOOTH DECAY. When a toothache is persistent and severe, highly sensitive to pressure or touch, and the surrounding gum is swollen, a TOOTH ABSCESS may be suspected. Toothaches generally indicate the need for a dental evaluation.

Torsion

Twisting of an object. Torsion is a factor in several medical conditions. For example, a torsion fracture, also called spiral fracture, refers to a bone that is broken because it has been twisted. Torsion also refers to the abnormal twisting of a testicle within the scrotum or of a loop of bowel in the abdomen; both conditions can prevent blood flow to those areas of the body, which can subsequently cause severe damage.

A condition called torsion dystonia is a postural disorder beginning in childhood at about 12 years old. In this debilitating disorder, affected children gradually become unable to perform the simplest of motor tasks and usually end up confined to wheelchairs.

Torticollis

A muscle spasm in the neck that produces a contraction of several muscles pulling the head to one side in an unnatural position. Also called wryneck, torticollis causes pain and stiffness in the neck. The condition may be due to a physical injury of the neck muscles, to a twisted position of the neck during sleep, or to exposure from extreme cold (such as an air conditioner). Certain tranquilizers may cause torticollis. In newborn infants, it is sometimes caused by neck muscle damage following a difficult birth. In children, torticollis can be caused by infected, swollen glands in the neck. The condition is diagnosed by physical examination. In adults and older children, physical therapy, massage, application of heat, a supportive collar, and the use of pain-killing medication may help control discomfort and restore function. This condition usually improves in 7 to 10 days without complications.

Tourette syndrome

An inherited, neurological disorder characterized by involuntary movements (motor tics) and vocalizations (phonic or vocal tics). Other disorders related to Tourette syndrome (TS) include OBSESSIVE-COMPULSIVE DISORDER (OCD), ATTENTION DEFICIT/HYPERACTIVITY DISORDER (ADHD), and chronic tic disorder.

The symptoms of this disorder generally begin before the age of 21 years and continue throughout a person's lifetime. The severity of symptoms ranges from mild to severe and disabling. The first signs of TS are usually facial tics, such as eye blinking. There may also be nose twitching and grimacing. In time, motor tics grow more extensive. They may come to include neck stretching, head jerking, foot stamping, and body twisting or bending.

The vocalizations of TS may include strange sounds and unacceptable words and phrases. A person with TS may repeatedly clear his or her throat, grunt, sniff, cough, bark, yelp, or shout. People may repeat the words of others (echolalia) or involuntarily shout obscenities (coprolalia).

There is no single medication to control TS. Drugs that may be helpful include haloperidol, pimozide, and clonidine. Other helpful measures include treatment of related behavioral disorders, psychotherapy, and biofeedback.

Tourniquet

A device used to stop severe bleeding. A tourniquet is usually made from a strong piece of cloth or bandage, wrapped around the blood pressure site nearest the wound but between the wound and the heart, and tightened by tying a knot or twisting it with a stick. Because the use of a tourniquet can be very dangerous, it should be used only when bleeding is life-threatening and uncontrollable by more conservative first aid.

Toxemia

Contamination or poisoning of the blood by toxic material, usually from bacteria but also from chemicals or hormones. Toxemia is popularly known as blood poisoning. See SEPTICEMIA for more information on bacterial contamination of the blood.

Toxemia can also refer to a condition that can affect some women late in pregnancy. See ECLAMPSIA and PREECLAMPSIA for details.

Toxemia of pregnancy

Disorders characterized by high blood pressure, tissue swelling, and protein in the urine of a pregnant woman. Severe toxemia of pregnancy occurs in late pregnancy, can lead to eclampsia and coma, and is considered a medical emergency. See also PREECLAMPSIA.

Toxic shock syndrome

A rare disorder that mostly occurs in menstruating women who use tampons. This dangerous condition has also been noted in association with contraceptive sponges, diaphragms, cervical caps, and (rarely) in people with wound infections. Symptoms include a sudden high fever (a temperature of 102°F or higher), headache, sore throat, aching muscles, vomiting, diarrhea, dizziness and fainting, and a rash resembling sunburn, especially on the palms of the hands and soles of the feet. The initial flulike symptoms can progress rapidly to a serious illness that can be fatal. Toxic shock syndrome is caused by strains of the *Staphylococcus* bacteria that are capable of producing certain toxins.

Immediate treatment with antibiotics and often hospitalization are needed. The patient may go into shock because the syndrome affects the mechanism that regulates blood pressure, which may drop quickly. Prompt treatment stops the infection, and death is rare. However, toxic shock syndrome tends to recur in those who have had this disorder in the past. Women who have had it

should not use tampons, cervical caps, or diaphragms.

Toxin

A poisonous substance. Toxins are usually proteins produced by living cells or organisms that are capable of causing disease when released into body tissues. Toxins are commonly produced by microorgansims such as bacteria; examples include the microorganisms that cause anthrax, cholera, dysentery, diphteria, and botulism.

Toxocariasis

An infection caused by the larvae of parasitic roundworms commonly found in the intestines of dogs and cats. Toxocariasis can take one of two forms known as ocular larva migrans and visceral larva migrans.

Most infections are mild and may not produce noticeable symptoms. If symptoms are present, they may include abdominal pain, liver enlargement, headache, weakness, lethargy, coughing and wheezing, and fever. In some rare cases, toxocariasis can produce severe disease and death. The form of toxocariasis called ocular larva migrans causes an eye disease that can result in blindness. This occurs when a microscopic worm enters the eye, producing inflammation and scarring of the retina. Partial loss of vision may be permanent with this infection. Visceral larva migrans occurs as a result of severe or repeated toxocariasis. This form causes swelling of the body's organs and affects the central nervous system. The symptoms of this form of the infection are caused by the migration of the worms through the body and include fever, coughing, asthma, and pneumonia.

A blood test can be used to diagnose toxocariasis, but most people recover without specific therapy. The more severe form of the infection is treated with antiparasitic medications and sometimes anti-inflammatory medication. Ocular larva migrans is more difficult to treat.

Toxoplasmosis

An infection caused by the single-celled parasite *Toxoplasma gondii*, which is widespread and carried by many people in the United States without symptoms. Toxoplasmosis occurs when the immune system cannot prevent the parasite from causing illness. The infectious parasite that causes toxoplasmosis spends most of its life cycle in cats. An infected cat can shed millions of the parasites every day in its stool. The infection is easily transmitted to other animals sharing an environment with cats. Humans typically become infected in one of two ways: when they have direct contact with cat feces, as when changing cat litter, and accidentally swallow parasites that have contaminated their hands; or when they ingest undercooked pork, lamb, or venison meat from infected animals.

Once ingested, the *Toxoplasma* parasites multiply within the cells that line the human digestive tract. The parasites may spread to other organs and structures in the body, including the brain, skeletal muscles, heart muscle, eyes, lungs, and lymph nodes. The parasites' spread is eventually stopped by the immune system of a healthy person.

Symptoms

The great majority of healthy people with normal immune defenses have no symptoms when they are infected with toxoplasmosis. If symptoms are present, they may include painless swelling of the lymph nodes, headache, malaise, fatigue, and low-grade fever. Less common symptoms may include muscle aches, sore throat, abdominal pain, a skin rash, or various symptoms related to nerve function.

In people who have AIDS or other forms of immune system impairment, the symptoms of toxoplasmosis are severe and related to brain function. They may include disturbances in mental functioning, disorientation, difficulty concentrating, or changes in behavior. There may also be disturbances in nerve function, including irregular movement, difficulty walking, difficulty speaking, and partial loss of vision. Fever, headache, and seizures may occur. If the infection affects the eyes, vision may be blurred, spots may appear in the field of vision, and the person's eyes may hurt and be extremely sensitive to light.

If a woman who is pregnant acquires toxoplasmosis within 6 to 8 weeks of becoming pregnant or during her pregnancy, her baby is at risk of being born with a congenital form of the disease. Congenital toxoplasmosis increases the risks of premature birth and fetal death. The baby may not have symptoms at birth, but signs of infection can be found in the infant's eyes during an eye examination.

Diagnosis and treatment

If a person has symptoms of toxoplasmosis, a doctor will take a history to determine the person's exposure to cats and whether the person is taking medications that suppress the immune system or has a condition that causes immune system impairment. During a physical examination, the doctor will check for swollen glands, eye damage, and signs of brain involvement.

A woman who is pregnant may undergo ultrasonography (see ULTRASOUND SCANNING) and AMNIOCENTESIS to diagnose congenital toxoplasmosis in the fetus. The newborn may undergo eye and neurologic examinations, CT scanning of the head, and a spinal tap to obtain cerebrospinal fluid for laboratory analysis.

Treatment is usually unnecessary in a healthy person whose symptoms are not severe or persistent. If the eyes are affected, pyrimethamine may be prescribed in combination with sulfadiazine or clindamycin. People who have weakened immune systems are treated with a combination of medications to destroy the *Toxoplasma* parasite. In cases of congenital toxoplasmosis in newborns, a combination of medications may be given for a minimum of 1 year.

Trabeculectomy

An operation to facilitate drainage of fluid (aqueous humor) from the front of the eye. Trabeculectomy is used to treat GLAUCOMA, a disease in which rising pressure inside the eyeball impairs vision. After the person has been given a local anesthetic, the eye surgeon removes a small portion of the blocked drainage system (trabecular meshwork) to allow better flow of the aqueous humor out of the eye, reducing internal pressure. The procedure is safe, and those who undergo it often subsequently need less

medication or no medication at all for glaucoma treatment. Trabeculectomy increases the risk of cataracts, and in some cases a second surgery is needed later to reopen the drain.

Trace elements

Minerals that are required by the body in very small quantities for good health. Trace elements include ZINC, IODINE, COPPER, CHROMIUM, sulfur, and SELENIUM. Along with other nutrients, these minerals ensure that the body functions properly.

Tracer

A substance used to mark and indicate the course of a chemical or biological process inside the body. A radioactive tracer refers to an element (called a radioisotope) that has the same atomic number as another with a different atomic weight. Radioisotopes exhibit spontaneous decomposition, which gives off radiation in the form of gamma rays. These rays can be detected with special instruments. Radioactive tracers are attached to biological compounds and injected into the body, where an image of their path can be produced.

Trachea

The windpipe, the airway that connects the pharynx (throat) with the bronchi, the two major tubes leading into the lungs. The trachea is about 4 inches long and slightly less than an inch in diameter. It begins at the larynx (voice box) and can be felt just under the skin below the larynx as a hard, ringed pipe. These rings are C-shaped cartilages that keep the trachea open and protect the airway against damage. The open area of the C-rings faces back toward the esophagus and is spanned by smooth muscle. This structure allows the trachea to stay open even as it flexes during swallowing. The interior of the trachea is lined with mucous membrane that helps trap tiny particles in inhaled air, thereby keeping the lungs and airway open. See RESPIRATORY SYSTEM.

Tracheostomy

A small opening, called a stoma, that is made by a tracheotomy, a surgical procedure through the neck and into the trachea, or windpipe. A tracheostomy usually involves the placement of a plastic tube into this opening to provide an airway and permit the removal of secretions from the lungs. The tube allows air to be pumped directly into the lungs and may be equipped with an inflatable cuff that makes speech possible by allowing air to pass over the vocal cords.

A tracheostomy can become neces-

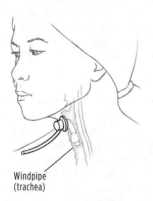

Windpipe
(trachea)

Living with a tracheostomy
Breathing through a tracheostomy tube is difficult at first, but most patients adapt within a few days. If the tube is in place permanently or for a long time, most people can learn to talk with training and practice.

sary as a result of diseases, conditions, or injuries that obstruct or interfere with breathing through the windpipe. These include long-term unconsciousness or coma, inherited abnormalities of the voice box or windpipe, severe injuries to the mouth or neck, a foreign body lodged in the airway, and the inhalation of a corrosive material, smoke, or steam.

Tracheotomy

Surgery involving the insertion of a tube through the neck and into the windpipe to keep the airway open. Tracheotomy may be performed as a nonemergency surgical procedure to allow a person to use a ventilator, or it may be done as an emergency, life-saving strategy when the windpipe is completely obstructed and breathing is not possible.

Trachoma

An eye infection caused by *Chlamydia trachomatis* bacteria. Trachoma causes inflammation of the cornea of the eye and clouding of vision. The eye becomes scarred, causing malformation of the eyelids and an abnormal inward growth of the eyelashes. The cornea, which is continually scraped by the eyelashes, hardens and becomes opaque, leading to a loss of vision. Trachoma is diagnosed by microscopic identification of the bacteria in scrapings from the eyes. Tetracycline and erythromycin are the antibiotics used to treat the infection. If the eyelids are deformed, surgery is required to restore normal appearance and function.

Traction

A treatment procedure that uses a pulling force to prevent or reduce muscle spasm, to keep a joint or other body part stationary, or to hold the ends of broken bones in place. Skin traction is a form of traction that uses dressings, belts, halters, boots, or straps that may be attached to an arm, the head, a leg, or the pelvis. Skin traction is noninvasive and may be done at home under medical supervision. It is used to treat muscle injuries such as muscle spasm, some bone fractures, slipped disks, and arthritic conditions.

Skeletal traction is used for severe injuries that demand longer periods of immobilization in the hospital. In the treatment of fractures, particularly of the thighbone, traction uses a pulley system of weights that are attached to the bone by a surgically implanted pin. The weights apply sufficient force to counteract the powerful thigh muscles and hold the bone fragments in a position of correct alignment while the fracture heals.

Tranquilizers

See ANTIPSYCHOTIC DRUGS; SEDATIVES.

Transcendental meditation (TM)

A simple program of meditation for reducing stress. Transcendental meditation is taught by qualified teachers in seven steps, beginning with the assignment to each student of a secret mantra, a word or phrase repeated over and over by the practitioner to induce a meditative trance.

Transcutaneous electrical nerve stimulation

See TENS.

Transdermal patch

See SKIN PATCH.

Transesophageal echocardiogram

An ultrasound image of the heart made by inserting a small device called a transducer into the esophagus (the tube that connects the throat to the stomach). An echocardiogram bounces ultrasound waves off the heart and into a machine that transforms the echoes into a computer-generated image. This allows doctors to see the heart while it is moving and to observe its main pumping chambers, the shape and thickness of the chamber walls, the valves, the outer covering, and the major vessels leading in and out of the heart. It is also possible to determine the volume and direction of blood flow through the heart. An echocardiogram is useful for assessing the size of the heart, its pumping strength, valve problems, damage to the heart muscle, abnormal blood flow patterns, structural abnormalities (such as enlargement of the heart, or cardiomegaly), and blood pressure in the artery leading to the lungs (see HYPERTENSION, PULMONARY).

Trans-fatty acids

Fats that are produced by the hydrogenation process that solidifies liquid oils for use in food products. Also known as trans fats, varying amounts of trans-fatty acids are present in stick margarine, crackers, cookies, doughnuts, deep-fried foods, and many processed fats. Like saturated fats, these substances contribute to increased levels of low-density lipoprotein cholesterol, promoting clogged arteries and increasing the risk of heart disease. The content of trans-fatty acids is now included on the Nutrition Facts panel of food labels. See also FATS AND OILS.

Transfusion

A procedure for infusing blood or blood components into a person's bloodstream. The blood may come from a different person than the one who receives it, or it may have been taken in advance from the recipient and stored for use later (see AUTOLOGOUS BLOOD DONATION). Blood transfusion is a highly effective therapy that has saved the lives of many people, and it is used to treat many diseases.

Transfusion between people with the same blood group usually succeeds. There are four principal blood groups: A, B, AB, and O. The blood groups are further divided by the presence or absence of the Rh factor (for rhesus, the name of the species of monkey in which the factor was discovered). Blood with the Rh factor is Rh-positive (+); blood without it is Rh-negative (–). The most common blood group among Americans is O+, followed in order by A+, B+, O-, A-, AB+, B-, and AB-.

Transfusion, autologous

Using the previously donated and stored blood of a person during surgery to replace any blood that is lost as a result of the procedure. An autologous transfusion replaces a standard blood transfusion, in which blood from a donor other than the patient is used, avoiding any risk that the donor blood is infected.

Some surgeons also use a technique known as an intraoperative autologous transfusion. Blood is suctioned from bleeding in the surgical wound; then, it is filtered and returned to the patient through a needle in a vein. This technique is highly effective and is being used more frequently now, especially in surgeries that involve the cardiovascular system, orthopedic problems, and ectopic pregnancies.

Transient ischemic attack

Also known as a TIA or a mini stroke, a brain disorder caused by a temporary interruption of blood supply to the brain. A TIA is caused by reduced blood flow (ischemia). Ischemia may in turn be the result of ATHEROSCLEROSIS (narrowing of the arteries) or emboli (clots that travel and lodge in blood vessels). A TIA results in a temporary loss in brain functions that may last from several minutes to several hours. A TIA that lasts for more that 24 hours is a STROKE.

Symptoms of a TIA usually occur rapidly. They may include numbness, tingling, weakness, speech difficulty, double vision, and loss of balance and coordination. Attacks are followed by full recovery. However, a transient ischemic attack may be a warning sign of the potential for a more serious stroke.

The goal of treatment is to prevent a stroke from occurring. This means appropriate treatment of underlying disorders, such as HYPERTENSION (high blood pressure), heart disease, and diabetes mellitus. The doctor may also recommend aspirin or other medications to reduce clotting. If the doctor thinks a TIA is caused by a significant narrowing in the carotid artery, surgery may be recommended to reduce the risk of future stroke.

Transplant surgery

A procedure in which a diseased organ or tissue is replaced with a healthy donor organ. The list of organs that can be transplanted includes the cornea, heart, lungs, kidney, liver, pancreas, small intestine, and bone marrow.

Because of advances in surgical techniques, the challenge of transplant surgery is less in connecting the donated organ to the recipient than in managing the tendency of the body to reject the donor organ as a foreign invader. Powerful medications called immunosuppressant drugs are given to the recipient before and after the surgery and must be continued throughout life. These medications decrease the ability of the immune system to attack the transplanted organ as an invader. Since immunosuppressant drugs decrease the ability of the body to fight infection, the transplant recipient is at greater risk for various kinds of opportunistic bacterial and fungal infections. To reduce this risk, transplant recipients take preventive doses of medications targeted against these pathogens and also take precautions to avoid exposure to communicable diseases.

Transposition of the great vessels

A birth defect in which the positions of the pulmonary artery and the aorta are reversed. As a result, blood circulates to and from the body without picking up oxygen in the lungs. Babies born with transposition of the great vessels survive only if an abnormal connection, such as a hole between the two upper heart chambers (atrial septal defect), allows oxygen-rich blood to reach the body. Transposition of the great vessels can be repaired surgically. Long-term outlook depends on the severity of the defect, and lifelong medical follow-up is required.

Transsexualism

Acting and presenting oneself as a member of the opposite sex, combined with strong feelings of discomfort in one's physical sex, for a period of at least 2 years. This rare disorder appears in both children and adults. The course of the disorder depends on when it begins. In boys, the disorder usually begins between 2 and 4 years of age and may be resolved by the time of adolescence. However, in a minority of cases the disorder continues into adulthood. These individuals usually seek sex-reassignment surgery as adults. If the disorder begins in late adolescence or adulthood, the degree of cross-gender identification is more changeable, and the individual is less likely to seek surgery as a solution. The course of the disorder in girls remains unclear.

The cause of gender-identity disorder is not fully understood. Treatment consists of family and individual psychotherapy. Sex-reassignment surgery is an option for some individuals, but emotional problems may continue after surgery.

Transvestism

Dressing in the clothing of the opposite sex as a way of becoming sexually excited, known popularly as "cross-dressing." The disorder occurs primarily among men who are generally heterosexual but may have had occasional homosexual encounters.

Trauma

Injury, damage, wound, or shock. Trauma is used both to describe any physical injury caused by external force or violence, such as an automobile accident, and to describe psychological damage caused by distressing circumstances.

Trauma emergencies are very serious, and the person should seek medical attention.

Trauma center

A hospital-based facility for the treatment of trauma. Trauma centers are specialized facilities designed to provide diagnostic and therapeutic services to people who have sustained a severe injury, or trauma.

Trauma surgery

Specialized surgery used in emergency care of severe injuries. Trauma surgery is used in cases of extreme injury to provide immediate care to persons who have sustained complex and life-threatening injuries. Traumatology is another name for trauma surgery.

Travel immunization

Vaccines for protection from disease for Americans traveling outside the United States. Travel immunization involves anticipating exposure to the infectious diseases endemic to a destination and the process of being vaccinated against those potential health hazards before a planned trip to a foreign country.

There are distinctions among the vaccinations intended for travelers. To enter some countries, certain vaccinations may be required by law. The Centers for Disease Control and Prevention maintains a web site that provides the latest recommendations in immunization for traveling. However, before scheduling travel immunization, a person should check with a personal physician who is familiar with his or her medical history.

Immunization during pregnancy has historically been avoided because of the potential risk of miscarriage and possible birth defects. This is a matter for discussion between a woman and her physician.

Traveler's diarrhea

See DIARRHEA, TRAVELER'S.

Trematode

A type of parasitic flatworm that includes the fluke. Trematodes can live in four different animal hosts in the course of their life cycle. During the first stage, pond snails are hosts to trematode eggs, which hatch inside the snail into tiny swimming trematodes that migrate out of the snail and into the pond water. They locate a tadpole host and burrow in, converting into a tough cyst that remains in the tadpole throughout the tadpole's life cycle. The tadpole undergoes metamorphosis to become a frog, and if there are many trematode cysts present, the frog may become deformed or grow extra legs. If the tadpole or frog is eaten by a garter snake, the snake then eats the trematodes and becomes a host for the parasite. In the snake, the trematode develops from a cyst into an adult that lays eggs. The eggs are eliminated from the snake's intestines at the bottom of the pond, where aquatic snails feed. Trematode eggs on the plants and algae that the snails eat begin their life cycle again inside the snails. Trematodes enter the human body if people eat contaminated snails or drink contaminated water.

Tremor

Involuntary, rhythmic muscle movement caused by alternate contraction and relaxation of the muscles. Tremor is the most common involuntary movement disorder. In many cases, it is a symptom of an underlying disease such as PARKINSON DISEASE. Other causes of tremor include MULTIPLE SCLEROSIS, STROKE, head injury, alcohol or drugs, the effects of aging, and emotional disorders.

There are many different types of tremors. Proper evaluation of tremors is necessary because appropriate treatment depends on accurate clinical diagnosis. Tests to determine the cause include blood tests and CT (computed tomography) SCANNING or MRI (magnetic resonance imaging) of the brain. Some tremors respond to drug treatment.

Trephine

A surgical instrument used for cutting a circular hole. The trephine is used to cut through bone, most commonly the skull during brain surgery. Another type of trephine is used to remove a circular section from the cornea, the outer covering of the eye.

TRH

Thyrotropin-releasing hormone; also known as protirelin or thyrotropin-releasing factor (TRF). TRH is a by-product of the hypothalamus, which stimulates the pituitary gland to produce and release TSH (thyroid-stimulating hormone). TRH production in the hypothalamus is stimulated when blood levels of the thyroid hormone thyroxine are low.

Trial, clinical

See CLINICAL TRIAL.

Trichinosis

A parasitic disease produced by eating undercooked or raw meat, usually pork or wild game, which contains the cysts of the parasitic roundworm called *Trichinella spiralis*. It is most likely to occur in the United States when the meat of wild animals (such as bears), is not cooked thoroughly before it is eaten. The cysts develop into adult roundworms in the human intestinal tract, where they produce many larvae that migrate to muscle tissue and form cysts.

Light infestations may not produce noticeable symptoms. Heavy infestations can cause severe symptoms and may result in heart failure. The early symptoms tend to occur in 1 or 2 days and include cramping, nausea, vomiting, and diarrhea. Headache, fever, chills, cough, itchy skin, and fatigue may follow the start of infestation. Muscle pain occurs due to the inflammatory response to the presence of the worm larvae in muscle tissue. The pain may be especially intense when breathing, chewing, or using the large muscles, and the diaphragm and rib muscles may be particularly painful. The person may have difficulty breathing, and muscle coordination may be impaired. During the larvae's migratory stage, there may be swelling in the face and around the eyes. If the larvae migrate to the heart muscle, it can become damaged. If trichinosis is suspected, diagnostic tests including blood tests to identify the parasite and a muscle biopsy to locate *Trichinella* cysts may be performed. There is no treatment for this disease once the larvae have invaded the muscles. Nonprescription pain relievers such as aspirin, other NONSTEROIDAL ANTI-INFLAMMATORY DRUGS, or acetaminophen may be used to relieve muscle pain. Mild to moderate infections usually improve within a few months. Fatigue, diarrhea, and weakness may persist for months.

Trichomoniasis

One of the common SEXUALLY TRANS-MITTED DISEASES (STDs), which causes a vaginal infection in women. Trichomoniasis can be transmitted to and from men by sexual contact. The infection can affect a man's urethra, usually without symptoms, and can be spread to other women via sexual intercourse. A woman who is pregnant can transmit the infection to her newborn during childbirth.

The organism that causes trichomoniasis can survive in a woman's vagina for years without symptoms. If symptoms are experienced, they may include a painful inflammation of the vagina, pain during sexual intercourse, redness and burning in the vagina, frequent and painful urination, abdominal pain, itching in the vagina and vulva, and an unusual vaginal discharge that has an odor and is yellow and frothy. These symptoms may increase in severity during a menstrual period. While symptoms in men are uncommon, they may include an unusual penile discharge, painful urination, inflammation and pain in the tip of the penis, and a tingling sensation inside the penis.

Trichomoniasis is treated with antibiotics, usually metronidazole. While the infection is being treated, unprotected sexual activity should be avoided. Sex partners should be informed of the infection so they can seek medical testing and treatment. Care should be taken to wash all washcloths, towels, bathing suits, underpants, and bed linens that have been in direct contact with a woman's genitals or with her hands after she has touched her vagina.

Tricuspid insufficiency

Failure of the tricuspid valve of the heart to close tightly, causing it to regurgitate (leak); also known as tricuspid regurgitation. The tricuspid valve connects the right atrium (upper chamber) of the heart with the right ventricle (lower chamber). Leakage from the right ventricle back into the right atrium reduces the flow of blood to the lungs. The tricuspid valve usually leaks because of enlargement of the right ventricle, a condition that can result from a number of diseases, including pulmonary hypertension (abnormally high blood pressure in the blood vessels in the lungs). In addition, the tricuspid valve can be damaged by rheumatic fever.

If tricuspid insufficiency occurs in the absence of pulmonary hypertension, it often produces no symptoms and does not require treatment. See PULMONARY HYPERTENSION, PRIMARY. Treatment of pulmonary hypertension or any other disease causing enlargement of the right atrium may resolve the tricuspid insufficiency. Surgery to repair or replace the valve may be necessary. See HEART VALVE SURGERY.

Trigeminal neuralgia

Also known as tic douloureux, a disorder of the trigeminal nerve that causes severe pain on one side of the face. When this major facial nerve is damaged or inflamed, sharp, stabbing pain can affect the cheek, lips, gums, or chin. A facial tic or twitching may accompany the pain. The pain of trigeminal neuralgia may be difficult to control. Medications such as carbamazepine or phenytoin may be helpful. In some cases, surgery is necessary.

Trigger finger

A locking of the finger in a bent position, caused by a constriction of the tendon sheath. Trigger finger is a form of TENOSYNOVITIS, an inflammation of the thin lining of the sheath that surrounds a tendon. Inflammation can be caused by overuse, trauma, or a bacterial infection. Trigger finger may be treated with medications such as NONSTEROIDAL ANTI-INFLAMMATORY DRUGS (NSAIDs) to relieve inflammation and swelling. If other treatments are ineffective, an injection of the corticosteroid cortisone may be considered. Surgical options include tendon release.

Triglycerides

A type of fat found in the blood and also the form in which excess fat is stored in tissue. Triglycerides constitute approximately 95 percent of fatty tissue. A high level of blood triglycerides increases the risk of heart disease, and excess body fat can lead to serious health problems such as high blood pressure, elevated cholesterol levels, ATHEROSCLEROSIS (arterial blockage by fat deposits), diabetes mellitus, and an increased risk of cancer. Most of the fats that Americans eat are triglycerides.

Trismus

Spasm of the chewing muscles in the jaw. Trismus, also called lockjaw, may be caused by a variety of abnormal conditions or diseases. It is also a result of dental infections, drug reactions, jaw fracture, mumps, or severe strep throat. Usually, a person who has trismus cannot open the mouth more than about 1 inch. It is often the first symptom of TETANUS. Treatment varies, depending on the cause.

Trisomy

A state in which an individual or a cell carries an extra chromosome. Normally chromosomes exist in pairs; in trisomy, there are three copies of a given chromosome. In humans, trisomy occurs when a cell carries 47 chromosomes instead of 46. For example, in trisomy 21, which causes DOWN SYNDROME, there is an extra chromosome 21. Trisomy causes a higher rate of miscarriage.

Trisomy 21 syndrome

Down syndrome; a genetic disorder involving an extra chromosome 21. Trisomy 21 syndrome is more common than Trisomy 18 syndrome. See DOWN SYNDROME.

Truss

A device worn to hold an intestine or other tissue in place when it protrudes through the abdominal wall. Trusses are also used to control the symptoms of a hernia in individuals who cannot have the operation to repair it for medical reasons or who refuse to have surgery.

Trypanosomiasis

A rare illness caused by the bite of an infected tsetse fly. There are two types of trypanosomiasis, named after the regions where they occur: West African trypanosomiasis, also called Gambian sleeping sickness, is caused by the parasite *Trypanosoma brucei gambiense* and occurs in western and central Africa; East African trypanosomiasis is caused by the parasite *Trypanosoma brucei rhodesiense* and occurs in parts of eastern and central Africa.

Both forms of infection cause serious symptoms including fever, headache, irritability, extreme fatigue, swollen lymph nodes, aching muscles and joints, skin rash, progressive confusion, personality changes, slurred speech, seizures, and difficulty walking and talking; death can result if not promptly treated.

Hospitalization and medication can effectively treat the infections if a correct diagnosis is made soon enough and treatment is begun early in the course of the illness.

Tryptophan

An amino acid that is a building block of NIACIN and SEROTONIN. Tryptophan is important for maintaining normal levels of proteins and normal growth in infants. Good dietary sources include meats, poultry, fish, eggs, nuts, peanut butter, brewer's yeast, and wheat germ.

TSH

Thyroid-stimulating hormone. TSH stimulates the production of the thyroid gland hormone THYROXINE and its release into the bloodstream. TSH secretion is regulated by TRH (thyrotropin-releasing hormone), a hormone produced by the hypothalamus.

Tubal ligation

A sterilization procedure for women in which the passage of eggs through the fallopian tubes is interrupted, using various methods. The goal is to block the eggs from traveling down the tubes to meet the sperm for fertilization. In the procedure, the tubes are looped and banded closed with rubber rings, pinched closed with metal or plastic clips, cut and tied off, or cauterized (burned) with an electric current and cut. A tubal ligation is intended to be a permanent method of birth control, and reversal procedures are complicated and costly and may be unsuccessful. Therefore, sterilization is intended for women who are certain they will not want to become pregnant in the future. A tubal ligation is performed in a hospital or outpatient surgical center with the patient usually under general anesthesia. Usually the patient can go home at the end of the day.

Tubal pregnancy

A pregnancy that develops in a fallopian tube. The vast majority of ectopic pregnancies (pregnancies that start outside the uterus) take place in the fallopian tubes. Tubal pregnancies occur when a scarred or damaged fallopian tube is open enough to permit a sperm to reach an egg and fertilize it, but not enough to allow the fertilized egg to travel to the uterus. The fertilized egg gets stuck in the narrow part of the tube and grows there. Symptoms include a missed period, pelvic pain, or abnormal vaginal bleeding within the first 8 to 12 weeks of pregnancy. Pains can be sudden and severe, sharp, and stabbing. The woman may feel dizzy or faint. Some women have no symptoms, or they may have light bleeding and assume they are miscarrying. Women with tubal pregnancies frequently do not realize they are pregnant.

Early detection of a tubal pregnancy is essential to prevent the rupture of the fallopian tube, which can be life-threatening. Diagnosis will be based on a vaginal examination, an ultrasound (see ULTRASOUND SCANNING) to determine the location of the embryo, and blood tests to measure the level of the hormone HUMAN CHORIONIC GONADOTROPIN (HCG).

Treatment may involve immediate surgery to remove the embryo and any damaged tissue in the fallopian tube. A laparoscope may be used to locate a tubal pregnancy and to remove it. If the fallopian tube is ruptured or bleeding, part or all of it is removed (see SALPINGECTOMY). Sometimes, surgery can be avoided by using a drug called methotrexate, which breaks down the tissue of the abnormal pregnancy so that the woman's body can absorb it.

Tuberculin skin test

The injection of a small amount of testing fluid, called tuberculin, under the skin to see if a reaction develops and to determine whether TUBERCULOSIS, or TB infection, is present. Tuberculin skin tests, which are also referred to as Mantoux tests, are examined and measured 2 to 3 days after the injection.

Tuberculin skin tests are generally performed when a person has been exposed to someone with infectious tuberculosis. It takes several weeks after a person has been exposed and become infected for the immune system to react to the tuberculin skin test.

Tuberculosis

An infectious bacterial disease that usually affects the lungs. Tuberculosis, or TB, may also involve other parts of the body in up to one third of all cases. The lymph nodes, urinary tract, bones, joints, the membrane that covers the brain (called the MENINGES), and the membrane that covers the digestive organs (called the PERITONEUM) may be affected. The bacteria that cause tuberculosis are transmitted from one person to another via contaminated fluid droplets that become airborne when an infected person coughs, sneezes, laughs, or talks.

Forms of tuberculosis include primary pulmonary tuberculosis, reactivation tuberculosis, and extrapulmonary tuberculosis. Primary pulmonary tuberculosis involves a portion of the lungs and nearby lymph nodes. It occurs most often in infants and children. In some children, the primary TB infection spreads from the lungs through the bloodstream to other areas of the body within 2 to 6 months, causing extrapulmonary tuberculosis.

Symptoms and diagnosis

A person with a primary tuberculosis infection generally has no symptoms of disease. The tuberculin skin test usually becomes positive within 3 months of contracting the infection. The symptoms associated with active TB infection vary depending on the specific form of disease.

More than half the children infected with primary pulmonary tuberculosis have no symptoms. Others may have a mild cough that persists, low-grade fever, night sweats, poor appetite, ongoing fatigue, and difficulty gaining weight.

Many times people manage to control the infection initially, but then the infection can reactivate after many years.

Symptoms of postprimary pulmonary tuberculosis may include fever, night sweats, weight loss, poor appetite, weakness, general fatigue, and coughing. The cough eventually causes discolored mucus. As the disease becomes severe, coughing may produce blood, there may be shortness of breath, and severe breathing problems may develop.

Symptoms of extrapulmonary tuberculosis are related to the body areas affected by the infection. When the lymph nodes are involved, the glands become swollen without pain at the sides and base of the neck. The nodes may eventually drain a thick, foul-smelling liquid. If the bones and joints are affected, there may be a curvature of the spine, producing a hunchback, or pain and swelling of a knee or hip, usually resulting in a limp. If the urinary tract is involved, there may be side pain, frequent urination, pain or discomfort on urination, and blood in the urine.

Tuberculosis is diagnosed on the basis of physical symptoms and results of the skin test. If the skin test results are positive, a chest X ray will be evaluated for signs of active TB in the lungs. Sputum and other body fluids may be cultured and examined in a laboratory for TB bacteria.

Treatment, prognosis, and prevention

Tuberculosis is usually treated with isoniazid, which may be given in combination with a second drug. Some strains of TB bacteria are resistant to these first-line medications and are treated with "second-line" medications, including ethionamide, cycloserine, and ofloxacin. It may be necessary to take these medications for as long as 18 months.

Tuberculosis can usually be cured by medication when the course of medication is followed for the full term, which may last as long as 6 months to 2 years. It is essential that TB medication be taken correctly and for the full term to prevent the bacteria from becoming resistant to the medication. Multi-drug resistant tuberculosis is a serious and dangerous form of TB infection that is much harder to treat and can be transmitted to others.

Tuberous sclerosis

A genetic condition characterized by nodular tumors in the brain and other organs. Tuberous sclerosis (TS) develops before birth and continues to progress over the lifetime of the affected individual. Although TS can affect all systems of the body, the abnormal growths most commonly occur in the brain, heart, skin, and kidney. Other organs that can be affected include the eye, bone, lung, and liver. TS leads to a variety of problems, including seizures, skin lesions, tumors, and mental retardation.

Symptoms of TS can vary from no signs of disease to severe symptoms involving one or more organs. The first symptom often may be patches of white skin, seen even on newborns, usually on the trunk and limbs. Older children with the disease develop a characteristic facial rash, particularly around the nose, chin, and cheeks. The rash begins as tiny red spots, which later become small lumps.

Lesions in the brain (injuries caused by abnormal tumor growths) are responsible for the most severe symptoms of TS. Children with TS often have mild to severe mental retardation. Behavior problems are common.

Symptoms involving other organs of the body are also possible. Tumors or cysts in the kidney are most often seen in adults and may cause severe bleeding and dysfunction. Growths in the heart are common in children with TS but rarely cause severe problems and tend to diminish as the child ages.

There is no cure for TS. Treatment is usually focused on the particular symptoms appearing in each case. EPILEPSY is treated with anticonvulsant medication to try to control seizures. Skin problems can be treated with laser techniques. Behavioral problems and mental retardation require psychological and educational treatments.

Tubes in ears

See MYRINGOTOMY.

Tuboplasty

A surgical procedure used to open and sometimes to rebuild fallopian tubes (see FALLOPIAN TUBE), where blockage has prevented conception.

Tularemia

An infectious disease caused by the bacterium *Francisella tularensis* (*F. tularensis*), which is found worldwide in more than 100 species of wild animals, birds, and insects. Tularemia, an acute illness of humans marked by a high fever, is acquired by contact with an infected animal, most commonly a rabbit or tick.

The infection has two forms: the more common form, ulceroglandular tularemia has localized symptoms, and the more lethal typhoidal tularemia involves symptoms that may affect the whole body.

In ulceroglandular tularemia, *F. tularensis* enters the body via a cut or abrasion on the person's skin or by a tick or insect bite. The eyes may become infected as the result of contact with infectious material from contaminated hands. However, in most cases of this illness, the means of transmission are unknown. Research is proceeding on the use of *F. tularensis* to spread tularemia as a form of bioterrorism.

Symptoms of ulceroglandular tularemia include ulcers at the infection site, enlarged lymph glands, headache, muscle pain, and fever. The illness can be effectively cured with antibiotic therapy. Tularemia, especially the typhoidal form, can cause death if it is not treated with appropriate antibiotics. A vaccine against tularemia is recommended for people who are at high risk.

Tummy tuck

A surgical procedure to remove excess skin and fat from the abdomen and to tighten the muscles of the abdominal wall; known medically as an abdominoplasty. The procedure is most successful in individuals who are in good physical health but have a deposit of excess fat and loose skin in the abdomen.

In a complete tummy tuck, the surgeon makes a long incision that runs from one hipbone, down to just above the pubic area, and up and across to the other hipbone. Another incision separates the navel from the surrounding tissue to allow its position to be moved in relationship to the skin. The skin is then separated from the underlying tissue, exposing the muscles of the abdomen. The muscles are pulled more closely together and stitched to hold them in place, firming the wall of the abdomen and narrowing the waist. The flap of skin is drawn down, the excess is cut way, and a new hole for the navel is made.

In a partial tummy tuck, the incision is smaller, and the skin is separated from the underlying tissue only up to the navel. The skin is then drawn down and trimmed, and the incision is sutured shut.

Tumor

A new abnormal growth of tissue in which the reproduction of cells is uncontrolled and escalating. Typically, the more rapid the growth, the more abnormal the cells. Tumors, also called neoplasms, can be benign or malignant. Benign tumors, such as warts and moles, are clumps of cells that resemble the tissue from which they develop but have reproduced and multiplied faster than normal. The cells of benign tumors never spread to other parts of the body.

Malignant tumors do not remain in well-defined clumps, but spread to nearby tissues and organs. The tumor cells also spread along tissue surface and through blood and lymph systems to distant parts of the body.

Tumor-lysis syndrome

A side effect of the rapid destruction and breakdown of a tumor, as with chemotherapy or radiation therapy, that can have dangerous, life-threatening effects. Certain bulky and fast-growing tumors that are very sensitive to treatment can shrink rapidly. The products of the breakdown of the tumor cells are rapidly released into the person's circulation, which can result in high levels of potassium that can affect the electrical rhythm of the heart or high levels of uric acid that can damage the kidneys. The syndrome can be anticipated in certain types of tumors and managed in advance to avoid harm to the person.

Tunnel vision

Sight that lacks vision to the sides and is tightly restricted to the center of the visual field. Tunnel vision can be caused by a number of eye diseases, including RETINITIS PIGMENTOSA and advanced chronic GLAUCOMA. It can also be caused by tumors of the pituitary gland, by strokes, and by mercury poisoning.

Turf toe

An irritation of the joint at the base of the first, or big, toe, which is usually caused by the toe being bent backward or jammed against the ground. Symptoms include pain and swelling of the toe and difficulty walking. Treatment consists of applying ice, taking pain relievers or anti-inflammatory medications, and elevating the foot.

Turner syndrome

A chromosomal abnormality characterized by short stature and infertility in females. In Turner syndrome the ovaries fail to develop, resulting in estrogen deficiency, which prevents development of secondary sexual characteristics, such as the breasts.

Turner syndrome is associated with a number of symptoms and is usually suspected in newborn babies and children by the appearance of physical symptoms such as a "caved-in" chest and puffy hands and feet at birth, short stature, low hairline, drooping eyelids, and absent or retarded physical development at puberty, including the failure to menstruate.

There is no cure for Turner syndrome. Treatment is usually supportive and may include prescribing growth hormone to improve growth rate and final adult height. Estrogen replacement therapy is usually started at age 12 or 13 to stimulate the development of secondary sex characteristics; it cannot, however, reverse the infertility associated with the syndrome. Women with Turner syndrome can sometimes become pregnant by having a donor egg implanted in the uterus.

Cardiac surgery is sometimes required to correct heart defects. There is also the at risk of developing high blood pressure, cataracts, arthritis, obesity, and diabetes mellitus. Most females with Turner syndrome are able to live full and satisfying lives.

Twelve-step program

A method of dealing with addiction that relies on self-help, peer counseling and support, abstinence, and spiritual awakening. The best-known twelve-step program is Alcoholics Anonymous (widely known as AA), founded by a recovered alcoholic in 1935. A number of similarly organ-ized recovery groups follow much the same approach, including Al-Anon (for the relatives and friends of people in recovery) and Narcotics Anonymous.

Twins

Two siblings resulting from the same pregnancy. Twins occur in about 1 percent of all births. Most twins are fraternal, meaning that each baby developed from a separate egg and sperm and has its own placenta and amniotic sac. Fraternal twins can be the same sex or different sexes, and they may not look alike. Identical twins are rare, occurring when one fertilized egg splits early in pregnancy and develops into two fetuses. Identical twins may share a single placenta, but each fetus usually has its own amniotic sac. They are always the same sex, with the same blood type, and they always look alike, with the same hair and eye colors.

Women who are pregnant with twins need special prenatal care. They often see their medical caregiver more often than usual and have more prenatal tests. They need to eat about 2,700 calories per day, more than they would if they were carrying one baby. Anemia is more common in women pregnant with twins, and it is important for the woman to take prenatal vitamins, iron supplements, and folic acid as prescribed.

Tympanometry

A test of the movement of the eardrum (tympanic membrane) to determine if there is fluid in the middle ear space and to measure the air pressure if there is no fluid. Tympanometry is not a hearing test and cannot measure a person's ability to hear. Rather, it is a diagnostic tool used to determine a possible cause of hearing loss or impairment. See also OTITIS MEDIA.

Tympanoplasty

A surgical procedure to treat hearing loss by repairing the eardrum (tympanic membrane) or by repairing or repositioning the tiny bones of the middle ear. Tympanoplasty is performed to eliminate an infection or repair a perforation of the eardrum and to repair the sound-transmitting structures of the middle ear. See OTITIS MEDIA.

Tympanum

The eardrum (tympanic membrane). The tympanum consists of a membrane in the ear canal between the outer ear and the middle ear. The eardrum resembles the head of a tiny drum. Sound waves cause the tympanum to vibrate. These vibrations stimulate the eighth cranial nerve, which transmits these impulses to the brain where they are interpreted as sounds. See EAR.

Typhoid fever

A bacterial infection most commonly caused by *Salmonella typhi*. Typhoid fever, also called enteric fever, is spread by eating or drinking food or water contaminated by fecal matter containing infectious bacteria. Once ingested, the bacteria multiply in the blood and spread from the intestines through the bloodstream to the intestinal lymph nodes, the liver, and the spleen.

Early symptoms may include fever, malaise, and abdominal pain. The temperature tends to increase and may go as high as 103°F, often with severe diarrhea. Weakness, debilitating fatigue, delirium, and an ill physical appearance may follow. In about half of cases, a rash of small, pink, flat lesions called "rose spots" appears on the abdomen and chest, usually during the second week of fever.

The illness is treated with antibiotics, intravenous fluids, and electrolytes given to combat dehydration. (See REHYDRATION FLUID, ORAL.) With treatment, the condition of a person with typhoid fever can improve within 5 days to 2 weeks.

Ulcer

A sore or wound on the skin or a mucous membrane.

Ulcerative colitis

See COLITIS.

Ulcer-healing agents

See ANTACIDS; HISTAMINE₂ BLOCKERS; PROTON PUMP INHIBITORS.

Ultrasound scanning

Also known as sonography or ultrasonography; a diagnostic screening technique that uses high-frequency sound waves to create images of internal body structures. Because ultrasound scanning does not involve exposure to ionizing radiation (as X rays do), it is a safe screening and di-

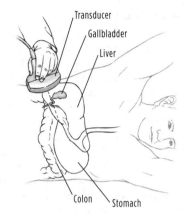

Having an ultrasound

A person getting an ultrasound scan (for example, of the gallbladder) lies on an examining table, and a technician runs a transducer over the area that is being examined. If the gallbladder contains gallstones, the solid stones will reflect sound waves differently than the bile fluid in the gallbladder.

agnostic technique that can safely be used in pregnant women and in children. During pregnancy, ultrasound is used to determine the age and rate of growth of the fetus and its position in the uterus. It can also be used to identify multiple pregnancies or a visible birth defect, and to determine the position of the placenta and the amount of amniotic fluid. Ultrasound scanning is also used to guide procedures such as LAPAROSCOPY, AMNIOCENTESIS, CHORIONIC VILLUS SAMPLING, and needle biopsies. See also DOPPLER ULTRASOUND.

Ultrasound treatment

The use of sound waves to produce heat internally to treat an injured joint or muscle and other musculoskeletal conditions. The deep heat promotes healing by increasing blood flow to the affected area. Ultrasound treatment is sometimes used in physical therapy.

Ultrasound, vaginal

An imaging method used to detect abnormalities of the female reproductive system. During this painless procedure, a long, thin wand called a transducer is inserted into the vagina; the transducer emits sound waves that bounce off the organ under study and produce an image of the organ on a video screen. Vaginal ultrasound is also used to evaluate a pregnancy at a very early stage, particularly to diagnose an ECTOPIC PREGNANCY.

Ultraviolet light

Invisible rays that occur naturally in sunlight. The ultraviolet light spectrum is divided into ultraviolet A (UVA), ultraviolet B (UVB), and ultraviolet C (UVC). UVA light is most responsible for the tanning and burning effects on the skin. Overexposure to ultraviolet light is associated with an increased risk of skin cancer, premature aging of the skin, suppression of the immune system, and cataracts.

Umbilical cord

A flexible, ropelike structure that connects the fetus to the placenta inside the uterus during pregnancy. The umbilical cord delivers nutrients from the mother to the fetus and eliminates waste from the fetus. The umbilical cord contains two arteries and one vein and is about 16 to 24 inches long. At birth, the umbilical cord is clamped and cut.

Umbilicus

The scar left on the abdomen when the umbilical cord falls off after birth; usually called the navel or belly button.

Unconscious

Unaware; lacking the ability to respond. A person who is unconscious does not respond when spoken to, touched, or stimulated in other ways. Any unconscious person who does not regain consciousness quickly requires emergency medical treatment.

Unsaturated fats

Dietary fats that come primarily from plants and fish rather than from animal sources and are divided into two groups: polyunsaturated and monounsaturated fats. See FATS AND OILS.

Urea

A by-product of the metabolism of protein in the liver; the principal waste product in urine. Urea is normally filtered from the blood by the kidneys and excreted in urine. An accumulation of urea in the blood, a condition called uremia, is a sign of KIDNEY FAILURE.

Uremia

An abnormal accumulation of urea and other metabolic waste products in the bloodstream. Uremia is caused by impaired kidney function and occurs when the kidneys are unable to filter the waste product urea from the blood. Symptoms of uremia include nausea, vomiting, loss of appetite, hiccups, weakness, itching, and mental confusion.

Ureters

The tubes that transport urine from each kidney to the bladder. See URINARY TRACT.

Ureteral colic

Severe pain in the back that occurs when one or more kidney stones become trapped in a ureter (one of two tubes that transport urine from the kidneys to the bladder).

Urethra

The tube that drains urine from the bladder out of the body. The urethra is much shorter in women than in men, which may be why women tend to experience many more urinary tract infections than men.

Urethral dilation

A surgical procedure to widen an abnormally narrow urethra (the tube that drains urine from the bladder). To perform the procedure, instruments of progressively larger sizes (called dilators) are inserted into the urethra to stretch the narrowed area. It is performed most often on men who have a URETHRAL STRICTURE.

Urethral discharge

Fluid (other than urine) such as pus expelled from the urethra. Discharge without blood is usually a symptom of a SEXUALLY TRANSMITTED DISEASE, such as GONORRHEA or CHLAMYDIA. Blood in the discharge may indicate a foreign object in the urethra, abnormal narrowing of the urethra (URETHRAL STRICTURE), or a tumor. An examination is needed to determine the cause and treatment.

Urethral stricture

Abnormal narrowing of the urethra (the tube that drains urine from the bladder). The problem is common in men but rare in women. Urethral stricture usually results from injury, sometimes as a side effect of surgery on the urinary tract, or infection. Symptoms include pain during urination, difficulty urinating, a weak urine stream, a need to urinate frequently, blood in the semen or urine, pain in the lower abdomen or pelvis, discharge from the urethra, or swelling of the penis. Left untreated, urethral stricture can block urine flow and cause kidney damage.

Treatment consists of widening the urethra with an expanding instrument called a dilator. If this is not successful, or if the stricture reoccurs, surgery may be recommended.

Urethral syndrome, acute

Irritation of the bladder that is not caused by infection; also known as noninfectious CYSTITIS. The condition is most common in women of childbearing age and rarely occurs in men. Possible causes include bubble baths, feminine hygiene sprays, sanitary napkins, spermicidal jellies, and sexual intercourse.

Symptoms may include pressure in the lower pelvis; painful urination; frequent, urgent need to urinate; decreased ability to hold urine (incontinence); having to urinate at night (nocturia); cloudy, bloody, or foul-smelling urine; pain during sexual intercourse; pain in the penis; pain in the side below the ribs; fatigue; and chills. The condition is usually treated with medication to control the symptoms and dietary changes such as avoiding fluids that can irritate the bladder (such as alcohol, caffeine, and citrus juices).

Urethritis, nongonococcal

A SEXUALLY TRANSMITTED DISEASE (STD) that causes inflammation of the urethra. Nongonococcal urethritis (NGU) is usually caused by *Chlamydia* bacteria, but may also be caused by types of *Ureaplasma, Mycoplasma,* and *Trichomonas* bacteria and the herpes simplex virus.

Because the symptoms of NGU tend to be mild or nonexistent, an infected person may not be aware of the infection and does not seek medical treatment. Without treatment, NGU can spread further into the reproductive tract.

When symptoms develop, they tend to occur gradually and intensify over a period of several days. In men, they may include a clear mucous discharge from the penis and redness around the urinary opening. Both men and women may experience frequent urination with pain or burning. Women's symptoms may include a vaginal discharge, abnormal menstrual bleeding, and discomfort in the anal or rectal area.

The bacteria that cause NGU can be detected in urine and in genital tract secretions. Antibiotics can treat NGU successfully. Infected people and their partners should abstain from sexual activity until the infection has cleared up.

Urethrocele

A condition in which the urethra bulges into the vagina. A urethrocele most often results from stretching of the pelvic muscles that support the vagina, rectum, and bladder, usually from childbirth. Symptoms may include a feeling of pressure or aching in the vagina, difficulty urinating, and difficulty with penetration during sexual intercourse.

A urethrocele can usually be detected by a doctor during a routine pelvic examination. Practicing KEGEL

EXERCISES (alternately contracting and relaxing the pelvic floor muscles) may help relieve the symptoms. Hormone replacement therapy may be recommended to some postmenopausal women to help reverse some of the weakening of pelvic support tissues that can occur from the loss of estrogen. Incontinence can be treated with medication; a plastic device called a pessary may be inserted to restore prolapsed organs to their normal position. When symptoms are severe enough to interfere with daily activities, urethroceles can be corrected surgically.

Uric acid

An organic acid containing nitrogen; the by-product of nucleic acid metabolism and a component of blood and urine. Normal amounts of uric acid are eliminated from the body in urine, but high amounts of uric acid can form solid crystals. If these solid crystals lodge in the joints and skin, they can cause a painful condition called GOUT. Uric acid crystals that form in the kidneys can cause KIDNEY STONES. Large amounts of uric acid are found in certain foods, particularly red meats, organ meats such as liver and kidney, anchovies, and some shellfish.

Urinalysis

Evaluation of a sample of urine to look for abnormal substances that could indicate a health problem; used to confirm a pregnancy. Urinalysis is also used to diagnose urinary tract infections and diabetes.

Urinary diversion

A surgical procedure that reroutes the flow of urine from the kidneys. Urinary diversion is usually performed when the bladder must be removed because of cancer or a birth defect. A number of surgical procedures can be performed, depending on the abnormality and the health of the person.

Urinary retention

Slow, hesitant, weak, or incomplete emptying of urine from the bladder. The disorder can be caused by several different conditions, including partial or complete blockage of the urinary tract by a calculus (stone), injury to the urethra (see URETHRAL STRICTURE), an enlarged prostate gland, cancer of the prostate, a birth defect, an infection, bladder muscle weakness, or a tumor. Left untreated, the condition can cause urine to back up into the kidneys and severely damage them. An examination by a doctor and various tests, such as a URINALYSIS, X rays, or CYSTOSCOPY, are needed to establish the cause. Treatment depends on the cause.

Urinary tract

The system of organs that filter out waste products and excess water from the bloodstream and expel it as urine. The major structures within the urinary tract are the KIDNEYS, the URETERS, the BLADDER, and the URETHRA. The kidneys filter blood. Waste materials and excess fluid filtered out of the blood collect first in each kidney, in a system of collecting ducts and storage areas. This fluid, urine, is composed of water, urea (the waste product), and sodium chloride. From each kidney, a slender tube called a ureter transports the processed urine from the kidneys to the bladder, a muscular sac that holds the urine until enough builds up to eliminate. When the bladder contracts, urine flows into the urethra and out of the body. In females, the urethral opening is located just above the vaginal opening; in males, the urethra runs the length of the penis and opens at the tip.

Urinary tract infections

Bacterial infections affecting the urinary tract. Urinary tract infections occur more frequently in women than in men. Symptoms include pain or a burning sensation while urinating, a frequent urge to urinate, pressure in the lower part of the abdomen, blood in the urine, and foul-smelling urine.

The most common urinary tract infection is CYSTITIS (infection of the bladder). Infection of the urethra (see URETHRITIS, NONGONOCOCCAL) often occurs at the same time. If bacteria travel up to the kidneys, PYELONEPHRITIS may result. Urinary tract infections are treated with antibiotics. The person may be referred to a urologist.

Urination, painful

Discomfort or burning during urination. The problem usually results from an infection in the urinary tract, although it may also be caused by inflammation of the prostate gland (PROSTATITIS) or a calculus or stone in the urinary tract. In women, it can be caused by a problem of the reproductive system such as cancer of the cervix. Diagnosis requires a physical examination and urinalysis to check for infectious microorganisms. Treatment depends on the cause.

Urine

Liquid waste produced by the kidneys, stored in the bladder, and eliminated from the body through the urethra. In humans, urine is made up of water, urea, salt, and uric acid. Urine is about 96 percent water and 4 percent solid waste. The average amount of urine excreted each day ranges from 40 to 80 ounces. Abnormal urine contains substances not usually present in urine and can be a sign of infection or disease.

Urine tests

Laboratory studies of a sample of urine to determine the health of the kidneys, bladder, and urinary tract or to help diagnose some disorders such as diabetes or kidney disease.

Urology

The branch of medicine that treats disorders of the urinary tract in both males and females and the reproductive system in males. A urologist is a physician who specializes in this discipline. See URINARY TRACT; REPRODUCTIVE SYSTEM, MALE.

Urticaria

See HIVES.

Uterus

A hollow, muscular organ of the female reproductive system, located in the center of the pelvis. The wall of the uterus is lined with tissue (called the endometrium) that builds up and sheds during each menstrual cycle (see MENSTRUATION). For pregnancy to occur, a fertilized egg implants in the wall of the uterus and develops into a fetus. The uterus is very elastic, able to expand to many times its original size during pregnancy. See also REPRODUCTIVE SYSTEM, FEMALE.

Uterus, cancer of the

Most uterine cancers are tumors involving cells in the uterine lining (endometrium). Symptoms include abnormal bleeding, spotting, or discharge from the vagina. Cancer of the uterus is rare before age 40 and most often occurs in women between ages 60 and 75.

A suspected cancer of the uterus can be evaluated by a number of tests, including ULTRASOUND SCANNING, ENDOMETRIAL BIOPSY, HYSTEROSCOPY, and D AND C. (A PAP SMEAR is not a reliable test for diagnosing uterine cancer.) Treatment for uterine cancer is usually a HYSTERECTOMY (surgical removal of the uterus) and a SALPINGO-OOPHORECTOMY (surgical removal of the ovaries and fallopian tubes). Some women are given RADIATION THERAPY after surgery. CHEMOTHERAPY may be used to treat cancer that has spread to other organs.

Uterus, prolapse of the

A condition in which the uterus drops down from its normal position into the vagina. Prolapse occurs when the ligaments holding the uterus in place are stretched by pregnancy and childbirth or are weakened after menopause due to loss of estrogen. Depending on the degree of prolapse, symptoms can include a lump or bulge in the vagina, a feeling of heaviness and discomfort, occasional backache, and stress incontinence (leaking of urine when a woman coughs or sneezes).

Prolapse poses little risk to general health. Treatment of a mild prolapse includes KEGEL EXERCISES to strengthen the pelvic muscles, weight loss to reduce pressure on the pelvis, and a high-fiber diet to prevent constipation. See also URETHROCELE.

Uterus, retroverted

A uterus that inclines downward and backward; also called a "tipped" uterus. This condition occurs in about 20 percent of women; in most cases, it causes no symptoms or problems and no treatment is required. A small percentage of women experience pain during sexual intercourse or menstruation. If symptoms are severe, surgery to adjust the position of the uterus may be recommended.

UV light

See ULTRAVIOLET LIGHT.

Uveitis

Inflammation of the uvea, the middle layer of the eye. The uvea includes the iris (the colored part of the eye), the ciliary body (which lies behind the iris), and the choroid (which supports the retina, the light-sensitive layer at the back of the eye). Since the uvea contains large numbers of blood vessels that nourish the eye, inflammation can threaten sight. Symptoms, which can come on suddenly or develop slowly, include sensitivity to light, blurred vision, pain, and redness. The disease has many possible causes, including viral infections. Treatment, which aims to relieve pain and preserve vision, may include corticosteroid medications in eye drops, pills, or injections, and antibiotics. Any underlying disease will also be treated.

Uvula

A small, fleshy mass at the back of the mouth that hangs from the soft palate above the back of the tongue. The uvula is made of muscle and connective tissue and is covered by a mucous membrane. Its function is not clear.

Vaccination

The process of stimulating the body's immune system to develop long-term protection against, or immunity to, certain diseases without actually having the disease. Introducing an inactivated form of specific disease-causing organisms stimulates the immune system to produce antibodies to fight the specific disease-causing organisms when a person is exposed to them.

Vaccinations are given on a recommended schedule from birth to age 16 to protect children from a number of serious, contagious infections. DIPHTHERIA, PERTUSSIS (whooping cough), MEASLES, and POLIO used to kill thousands of American children each year but routine childhood vaccinations have virtually eradicated these diseases in the United States. Most vaccinations are given by injection. The risk of having a reaction to a vaccination is much lower than the health risks involved in having the infection. Serious reactions to vaccinations are rare. The most common side effect is soreness or swelling at the site of the injection. Vaccines are available to protect against diphtheria, TETANUS, and pertussis (together in an injection referred to as aDTP); HEPATITIS B

(HBV); polio; HAEMOPHILUS INFLUENZAE type B (Hib); measles, MUMPS, and RUBELLA (MMR); poliovirus (IPV); pneumococcal bacteria infections (PCV and PPV); INFLUENZA; and CHICKENPOX (varicella). See also VACCINE; TRAVEL IMMUNIZATION.

Vaccine

A preparation introduced into the body to stimulate an immune response to provide future protection against, or immunity to, certain infectious diseases. Vaccines contain killed or weakened forms of infectious organisms or particles of an infectious organism that stimulate the immune response without producing an actual infection.

Vacuum extraction

A procedure that uses suction to pull a baby down the birth canal during a vaginal delivery that is difficult or prolonged. A metal or plastic cap is attached to the baby's scalp and connected to a vacuum pump. Vacuum extraction is used instead of a FORCEPS DELIVERY if the mother is exhausted or has a heart condition, or when the baby begins to show signs of distress.

Vagina

A muscular tube about 5 inches long that extends from the neck of the uterus (cervix) to the external genital area in females. The vagina is the passageway to the internal reproductive organs. See REPRODUCTIVE SYSTEM, FEMALE.

Vaginal bleeding, abnormal

Bleeding from the vagina at times other than during a menstrual period, or bleeding during a period that is heavier than usual. In women of reproductive age, causes of abnormal vaginal bleeding can include the use of birth control pills; hormonal imbalances; infections of the reproductive system, including SEXUALLY TRANSMITTED DISEASES; an ECTOPIC PREGNANCY; and miscarriage. Abnormal bleeding can also result from scars, tumors, fibroids, or other abnormal tissue in the uterus or cervix; or by cysts on the ovaries.

Irregular periods are common during the years before menopause. Treatment depends on the cause of the bleeding.

Vaginal ultrasound

See ULTRASOUND, VAGINAL.

Vaginal vault prolapse

A condition in which the top of the vagina loses its support and drops, usually following a HYSTERECTOMY. The weakening of the tissues supporting the pelvic organs usually results from pressure on the organs during pregnancy and childbirth or from loss of estrogen after menopause. Symptoms include a feeling of heaviness in the vagina, aching in the lower abdomen or lower back, and bulging of organs against the vaginal wall. The diagnosis of vaginal vault prolapse requires a pelvic examination. Treatment may include KEGEL EXERCISES to strengthen the pelvic muscles, a pessary (a device inserted into the vagina to support the pelvic organs), or surgery to strengthen pelvic support.

Vaginismus

Involuntary spasms of the muscles of the vagina, making sexual intercourse uncomfortable, difficult, or impossible. A woman with vaginismus may also be unable to tolerate a pelvic examination or the insertion of a tampon. Past traumatic sexual experiences may lead to vaginismus in some women. Doctors usually refer affected women to a sex therapist for treatment that combines education and counseling with behavioral exercises such as KEGEL EXERCISES (which improve voluntary muscle control).

Vaginitis

A common condition characterized by inflammation of the vagina, usually resulting from an infection. Other causes include irritation from products such as soaps and the reduction in estrogen after menopause. Common symptoms include irritation, redness, or swelling of vaginal tissues. Vaginitis can also cause a discharge, itching, odor, or a burning sensation. For a diagnosis, a sample of vaginal discharge is examined under a microscope. Treatment depends on the cause, and may include oral medication or a cream or gel that is applied to the vagina. The risk of vaginitis can be reduced by using condoms during sexual intercourse, washing diaphragms and cervical caps carefully after each use, and avoiding feminine hygiene sprays, deodorant tampons, and douches.

Vaginitis, atrophic

Inflammation of the vagina usually resulting from the reduction in estrogen after menopause that can cause the walls of the vagina to become drier, thinner, less elastic, and more likely to bleed. Vaginal dryness can cause irritation, burning, or itching and a feeling of pressure, all of which can interfere with a woman's sexual enjoyment. To relieve the symptoms, treatment may involve topical hormonal creams (inserted vaginally) or hormone therapy to restore estrogen levels.

Vaginosis, bacterial

Inflammation of the vagina caused by bacteria; the most common vaginal infection. See VAGINITIS.

Vagotomy

A surgical procedure in which the vagus nerve is cut to reduce acid production in the stomach. The vagus nerve, a major nerve that extends from the brain to most of the other major organs, controls production of stomach acid in addition to many other activities. A vagotomy is performed when a peptic ulcer (see PEPTIC ULCER DISEASE) fails to respond to medication or less invasive treatment or when complications such as bleeding or obstruction develop. The procedure is normally combined with a pyloroplasty (surgical widening of the pylorus, the stomach outlet to the intestine). In some cases, a vagotomy is done with a partial gastrectomy (surgical removal of part of the stomach). Advances in the treatment of ulcer disease have dramatically reduced the need for this procedure.

Valsalva maneuver

An exercise that doctors use to diagnose and treat abnormal heart rhythms and relieve chest pain. In the Valsalva maneuver, a person tries to exhale while keeping his or her mouth and nose closed. The maneuver is sometimes used with echocardiography (ultrasound examination of the heart).

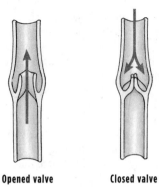

Opened valve   **Closed valve**

One-way flow
A valve in a vein opens when the muscles in the wall of the vein contract and cause pressure to build behind the valve. When the muscles relax and the pressure decreases, the valve closes and prevents backflow.

Valve

A structure in some body parts that allows fluid to flow in one direction. Valves are important to the function of the heart, the veins, and the lymphatic system. Valves consist of cusps, or flaps, that fasten to the walls of the body part. When blood or lymphatic fluid flows through the valves in the proper direction, the cusps stay open; if the fluid flow is reversed, the cusps become filled with liquid and expand to block the backflow.

Valve replacement

See HEART VALVE SURGERY.

Valvotomy

An open-heart surgical procedure in which a damaged heart valve is cut in order to open it; also known as a valvulotomy. See HEART VALVE SURGERY.

Valvular heart disease

Any dysfunction or abnormality affecting one or more of the valves that control blood flow into, out of, and inside the heart. Several kinds of problems can affect the valves. Incompetence, or regurgitation, occurs when a valve leaks (see AORTIC INSUFFICIENCY; MITRAL INSUFFICIENCY; TRICUSPID INSUFFICIENCY). Narrowing or partial blockage of a valve is called valvular stenosis (see STENOSIS, VALVULAR). Atresia is a serious condition in which a valve fails to develop properly and is closed at birth; it can affect any of the valves. Prolapse refers to abnormal bulging of the valve when the heart contracts.

Valvuloplasty

A minimally invasive, nonsurgical procedure for treating stenosis (narrowing) of a heart valve; also known as balloon valvuloplasty. For a valvuloplasty, the doctor makes a small incision, usually into the groin, to expose an artery or vein, and then threads a catheter (thin tube) through the blood vessel into the heart. When the catheter reaches the narrowed valve, a balloon at its tip is inflated to open the narrowed valve. The balloon is then deflated and the catheter is withdrawn. Valvuloplasty is used most often to treat stenosis of the mitral valve (see MITRAL STENOSIS).

Varicella

See CHICKENPOX.

Varices

Enlarged, twisted, winding veins, arteries, or lymphatic vessels; singular, varix. See VARICOSE VEINS.

Varicocele

Enlarged veins along the spermatic cord, or vas deferens, the tubular structure that suspends the testicles and transports sperm cells. Abnormal valves in the veins cause blood to back up and stretch the veins, disrupting normal blood flow. Varicoceles often develop slowly and usually are painless. They are most likely to develop on the left side of the scrotum in men between ages 15 and 25 and are a common cause of infertility in men. In an older man, the sudden appearance of a varicocele can be a sign of a kidney tumor affecting the renal vein and altering blood flow from the scrotum.

Varicose veins

Enlarged, twisted, stretched veins, usually close to the surface of the skin and visible as soft, bluish, bulging curves. Varicose veins are most likely to affect the feet and legs, can cause the legs to ache, and can bleed if injured. When deep veins are involved, the leg may swell and skin ulcers may develop, usually near the ankles. The skin typically turns brown before a skin ulcer appears. People with varicose veins should avoid sitting or standing for long periods. Elevating the legs at least 12 inches above the heart at the end of the day helps relieve swelling. If an ulcer appears, it should be treated by a doctor to prevent infection and GANGRENE (death of the tissue). Mild to moderate varicose veins can be treated with laser therapy or sclerotherapy (the injection of a solution into the veins to decrease blood flow to an affected area).

Vas deferens

In males, a narrow, coiled tube that carries sperm from the epididymis (a connecting duct) and testicles through the prostate gland and into the urethra during ejaculation. The vas deferens, about 2 feet long, is also

known as the spermatic cord. See RE-
PRODUCTIVE SYSTEM, MALE.

Vascular dementia

A form of DEMENTIA caused by a series of small strokes (damage to brain
tissue from an interruption in the
blood supply to the brain). Vascular
dementia is also known as multi-
infarct dementia. High blood pressure
is the primary cause. The symptoms
tend to occur and progress in steps.
There may be only mild weakness in
an arm or leg, slurred speech, or temporary dizziness or confusion. The
condition then progresses as each
stroke occurs, in contrast with the
steady progression of symptoms in
ALZHEIMER'S DISEASE. In addition to
confusion and short-term memory
problems, symptoms may include decreased judgment and understanding, disorientation, impaired speech,
an inability to name objects, and difficulty concentrating. Affected people may have some improvement
after a stroke but then symptoms
worsen again after another stroke.

A diagnosis of vascular dementia,
which can be difficult to distinguish
from Alzheimer's disease, is based on
a physical examination including a
neurological examination, a full medical history, and test results. The imaging studies may show areas of
damaged brain tissue consistent with
damage from stroke. Treatment,
which focuses on reducing the risk of
future strokes, includes controlling
underlying conditions such as high
blood pressure and type 2 diabetes.

Vascular surgery

Surgery performed on the blood vessels. Examples include CAROTID EN-
DARTERECTOMY and THROMBECTOMY.

Vasculitis

Inflammation of a blood vessel. Vasculitis can result from an allergic reaction to a drug or foreign substance
(allergic vasculitis) or from inflammatory diseases such as RHEUMATOID
ARTHRITIS or systemic lupus erythematosus (see LUPUS ERYTHEMATOSUS,
SYSTEMIC) that scar blood vessels and
can impair blood flow to a part of the
body.

Vasectomy

A sterilization procedure for men
that cuts and seals off the vas deferens, the small tubes that transport
sperm from the testicles. A vasectomy has no effect on sexual desire or
performance. Although a vasectomy
can sometimes be reversed, it should
be considered a permanent form of
sterilization. Serious complications
from the procedure are unusual.
There is a small risk of infection, excessive bleeding during recovery, or
blood collecting in the scrotum. In
rare cases, the two ends of the vas deferens rejoin and fertility is restored.

A vasectomy does not result in
immediate infertility because some
sperm cells remain in the reproductive system, particularly in the seminal vesicles. Until these sperm cells
are ejaculated or die, the man is still
fertile. Until two consecutive counts
show no sperm cells, the man and his
partner should use an alternate form
of contraception.

In some cases, a vasectomy can be
reversed in a procedure called a
vasovasostomy. In vasovasostomy, a
surgeon uses a powerful operating
microscope to see and repair the tiny
structures in the vas deferens. Most
men who have a vasovasostomy are
able to ejaculate sperm cells, but only

about half are able to produce a pregnancy.

Vasoconstriction

Narrowing (constriction) of a blood vessel, which can slow or stop blood flow. The autonomic nervous system controls the smooth muscle in blood vessel walls that constricts the blood vessel. The body uses vasoconstriction and vasodilation to help distribute blood throughout the body.

Vasodilation

The relaxing and widening (dilation) of blood vessels, which increases blood flow. Certain medications used to treat HYPERTENSION (high blood pressure) achieve their effect through vasodilation. As the blood vessels relax, they offer less resistance to the flow of blood, and blood pressure drops.

Vasodilators

Drugs that widen blood vessels by relaxing blood vessel walls. Vasodilators are used to treat congestive heart failure (see HEART FAILURE, CONGESTIVE) by reducing the workload of the heart and by lowering blood pressure to increase the supply of oxygen and blood to the heart. These drugs are also used to treat HYPERTENSION.

Angiotensin-converting enzyme (ACE) inhibitors

A group of vasodilators that block an enzyme needed to produce a substance that causes blood vessels to constrict or narrow.

Angiotensin II
Receptor blockers (ARBs)

For people who need something stronger than an ACE inhibitor, ARBs completely block the effects of angiotensin on the blood vessels.

Nitrates

Vasodilators that work by relaxing or dilating blood vessels to increase the flow of blood and oxygen to the heart and heart muscle. Nitrates are used to treat chest pain associated with ANGINA.

Vasopressin

See ADH.

Vasospasm

The constriction or narrowing of blood vessels as a result of contraction of the smooth muscle in blood vessel walls. Cerebral vasospasm is a common complication of a subarachnoid hemorrhage (bleeding into the space between the brain and the arachnoid membrane; see HEMORRHAGE, SUBARACHNOID). If the blood vessels in the brain narrow to the point of limiting blood flow, there is an increased risk of tissue damage and death.

Vector

A public health term for an animal, arachnid (such as a tick), or insect (such as a mosquito) that can transmit a disease-causing microorganism to people. Vectors can transmit viruses, bacteria, protozoa, and worms from one host to another. The most common diseases transmitted by infected vectors include ROCKY MOUNTAIN SPOTTED FEVER and LYME DISEASE (which are carried by ticks) and MALARIA (which is carried by mosquitoes).

Vegetarianism

A diet that emphasizes plant foods and restricts some or all animal foods. There are three types of vegetarians: lacto-ovo-vegetarians, lacto-vegetarians, and vegans. Lacto-ovo-vegetarians consume milk, cheese, yogurt, and eggs along with plant foods. Lacto-vegetarians consume milk, cheese, and yogurt but no egg products. Vegans eat no animal products at all.

Vegetative state

A condition in which a person has lost cognitive neurological function and awareness but retains noncognitive (automatic) functions and a sleep-wake cycle. A persistent vegetative state sometimes follows a COMA. The prognosis depends on the nature and cause of the neurological damage. Some people regain a certain amount of awareness after a vegetative state. Others remain in this condition for many years without recovering. PNEUMONIA is the most common cause of death for people who are in a vegetative state.

Veins

Blood vessels that carry deoxygenated blood back to the heart. Veins complete the circulation of the blood that begins in the arteries, which transport oxygenated blood from the heart to the rest of the body. Unlike arteries, veins do not pulse; they depend on the movement of muscle surrounding them to push the blood along. Veins in the arms and legs (but not in the head, neck, or torso) have one-way valves that allow the blood to flow only in one direction. See CARDIOVASCULAR SYSTEM.

Vena cava

One of the two largest veins in the body. The superior vena cava starts at the top of the chest and carries blood from the head, neck, arms, and chest to the heart, entering the heart at the right atrium. The inferior vena cava begins in the lower abdomen and transports blood from the legs, pelvis, and abdomen, entering the heart at the right atrium. See CARDIOVASCULAR SYSTEM.

Venipuncture

The puncture of a vein through the skin with a stylet or a steel needle attached to a syringe or catheter. Venipuncture is performed to withdraw blood, inject a medication, start an intravenous infusion, or inject a radioactive substance for body imaging techniques.

Ventilation, mechanical

The use of a machine to take over a person's breathing if he or she cannot breathe independently; it can be used temporarily or permanently. Mechanical ventilation maintains the correct balance of oxygen and carbon dioxide in the body.

Ventilator

A machine designed to provide proper gas exchange (ventilation) in the body for people who are unable to breathe independently. Mechanical ventilators consist of a system for pumping air combined with a control panel that monitors and adjusts the air delivery system. Ventilation tubing is connected to a humidifier (to prevent the lungs from drying out) and to the person receiving ventilation via an endotracheal tube, tracheostomy, or mask.

Ventricle

A small functional space or cavity in an organ, particularly the heart and brain.

Ventricular ectopic beat

A heart rhythm abnormality in which the ventricles (the lower chambers of the heart) contract before the atria (the upper chambers of the heart); also known as premature ventricular contractions. Some people with the condition experience it as a wildly fast, galloping heartbeat (palpitations), which can be frightening and startling. Other people have no noticeable symptoms. Ventricular ectopic beat has a number of possible causes, including anxiety and stress, fatigue, alcohol, caffeine, and electrolyte imbalance.

A person experiencing frequent or worsening ventricular ectopic beats, particularly if accompanied by chest pain, should see a doctor. Medications such as BETA BLOCKERS, which block the stress response, may be prescribed. In severe cases, a procedure called ABLATION THERAPY is used to eliminate the abnormal tissue that is causing the arrhythmia.

Ventricular fibrillation

Rapid, weak, uncontrolled quivering of the ventricles (the lower chambers of the heart), reducing the amount of blood the heart pumps. Ventricular fibrillation is a medical emergency requiring immediate medical treatment. If a normal heartbeat cannot be reestablished within a few minutes, death will result. Defibrillation, the administration of an electric shock to the heart, is given to reestablish a normal rhythm.

Ventricular fibrillation occurs sud-

denly, sometimes preceded by feelings of light-headedness. Other warning signs can include palpitations, fatigue, weakness, shortness of breath, and chest pain. The person faints because the oxygen supply to the brain is insufficient. Anyone who survives an episode of ventricular fibrillation needs to be examined by a doctor to determine the cause.

Treatment depends on the cause. Medications can be used to control heart rhythm. An electronic device (called an internal cardioverter defibrillator), which monitors the heart for arrhythmia and administers an electrical shock if ventricular fibrillation occurs, may be permanently implanted in the chest. Many public places now make automated external defibrillators (AEDs) available for use even by nonmedical people who have had no prior training.

Ventricular tachycardia

See TACHYCARDIA, VENTRICULAR.

Vernix

A greasy, white coating on the skin of newborns. The vernix protects the skin of the fetus inside the uterus.

Verruca

See WARTS.

Version, external

A procedure in which a doctor attempts to reposition a fetus in the uterus to avoid a breech delivery by applying slow, steady pressure to the pregnant woman's abdomen. If a fetus is in a breech presentation (buttocks or feet first instead of head first) after the 36th week of pregnancy, external version may be used to turn the head of the fetus downward.

Vertebra

One of the ringlike bones that make up the spine. A cushion of fibrous cartilage with a gelatinous center (called a disk) lies between each vertebra except the first two below the skull and the last two, the sacrum and coccyx (tailbone). The disks allow each vertebra to move as a unit, giving the spine some flexibility.

Vertigo

For symptom chart, see DIZZINESS, page xx.

The sensation of loss of balance, unsteadiness, disorientation, dizziness, or faintness produced by an illusion of movement, either of one's surroundings or one's body. Vertigo is often accompanied by nausea, vomiting, headache, or sweating, usually with no change in mental status. Vertigo is a symptom of a disorder, usually of the organs of balance in the inner ear.

Inflammation, infection, or a disorder of the semicircular canals of the labyrinth (the organ of balance in the inner ear) can also cause vertigo. Some medications may cause vertigo. MENIERE DISEASE may be the cause of ongoing episodes of vertigo. Tumors that develop in the balance or hearing nerves can cause vertigo with accompanying hearing loss and TINNITUS (hearing ringing in the ears). Treatment of vertigo depends on the cause. Many of the underlying disorders can be treated medically or surgically.

Vertigo, benign positional

Sudden, short episodes of dizziness brought on by a change in the position of the head or body. Benign positional vertigo, also called benign paroxysmal positional vertigo (BPPV), results when small crystals of calcium carbonate collect within a part of the inner ear that is responsible for balance. In half of all cases, the cause is unknown. BPPV produces intermittent symptoms that may include lightheadedness, loss of balance, and nausea in addition to dizziness. Rapid, involuntary eye movements may accompany the dizziness. Episodes of BPPV may appear intermittently for several weeks, disappear, and return again.

An otolaryngologist or neurologist usually diagnoses BPPV based on a person's history, a physical examination, and the results of hearing tests and tests of the vestibular system (the system in the inner ear responsible for balance).

Treatment may be postponed for 6 months to see if the symptoms decrease in intensity or disappear, which often occurs. The nausea can be controlled with motion sickness medication. Various physical maneuvers (such as the Epley maneuver) and exercises may be performed with a doctor's guidance to help relieve the symptoms. If these maneuvers or exercises do not eliminate the symptoms, surgery on the back of the ear may be recommended.

Vesicle

A small pouch, sac, or hollow organ, usually filled with fluid; examples include blisters and the seminal vesicles (located behind the bladder in males).

Vestibulitis

Recurring inflammation of the external genitals in females. The most common symptoms are a burning sensation around the opening of the vagina and extreme pain during sexual intercourse. Some women find it painful to insert tampons. Vestibulitis often disappears suddenly and then reappears a few months later. It can become chronic and persistent. The most common causes of vestibulitis are chemical irritants, such as soap, deodorant, shampoo, bubble bath, and fabric softener. Depending on the source of the inflammation, treatment may include antibiotics or other medication.

Villus

A tiny hairlike or fingerlike vascular projection present on a mucous membrane. Villi are present in all three sections of the small intestine, but are largest and most numerous in the duodenum and jejunum (the first and second parts of the small intestine), where most of the absorption of food takes place. See also CHORIONIC VILLI.

Violence, family

The physical attack or abuse of one family member by another; also called domestic violence. Violence that occurs in families includes partner abuse (see ABUSE, PARTNER), elder abuse (see ABUSE, OF OLDER PEOPLE), child abuse (see ABUSE, CHILD), and child neglect. All of these acts are crimes.

Virilism

A condition caused by excessive production of the male hormones (androgens). See ADRENAL HYPERPLASIA, CONGENITAL; ADRENOGENITAL SYNDROME.

Virilization

The development of masculine characteristics in a woman caused by over-production of the male sex hormones (androgens) by the ovaries or by the adrenal glands. In postmenopausal women, the condition may result from ovarian cancer. Virilization can cause excessive body hair growth, deepening of the voice, increased muscle mass, and acne. In premenopausal women, menstrual periods may stop. Synthetic gonadotropin-releasing hormone (GNRH) may be administered to treat some forms of virilization caused by an ovarian tumor.

Viruses

Infectious microorganisms that are found in all life forms, including humans, animals, plants, fungi, and bacteria. Each viral unit, or virion, consists of a strand of ribonucleic acid (RNA) or deoxyribonucleic acid (DNA). No virus contains both RNA and DNA, a characteristic that distinguishes viruses from all other cells. The virion is enclosed in a protein shell of one or two layers, called a capsid. Some viruses are coated with another layer called a viral envelope.

Viruses are parasites because they are not independently capable of vital activities, such as growth, metabolism, and reproduction. Viruses need to invade living cells and take over their internal processes in order to survive and reproduce. To enter a cell, a virus must first attach itself to the cell's surface. This is possible only if the cell has specific protein receptor sites for the particular virus to attach to on its surface.

The severity of a viral infection depends on the body's response to it. Because different viruses affect different tissues, structures, and organs in different ways, they produce various kinds of illnesses. INFLUENZA, RA-

BIES, SMALLPOX, MUMPS, MEASLES, herpes simplex, POLIO, HIV, and warts are examples of viral infections.

Several tests are available for diagnosing viral infections. An IMMUNOASSAY is a blood test that detects specific antibodies in the blood that fight a specific virus. Another test uses antigens (fragments of disease-causing protein substances that trigger the body's immune response; see ANTIGEN) to detect the presence of antibodies produced by the body to fight the specific infecting virus. The enzyme-linked immunosorbent assay (see ELISA TEST) uses prepared antigens to detect antibodies to a specific virus.

Viruses cannot be easily grown in the laboratory (cultured), so indirect methods are sometimes used to detect them. One diagnostic technique uses active cells grown in a solution of nutrients. When blood or other body fluid samples are added to the cells, they may cause changes in the cells that are associated with the presence of specific viruses in blood or body fluids.

Viruses are difficult to treat because they reproduce quickly. Also, because they incorporate their own genetic material into the genetic material of the host cell, medications that are intended to destroy a virus may also destroy the cell it has invaded. Most antiviral medications work by inhibiting the reproduction of the virus. Some antiviral medications prevent viruses from penetrating host cells.

Vision

The ability to see provided by the eyes and brain working together. Light enters the eye through the cornea (the clear outer covering of the eye), which, along with the lens, focuses it on the retina (the light-sensitive layer at the back of the eye). The retina contains nerve cells known as rods and cones that respond to different aspects of light. Cones perceive color and are sensitive to detail. Rods are insensitive to color, but very responsive to dim light and movement. Since the retina has many more rods than cones, the eye can see even in darkness, but it perceives color and detail best in bright light.

The electrical signals generated by the retina pass through the optic nerve, which follows a pathway leading to the visual cortex in the back of the brain. The visual cortex makes sense of incoming visual information. Since the eye contains only one lens, the image it receives is upside down; the brain then puts it right-

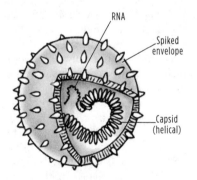

Structure of an influenza virus

Viruses come in many varieties, but they all have an outer coating (capsid) composed of units of protein and a nucleus that contains genetic material (DNA or RNA). Scientists classify them according to the shape of the capsules and the type of genetic material they contain. The virus shown above is an RNA influenza virus with an helical capsid in a spiked envelope.

side up and joins the images of both eyes to provide depth perception and binocular vision.

Vision tests

A variety of examinations used to determine how well a person can see. Vision tests are often combined with a physical examination of the eye. See EYE, EXAMINATION OF. Vision tests check for visual acuity (the sharpness of vision), refraction (which determines the correct prescription for glasses or contact lenses), blind spots, color perception, and visual field (the total area a person can see when looking straight ahead).

Visual field

The total area a person can see when looking straight ahead. A normal visual field is 180 degrees, or a half-circle. The visual field is measured in a standard eye examination (see EYE, EXAMINATION OF). Visual field testing is useful for diagnosing and evaluating diseases that can limit or impair the field of vision, such as GLAUCOMA, MULTIPLE SCLEROSIS, STROKE, or a tumor in the brain.

Visual field defect

A blind spot in the normal range of vision. Visual field defects caused by migraines are temporary; most others are persistent. Visual field defects have a number of possible causes. Overall narrowing of the range of vision can be caused by GLAUCOMA (abnormal pressure within the eye). A blind spot in the center of vision may come from swelling of the optic nerve or an abnormality of the macula. Defects that affect one half or one quarter of the visual field in each eye

are usually caused by strokes or tumors in the brain.

Visualization

Use of the imagination to heal the body. Visualization uses imagery to help relieve pain, speed healing, and promote mental and physical health. Images can be visual, auditory, sensory (touch), olfactory (smell), and gustatory (taste).

Vital sign

A critical measurement of body function. Vital signs include blood pressure, temperature, pulse rate, and respiratory rate.

Vitamin A

Retinol, a fat-soluble vitamin important for healthy eyes, skin, hair, and mucous membranes. Vitamin A is also essential for proper growth and reproduction, as well as normal bone development. Carotenes, which are building blocks of vitamin A, are antioxidants that prevent free-radical-induced changes that damage cells. Beta-carotene, a carotene found in plants, is converted into vitamin A by the liver.

Good dietary sources of vitamin A include fish-liver oil, egg yolks, milk, cheese, and butter. Low-fat milk and ready-to-eat cereals are also fortified with vitamin A. Vitamin A can be derived from carotenes in fruits and vegetables. Beta-carotene is found in orange-colored produce such as carrots, cantaloupe, papaya, sweet potatoes, and pumpkin; dark green, leafy vegetables such as spinach and kale; and deep yellow vegetables such as winter squash.

A deficiency of vitamin A can cause night blindness, dry eyes, eye and respiratory infections, skin problems, and slow growth and bone deformities in children. Health conditions that may increase the body's need for vitamin A include CYSTIC FIBROSIS, chronic diarrhea, a serious injury, liver disease, malabsorption, pancreatic disease, or a chronic illness.

Vitamin B

A group of water-soluble vitamins that is important to good health. B vitamins help the body metabolize carbohydrates, fats, and protein and build red blood cells and are important for nerve and muscle function. Good dietary sources of B vitamins include meats, dairy products, nuts, grains, and leafy green vegetables. B deficiency diseases depend on which B vitamin is deficient. For example, folic acid deficiency in pregnant women increases the risk of a NEURAL TUBE DEFECT in the fetus, and niacin deficiency can result in pellagra (a nutritional disorder). A lack of B vitamins can cause anemia.

Among the B vitamins are vitamin B1 (thiamin), which is essential for energy production from carbohydrates and nerve and muscle function, including function of the heart muscle; vitamin B2 (riboflavin), which is important in the metabolism of carbohydrates, fats, and protein; vitamin B3 (niacin), which improves blood circulation by dilating arteries and is important for a healthy gastrointestinal tract, nervous system, skin, and sex hormones; vitamin B6 (pyridoxine), which helps the body use protein; folic acid, which is essential for growth, cell repair, a healthy pregnancy, and good cardiovascular function; and vitamin B12 (cyanocobalamin), which is es-

sential to the development of red blood cells.

Vitamin B12 deficiency

A deficiency of vitamin B12 due to the absence of the vitamin or decreased ability of the body to absorb the vitamin. A deficiency can result from diets that exclude all animal products and is also associated with various autoimmune disorders, especially those involving the thyroid, parathyroid, and adrenal glands. This deficiency can also develop if stomach acid is not produced in sufficient amounts. Other conditions that can inhibit the body's absorption of vitamin B12 include CELIAC DISEASE, CROHN DISEASE, WHIPPLE DISEASE, intestinal worms, structural defects of the intestinal system, surgical removal of the stomach, poisoning with corrosive substances, and TUBERCULOSIS. A vitamin B12 deficiency can cause pernicious anemia (see ANEMIA, PERNICIOUS), a disease in which red blood cells are abnormally formed. Treatment of pernicious anemia is with lifelong injections of vitamin B12 or very high doses of oral vitamin B12. Other forms of B12 deficiency that do not involve a lack of intrinsic factor may be treated with oral vitamin B12 supplements.

Vitamin C

Ascorbic acid, a water-soluble antioxidant vitamin involved in fat metabolism, the development of connective tissue, immune function, wound healing, and iron absorption. Vitamin C is necessary for healthy bones, teeth, and skin. A deficiency of vitamin C can lead to scurvy, a condition characterized by fatigue, muscle weakness, joint and muscle aches, bleeding gums, and a rash on the legs. Many fresh fruits and vegetables are rich in vitamin C, including citrus fruits such as oranges, lemons, limes, and grapefruit; green vegetables such as broccoli and kale; and berries, tomatoes, potatoes, and green peppers. Juices and cereals are often fortified with vitamin C. High doses of vitamin C supplements can cause diarrhea and, in some people, can cause or worsen GOUT or lead to the development of kidney stones.

Vitamin D

Cholecalciferol, a fat-soluble vitamin essential for the formation of bones and teeth and for the absorption of calcium and phosphorus. A deficiency of vitamin D can cause bone diseases such as OSTEOPOROSIS and RICKETS. Good dietary sources of vitamin D include organ meats, fish liver oils, egg yolks, and saltwater fish such as salmon, sardines, and herring. Because relatively small amounts of vitamin D are naturally available, dairy products, cereals, and breads are usually fortified with it. Exposure to sunlight enables the skin to manufacture vitamin D. As little as 10 minutes of exposure to sunlight may produce sufficient quantities of vitamin D to maintain bone strength.

Vitamin E

Tocopherol, a fat-soluble antioxidant vitamin that helps form red blood cells, muscles, and lung and nerve tissue. Vitamin E is also important in reproduction. Vitamin E is composed of eight related compounds: four tocopherols and four tocotrienols. Alpha tocopherol is the main type of vitamin E in the body. Foods such as veg-etable oils, whole grains, wheat germ, nuts, and leafy green vegetables are good sources of vitamin E. Most ready-to-eat cereals are also fortified with vitamin E. People who are taking anticoagulant drugs need to be careful about taking large doses of supplemental vitamin E because it can increase the risk of bleeding. Many people take vitamin E supplements to reduce their risk of heart disease, although studies have not shown conclusively that there are benefits.

Vitamin K

A fat-soluble vitamin essential for blood clotting. It may also have a role in preserving the strength of bones. Good dietary sources of vitamin K include leafy green vegetables such as spinach, lettuce, and cabbage; liver; egg yolks; cauliflower; grain products; potatoes; fruits; and low-fat milk and cheese. Vitamin K is also synthesized by bacteria that normally reside in the large intestine. Prolonged use of antibiotics can lead to a vitamin K deficiency if dietary intake is not increased to compensate for the reduced amounts obtained from intestinal bacteria. A vitamin K deficiency can result in potentially fatal bleeding in the event of an injury.

Vitamin supplements

Usually over-the-counter preparations that contain one or more vitamins. Many doctors recommend a daily multivitamin-mineral for everyone, especially older people who often do not eat enough; women who are breast-feeding, pregnant, or planning to become pregnant; people with a chronic illness; or vegetarians and people on a low-calorie diet. Taking vitamin supplements is not as effective as getting vitamins from a variety of foods, and taking large doses of some vitamins can be toxic.

Vitamins

Chemical compounds that are essential for normal functioning of the body. Vitamins regulate chemical processes in the body and have a role in maintaining health and preventing disease. A deficiency of vitamins can lead to a wide range of diseases, from birth defects (caused by a folic acid deficiency) to scurvy (caused by a lack of vitamin C). Vitamins can be water-soluble or fat-soluble. Water-soluble vitamins mix easily in the blood. The body is able to store only small amounts of these vitamins, most of which are excreted in urine and sweat. For this reason, water-soluble vitamins must be replaced daily. The water-soluble vitamins are vitamin C and the B complex vitamins—including thiamin (B1), riboflavin (B2), niacin (B3), pyridoxine (B6), cyanocobalamin (B12), folic acid, and biotin. The fat-soluble vitamins—A, D, E, and K—are found in fats and oils in foods and are stored in the body's fat cells. If a person takes too many fat-soluble vitamins, the vitamins can build up in the body and have harmful effects.

Vitiligo

A skin disorder characterized by patches of white skin resulting from loss of pigment cells (melanocytes). Although its exact cause is unknown, vitiligo is believed to have an autoimmune component in which the immune system mistakes the melanocytes for invading microorganisms and destroys them. Although most people with vitiligo are generally in good health, they are at increased risk of developing thyroid dysfunction, vitamin B12 deficiency, diabetes, and alopecia areata (a temporary loss of patches of hair). There is no cure for vitiligo, but treatments are available.

Any part of the body can be affected by vitiligo but common sites are around the eyes, nose, and mouth; on the hands and genitals; and in injured areas. Some people experience increased loss of pigment after emotional or physical stress.

Treatment involves trying to restore normal pigment to the affected areas (repigmentation) or to destroy the remaining pigment (depigmentation) to make the skin color uniform. Treatment depends on the severity of the disease. Treatment to repigment the skin includes topical corticosteroids and the drug psoralen plus ultraviolet A (puva), which is a form of phototherapy (treatment with light). Surgical therapies for repigmentation include skin grafts, tattooing, and melanocyte transplants.

Vitrectomy

A surgical procedure in which the normally clear, jellylike liquid (vitreous) inside the eye is removed and replaced with a salt solution. The surgery is performed when blood has leaked into the vitreous and clouded vision or to treat retinal disorders. The surgeon makes a small incision in the white of the eye (sclera) and inserts an instrument that draws out the cloudy fluid and replaces it with a clear salt solution. Vitrectomy can be performed under local or general anesthesia and

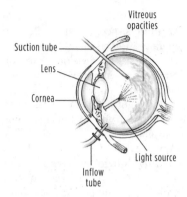

Vitreous
opacities

Suction tube

Lens

Cornea

Light source

Inflow
tube

Clearing clouded vision

Vitrectomy is an advance in eye surgery in which vitreous humor that has been clouded with blood is suctioned out and replaced with a clear salt solution. The procedure makes more space in the eye and clears the vision.

may require an overnight hospital stay. Vision following a vitrectomy can be greatly improved.

Vitreous hemorrhage

Bleeding into the clear, jellylike liquid (vitreous) inside the eye. Minor bleeding can cloud vision; heavier bleeding can produce a mass of red or black lines and very dark vision. If the blood is not absorbed on its own, vitreous hemorrhage is treated with a VITRECTOMY. After vitrectomy, laser surgery (see PHOTOCOAGULATION) may be performed to cause the abnormal blood vessels to regress.

Vitreous humor

The transparent jellylike substance that fills the eyeball; also called the vitreous body. In medicine, the term humor refers to a fluid or semifluid.

VLDL

Very-low-density lipoprotein, a type of lipid (fat) and protein complex made by the liver and transported in the blood. Elevated levels of VLDL in the blood are associated with high triglyceride levels, a buildup of plaque in the arteries, and an increased risk of ATHEROSCLEROSIS and heart disease. See CHOLESTEROL.

Vocal cord nodules

Noncancerous growths of the epithelium (mucous membrane covering) on the surface of the vocal cords. The vocal cords are folds of mucous membrane draped over a ligament and muscle that extend from the wall of the larynx (voice box). The nodules are usually located on both sides of the vocal cords. The most common symptom is hoarseness and, possibly, a breathy sound to the voice. The nodules are the result of irritation and inflammation of the mucous membrane.

If rest does not improve the voice, the nodules may be surgically removed. However, with ongoing misuse or overuse of the voice, the nodules tend to return.

Vocal cord paralysis

The inability of one or both vocal cords to move because of damage to the nerves that control the muscles of the larynx or damage to the brain. Opening and closing of the vocal cords have a vital role in speech, swallowing, and breathing. Any impairment in their ability to move can affect these essential functions. The cartilage that attaches the vocal folds may become locked in place and restrict movement of the folds. Accumulated scar tissue can also prevent the vocal folds from moving normally.

In some cases, the voice returns

without treatment during the first year after damage. During this time, the person is given voice therapy, which may involve exercises to strengthen the vocal cords or improve breath control during speech. If one of the vocal cords is immobilized, the condition may be treated with surgery (medialization thryoplasty), implants, or injections. Medialization thryoplasty, which is effective and painless, involves making a small incision through the skin near the larynx, removing a small piece of the cartilage, and inserting a small block of silicone into the cartilage to help the vocal folds close.

If both vocal cords are paralyzed, treatment aims at surgically opening the airway and restoring breathing.

Vocal cords

Two folds of mucous membrane overlying two vocal ligaments in the larynx (voice box) that vibrate to produce the sounds of speech. See SPEECH MECHANISM. Most of the time the vocal cords lie apart, forming a triangle-shaped opening through which air passes for breathing. The cords also close automatically during swallowing to prevent food from going down the trachea instead of the esophagus.

Voice box

See LARYNX.

Voice, loss of

Inability of the larynx (voice box) to produce normal speech. A person can lose his or her ability to speak when the nerve supply that normally pushes the two vocal cords together is damaged or destroyed. The most common causes of voice loss are viral infections and overuse of the voice. The voice usually returns to normal when the infection clears up or the person uses his or her voice less. Nerve loss can be caused by a stroke, throat cancer or its treatments, or an injury to the throat or neck. Usually, when it becomes impossible to speak, breathing is also restricted, and there is a risk of choking when swallowing. When the loss of voice is severe and prolonged, surgery may be required. See also VOCAL CORD PARALYSIS.

Volvulus

A condition in which a loop of the intestine becomes knotted or twisted. Volvulus can obstruct the intestine (see INTESTINE, OBSTRUCTION OF), trapping gas and stool that can cause abdominal swelling, pain, and vomiting. If the blood supply is cut off, the intestine can die (gangrene). Volvulus is usually diagnosed with imaging studies such as X rays. When the problem develops in the small intestine, only surgery can provide a definitive diagnosis. However, volvulus most frequently occurs in the S-shaped lower portion (sigmoid) of the large intestine (colon). Doctors are often able to treat this condition with a SIGMOIDOSCOPY or BARIUM ENEMA. In recurring cases of volvulus in the sigmoid colon, or when the problem develops elsewhere in the intestine, more extensive abdominal surgery may be required.

Vomiting

For symptom chart, see NAUSEA OR VOMITING, page xxv.

The forceful, involuntary ejection of stomach contents through the mouth. Unless vomiting is recurring, prolonged, painful, or contains blood (see VOMITING BLOOD), it is usually not a sign of a serious problem. Doctors advise people with nausea and vomiting to not eat anything until their symptoms subside. To prevent dehydration, small amounts of nonalcoholic fluids, such as water or weak tea, should be consumed. After 24 hours, a normal diet can be resumed. If vomiting is violent or persistent, medical attention should be sought.

Vomiting blood

A symptom of a disorder in the digestive tract. Also known as hematemesis, vomiting blood can result from excessive vomiting or from excessive consumption of alcohol. It can also be a sign of potentially life-threatening internal bleeding, so it should not be ignored. Blood in vomit can be red or, when digested by the stomach, it can resemble coffee grounds. An individual who vomits blood should call a doctor. If other symptoms, such as chills, sweating, weakness, or dizziness, are present, immediate medical attention is required.

Vomiting in pregnancy

Nausea and vomiting in pregnancy are attributed to changing hormone levels. See MORNING SICKNESS.

von Willebrand disease

An inherited chronic bleeding disorder. Von Willebrand disease (VWD) is a platelet disorder caused by a defect in a clotting factor known as von Willebrand factor (a protein that is essential for the formation of blood clots). A deficiency of the factor impairs the aggregation of platelets at the site of a wound, which delays or prevents the formation of blood clots

needed to stop bleeding. Factor VIII, a substance in blood that is necessary for clotting, may be reduced in people with VWD because von Willebrand factor serves as a carrier for factor VIII.

Symptoms can vary in severity from person to person. While the severest form of the disease is rare, milder forms are common. Affected children have frequent nosebleeds that are severe enough to require visits to a doctor or emergency department. Affected females experience very heavy bleeding during menstrual periods.

Unlike people with HEMOPHILIA, people with VWD do not usually bleed into joints and muscles. Because it is a disorder of the platelets, VWD causes bleeding into mucous membranes of the mouth, nose, intestine, or uterus. Many people with VWD must take a drug that stimulates the release of von Willebrand factor and factor VIII from the walls of blood vessels. Transfusions of plasma or cryoprecipitate (a concentrate of clotting factor derived from human blood) may also be given.

Vulva

The external female genitals. See REPRODUCTIVE SYSTEM, FEMALE.

Vulva, cancer of the

Cancer involving the vulva (the external female genitals). Most cases (nearly 90 percent) are SQUAMOUS CELL CARCINOMAS (a type of skin cancer); about 5 percent are melanoma (another type of skin cancer). The most common symptom of cancer of the vulva is persistent itching. Lumps may appear on the labia, the clitoris, or the perineum (the area between the anus and the vagina). Burning, pain, discharge, or bleeding may occur. If the cancer becomes invasive, a large mass may develop on the vulva or in the groin. When the cancer is a melanoma, it usually appears on the clitoris and the outer labia as brown, black, or blue-black lumps or patches.

Treatment depends on the extent of the cancer. If the area of cancerous tissue is small, a cream containing a chemotherapy agent can be applied directly to the vulva. Larger areas of cancerous tissue may need to be surgically removed (vulvectomy). If the cancer has spread to the lymph nodes, RADIATION THERAPY after surgery is usually recommended.

Vulvectomy

Surgical removal of the vulva (external female genital area) and the lymph nodes in the groin. A vulvectomy is the most common and effective treatment for cancer of the vulva. Sexual intercourse is possible after a vulvectomy, although some women are not able to achieve orgasm because much of the sexually sensitive tissue of the clitoris has been removed.

Vulvitis

Inflammation of the vulva (external female genitals). Vulvitis usually causes redness, swelling, and itching of the labia (lips) and other parts of the vulva. If vulvitis becomes chronic, scaly whitish sore patches may develop on the skin along with blisters that burst and crust over, and a woman may have a foul-smelling vaginal discharge. Diagnosis requires a pelvic examination and various tests to rule out more serious conditions.

The irritation may be treated with soothing baths with baking soda or warm boric acid compresses. Over-the-counter hydrocortisone creams can be used to relieve the itching. If vulvitis does not respond to these measures, a doctor will need to evaluate and treat the condition. See also VESTIBULITIS.

Vulvovaginitis

Inflammation of the vulva (the external female genitals) and the vagina. Symptoms include redness, itching, and soreness of the vulva and vagina, sometimes accompanied by a vaginal discharge.

Vulvovaginitis can be caused by infectious microorganisms such as yeast, a skin allergy, pinworms, and, in children, bed-wetting. Repeated sexual intercourse over a short period of time can also lead to vulvovaginitis. A diagnosis can usually be made through microscopic examination of a sample of vaginal discharge. Treatment can range from soothing baths and improved personal hygiene to vaginal antibiotic creams.

Waist-to-hip ratio

A tool used to assess fat distribution and health risk. Waist-to-hip ratio is calculated by measuring waist and hip circumferences and then dividing the waist measurement by the hip measurement. The waist-to-hip ratio indicates whether a person carries more weight around the abdomen or around the hips and thighs. People who tend to store fat around the abdomen tend to have elevated levels of harmful low-density lipoprotein (LDL) cholesterol, which causes fatty plaque deposits to accumulate on artery walls (see ATHEROSCLEROSIS). A healthy waist-to-hip ratio is 0.8 for women and 0.95 for men. See also BODY MASS INDEX.

Walking aids

Assistive devices, such as walkers, crutches, canes, and prostheses, that can help people whose walking ability is impaired. Walking aids can help people who have muscle weakness, poor flexibility, poor balance, degenerative diseases, or injuries that make it difficult to get around. To determine whether an individual can benefit from a walking aid, a doctor usually refers him or her to a physical therapist. The physical therapist evaluates the person's balance, strength, and range of movement and makes recommendations. Once a walking aid is selected, the therapist instructs the person in how to use it properly. See also PROSTHESIS.

Walking, delayed

When a child has not developed the ability to walk within the normal age range. Although each child has his or her own rate of development, babies normally become able to bear some weight on their legs by 7 months. The inability to walk by the age of 18 months is generally considered de-layed motor or movement development (see DEVELOPMENTAL DELAY), and a complete medical and developmental evaluation is necessary to determine the cause. Affected children are usually referred to a pediatrician who specializes in developmental problems.

Warts

See HUMAN PAPILLOMAVIRUS.

Waterborne infections

Infections acquired by contact with or ingestion of contaminated water. Waterborne infections include SALMONELLA, GIARDIASIS, CRYPTOSPORIDIOSIS, E. COLI, and SHIGELLOSIS.

Weaning

The gradual transition from getting nourishment from the breast or bottle to drinking from a cup. There is no right or wrong time to make this transition, but most doctors recommend weaning babies from the breast or bottle after the first birthday. (Solid foods are usually started between 4 and 6 months.) Breast milk or formula should be given to babies until their digestive system matures, at around age 1. After age 1, cow's milk can be introduced. Giving cow's milk before age 1 can be harmful because a child's kidneys cannot yet excrete the excess calcium and phosphorus that are present in cow's milk. See also FEEDING, INFANT.

Wegener granulomatosis

An autoimmune disorder that causes inflammation in blood vessels and damages the walls of small and medium-sized arteries and capillaries. Wegener granulomatosis is potentially life-threatening because it can impede the blood supply to tissues supplied by the damaged arteries. The disorder occurs most often in people who are in their 40s or 50s and, without treatment, is almost always fatal.

The lungs, kidneys, upper airways (including the sinuses, windpipe, and nose) are usually affected. About 60 to 80 percent of people with Wegener granulomatosis have chronic nasal and sinus problems and persistent congestion with discolored nasal discharge, frequent nosebleeds, and sores or crusting inside the nose. When the lungs are involved, people may have shortness of breath, wheezing, and a cough. Other symptoms include fever, weakness and fatigue, weight loss, night sweats, joint pain, and muscle aches. Kidney involvement occurs in approximately 75 percent of affected people.

A preliminary diagnosis is based on a complete physical examination and a history of persistent symptoms of SINUSITIS, RESPIRATORY TRACT INFECTIONS, or respiratory allergies. To confirm the diagnosis, a biopsy may be taken from affected tissues in the sinuses, lung, or kidney.

Treatment is usually two medications, the corticosteroid prednisone to reduce inflammation and low-dose oral cyclophosphamide to suppress the errant immune activity. About 90 percent of people improve with therapy; however, cyclophosphamide can have serious side effects, including an increased risk of cancer.

Weight training

The use of free weights or weight machines to increase muscle strength.

Weight training also increases bone strength and may help prevent bone loss associated with aging. To build strength in the muscles, the weights must challenge the muscles. The ideal weight is one that painlessly exhausts the muscles after 12 to 20 repetitions of an exercise. Lighter weights can build muscle endurance but have less effect on strength. Proper technique is important for preventing injuries when lifting weights. A certified professional instructor or trainer should demonstrate how to lift free weights or use weight machines correctly when a person begins a weight-lifting program. See also EXERCISE, RESISTANCE; EXERCISE, STRENGTHENING.

Weight-bearing exercise

See EXERCISE, WEIGHT-BEARING.

Weil disease

An infection or parasitic disease produced by the bacteria *Leptospira*. Weil disease is a severe form of leptospirosis that is characterized by severe dysfunction of the liver and kidneys. The infection causes excessive bleeding inside the body and is potentially fatal. It is contracted by ingesting or swimming in water contaminated with the infected urine of wild or domestic animals (including rats, cats, and dogs) who shed the bacteria in their urine. The infection is treated with antibiotics.

Wernicke encephalopathy

Also known as Wernicke disease, a life-threatening brain disorder characterized by confusion, an unsteady gait, and abnormal eye movements. Wernicke encephalopathy most commonly occurs in chronic alcoholics as

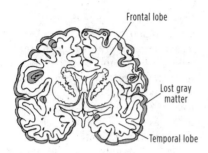

Frontal lobe

Lost gray matter

Temporal lobe

Loss of brain tissue
A deficiency of the B vitamin thiamin reduces the body's ability to metabolize glucose to supply the brain, and results in a loss of brain tissue. The damage is generally evident by changes in appetite, emotional response, and memory. The tint shows the grey matter that is lost.

a result of vitamin B1 (thiamin) deficiency. The disorder can cause damage to nerves throughout the body. Untreated, it can be fatal.

Symptoms of Wernicke encephalopathy include confusion, memory loss, inattention, delirium, disorientation, and drowsiness. Poor balance and coordination make walking difficult. Often a person has abnormal eye movements, such as double vision and jerking of the eyes. Wernicke encephalopathy is often accompanied or followed by KORSAKOFF PSYCHOSIS (also known as Korsakoff syndrome), which involves impairment of memory and cognitive skills. The combination of Wernicke encephalopathy and Korsakoff psychosis is known as Wernicke-Korsakoff syndrome.

Prompt administration of vitamin B1 is essential. Without it, the disorder can progress to stupor, coma, and death. Hospitalization is usually required to bring the symptoms under control. The results of treatment vary from person to person.

West Nile virus

A virus transmitted by mosquitoes that can cause severe cases of EN-CEPHALITIS. The majority of infections (80 percent) do not cause symptoms but, among people who are sick enough to require hospitalization, the death rate is higher than 10 percent. Mild infections cause fever, fatigue, enlarged lymph nodes, eye pain, stomach pain, muscle ache, and headache. A rash may develop in children. A diagnosis of West Nile virus is made with blood tests. There is no specific antiviral therapy for the infection, but regular use of insect repellant can help prevent mosquito bites.

Wheal

See HIVES.

Wheezing

A high-pitched, whistling sound made when air passes over a partial obstruction in the airways. ASTHMA is the most common cause of recurring wheezing. But it can also be caused by other conditions, such as CHRONIC OBSTRUCTIVE PULMONARY DISEASE (COPD), congestive heart failure (see HEART FAILURE, CONGESTIVE), a tumor in the airways, or a foreign particle, such as a piece of food, lodged in an airway.

Whiplash

An injury to the cervical vertebrae (neck bones) or adjacent soft tissues (muscles, ligaments, disks, and tendons) that occurs from a sudden, accelerated, jerking movement of the head and neck or by a rapid back and forth movement of the head or neck. Whiplash often occurs to passengers of cars involved in rear-impact or head-on collisions. It causes pain and stiffness in the neck. It is generally treated with anti-inflammatory and pain-relieving medication and often improves with time. In some cases, a rigid collar covered with soft material, called a cervical collar, is worn around the neck to support the injured area. Physical therapy, including deep heat and traction, is also prescribed. Occupational therapy may be necessary, too.

Whipple operation

A surgical procedure to remove cancer in the head of the pancreas. The procedure removes the head of the pancreas, a portion of the bile duct, the gallbladder, and the duodenum (the first section of the small intestine). A tumor that develops in the head of the pancreas often causes jaundice because it blocks the common bile duct, preventing secretions produced by the liver and stored in the gallbladder from entering the small intestine. The Whipple operation can provide a cure only for localized cancers.

Whipworm infestation

Infestation with the roundworm *Trichuris trichiura*, called the human whipworm; also called trichuriasis. In the United States, whipworm infestations occur in some southern states. The eggs of the roundworms are found in the soil and are transmitted to humans when food or a person's hands come in contact with contaminated soil and the worms are ingested. Adult whipworms infest the human colon, where the females then lay their eggs.

A person with a whipworm infestation usually does not have symptoms. Heavy infestations may cause gas-

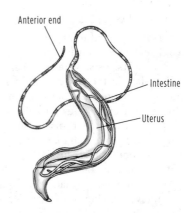

Anterior end

Intestine

Uterus

Parasitic roundworm
A whipworm, so named for its long, whiplike tail, is about 1/25 of an inch (1 mm) long. The whipworm lives in the large intestine, and the female lays from 3,000 to 20,000 eggs per day. The eggs pass from the body in stool.

trointestinal problems and sometimes slowed growth in children. If symptoms occur, they may include abdominal pain, diarrhea, and REC-TAL PROLAPSE. The infestation is diagnosed by identifying the worm eggs in feces under a microscope. Antiworm medications, including mebendazole and albendazole, are the usual treatment.

White matter

Brain tissue containing myelinated nerve fibers. White matter carries information between nerve cells in the brain and spinal cord. White matter is found in the inner portion of the cerebrum, the area of the brain where thought and other higher brain functions take place.

Whitehead

A small, hard, painless, white blemish on the skin that results when a hair follicle becomes blocked with an oily substance called sebum.

Whitlow, herpetic

An intensely painful infection of the hand that causes blisters on one or more fingers, usually on the palmside surface of the area of the finger closest to the fingertip. Herpetic whitlow is most often caused by herpes simplex virus 1, but may also be caused by herpes simplex virus 2. The infection is transmitted by contact with infected body fluids.

A clinical history usually reveals a recent fever and illness that preceded the blisters on the finger by a few days. Previous similar outbreaks on the same finger may indicate a recurring or reactivated infection. Diagnostic tests may include the Tzanck test (which evaluates a smear scraped from the base of a blister) or microscopic examination of fluid from the blisters. The infection often improves without treatment. Painful symptoms can be treated. In some cases, the blisters are treated by a doctor to relieve the pain and swelling.

Whooping cough

See PERTUSSIS.

Will, living

A legal document that describes a person's wishes regarding medical treatment when he or she is terminally ill or unable to make decisions independently. See ADVANCE DIRECTIVES.

Wilms tumor

A cancerous tumor of the kidneys that occurs mainly in children. The tumor may develop in fetal tissue, but most often occurs at about age 3. The cancer is curable in most cases. It is associated with some congenital defects such as urinary tract abnormalities and enlargement of one side of the body. Although it generally remains localized, the tumor can become large and spread to other tissues.

The first sign of Wilms tumor is usually a large lump in the belly and a swollen abdomen. Some children may have abdominal pain, fever, blood in the urine, or swelling in the legs.

The diagnosis is confirmed with a biopsy of tissue taken from the affected kidney. Treatment depends on the stage of the cancer, the tumor size, and the child's age and general health. The most common treatments are surgery to remove the tumor and part of all of the kidney, chemotherapy, and radiation.

Wilson disease

A genetic disorder that causes copper to accumulate in several organs of the body, particularly in the brain, eyes, kidneys, and liver. Wilson disease is essentially a disease of copper poisoning. Normally, the body is able to eliminate excess copper, which is present in most foods. But people with Wilson disease cannot eliminate copper, and it begins to accumulate in the body immediately after birth.

Symptoms, which usually appear between ages 6 and 20, include jaundice, abdominal swelling, vomiting of blood, and abdominal pain. Some people have neurological symptoms such as difficulty walking, talking, and swallowing. Some people have depression. Women with Wilson disease may have irregular menstrual periods, multiple miscarriages, or infertility.

Without treatment, Wilson disease is fatal. Liver damage can occur before symptoms develop. Treatment consists of medications such as penicillamine or trientine, which remove excess copper by increasing its excretion in urine. Another medication for treating Wilson disease is zinc acetate, which blocks the absorption of copper in the intestinal tract, reducing accumulated copper and preventing further accumulation. Any of these medications must be taken for life.

Wisdom teeth

The third molars, or the last back teeth in the upper and lower jaws. Most people have four wisdom teeth: one on each side of the upper and lower jaws. Wisdom teeth are the last of the permanent teeth to come in, usually when a person is between the ages of 17 and 23 years. However, there is often insufficient space for these last teeth to develop and emerge from the gums after all the permanent teeth are in place. If a wisdom tooth has not fully erupted by the time a person is 25 years old, the tooth is generally considered to be impacted.

Withdrawal method

See COITUS INTERRUPTUS.

Withdrawal syndrome, alcohol

The physical and psychological symptoms that result when a person who is dependent on alcohol suddenly stops drinking. See ALCOHOL DEPENDENCE; DELIRIUM TREMENS.

Withdrawal syndrome, opiates

The physical and psychological symptoms that result when someone who is dependent on morphine, heroin, or another opiate stops using the substance. Symptoms can vary from person to person but the syndrome usually begins about 6 to 12 hours after the last opiate dose. Symptoms during the first 24 hours include restlessness, watering of the eyes, runny nose, yawning, heavy sweating, goose bumps, restless sleep, and dilation of the pupils. As time passes, these symptoms become more severe.

The symptoms usually peak between 36 and 72 hours after withdrawal and gradually diminish. Withdrawal symptoms usually end in about 5 to 7 days, although cravings for the drug may continue for months. Opiate withdrawal is usually treated in a clinical setting (see DETOXIFICATION PROGRAMS) by administering controlled doses of the synthetic opiate methadone to reduce symptoms.

Wolff-Parkinson-White syndrome

Episodes of rapid heart rate caused by an extra, abnormal electrical conduction pathway between the upper and lower parts of the heart; also known as pre-excitation syndrome. In a healthy heart, the electrical signals that trigger a heartbeat follow a specific route from the atria (upper chambers) to the ventricles (lower chambers). In Wolff-Parkinson-White syndrome, the electrical signals instead travel along an accessory pathway known as the Kent bundle, which can cause the heart to beat abnormally fast, more than 100 beats per minute (see TACHYCARDIA). Other symptoms can include lightheadedness, palpitations (an uncomfortably rapid heart rate), and syncope (fainting). Symptoms, which usually appear between ages 10 and 50, can vary in severity from person to person, ranging from nonexistent to disabling.

Most people with Wolff-Parkinson-White syndrome have no other heart problem, but some people have MITRAL VALVE PROLAPSE (MVP), CARDIOMYOPATHY (impaired heart muscle function), or Ebstein anomaly (a rare condition in which the tricuspid valve is deformed and misplaced). If Wolff-Parkinson-White syndrome causes no symptoms, treatment is not needed. When symptoms are present, medication that coordinates the electrical signals of the heart is sometimes successful in controlling episodes of tachycardia. Another approach involves a minimally invasive procedure that destroys the abnormal conduction pathway (see ABLATION THERAPY).

Wound

A break or opening in the skin. Types of wounds include cuts, punctures, and tears.

Wrinkles

Skin damage ranging from fine lines to deep furrows. Wrinkles have three primary causes: aging, sun exposure, and smoking. With age, the skin becomes thinner and produces less oil. Collagen and elastin, fibrous proteins in the dermis (the middle layer of skin), normally provide the skin with strength and elasticity. These fibrous proteins tend to weaken with age. Repeated sun exposure and smoking also can damage the fibers, leading to premature wrinkling and sagging.

A variety of drugs and procedures can be used to reduce the appearance of fine lines and deep wrinkles. In addition to over-the-counter moisturizers containing sunscreen, helpful topical products include retinol, tretinoin (a vitamin A derivative), and alpha-hydroxy acids (naturally occurring acids in fruit and milk). Higher concentrations of alpha-hydroxy acids are used in chemical skin peels. Skin-rejuvenation procedures include botulinum toxin injections and collagen injections that make wrinkles disappear temporarily, dermabrasion (removal of the surface layer of skin by high-speed sanding), laser resurfacing (which uses a powerful beam of pulsing light to vaporize unwanted skin tissue), and traditional plastic surgery. While medications and surgery can help reduce wrinkles, these procedures can carry risks.

Wrist

The area where the hand joins the arm. The wrist is a complex arrangement of joints between eight wrist bones (carpals in two rows of four bones each), two bones in the lower arm (radius and ulna), and five bones in the palm (metacarpals).

Wristdrop

A type of paralysis characterized by an inability to extend or lift the wrist resulting from damage to the radial nerve (the nerve that supplies the arm, forearm, and hand).

X chromosome

The female sex chromosome, which, along with the male Y chromosome, determines sex in humans and most animals. Everyone has two sex chromosomes—either two X chromosomes or an X and a Y. Having two X chromosomes makes a person female; having an X and a Y chromosome makes a person male.

X rays

Electromagnetic waves generated by an electrical current that passes through an X-ray tube and produces a beam of ionizing radiation that can pass through the body to form an image on film or on a digital screen. Because soft body structures are less dense, a greater amount of radiation passes through them, and more radiation reaches the film (the film is exposed to larger amounts of X rays). Soft body tissues appear dark on X-ray film. Because bones are denser than soft tissue, they absorb more radiation, and a lesser amount passes through them. Bones leave the film only slightly exposed and appear light or white on the X-ray film. X rays are performed on different parts of the body for various diagnostic purposes. For example, a chest X ray may be performed to look for evidence of PNEUMONIA, TUBERCULOSIS, or fluid in the lungs or to evaluate the size of the heart. Chest X rays are often performed before major surgery, but they are no longer given during routine checkups.

Xanthelasma

A yellow-orange bump beneath the surface of the skin (xanthoma) on the eyelids made of cholesterol deposits. Xanthelasmas are associated with an elevated blood cholesterol level. Although they may be unsightly, xanthelasmas are painless and are not cancerous. If the growths become bothersome, they can be surgically removed or treated with applications of trichloroacetic acid.

Xanthoma

A yellow-orange nodule (solid mass of tissue) with sharply defined borders beneath the surface of the skin. Xanthomas commonly appear on the elbows, hands, feet, knees, and buttocks. Growths range in size from small to more than 3 inches in diameter. Although they may be unsightly, xanthomas are painless and noncancerous. They most frequently affect people with elevated blood cholesterol levels or genetic cholesterol disorders. The goal of treatment is to manage any underlying disorders, such as diabetes, CIRRHOSIS, or HYPERCHOLESTEROLEMIA. Reducing triglyceride and cholesterol levels can help reduce the occurrence of xanthomas. If the growths become bothersome, they can be removed surgically. See also CHOLESTEROL.

Xanthomatosis

A condition in which fatty deposits accumulate in the brain, skin, internal organs, and tendons. Fat deposits that accumulate in the linings of the blood vessels (see ATHEROSCLEROSIS) can narrow the blood vessels and reduce the blood supply to organs.

Xenograft

A procedure in which tissue from a donor is grafted or transplanted into another species. A commonly performed xenograft replaces diseased human heart valves with heart valves from pigs. Pigs are used as donor animals because their internal organs are approximately the same size as human organs.

Xerophthalmia

Abnormal dryness and thickening of the exposed outer layer of the eye as a result of a deficiency of vitamin A (beta-carotene) in the diet or as a result of disease. Xerophthalmia can lead to serious vision loss, which begins with difficulty seeing in dim light (night blindness) and progresses to ulceration of the clear covering of the eye (cornea).

X-linked characteristic

A trait associated with a gene on the X sex chromosome. Any trait associated with a gene on the X chromosome will almost always be expressed in males, who have only one X chromosome. Women who inherit an X-linked disease gene are usually not affected by the disease because they have two X chromosomes and have a healthy copy of the gene on the other X chromosome (which overrides the effects of the disease gene). X-linked genetic disorders are often passed from mothers (who are unaffected) to sons.

Y chromosome

The male sex chromosome, which, along with the female X chromosome, determines sex in humans and most animals. Everyone has two sex chromosomes—either an X and a Y or two X chromosomes. Having an X and a Y chromosome makes a person male; having two X chromosomes makes a person female.

Yeast infections

A common vaginal infection usually caused by an overgrowth of the *Candida* fungus that is commonly present in the vagina. Symptoms include intense itching, burning, and redness in the vaginal area. A thick cottage cheese-like discharge is frequently present. Some women with yeast infections experience pain during sexual intercourse or a burning sensation during urination.

The doctor may prescribe suppositories or creams to use in the vagina or oral medication. Over-the-counter medications are available but should not be used by women who have never had a yeast infection diagnosed by a doctor and who are unfamiliar with its symptoms.

In children, yeast infections can cause diaper rash. THRUSH is a yeast infection that affects the mouth.

Yellow fever

A viral infection that varies in severity and occurs in two forms. Urban yellow fever is acquired when a person is bitten by a certain species of mosquito that has become infected by biting an infected person. Jungle yellow fever, also called sylvatic yellow fever, is transmitted by mosquitoes that have fed on infected wild primates. The infection is found mostly in central Africa and in tropical areas of South America. The illness can be very mild with symptoms limited to fever and headache within 48 hours of infection, or it can be severe or fatal. Although the infection occurs rarely in travelers, visitors must meet requirements for vaccination against yellow fever before entering countries where it is endemic, such as India.

Yoga

An ancient holistic Indian system that uses controlled breathing, specific body postures, and meditation to achieve a state of balance and harmony between the body and the mind; a philosophy and way of life. Yoga exercises, or postures, stretch muscle groups in the body while gently squeezing internal organs. Breathing techniques are practiced before and during exercise to help focus the mind. Yoga can be a useful relaxation technique and may provide health benefits such as lowering blood pressure and respiratory rate. See also MIND-BODY MEDICINE.

Z

Zenker diverticulum

An abnormal pouch of tissue that forms at the juncture of the pharynx (lower part of the throat) and the esophagus (the muscular tube that connects the throat to the stomach). Zenker diverticulum is a common type of ESOPHAGEAL DIVERTICULUM. The condition is usually diagnosed by an upper gastrointestinal (GI) series (an X-ray procedure that is also called a BARIUM SWALLOW). Zenker diverticulum may not require treatment. However, because food can become trapped in the diverticulum and inhaled, a doctor may recommend surgery to correct the problem.

ZIFT

Zygote intrafallopian transfer; an ASSISTED REPRODUCTIVE TECHNOLOGY, or infertility treatment, in which fertilized eggs (zygotes) are placed in a fallopian tube, usually using LAPAROSCOPY. The initial steps are similar to IN VITRO FERTILIZATION (IVF), in which the eggs are retrieved from the woman and fertilized outside the body (in vitro). The resulting fertilized eggs are transferred into one of the woman's fallopian tubes to allow the cells of the early embryo to divide in a natural environment. As IVF success rates have improved, the need for ZIFT has declined.

Zinc

A mineral essential for cell production, normal growth and development, tissue repair and growth, and production of sperm and testosterone. Zinc is found in meats, poultry, eggs, milk, yogurt, oysters, nuts, legumes, and whole-grain cereals. There is some evidence that over-the-counter zinc supplements may shorten the duration of cold symptoms.

Zone therapy

A form of pressure point massage of the feet and hands designed to reduce and relieve pain. Zone therapy is based on the idea that the body is divided into 10 equal energy channels: five on each side and each containing its own "bioelectrical energy" that travels from the toes to the brain to the fingers. Pain relief is achieved by pressing the joints of toes and fingers in the appropriate zone. Zone therapy is used by chiropractors and osteopaths who, whenever possible, prefer not to use pain-relieving drugs. See REFLEXOLOGY.

Zoonosis

A disease that can be transmitted from animals (usually mammals) to humans. Examples include RABIES (which can be transmitted from an infected dog or cat to a person through a bite), TOXOPLASMOSIS (carried by cats), and roundworm infestations (see ROUNDWORMS). Ticks can transmit diseases such as ROCKY MOUNTAIN SPOTTED FEVER and LYME DISEASE from animals to people. ENCEPHALITIS is transmitted by mosquitoes to humans from infected birds, rodents, bats, and rabbits. HISTOPLASMOSIS occurs in humans who have contact with soil contaminated with the feces of infected bats or birds. MAD COW DISEASE is a fatal disease caused by ingesting meat from infected cattle.

Z-plasty

A surgical technique to make a scar less noticeable by partially removing and repositioning it. The technique also helps relieve tension on the skin caused by a scar that has contracted during healing.

Zygote

A fertilized egg; the cell formed by the union of a male sex cell (sperm) and a female sex cell (egg). A zygote is a single cell with a full set of genetic material that provides the instructions for it to divide and develop into an embryo.

Zygote intrafallopian transfer

See ZIFT.

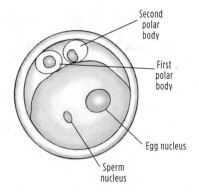

Egg and sperm

Labels: Second polar body, First polar body, Egg nucleus, Sperm nucleus

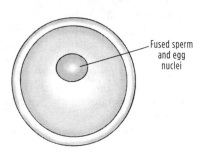

Zygote

Label: Fused sperm and egg nuclei

Fusion of sperm and egg
A zygote is formed when a sperm penetrates an egg, and the nucleus of the sperm (which carries 23 chromosomes) and the nucleus of the egg (which carries 23 chromosomes) fuse. The resulting cell has one nucleus with 46 chromosomes—a unique combination of genetic material.

INDEX

Note: page numbers in *italics* indicate illustrations.

A

Jews, Tay-Sachs disease,
675–676
Jock itch, 219, 404–405
Joint, 405
  arthrodesis, 64
  aspiration, 405
  contracture, 191
  degeneration, Charcot, 159
  dislocation, 229
  gout, 315–316
  hip replacement, 406
  injection, 405–406
  knee replacement, 406
  mice, 167
  neuropathic, 501
  pain, backache and, x
  replacement, 406
  replacement, arthritis and,
  64
  sacroiliac, 611
  seven types of, 405
  synovial membrane, syn-
  ovium, 670, 671
Joint disease, degenerative.
  See Osteoarthritis
JRA. *See* Juvenile rheumatoid
  arthritis
Jugular vein, 407
Jumper's knee, 407
Juvenile rheumatoid arthritis,
  407–408, 657
  bow legs and, 116

K

Kala-azar, 425–426
Kallmann syndrome, 374
Kaposi sarcoma, 408
  AIDS-related, 19
Karyotyping, 169, 408
Kawasaki disease, 408–409
Kegel exercises, 207, 208,
  409
Keloid, 409
Keratectomy, photorefractive,
  548
Keratin, 321, 411
Keratitis, herpes, 350
Keratoacanthoma, 409
Keratoconjunctivitis, 410
Keratoconus, 410

Keratomileusis, laser in situ.
  See LASIK
Keratoplasty
  conductive, 410–411
  penetrating, 411
Keratosis, 411
  actinic, 9
  seborrheic, 620
Keratotomy, radial, 583–584
Kerion, 411
Ketoacidosis, 7, 411
Ketones, 412
Ketoprofen, 55
Ketosis, 412
Keyhole surgery, 45
Kidney, *412*, 412–414,
  496–498, 593–595
  anuria (lack of urine production), 55–56
  artificial, 65
  biopsy, 412
  cancer, 412–413
  cancer, renal cell carcinoma,
  593–594
  cortex, 412
  cyst, 413, 560
  diabetes insipidus, 221
  failure, 413
  failure, hemodialysis,
  339–340
  failure, hemolytic-uremic
  syndrome, 227
  failure, renal diet, 594
  function tests, 413
  function tests, BUN (blood
  urea nitrogen), 108
  glumerulonephritis,
  310–311
  hemodialysis, 339–340
  imaging, 413–414
  infections, viii
  inflammation, 496
  inflammation, pyelonephritis, 581–582
  medulla, 412
  pelvis, 412
  polycystic, 560–561
  renal vascular hypertension, 595
  stones, 414
  stones, lithotripsy, 436

  stones, renal colic, 594
  stones, symptoms of, viii
  surgical removal (nephrectomy), 496
  transplant, 414
  urine drainage tube
  (nephrostomy), 498
  Wilms tumor, 746
Kilocalories, 138, 414
Kleptomania, 414
Klumpke paralysis, 414–415
Knee, 415
  Baker cyst, 80–81
  joint, chondromatosis,
  167–168
  jumper's, 407
  ligament injuries, 434
  replacement, 406
  runner's, 610–611
Kneecap, patellar tendinitis,
  535
Knock-knees, 415
Korsakoff psychosis, 415, 744
Kyphosis, 415

L

La Leche League, 126
Labia, 415–416
Labia majora, 596
Labor, 416
  amnio fusion, 31
  false (Braxton Hicks contractions), 120–121
  final stage (afterbirth), 16
  induction of, 191, 386
  induction of, after fetal
  death, 2
  induction of by amniotomy,
  32
  preterm, 153, 568
  stages of, 416
  uterine contractions, 191
Labyrinth, Meniere disease,
  459
Labyrinthitis, *416*, 416–417
  symptoms of, xxi, xxvii
Laceration, 417
Lacrimal apparatus, 417
Lacrimal gland, 417
  Sjögren syndrome, 635